P9-BZK-327

$$Q = SV \times HR$$

oxygen

$$HRmax = 220 - age$$

RQ

fatigue RER

stress

mmHg

$$VO_2max$$

FUNDAMENTAL PRINCIPLES OF

Exercise Physiology

For Fitness, Performance, and Health

FUNDAMENTAL PRINCIPLES OF

Exercise Physiology

For Fitness, Performance, and Health

Robert A. Robergs, Ph.D., FASEP

Center for Exercise and Applied Human Physiology
The University of New Mexico
Albuquerque, New Mexico

Scott O. Roberts, Ph.D., FACSM, FAACVPR

Department of Physical Education, Health Education, and Leisure Services
Central Washington University
Ellensburg, Washington

Boston   Burr Ridge, Il   Dubuque, IA   Madison, WI   New York   San Francisco   St Louis
Bangkok   Bogotá   Caracas   Lisbon   London   Madrid
Mexico City   Milan   New Delhi   Seoul   Singapore   Sydney   Taipei   Toronto

Lake Superior College Library

McGraw-Hill Higher Education

A Division of The **McGraw-Hill** Companies

FUNDAMENTAL PRINCIPLES OF EXERCISE PHYSIOLOGY:
FOR FITNESS, PERFORMANCE, AND HEALTH

Copyright © 2000 by The McGraw-Hill Companies, Inc. All rights reserved. Printed in the
United States of America. Except as permitted under the United States Copyright Act of 1976,
no part of this publication may be reproduced or distributed in any form or by any means, or
stored in a data base or retrieval system, without the prior written permission of the publisher.

 This book is printed on recycled, acid-free paper containing 10% postconsumer waste.

1 2 3 4 5 6 7 8 9 0 QPD/QPD 0 9 8 7 6 5 4 3 2 1 0

ISBN 0–8016–7907–9

Vice president and editorial director: *Kevin T. Kane*
Publisher: *Edward E. Bartell*
Executive editor: *Vicki Malinee*
Senior developmental editor: *Michelle Turenne*
Senior marketing manager: *Pamela S. Cooper*
Senior Project manager: *Jayne Klein*
Production supervisor: *Enboge Chong*
Design manager: *Stuart D. Paterson*
Senior photo research coordinator: *Carrie K. Burger*
Senior supplement coordinator: *Candy M. Kuster*
Compositor: *GTS Graphics, Inc.*
Typeface: *10/12 Times Roman*
Printer: *Quebecor Printing Book Group/Dubuque, IA*

Cover/interior designer: *Maureen McCutcheon*
Cover image: (top) *The Image Bank,* (bottom) *FPG International*

The credits section for this book begins on page 473 and is considered an extension of the
copyright page.

Library of Congress Cataloging-in-Publication Data

Robergs, Robert A.
    Fundamental principles of exercise physiology: for fitness, performance,
and health / Robert A. Robergs, Scott O. Roberts. — 1st ed.
        p.   cm.
    Includes index.
    ISBN 0–8016–7907–9
    1. Exercise—Physiological aspects. I. Roberts, Scott.
II. Title.
QP301.R547   2000
612'.044—dc21
                                                    99–15122
                                                       CIP

www.mhhe.com

BRIEF CONTENTS

CONTENTS

FOCUS BOXES

To provide students with greater depth of coverage of important topics, focus boxes are included in the text to present additional content that supplements the main narrative. The focus boxes can be found on the following pages:

PREFACE

Exercise physiology is a discipline that has experienced enormous growth during the last decade. Most university programs that offer both undergraduate and graduate exercise science or related degrees offer more than one exercise physiology course.

Who Is This Text Written For?

Typically, one course provides an introduction to exercise physiology and covers the basic content. This introductory course is useful for students of other majors, such as physical education, athletic training, biology, nursing, health, or nutrition. In addition, this course serves as a means to present the fundamentals of exercise physiology to exercise science majors, thereby allowing a second more advanced class to serve the needs of more contemporary research topics within exercise physiology.

During the writing of our "advanced" text *Exercise Physiology: Exercise, Performance, and Clinical Applications*, it was always our intent to follow it with a text that was obviously intended for an introductory study of exercise physiology. This was based on the current need of many instructors to recommend one text for their lower-level course and another for the advanced course. Conversely, some instructors may use just one book. In either case, the student is in an undesirable situation in which he or she must buy two very different texts from different authors, or use one "middle of the road" text for both classes. We wrote our first text as an advanced book because this approach was needed the most in exercise physiology. Its format also provided us with an organizational structure to follow for an introductory-level book.

It was important to keep a consistent structure and format between the books. You will see that *Fundamental Principles of Exercise Physiology: For Fitness, Performance, and Health* differs in the scope of topics covered, as well as the depth of explanation and presentation of specific topics in exercise physiology. Nevertheless, the theme of acute and chronic adaptations to exercise has been retained, as is fundamental content for the chapters concerning metabolism, cardiovascular and pulmonary physiology, neuroendocrinology, training, measurement of capacities, and environmental physiology. These similarities support an easy transition between the two books as the student progresses to a more advanced study of exercise physiology.

As with all textbooks, we do not believe that we have succeeded in producing ideal versions of both texts in their first editions. We recognize that there is always room for improvement in striving to achieve the balance of content and writing level that results in the "ideal" content and structure. However, on the basis of the positive responses to our first book, we believe that the originality of our approach will be equally suitable, if not more so, for a fundamental study of the discipline.

What Is the Academic Level?

As with our first book, we believe strongly that exercise physiologists, no matter what their final degree, must be educated in a manner that *does not undercut the academic standards and advanced content* of the discipline of exercise physiology or the competency and knowledge of exercise physiologists. The standards of exercise physiology and the education and training of future exercise physiologists begins at a fundamental level. *Fundamental Principles of Exercise Physiology: For Fitness, Performance, and Health* should better prepare students to be successful in more advanced study. An adequately prepared undergraduate student who has taken prerequisite classes in human physiology, introductory organic chemistry and biochemistry, human anatomy, kinesiology, and/or biomechanics will have no difficulty in reading and understanding the content of this textbook.

What Makes This Text Unique?

There are many existing textbooks on exercise physiology. The format and structure of some of these texts date back to the 1970s, and reveal the strong connection that existed at that time between exercise physiology, sport, athletic performance, and the discipline of physical education. A few of the texts are known for their more advanced presentation of material, some present too much material, and others present material unrelated to the physiology of exercise.

Improving current texts means not just doing things differently, but making changes in content and presentation that are logical improvements to the study of exercise physiology. Textbooks in exercise physiology have traditionally divided content based on systems physiology, and presented specific examples of how exercise affects physiology. This structure required the presentation of all there is to know about a particular measure in exercise physiology in one section. In doing this, texts present both pure physiology and applied physiology, integrate other physiological systems, and reveal how the measured variable changes with training when the student may be struggling with simply understanding the concept. This trait is more a problem for a fundamental or introductory study of exercise physiology than it is for more advanced study. Therefore, our introductory exercise physiology textbook will benefit from the structure adopted in our first book.

We strongly believe that a text is needed that represents a new approach to the knowledge base in exercise physiology, and that recognizes the development of the field as we enter the twenty-first century. As with our first book, this text uses acute and chronic adaptations to exercise as consistent organizational themes. In addition, by offering an introductory text complementary to our advanced book, we provide a sequence of textbooks for the student of exercise physiology. Our two-book approach better reflects the future of exercise physiology: a future based on academic program accreditation, a nationwide certification exam that is currently being developed by the American Society of Exercise Physiologists (ASEP), and heightened standards of education and professional practice that reflect the professional quality of the discipline and graduates of exercise physiology.

How Does This Text Meet the Future of Exercise Physiology and the Future Needs of Student Populations?

The future of exercise physiology is now being directed by the American Society of Exercise Physiologists (ASEP). In the first years of the new millennium, administrators and professors of college and university academic programs in exercise science and exercise physiology will have the choice of remaining separate, or aligning with ASEP in the professional development of exercise physiology. Academic program administrators and professors will be able to adhere to the course requirements of ASEP program accreditation, and for the first time have direction in how to prepare students to become exercise physiologists, as well as justify their academic programs to higher-level university administrators. These developments will stimulate change in the academic content of courses and, therefore, require change in the academic content of many textbooks.

Fundamental Principles of Exercise Physiology: For Fitness, Performance, and Health and its complementary advanced book provide academicians and students alike with a fresh approach to the academic content of exercise physiology. The content of exercise physiology has been divided into two books based on topical difficulty and level of rigor. The two books provide academicians with more flexibility in how they

teach courses in exercise physiology, and thereby better prepare students to be professional exercise physiologists. As already explained, this twofold approach to the study of exercise physiology is complementary with academic programs currently teaching exercise physiology as separate "fundamental" and "advanced" courses. The growing knowledge and skills base of exercise physiology warrants that this approach be developed by those academic programs training professional exercise physiologists. Therefore, our "fundamental" text will successfully educate students to study more "advanced" exercise physiology in later courses.

Organization

This text is written in five parts followed by a section of appendices which organize the knowledge base of exercise physiology.

Part 1: Energy, Metabolism, Work, and Power concisely presents the biochemical and physical principles which are fundamental to the study of exercise physiology.

Part 2: Systemic Responses to Exercise presents systems physiology and shows how each system acutely and chronically adapts to exercise.

Part 3: Methods to Improve Exercise Performance covers topics that are known to either improve or impair exercise performance.

Part 4: Measurements of Fitness and Exercise Performance explains how researchers measure endurance and intense exercise capacities, lung function, body composition, and use exercise in the clinical evaluation of cardiovascular disease.

Part 5: Special Topics within exercise physiology presents concise chapters describing the latest research findings of high-interest applied topics of exercise physiology and biochemistry, such as growth and development, aging, gender issues, environmental physiology, weight control, and health and disease.

Appendixes: The appendixes include professional issues in career opportunities, Internet sources, conversion units, gas volumes and indirect calorimetry, energy expenditure, recommended dietary allowances, the Canadian food guide, and nutrient recommendations for Canadians.

Unique Features

This text presents material in a unique format, and also includes material on topics not typically presented in an exercise physiology text. These unique features are as follows:

■ The level of presentation and content is written specifically to address the introductory student. Every effort has been given to present an appropriate amount of topical coverage and detail, including analysis by reviewers of introductory exercise physiology courses. For example, systems physiology is carefully presented to show how it is suited for the fundamental study of exercise physiology. At the same time, sufficient coverage of selected material is provided to satisfy the inquisitive mind of even the most advanced undergraduate student.

■ Examination of immediate and long-term responses to exercise for health and fitness focuses on how the individual adapts to exercise.

■ An introductory presentation of the current status of exercise physiology in today's society is offered, with special reference to issues in the development of the professional status of exercise physiology. This content also extends into appendix A which discusses career opportunities that an undergraduate degree in exercise science/physiology can provide the student.

■ Internet resources are described in appendix B. A brief description of pertinent websites also appears at the end of each chapter.

■ Calorimetry and ergometry are presented in chapter 4 with more complete coverage of the limitations and applications of the procedures, and with an emphasis that reflects the importance of these topics in the knowledge and skill competencies of exercise physiologists.

■ Muscle contraction and neuromuscular function are presented together in chapter 5 to better emphasize the connections between skeletal muscle contraction and both central and peripheral neural function.

■ Each of the chapters on neuromuscular, cardiovascular, pulmonary, and endocrine function during exercise include coverage of acute and chronic adaptations.

■ Emphasis has been given to carbohydrate nutrition before, during, and after exercise in chapter 11. Explanations of the research on micronutrients, and alternative macronutrients such as amino acids and fat, have also been provided to familiarize the student with the diverse influence of macro- and micronutrients on metabolism and substrate use during exercise.

■ Chapter 16 summarizes the clinical applications of exercise physiology.

■ Separate chapters overview the emerging fields of pediatric (growth and development) exercise physiology, and exercise and aging are covered in chapters 17 and 18.

■ The topics of exercise at altitude and exercise in hot or humid environments are extensively detailed in chapter 19.

■ Gender differences during and in response to exercise are combined in chapter 20.

■ Focus boxes in every chapter include additional information to support the main narrative such as exercise and asthma.

■ Applications conclude every chapter and provide brief situations to which students can apply the content just learned.

■ Full color is throughout the design of the text and in the illustration program to enhance the teaching-learning process.

Pedagogy

Numerous pedagogical tools are included in every chapter to enhance the learning process. These include chapter objectives, key terms, definition boxes (with pronunciation guides when appropriate), focus boxes, websites, bulleted chapter summaries, study questions, application questions, thorough references, and recommended readings. Additionally, a comprehensive glossary concludes the text.

The references cited in each chapter represent recent research, with many references published as recently as 1998. References dating back to the early twentieth century in some chapters provide a historical development of a topic, and most chapters also include references that date back to the 1970s. This should not be viewed as outdated material because many important studies of the physiology and muscle biochemistry of exercise were completed during the 1960s and 1970s. When these findings are relevant to the textual discussion, original research has been recognized.

Finally, helpful reference and conversion materials are located inside the front and back covers of the text for convenience of use.

Ancillaries

Instructor's Manual and Test Bank   Developed specifically for this text, the *Instructor's Manual* includes chapter overviews, learning objectives, discussion questions, class activities, and a comprehensive test bank of multiple-choice, true-false, matching, and essay questions. The manual is also perforated and three-hole punched for convenience of use.

Computerized Test Bank   A computerized version of the test bank for the *Instructor's Manual* is available for both IBM and Macintosh to qualified adopters. This software provides a unique combination of user-friendly aids and enables the instructor to select, edit, delete, or add questions, and construct and print tests and answer keys.

Visual Resource Library (VRL)   A CD-ROM of approximately 300 carefully selected images and lecture content slides allows instructors to create their own unique presentations by directly importing into any graphics or multimedia application, as well as making slides, PowerPoint presentations, or overhead transparencies. Organized by title, subject, and key word search for convenience of use. Available to qualified adopters.

Web Resources

McGraw-Hill's Exercise Physiology Supersite   The *Exercise Physiology Supersite* provides a wide array of information for instructors and students, from text information to the latest technology. It includes professional organization, convention, and career information. Visit the website at www.mhhe.com/hper/physed/exercisephys

Additional features of the supersite include:

Up close and personal   This link identifies who works on the exercise physiology list at McGraw-Hill, which conventions are attended, how to become a reviewer, and how to submit a book proposal.

By the book   To log onto the Robergs/Roberts *Fundamental Principles of Exercise Physiology* homepage, see the description and website address below. Link to the on-line catalog to find the perfect text or ancillary for your course.

Personalize your course   This includes sample simulations, journal articles, and additional features to assist in preparing for the profession of exercise physiology.

Especially McGraw-Hill   This links to other resources McGraw-Hill has to offer.

Fundamental Principles of Exercise Physiology HomePage
Developed specifically for *Fundamental Principles of Exercise Physiology,* a PowerPoint presentation has been prepared by Robert A. Robergs, Ph.D., and can be downloaded from this homepage. These presentations are organized by chapter, and contain the majority of graphic art used in the text.

Additionally, links to PageOut and PageOut Lite, our web-based programs which can be used to help create your own website, are included here. Visit the *Fundamental Principles of Exercise Physiology* homepage at www.mhhe.com/hper/physed/robergs_fund.

Acknowledgments

Special thanks are directed to Lisa Stolarcyk, Ph.D., who assisted in the proofreading of the first book, and followed this service into this fundamental version of our approach to the study of exercise physiology. Thanks also must be given to Don O'Connor for his hard work in preparing much of the complex artwork throughout both books.

Heidi K. Byrne
SUNY: Brockport
Gary A. Dudley
The University of Georgia

Blanche W. Evans
Indiana State University
Stephen C. Glass
Wayne State College (NE)

Dan Hostager
Upper Iowa University
Kimberly Hyatt
Weber State University (UT)
Peter W. Iltis
Gordon College (MA)
Gary Kastello
Winona State University (MN)
Vicki Kloosterhouse
Oakland Community College Highland Lakes Campus (MI)
Thomas G. Manfredi
The University of Rhode Island
Susan Muller
Salisbury State University (MD)
Vincent J. Paolone
Springfield College (MA)
David Petrie
Gettysburg College (PA)

Janice L. Radcliffe
The University of Oregon
Michael E. Rodgers
Wichita State University
Brent C. Ruby
The University of Montana
Janet M. Shaw
The University of Utah
Thomas E. Temples
North Georgia College and State University
Luke E. Thomas
Northeast Lousiana University
Robert Thomas
Atlantic Union College (MA)
Maridy Troy
The University of Alabama-Tuscaloosa
Michael Turner
University of North Carolina-Charlotte

First Draft Reviewers

William S. Barnes
Texas A&M University
Stanley P. Brown
The University of Mississippi
Julie Felix
Virginia Tech State University
Dan Fitzsimons
The University of Wisconsin-Madison
Ethel M. Frese
Saint Louis University (MO)

Robert Gotshall
Colorado State University
Douglas S. King
Iowa State University
Jeffrey A. Potteiger
The University of Kansas
Carol D. Rodgers
The University of Toronto
Serge P. von Duvillard
William Paterson College (NJ)
James L. Webb
California Polytechnic State University–San Luis Obispo

We would like to acknowledge and thank our reviewers whose comments, suggestions, support, and enthusiasm were valuable to us in improving the manuscript.

We appreciate everyone's efforts to improve the educational quality, scientific accuracy, and presentation of this book. Their suggestions for making this book better were more valuable to and respected by us than they could ever imagine.

As relatively young authors, our knowledge base and professional development can be easily traced to several individuals who have had a large impact on our lives. Many of these individuals were recognized in our first book. However, they all need to be recognized again, and the roles of additional individuals in our professional development since the publication of our first book must also be included.

From Robert A. Robergs

I am eternally grateful to the academic guidance and inspiration provided by the following individuals:

Alan Morton, Ph.D., formerly of the University of Western Australia
Paul Ribisl, Ph.D., Wake Forest University
David Costill, Ph.D., formerly of Ball State University
William Fink, formerly of Ball State University
Clyde Williams, Ph.D., Loughborough University, England
Vivian Heyward, Ph.D., University of New Mexico

My understanding of exercise physiology and desire to conduct research can be traced back to reading the research of exercise physiologists and physiologists such as Lars Hermannsen, Bengt Saltin, Phil Gollnick, David Costill, Eddie Coyle, George Brooks, Jack Wilmore, Karlmann Wasserman, Lawrence Spriet, Peter Wagner, and Howard Greene.

My research progress and development at the University of New Mexico has been aided by collaboration with the following physicians and scientists: Paul Montner, M.D., David James, M.D., Milton Icenogle, M.D., Eichi Fukoshima, Ph.D., Jack Leoppky, Ph.D., Bill Brooks, Ph.D., and Debra Waters, Ph.D.

Many of you are probably aware of my commitment to the professional development of exercise physiology. I am indebted to the professional example provided by Tommy Boone, Ph.D., M.P.H., who was instrumental in founding the American Society of Exercise Physiologists (ASEP). He provides an example of the professional competencies of all exercise physiologists, both in the United States and around the world. Thank you, Tommy.

Unending thanks are directed to my family in Australia who supported my departure for the United States in 1985, and have remained in full support ever since. Thank you Mum, Dad, and Helen, as well as my nieces whom I see far too little of: Casey and Deanne. I am always with you in spirit.

Finally, I need to express love and thanks to Sharon, my wife; Bryce, my stepson since he was 2 years of age; and my new son Dane who was born at 6:14 a.m. on April 23, 1999. Sharon and Bryce, I have shared my life with both of you since 1990. My success and productivity is nurtured by your love, understanding, and support.

From Scott O. Roberts

I am especially grateful to my friends and colleagues at Texas Tech University, particularly Jaclyn Robert, Ph.D., and Elizabeth Hall, Ph.D.

Also, many thanks to the reviewers who provided immensely valuable comments and suggestions in the development of this text. And to Michelle Turenne, our developmental editor for both books, for being so patient.

Last, heartfelt love and appreciation to my wife Julia and our children Andrew, Daniel, and Michael for their love and support.

Robert A. Robergs
Scott O. Roberts

*F*undamental Principles of Exercise Physiology: for Fitness, Performance, and Health provides basic information about the impact of exercise upon fitness and health for the introductory student in an exciting presentation. Practical features include content application exercises, very basic information about exercise physiology in the clinical setting, professional issues pertaining to career opportunities, helpful web site information, and how to use the Internet most effectively.

Color Presentation

Full color is included throughout the design of the text and in the photographs and artwork for a presentation that is both instructional and visually exciting.

Pedagogical Aids

This page is designed to graphically illustrate how to use the study aids included within the text to your best advantage.

Chapter Opening Features

■ *Chapter objectives* identify the goals to be accomplished after completing each chapter.
■ *Key terms* are listed at the beginning of each chapter and are boldfaced in the text for easy identification of important new words.

Focus Boxes

Focus boxes present related studies as well as practical information to supplement the presentation.

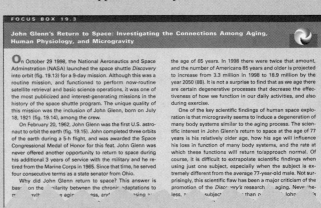

FOCUS BOX 19.3

John Glenn's Return to Space: Investigating the Connections Among Aging, Human Physiology, and Microgravity

On October 29 1998, the National Aeronautics and Space Adminstration (NASA) launched the space shuttle *Discovery* into orbit (fig. 19.13) for a 9-day mission. Although this was a routine mission, and functioned to perform now-routine satellite retrieval and basic science operations, it was one of the most publicized and interest-generating missions in the history of the space shuttle program. The unique quality of this mission was the inclusion of John Glenn, born on July 18, 1921 (fig. 19.14), among the crew.

On February 20, 1962, John Glenn was the first U.S. astronaut to orbit the earth (fig. 19.15). John completed three orbits of the earth during a 5-h flight, and was awarded the Space Congressional Medal of Honor for this feat. John Glenn was never offered another opportunity to return to space during his additional 3 years of service with the military and he retired from the Marine Corps in 1965. Since that time, he served four consecutive terms as a state senator from Ohio.

Why did John Glenn return to space? This answer is bas[ed] on the [sim]ilarity betwe[en] the chronic [a]daptations to [micro]grav[ity the] agin[g proc]ess, and [decrea]sing h[...]

the age of 65 years. In 1998 there were twice that amount, and the number of Americans 85 years and older is projected to increase from 3.3 million in 1998 to 18.9 million by the year 2050 (88). It is not a surprise to find that as we age there are certain degenerative processes that decrease the effectiveness of how we function in our daily activities, and also during exercise.

One of the key scientific findings of human space exploration is that microgravity seems to induce a degeneration of many body systems similar to the aging process. The scientific interest in John Glenn's return to space at the age of 77 years is his relatively older age, how his age will influence his loss in function of many body systems, and the rate at which these functions will return to/approach normal. Of course, it is difficult to extrapolate scientific findings when using just one subject, especially when the subject is extremely different from the average 77-year-old male. Not surprisingly, this scientific flaw has been a major criticism of the promotion of the *Disc[overy]*'s research [on] aging. Neve[rthe]less, [using a] subject [older] than [norma]l, John [...]

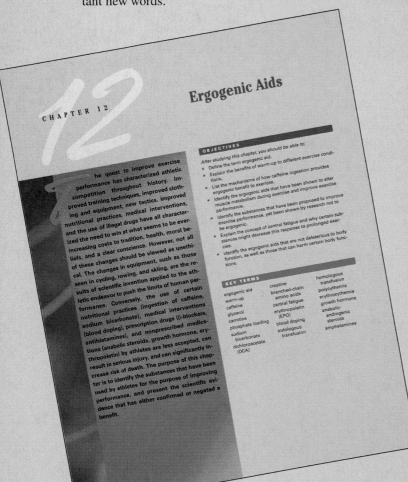

CHAPTER 12

Ergogenic Aids

OBJECTIVES

After studying this chapter, you should be able to:
* Define the term ergogenic aid.
* Explain the benefits of warm-up to different exercise conditions.
* List the mechanisms of how caffeine ingestion provides ergogenic benefit to exercise.
* Identify the ergogenic aids that have been shown to alter muscle metabolism during exercise and improve exercise performance.
* Identify the substances that have been proposed to improve exercise performance, yet been shown by research not to be ergogenic.
* Explain the concept of central fatigue and why certain substances might decrease this response to prolonged exercise.
* Identify the ergogenic aids that are not deleterious to body function, as well as those that can harm certain body functions.

KEY TERMS

ergogenic aid
warm-up
caffeine
glycerol
carnitine
phosphate loading
sodium bicarbonate
dichloroacetate (DCA)

creatine
branched-chain amino acids
central fatigue
erythropoietin (EPO)
blood doping
autologous transfusion

homologous transfusion
polycythemia
erythrocythemia
growth hormone
anabolic-androgenic steroids
amphetamines

he quest to improve exercise performance has characterized athletic competition throughout history. Improved training techniques, improved clothing and equipment, new tactics, improved nutritional practices, medical interventions, and the use of illegal drugs have all characterized the need to win at what seems to be ever-increasing costs to tradition, health, moral beliefs, and a clear conscience. However, not all of these changes should be viewed as unethical. The changes in equipment, such as those seen in cycling, rowing, and skiing, are the results of scientific invention applied to the athletic endeavor to push the limits of human performance. Conversely, the use of certain nutritional practices (ingestion of caffeine, sodium bicarbonate), medical interventions (blood doping), prescription drugs (β-blockers, antihistamines), and nonprescribed medications (anabolic steroids, growth hormone, erythropoietin) by athletes are less accepted, can result in serious injury, and can significantly increase risk of death. The purpose of this chapter is to identify the substances that have been used by athletes for the purpose of improving performance, and present the scientific evidence that has either confirmed or negated a benefit.

Illustration Program

Instructional *full-color illustrations and photographs* enhance learning with an exciting visual appearance.

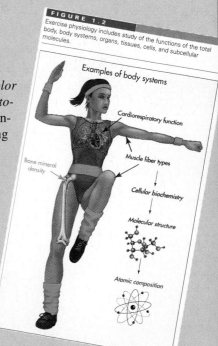

FIGURE 1.2

Exercise physiology includes study of the functions of the total body, body systems, organs, tissues, cells, and subcellular molecules.

Examples of body systems

Cardiorespiratory function

Muscle fiber types

Cellular biochemistry

Molecular structure

Bone mineral density

Atomic composition

oxygen

$$Q = SV \times HR$$

$$HRmax = 220 - age$$

RQ

fatigue   RER

stress

mmHg

VO_2max

Energy, Metabolism, Work, and Power

CHAPTER 1

An Introduction to Exercise Physiology

xercise and physical activity are daily parts of most people's lives. We become physically active when we get out of bed, walk, climb stairs at work or school, run to catch a bus or train, and participate in sports and athletics. Ever since we were children, we have been directed to participate in organized physical activity, or exercise, and have learned how to enjoy participation in exercise-related activities. Exercise is a vital part of our sports participation, and those of us who play organized sports, or participate in recreational athletic activities, use exercise in an organized manner to train our bodies to do better, or at least to better tolerate the demands we place on them. Medical-related research now informs us that exercise is not only a recreational pursuit, but also essential to the health and well-being of our minds and bodies. Not surprisingly, the importance of exercise in the prevention of illness has fueled a large industry that "sells" exercise-related knowledge and equipment to the community. Now, more than ever, the average consumer who is concerned with his or her health must know more about how exercise influences the body. The purpose of this chapter is to introduce the science of exercise physiology as a complex and advanced field of inquiry. In addition, the academic scope of the discipline, applications of the knowledge, and future employment opportunities for students who seek a future in exercise-related markets will be identified.

OBJECTIVES

After reading this chapter, you should be able to:

- Define the terms exercise, physical activity, training, and exercise physiology.
- Explain the academic preparation needed prior to studying exercise physiology at the undergraduate level.
- List many of the topical areas included in exercise physiology.
- Be aware of the efforts currently in place to professionalize exercise physiology, and the reasons why this process is being undertaken.
- Understand the different ways scientists conduct research in exercise physiology.
- Recognize several names of scientists who have contributed to the academic and research base in exercise physiology.
- Enter an academic library and know which research journals to inspect for research or review articles that pertain to exercise physiology.

KEY TERMS

exercise
physical activity
physical fitness
exercise training
acute adaptations
chronic
  adaptations

exercise
  physiology
profession
pure research
applied research
clinical research
human subjects
  research

animal research
experimental
  research
comparative
  research
epidemiological
  research
journals

Important Definitions

What Is Exercise?

Before discussing the field of exercise physiology, the concept of **exercise** must first be defined and explained. When we contract skeletal muscle to cause movement, or maintain a given posture, it is generally explained that we are being *active*. This is in contrast to being *inactive*, where we are not voluntarily contracting our skeletal muscles. The Webster's dictionary provides three important definitions of exercise: (1) ". . . regular or repeated use of a faculty or body organ," (2) ". . . bodily exertion for the sake of developing and maintaining physical fitness," (3) ". . . something performed or practiced in order to develop, improve, or display a specific power or skill" (26). The term *exercise* can therefore be used to denote activity that is performed for the purpose of improving, maintaining, or expressing a particular type of physical fitness.

The organized and purposeful implications of exercise that separate it from activity is a complication. When walking down the street to mail a letter, we are being active, but simply because we are performing this act for a task rather than for physical fitness means that it does not suit the previous definitions of exercise. Similarly, when workers lift objects or are forced to exert themselves with repeated periods of muscular contraction (e.g., furniture movers, farmers, construction workers, landscapers), they are active yet once again are not truly exercising. This definitional inadequacy of exercise has caused the term **physical activity** to be more widely used. Physical activity pertains to the activity performed by the body for purposes other than the specific development of physical fitness. Ironically, research has shown that physical fitness is improved from regular physical activity, just as it is from exercise. Thus, individuals who are physically active in general lifestyle and vocation can be physically fit without necessarily completing what we know to be exercise. However, as will be revealed in many of the chapters of this text, the trend in today's developed societies is for a lifestyle that is becoming less and less physically active, thereby requiring more and more exercise to develop and maintain physical fitness.

What Is Physical Fitness?

Just as exercise is a vague term, physical fitness is also vague and requires definitional clarification. To be fit means to be suited to a given stress. Consequently, the concept of fitness must be applied to specific stresses. Thus **physical fitness** concerns being fit for physical activity. As there are many types of physical activities, varying in each of the muscles used, forces developed, and durations of use, there are also multiple forms of physical fitness. The components of fitness are explained in focus box 1.1.

Individuals can therefore speak of physical fitness related to muscular strength, muscular power, muscular endurance, cardiorespiratory endurance, flexibility, body composition, and agility. As will be discussed in the chapters concerning metabolism, training, and nutrition, these divisions of physical fitness are useful for furthering our understanding of how the body supports the energy needs of muscle contraction and how we can organize exercise by training to improve specific components of physical fitness.

What Is Exercise Training?

It should be becoming clear that exercise can be performed in an organized manner for the development of specific components of physical fitness. The repeated use of exercise to improve physical fitness is termed **exercise training**. This concept is important for two reasons. First, it reveals that given exercise sessions must exert a stimulus for improvement in components of physical fitness. Second, the body must therefore be able to actually improve in certain functions when routinely exposed to exercise. These distinctions in the time of how the body responds to exercise is useful for the study of exercise physiology. For example, the body experiences immediate responses to exercise that must vary with the type of exercise performed. Such immediate responses are termed **acute adaptations**, and these function to help the body tolerate the exercise or physical activity. The performance of exercise by the body can also stimulate many body functions and structures to change, and to have these changes be retained even after the exercise is completed. For example, lifting heavy objects will eventually cause muscles to become stronger and larger; routinely walking or jogging will cause improved capacities of the active muscles to consume oxygen and release energy, and increase the total volume of the blood. In being retained from one exercise session to another, thereby being more long term or chronic in nature, these adaptations are referred to as **chronic adaptations**. Chronic adaptations may require several weeks to develop (e.g., improved muscle size), whereas others may take only several days (e.g., improved abilities to

---

exercise activity that is performed for the purpose of improving, maintaining, or expressing a particular type of physical fitness

physical activity the activity performed by the body for purposes other than the specific development of physical fitness

physical fitness a state of bodily function that is characterized by the ability to tolerate exercise stress

exercise training the repeated use of exercise to improve physical fitness

acute adaptations the immediate structural and functional responses to exercise that function to help the body tolerate the exercise or physical activity

chronic adaptations the changes in body structure and function that are retained after the exercise is completed

FOCUS BOX 1.1

The Components of Physical Fitness

Physical fitness is a state of bodily function that is characterized by the ability to tolerate exercise stress. As exercise stress can range from simply walking down the street, to running a 4-min mile, or lifting hundreds of kilograms in weight, there must be versatility in how physical fitness is defined. Such versatility comes from the multiple components of physical fitness, with specific components more important to specific exercises, sports, or physical activities than others. The components of physical fitness are listed below.

- *Muscular strength:* the capacity of muscles to generate force during contractions.
- *Muscular power:* the capacity of muscles to generate force during fast contractions.
- *Muscular endurance:* the capacity of skeletal muscles to sustain repeated contractions.
- *Cardiorespiratory endurance:* the capacity of the lungs to exchange gases, and the heart and blood vessels to circulate blood around the body.
- *Flexibility:* the ability to maximize joint range of motion.
- *Body composition:* the proportions of the body comprised of fat, mineral, protein, and water. Most laboratories quantify the body into lean (protein, mineral, and water) and fat components.
- *Agility:* the ability to change direction rapidly while moving.

For physical activities or exercises demanding the movement of heavy objects, the components of muscular strength and power are important in order to enable a person to tolerate these demands (fig. 1.1). Conversely, the need to run long distances requires the development of muscular endurance, cardiorespiratory endurance, and perhaps a favorable body composition that is low in body fat (25). The contemporary or classical dancer needs to be highly flexible, agile, have above average muscle power and endurance, and also have a body composition low in fat.

Based on the previous examples, the weight lifter, basketball player, and dancer would all be classified as being physically fit for their activities, but perhaps not for each other's activities. The weight lifter would not be physically fit for dancing, and the basketball player would not be physically fit for weight lifting. Once again, the specificity of physical fitness must be understood and appreciated.

FIGURE 1.1

The components of physical fitness portrayed in the weight lifter, modern dancer, and basketball player.

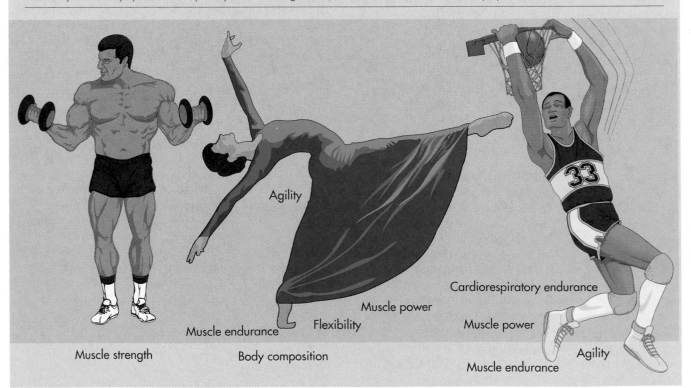

consume oxygen) or may occur after as little as one or two exercise sessions (e.g., increased blood volume).

What Is Exercise Physiology?

As already indicated, exercise and physical activity have multiple implications to body structure, function, and health. Not surprisingly, this important and expanding field of science and education is combined in a scientific discipline termed **exercise physiology**. By definition, exercise physiology is a discipline involving the study of how exercise alters the structure and function of the human body. Such a broad definition is problematic, as academic and research inquiry of exercise and the structure and function of the human body can be done at the level of the total body, body systems, organs, tissues, cells, and subcellular molecules (fig. 1.2)(5). For example, exercise obviously increases the energy used

by the body, which is important for weight control and the loss of body fat. In increasing energy expenditure, exercise invokes increased functions of the systems of the body—cardiovascular, respiratory, neuromuscular, musculoskeletal, neuroendocrine, immune, and so on. In our quest to further understand how exercise influences each of these systems, research has been done to understand how exercise specifically alters the *morphology* and function of body tissues. A notable example of this diverging level of inquiry applies to skeletal muscle. Exercise increases skeletal muscle contraction, and exercise training can change the appearance and function of skeletal muscle. To understand this, researchers study how exercise influences the activity and concentration of enzymes of metabolism, how exercise can alter the synthesis of muscle proteins, and the role of hormones and nerves in regulating these changes.

The Developing Field of Exercise Physiology

An interesting means to evaluate how the importance of exercise physiology has developed over the latter part of the twentieth century is to compare academic programs that incorporate the science of exercise physiology into their course offerings. Such a comparison is provided in figure 1.3. During the 1970s, exercise physiology was one of many core courses in physical education. At that time, the main employment options for graduates of physical education were in teaching, coaching, corporate fitness, community recreation programs, and fitness clubs. Today the academic structure comprising exercise physiology courses is totally different. Students from diverse backgrounds with equally diverse intended careers are taking classes in exercise physiology. Ironically, despite the recognized importance of exercise in the medical community, most medical programs throughout the United States do not require completion of a course in exercise physiology, yet it may not be long before this changes (focus box 1.2).

The Current Status of Exercise Physiology as a Discipline and Profession

Today exercise is used as a therapy during rehabilitation from injury and illness, and as a preventive strategy to combat atherosclerotic cardiovascular disease. Table 1.1 lists the various disciplines that use exercise as a condition from which to further evaluate physiological or cellular function. The medical interest in exercise physiology is developing a specialized subdiscipline, clinical exercise physiology, and textbooks are being written to satisfy this need.

Exercise, or the lack of it, is now recognized as an independent risk factor for cardiovascular disease. Although it is

---

FIGURE 1.2

Exercise physiology includes study of the functions of the total body, body systems, organs, tissues, cells, and subcellular molecules.

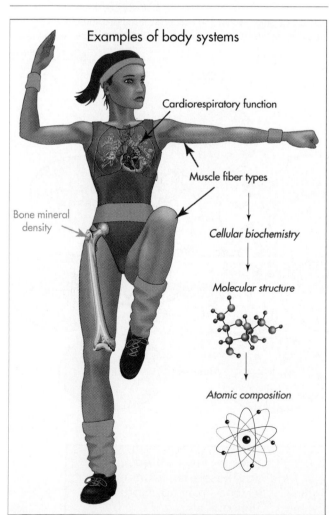

Examples of body systems

Cardiorespiratory function

Muscle fiber types

Bone mineral density

Cellular biochemistry

Molecular structure

Atomic composition

---

exercise physiology the study of how exercise alters the structure and function of the human body

TABLE 1.1

The academic disciplines that use exercise to further evaluate human function or as a clinical diagnostic tool

DISCIPLINE/TOPIC	EXAMPLE APPLICATIONS
Anatomy	The role of exercise in changing body composition
	Most accurate laboratory and field methods to estimate body composition
Biochemistry	Metabolic responses to muscle contraction and training
Biology	Alterations to the morphology of muscle after training
Biomechanics	Kinetics and kinematics of movement
Cardiology	Diagnostic, rehabilitative, and preventive uses
Endocrinology	Diabetes research
Immunology	Immune responses; treatment of individuals with AIDS
Nephrology	Reversal of cardiovascular risk factors
	Effects of exercise on renal function
Neurology	Effects of exercise on nerve function
Nutrition	Macro- and micronutrient needs during exercise
Occupational therapy	Injury rehabilitation/prevention
Orthopedics	Effects of exercise on bone remodeling
Physical therapy	Injury rehabilitation/prevention
Psychiatry	Stress reduction
Pulmonology	Respiratory muscle training

FIGURE 1.3

During the 1970s, exercise physiology was one of many core courses in physical education. Today the academic structure comprising exercise physiology courses must be suited to educating and training students from a diverse background for an equally diverse number of careers.

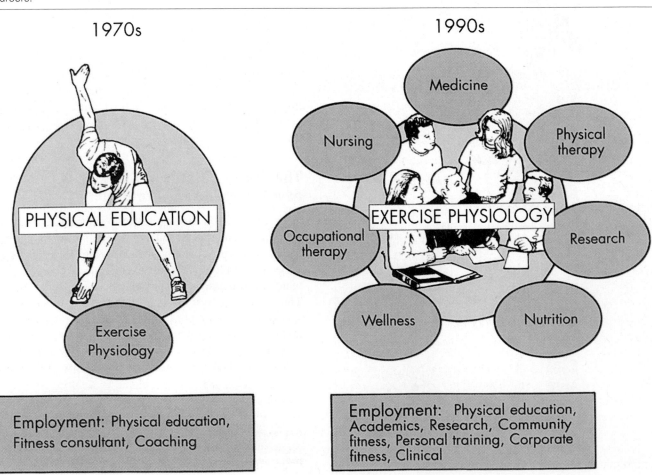

FOCUS BOX 1.2

Clinical Applications of Exercise Physiology

During the 1960s and 1970s, research findings were presented that indicated the potential for exercise to aid not only the athlete, but also the average citizen. Athletes were healthier than the average citizen, had fewer signs of degenerative diseases, and arguably had a higher quality of life. Indirect research evidence linked these differences to the adaptations of the body to continued exercise stress. Nevertheless, medical and public sentiment was skeptical because those who exercised regularly in Western societies during these dates were generally regarded as eccentric or antisocial. Despite the research indicating the benefits of exercise, the medical community was still lethargic about accepting the roles of exercise in preventive and rehabilitative medicine. However, with the vocalization of those medical doctors who were "hooked on exercise," such as George Sheehan and Kenneth Cooper, the medical community began to reinforce the health-related benefits of physical activity and exercise.

A significant development that catalyzed the medical recognition of the importance of exercise was the growing voice of the members of the American College of Sports Medicine (ACSM) (1), which was founded in 1954. These members comprised scientists and practitioners from fields such as physical education, exercise physiology, pure physiology, medicine, nutrition, and physical therapy, thereby fostering improved information exchange among the disciplines having an interest in how the body responds to exercise. In conjunction with the known deteriorating fitness of the children of most Western societies, with those of the United States being a notable example, and the increasing incidence of and mortality from coronary artery disease, the role of exercise in health maintenance and disease prevention was given increased attention (7, 18, 24).

Exercise was shown to lower serum cholesterol concentrations, and the known reductions in body fat and total body weight that accompany regular exercise with a healthy diet was also shown to decrease the risk for diabetes, hypertension, and musculoskeletal deterioration (1). The rest of the story will be presented in several of the chapters of this book. However, it is clear that exercise in today's society is more than a recreation. Two comments are brought to mind from two knowledgeable scientists. The first is from Covert Bailey, who has claimed that if exercise could be packaged into a pill, it would be the most prescribed medication in all of history. The second comment is from Åstrand's textbook (3), which identified the irony of the medical recommendation of requiring a physical examination prior to commencing an exercise training program. Åstrand stated that this reasoning is backward, for if a medical examination is required, it should be for all those individuals who refuse to regularly partake in physical activity! Åstrand's commentary, made prior to 1970 may make him a prophet, as it may not be long before insurance companies allow deductions for those individuals who give proof of regular physical activity!

---

difficult to precisely estimate the exact contribution of exercise to health and well being, evidence indicates that regular physical activity and exercise will increase longevity and decrease risk of death from cardiovascular disease (1, 4, 14, 17, 18, 24).

Prerequisite Study for Exercise Physiology

To complete a thorough study of exercise physiology, a student is required to understand anatomy, systems physiology, cellular biology, chemistry and biochemistry, and molecular biology.

A typical course schedule of classes in undergraduate exercise science is presented in table 1.2. These classes represent the core content of the undergraduate program in exercise science at the University of New Mexico. Table 1.2 also lists the prerequisite classes for graduate study in exercise science at the University of New Mexico. Not all universities offer the same classes, or have the same prerequisites, yet the trend for increased science and math preparation for an exercise physiology student is representative of most university programs.

As indicated in table 1.2, the study of exercise physiology requires academic knowledge in a number of disciplines. To be a successful exercise physiologist you must be a muscle physiologist, metabolic biochemist, cardiovascular physiologist, pulmonary physiologist, endocrine physiologist, environmental physiologist; you must also be proficient in understanding exercise training, exercise and weight control, body composition, nutrition, health, and clinical applications of exercise. A cardiovascular physiologist with an interest in exercise is not an exercise physiologist. Nor is a biochemist with an interest in how exercise alters muscle biochemistry, a nutritionist who is interested in the nutritional demands of exercise, or a pulmonologist who conducts exercise tests to better assess alterations in obstructive pulmonary disease. Without the knowledge of how exercise influences multiple physiological systems, a person would be extremely handicapped in appreciating the full impact exercise has on the human body. The multifaceted content of exercise physiology is a trademark of the discipline, and increases the academic and research difficulties of exercise physiologists. It is unfortunate that most other professions do not give exercise physiologists the academic and research respect they deserve. However, as indicated in appendix A, this trend is rapidly changing for the better for exercise physiology and exercise physiologists.

TABLE 1.2

An example of courses required for study of exercise science, with an emphasis on exercise physiology

COURSE AND DESCRIPTION

Undergraduate Program
Introductory Nutrition
Biology for the Health Sciences
General Chemistry and Laboratory
Introductory Biochemistry and Laboratory
Public Speaking
Introductory Math and Statistics
Human Anatomy and Physiology and Laboratory
First Aid
Tests and Measurements in Physical Education
Kinesiology
Motor Learning and Performance
Nutrition and Exercise
Athletic Injuries
Introductory Exercise Physiology
Fitness Assessment and Exercise Prescription
ECG Interpretation
Graded Exercise Testing
Weight Training and Physical Conditioning
Sports and Fitness Management
Statistics
Scientific Writing
Physical Defects and Exercise
Physical Activity and Aging
Advanced Exercise Physiology
Health Promotion

Prerequisites for a Master's Degree
Organic Chemistry
Biochemistry
Physics
Introductory Exercise Physiology
Kinesiology
Fitness Assessment and Exercise Prescription
Statistics
Scientific Writing

Prerequisites for a Ph.D.
as for a master's degree, and also
Advanced Exercise Physiology
Cell Biology
Research Experience[*]
Public Speaking Experience[†]

[*]Often this is in the form of a master's thesis.

[†]Either in a class, or documentation of a formal presentation.

Employment and Professional Issues

Despite the importance of knowing how exercise influences the body, and therefore the importance of the discipline of exercise physiology, until very recently the **profession** of exercise physiology had not been developed. This is a surprising deficiency of the discipline and profession of exercise physiology.

As an introductory student to exercise physiology, these facts may surprise you. However, the simple truth is that until 1997 there was no organization that functioned to develop the professional needs of exercise physiologists. The organization that now functions to do this is the American Society of Exercise Physiologists (ASEP)(2). Until the foundation of ASEP, the American College of Sports Medicine (ACSM) seemed to represent the main organization that exercise physiologists "pledged allegiance" to. However, by definition and their stated missions, ACSM is not a professional organization for exercise physiologists (20).

What do these issues mean to you as a student of exercise physiology? Well, unlike other allied health disciplines and professions, such as nursing, physical therapy, pulmonary therapy, or athletic training, there is no course accreditation or postgraduation certification exam to decree that a person is in fact an exercise physiologist. Of course, there are job descriptions for exercise physiologists in our hospitals, universities, fitness establishments, and corporate businesses. However, without organized course accreditation and/or certification, *almost anybody with a sincere interest in exercise or sports could market himself or herself as an exercise physiologist.* Furthermore, specific certification courses offered by such organizations as the ACSM, the National Strength and Conditioning Association, and the International Association of Fitness Professionals (IDEA), although superficially appearing to add credibility to exercise physiology-trained individuals, actually increase the likelihood that non–exercise science trained individuals will gain certification and will compete in the workforce for jobs that university-trained exercise physiologists (from an exercise science related program as detailed in table 1.2) are far better qualified to do. The American Society of Exercise Physiologists is working hard to develop national and international standards for course accreditation, and at developing a national certification exam so that exercise physiologists can finally be recognized for the quality scientists and educators they are (2).

The need to recognize exercise physiology as a profession is important to the future of exercise science courses in the universities of the United States and other countries of the world. For example, in the United States currently recognized allied health professions are lobbying to obtain sole responsibility for exercise-related testing in medical surroundings. Physical therapists, nurses, and nutritionists, although trained by Ph.D.-educated exercise physiologists, are claiming that it is they who are responsible for providing the knowledge base and skills for those who want to learn how exercise influences the human body. This means that tomorrow's jobs in clinical exercise testing, the nutrition of exercise, the rehabilitation of individuals with known disease, and perhaps university education will be taken away from those trained in exercise science and will be given to physical therapists, nutritionists, nurses, and pure physiologists with an interest in exercise. This means fewer jobs for you if you want to become an exercise physiologist, no matter what level of qualification (B.Sc. to Ph.D.)!

Of course, ASEP is functioning to prevent these dire forecasts from happening. Because you represent a potential exercise physiologist candidate, you need to empower yourself to be recognized for your training, knowledge, and competencies. Many exercise physiologists of all levels of education believe that they are worthy of receiving professional recognition. It is the hope of these people that they, as well as yourself, will one day be known by the medical and lay communities alike as exercise physiologists, and for the important function exercise physiologists play in today's and tomorrow's societies.

Given the previous description, what then is the potential for employment as an exercise physiologist? The answer depends on the degree you obtain. For undergraduates, current employment is focused toward completing additional teacher certification to become a physical education teacher. However, for many programs within the United States, most students do not pursue teaching but venture into private business as personal trainers, consult or work for fitness centers, and some even work in hospital settings as exercise test technicians within cardiac rehabilitation programs. Nevertheless, the feedback that the current undergraduate-qualified exercise physiologists provide does not paint a "pretty picture" of life as a B.Sc.-qualified exercise physiologist. For example, expressions that have been used in the newsletter of ASEP consist of "I've found that we [exercise physiologists] are not taken seriously," "we have to justify who we are and what we do on a regular basis," and "I am frustrated with people who think I am an aerobics instructor (with a lot of education)"(2).

Similar difficulties in nonuniversity professorial employment as an exercise physiologist exist for M.Sc.- and Ph.D.-trained individuals. It appears that not having course accreditation and certification as an exercise physiologist decreases the recognition of the competencies of exercise physiologists, resulting in limited employment opportunities and poor working conditions for already-employed exercise physiologists.

Another important question that deserves an answer in this chapter is, Why would people strive to pursue undergraduate and graduate training in exercise physiology if there is limited recognition of and professional respect for exercise physiologists? It is difficult to provide single answers to this question, because everybody is different. However, an overriding scenario is that the knowledge base and skills inherent in the training to become an exercise physiologist are so interesting and functionally important to all individuals that many students just "follow their hearts" and fulfill personal needs to become exercise physiologists. Many people place their faith in the fact that future events will reveal the importance of their talents and that one day exercise physiology will be a true profession, and employment opportunities will be better than they are today. For many, the improvements of professionalization are happening with the presence and growth of ASEP. The future direction of exercise physiology is now in the hands of exercise physiologists, and that can only be a positive development.

Research of Exercise Physiology

As with study of any scientific discipline, an appreciation of how research is conducted to develop the field, who conducts this research, and where it is published are very important. The student needs to be aware that a textbook cannot provide everything, and especially the latest research findings. Textbook material always needs to be supplemented with recent research findings. As a student in exercise physiology, you need to develop an inquisitiveness to seek out recent research, compare results and topics with information presented in textbooks, and combine both to frame your philosophy and understanding of the discipline.

Figure 1.2 indicated the different levels of inquiry in exercise physiology. There are many researchers who have focused on specific topics, and these are summarized in table 1.3. Of course, with today's computer-assisted library research tools, these names can be entered into a search of journal articles (e.g., "Medline" search) to reveal what articles have been published by a given researcher and provide the journals and dates of publication. This would be a useful exercise for you to do to better acquaint yourself with the research of exercise physiology.

Types of Research

The research of exercise physiology can be classified several ways (fig. 1.4). Brooks (6) classified research by purpose, with **pure research** representing research for the purpose of further understanding physiology, and **applied research** representing application of pure research findings to further understand exercise (9). Pure research is also referred to as *basic research*. For example, based on figure 1.2, pure research in exercise physiology would be the measurement of variables that contribute to muscular strength. This knowledge could then be applied to determine the best training for strength improvement, the extent of gender differences in strength, the influence of nutrition on strength development, and the potential for strength development in the elderly.

There is also **clinical research** in exercise physiology. Clinical research is a subdivision of applied research, and is defined as research conducted with application to medicine

---

profession an occupation that requires special education and training

pure research research for the purpose of further understanding physiology

applied research application of pure research findings to further understand exercise

clinical research research conducted with application to medicine or clinical practice

TABLE 1.3		
The names of prominent researchers in exercise-related topics since the 1970s		
NAME	RESEARCH INTERESTS	RESEARCH AFFILIATION*
Skeletal Muscle		
Molecular biology/histology		
	Ken Baldwin	U.C.–Irvine (U.S.)
	Frank Booth	University of Texas–Houston
	Phil Gollnick	Deceased (U.S.)
	David Costill	Now retired (U.S.)
CHO and lipid metabolism		
	David Costill	Now retired (U.S.)
	Eddie Coyle	University of Texas–Austin (U.S.)
	Bengt Saltin	Karolinska Institute (Sweden)
Metabolic biochemistry		
	George Brooks	U.C.–Berkeley (U.S.)
	Clyde Williams	Loughborough University (U.K.)
	Ronald Terjung	University of Missouri (U.S.)
	Eric Hultman	Queen's Medical Center (U.K.)
	Kent Sahlin	Karolinska Institute (Sweden)
Training adaptations		
	Bengt Saltin	Karolinska Institute (Sweden)
	John Holloszy	University of Washington–St. Louis (U.S.)
	Phil Gollnick	Deceased (U.S.)
Muscular strength and power		
	William Kraemer	Pennsylvania State University (U.S.)
	James MacDougall	McMaster University (Canada)
Pulmonary Function/Gas Exchange/ Ventilation		
	Jerry Dempsey	University of Wisconsin (U.S.)
	Richard Hughson	University of Waterloo (Canada)
	Peter Wagner	University of California–San Diego (U.S.)
	Brian Whipp	St. George's Hospital Medical School (U.K.)
	Karlman Wasserman	Harbor–UCLA Medical Center, CA (U.S.)

*Note: The university locations of these researchers were correct at the time of publication, but may have changed since then.

or clinical practice. For example, research of exercise training and its effects on serum cholesterol can be classified as clinical research, as can research of how certain drugs prescribed to individuals with heart disease affect their tolerance of exercise.

Research can also be classified by type of subject. Pure and applied research can be conducted using human subjects or by using animals. **Human subjects research** has the best application to human physiology; however, for ethical reasons, not all questions can be answered when using human subjects. For example, certain research methods, such as the use of radioactive molecules, can be questioned for application to human subjects. In addition, human subjects are not suited to pure research that attempts to isolate specific tissues or organs. A common model used in **animal research** for studying muscle metabolism during exercise is the rat hindlimb. Researchers can control blood flow, the content of the blood, and exercise by artificial electrical stimulation to

develop conditions that they know will best answer their questions. Mongrel dogs are also used for similar purposes, and especially to research the function of the liver during exercise.

Finally, research can also be classified by the type of design used. The differences are very important; the design of a study can be very significant in determining the validity of results and their application to the community. An important type of research is called **experimental research**. Experimental research involves researcher control of a variable between two or more groups of subjects. The best example of this type of research in exercise physiology involves research into how training influences certain body functions. The subjects are studied prior to training, and are then placed into groups that either train or do not train. After a period of time, the two groups are studied again, and the results are compared between the two groups to detect any differences (12). This research can be done another way, using **comparative research**. With this approach, rather than select sub-

TABLE 1.3

The names of prominent researchers in exercise-related topics since the 1970s

NAME	RESEARCH INTERESTS	RESEARCH AFFILIATION*
Bone Metabolism		
	Barbara Drinkwater	Pacific Medical Center–Seattle (U.S.)
Carbohydrate Ingestion During Exercise		
	Carl Gisolfi	Iowa State University (U.S.)
	David Costill	Now retired (U.S.)
	Eddie Coyle	University of Texas–Austin (U.S.)
Body Composition		
	Timothy Lohman	University of Arizona (U.S.)
	Vivian Heyward	University of New Mexico (U.S.)
Exercise and Health		
	Steven N. Blair	The Cooper Institute for Aerobics Research, TX (U.S.)
	William L. Haskell	Stanford University, CA (U.S.)
	Ralph Paffenbarger	Stanford University, CA (U.S.)
Cardiovascular Function During Exercise		
	Jere Mitchell	Harry S. Moss Heart Center (U.S.)
	Larry Rowell	University of Washington–Seattle (U.S.)
	Jack Wilmore	Texas A&M University (U.S.)
Fluid Balance and Exercise		
	J. Greenleaf	Ames Research Center, CA (U.S.)
	Timothy Noakes	University of Capetown (S. Africa)
	David Costill	Now retired (U.S.)
Environmental Physiology		
	Charles Houston	Retired
	Ethan Nadel	Yale University, New Haven, CT (U.S.)
	Michael Sawka	NATIC (U.S.)
	John Sutton	Deceased (Australia)

FIGURE 1.4

The multiple classifications of research.

Pure and applied
Exercise physiology research

Animal or Human subjects

Experimental
   Pure (Basic)
   Applied
   Clinical
Cross sectional
   Epidemiological
   Causal Comparative
   Predictive
   Explanatory
Descriptive
Observational

jects and control the exercise they do, researchers find subjects who are already exercise training the way they like, and another group of subjects who are not exercise training. The subjects are studied, and the results are compared (11). Where possible, *experimental research is always a better method than comparative research*, because the results are more likely to be the result of researcher control of a variable, rather than some unknown variable(s). For example, is the ability of marathon runners to consume oxygen during

human subjects research research performed with humans as subjects

animal research research performed with animals as subjects

experimental research research performed that involves the control of a factor, or factors, that will influence an outcome

comparative research research based on comparing one or more groups of individuals for certain characteristics

running solely due to their training, or are some other variables involved? We know from experimental research that other variables are involved, such as the genetically determined traits of high slow-twitch muscle fiber proportions, body frame, and relatively large heart sizes and other cardiovascular functional capacities.

A final type of research design, often used in clinical research, needs to be explained. When researchers collect data on hundreds, or even thousands of subjects, data can be analyzed to reveal trends or associations between variables. For example, research from the Framingham study on the risk factors for cardiovascular disease revealed the importance of high blood cholesterol, cigarette smoking, and high blood pressure to the risks of developing and dying from heart disease (24). Obviously, experimental human subjects research cannot be done because this would require forcing people to smoke, develop high blood pressure and blood cholesterol, and thereby have an increased risk of premature death! Thus, this form of large-scale comparative research is conducted and is termed **epidemiological research**. Epidemiological research has better control than simple comparative research because a large number of variables are studied, allowing the use of statistical techniques that can "control" how certain variables relate to others. Epidemiological research has been invaluable in evaluating the importance of exercise in the prevention and treatment of the different types of cardiovascular diseases (4, 14, 18, 24).

Journals that Publish Exercise Physiology Research

Research is published in special reports called **journals**. Unlike books, journals are published at regular intervals (usually monthly) for the purpose of revealing research findings to the scientific and lay communities. Many articles from journals are listed in the reference section of this chapter. Publication of research in journal articles is meant to be a relatively fast procedure. Compared to a textbook which may take 2 to 3 years to develop and publish, research and subsequent publication in a journal may take between 1 to 1½ years. Clearly, data in journals are published more rapidly than in books, but journals are still a relatively slow means of information dispersal. This is why many scientific organizations conduct meetings to present more recent research, which may be between 6 months to 1 year old. Nevertheless, journal articles are superior to research presented at meetings because they are stringently reviewed by other researchers who have expertise in the topic researched, termed *peer reviewed*. If research or the written presentation of the research is flawed or does not contribute new and important knowledge to a field, it is rejected by the reviewers and not published. The peer review process is an attempt to ensure quality research publications and the unhindered growth of knowledge on a particular topic (19).

The importance of exercise to the function of almost all body systems and to the general health and well-being of the body (see focus box 1.2) has caused exercise-related research to be published in an increasingly diverse number of

TABLE 1.4
Journals that publish exercise-related research and reviews

Acta Physiologica Scandinavia
American Journal of Clinical Nutrition
American Journal of Physiology
American Journal of Sports Medicine
Biochemistry
Canadian Journal of Applied Sports Sciences
Circulation
European Journal of Applied Physiology
International Journal of Sports Medicine
International Journal of Sports Nutrition
Journal of Applied Physiology
Journal of Biochemical Research
Journal of Biochemistry
Journal of Clinical Investigation
Journal of Exercise Physiology (online)
Journal of Physiology
Journal of Sports Medicine and Physical Fitness
Journal of Sports Sciences Research
Journal of Strength and Conditioning Research
Medicine and Science in Sports and Exercise
Metabolism
Pediatric Exercise Science
Pflugers Archives
Physiological Reviews
Professionalization of Exercise Physiology (online)
Research Quarterly for Exercise and Sport
Sports Medicine
The Physician and Sports Medicine

journals. A representative sampling of these journals is provided in table 1.4.

Just as a computer search of authors is rewarding, so is a computer search of article titles by journal. If you do not have access to computer-assisted searches, you should go to your library and sample the contents of many of these journals. This is another excellent exercise to become more acquainted with the research published in exercise physiology.

The New Frontiers of Exercise-Related Research

In the last 50 years, tremendous achievements have been possible in both pure and applied research because of the application of new or improved research techniques, or the application of techniques to new conditions. The percutaneous needle biopsy technique to sample human skeletal muscle before, during, and after exercise is an example of a revolutionary advancement that influenced both exercise physiology and muscle biochemistry research from the late 1960s to today (9, 23).

In recent years, advances in our understanding of exercise physiology similar to those from muscle biopsy have been made because of additional new equipment, technologies, and research techniques. The use of stable isotopes to study cellular metabolism in humans during rest, exercise, and postexercise conditions has contributed to our further understanding of substrates used during exercise (21, 22) (see chapter 6). Similarly, noninvasive techniques such as magnetic resonance (MR) imaging and MR spectroscopy (fig. 1.5) are providing insight into the function and adaptablity of skeletal muscle metabolism at different exercise intensities (8, 10). Finally, the improved application of computers and electronics to exercise equipment and measurement instruments (fig. 1.6) is improving the quantity of data that can be collected and analyzed from research, and is expanding the ability of researchers to ask and answer additional questions (13, 15, 16, 23).

The future of research in exercise physiology is more and more dependent on the use of sophisticated equipment and the academic and research skills that span applied approaches, as well as the pure fields of molecular biology, biochemistry, neurophysiology, cardiology, pulmonary physiology, and endocrinology. The enormous volume of exercise-related research published in journals (table 1.4) makes the acquisition of a broad knowledge base a more difficult task, and the future of the field more challenging and, hopefully, more rewarding.

As you begin your study of exercise physiology, be aware that the field is continually growing. Realize that your prerequisite study in human anatomy and physiology is ex-

tremely important, and that further knowledge of pure human physiology and biochemistry can only help you to become a better exercise physiologist. If you are studying exercise physiology as part of prerequisite study for careers in physical therapy, medicine, nursing, or other health-related occupations, this book will be a valuable resource in how you can apply exercise physiology to your vocation.

FIGURE 1.6

A photograph of a subject maximally contracting skeletal muscles on a computerized resistance machine that can quantify forces and velocities of muscle contraction at multiple joint angles during dynamic contractions.

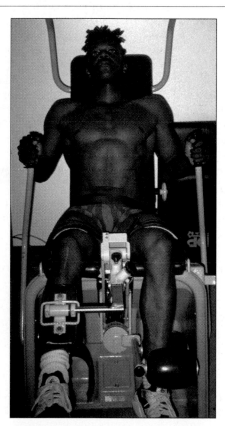

FIGURE 1.5

A photograph of a typical large bore magnet used for the study of forearm or lower-limb muscle metabolism during exercise, or in recovery from exercise. This equipment uses the noninvasive and harmless technique of magnetic resonance to quantify concentrations of certain molecules within living tissue.

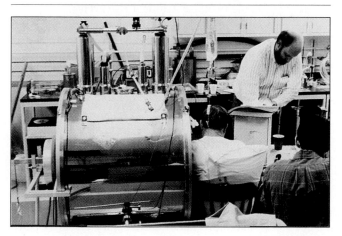

epidemiological research research using large numbers of subjects that attempts to establish relationships between multiple characteristics

journal a publication that presents results from research

WEBSITE BOX

Chapter 1: An Introduction to Exercise Physiology

The newest information regarding exercise physiology can be viewed at the following sites.*

css.edu/users/tboone2/asep/toc.htm
   American Society of Exercise Physiologists
csep.ca
   Canadian Society for Exercise Physiology
sportsci.org/
   Information resource for all disciplines within exercise and sport science.
nor.com.au/business/aaess/home.htm
   Australian Association of Exercise and Sport Science
acsm.org/
   American College of Sports Medicine
gssi.web.com/membership/toc-sse.html
   Gatorade Sports Science Index—lists all publications of the Gatorade Sports Science Exchange.
cortland.edu/www/libwww/exercise_physiology.html
   Provides directions for library research of topics within exercise physiology.

livjm.ac.uk/sports_science/exerphys.htm
   Provides links to other sites related to exercise physiology.
tees.ac.uk/sportscience/
   Provides lecture notes for the sport science degree at the University of Teesside, England. Use this site for additional content on many of the chapters in this text.
arfa.org/index.htm
   Excellent site providing comprehensive information on many topics within exercise physiology.
wso.williams.edu/~sbennett/exer.html
   Provides links to other sites related to exercise physiology.

*Unless indicated, all URLs preceded by http://www.

Note: These URLs were valid at the time of publication but could have changed or been deleted from Internet access since that time.

SUMMARY

- The term **exercise** can be used to denote activity that is performed for the purpose of improving, maintaining, or expressing a particular type of physical fitness. **Physical activity** pertains to the activity performed by the body for purposes other than the specific development of physical fitness.

- The components of **physical fitness** include muscular strength, muscular power, muscular endurance, cardiorespiratory endurance, flexibility, body composition, and agility.

- The repeated use of exercise to improve physical fitness is termed **exercise training**. The body experiences immediate responses to exercise that vary with the type of exercise performed. Such immediate responses are termed **acute adaptations**, and these function to help the body tolerate the exercise or physical activity. **Chronic adaptations** may require several weeks to develop (e.g., improved muscle size), whereas others may take only several days (e.g., improved abilities to consume oxygen) or may occur after as little as one or two exercise sessions (e.g., increased blood volume).

- By definition, **exercise physiology** is a discipline involving the study of how exercise alters the structure and function of the human body. To be an exercise physiologist requires knowledge of how all systems of the body respond to exercise and therefore involves considerable study. However, an unfortunate fact is that exercise physiology is not currently a recognized **profession**, and only since 1997 has there been an organization in the United States (American Society of Exercise Physiologists, ASEP) that exists to serve the professional needs of exercise physiologists.

- **Pure research** represents research for the purpose of further understanding physiology, and **applied research** represents the application of pure research findings to further understand exercise. **Clinical research** is a subdivision of applied research and is defined as research conducted with application to medicine or clinical practice. **Human subjects research** has the best application to human physiology; however, for ethical reasons, not all questions can be answered when using human subjects and therefore **animal research** is performed.

- Research can also be classified by the type of design used. An important type of research is called **experimental research**. Experimental research involves researcher control of a variable between two or more groups of subjects. **Comparative research** involves the study of two different groups of subjects who already differ in the variable at question. Where possible, *experimental research is always a better method than comparative research*, because the results are more likely to be the consequence of researcher control of a variable, rather than some unknown variable(s). **Epidemiological research** is another form of comparative research, but researchers study a large number of variables, and some of these are used to control which subjects are compared to other subjects.

▪ Research is published in special reports called **journals**. Unlike books, journals are published at regular intervals (usually monthly), for the purpose of revealing research findings to the scientific and lay communities.

▪ In the last 50 years, tremendous achievements have been possible in both pure and applied research because of the application of new or improved research techniques, or the application of techniques to new conditions. Examples are the percutaneous needle biopsy technique, the use of stable isotopes, magnetic resonance (MR) imaging and MR spectroscopy, and the improved quality and application of computers and electronics.

STUDY QUESTIONS

1. Define the terms exercise, physical activity, physical fitness, exercise training, and exercise physiology.

2. Why is participation in exercise becoming more important in today's society?

3. Explain the components of physical fitness and provide an exercise example that involves the development of many of these components.

4. What are acute and chronic adaptations to exercise?

5. What might be some of the benefits of the professionalization of exercise physiology? Are there any detriments?

6. Use the terms pure research, applied research, clinical research, human subjects research, animal research, and epidemiological research to explain how research can be conducted in exercise physiology.

7. Be able to mention the names and identify the research topic(s) of important researchers in exercise physiology.

8. List several journal names that publish research of exercise physiology.

9. How is improved technology influencing the research in exercise physiology?

APPLICATIONS

1. Visit your library and find one of the journals listed in table 1.4. Locate a recent issue of the journal and one of the earliest issues shelved. Make a list of the topics published in the recent and oldest issues and compare them. Are there differences? Try to explain why the recent topics may be more or less meaningful in application than the older topics.

2. Evaluate your own fitness. Which components would you improve if you could, and why?

3. Surf the Internet and find and read the contents of the following websites: American College of Sports Medicine, American Society of Exercise Physiologists,

Canadian Society of Exercise Physiology, *Journal of Applied Physiology* (American Physiological Society).

4. Do a computer search for the following:

   a. Recent research completed by one of the authors listed in table 1.3

   b. Recent research completed on an exercise-related topic that interests you

5. Explain why the academic content of exercise physiology is gaining increasing recognition in the medical community.

REFERENCES

1. American College of Sports Medicine. *ACSM's guidelines for exercise testing and prescription,* 5th ed. Williams & Wilkins, Baltimore, 1995.

2. American Society of Exercise Physiologists. Website, http://www.css.edu/users/tboone2/asep/toc.htm.

3. Åstrand, P. O. *Textbook of work physiology: Physiological bases of exercise.* McGraw-Hill, New York, 1970.

4. Blair, S. N., K. W. Kohl, N. F. Gordon, and R. S. Paffenbarger, Jr. How much physical activity is good for health? *Ann. Rev. Public Health.*13:99–126, 1992.

5. Boone, T. I know you're an exercise physiologist, but what do you do? *Profess. Exerc. Physiol.* 1(3): http://www.css.edu/users/tboone2/asep/pro9.htm.

6. Brooks, G. A. *Basic exercise physiology.* American College of Sports Medicine 40th anniversary lectures. American College of Sports Medicine, Indianapolis, 1994, pp. 15–42.

7. Chapman, C. B., and J. H. Mitchell. The physiology of exercise. *Scientific American* 212:88–96, 1965.

8. Cheng, H. A., R. A. Robergs, J. P. Lettelier, M. V. Icenogle, and L. Haseler. Changes in muscle transverse relaxation and muscle acidosis during forearm exercise and recovery. *J. Appl. Physiol.* 79(4):1370–1378, 1995.

9. Costill, D. L. *Applied exercise physiology.* American College of Sports Medicine 40th anniversary lectures. American College of Sports Medicine, Indianapolis, 1994, pp. 69–80.

REFERENCES

10. Fleckenstein, J. L., D. Watamull, D. D. McIntire, L. A. Bertocci, D. P. Chason, and R. M. Peshock. Muscle proton T2 relaxation times during work and during repetitive voluntary exercise. *J. Appl. Physiol.* 74(60):2855–2859, 1993.

11. Gollnick, P. D., R. B. Armstrong, C. W. Saubert, W. L. Sembrowich, R. E. Shepherd, and B. Saltin. Enzyme activity and fiber composition in skeletal muscle of untrained and trained men. *J. Appl. Physiol.* 33:312–319, 1972.

12. Gollnick, P. D. Metabolism of substrates: Energy substrate metabolism during exercise and as modified by physical training. *Federation Proc.* 44:353–357, 1985.

13. Hill, A. V. Muscular exercise, lactic acid, and the supply and utilization of oxygen. *Quart. J. Med.* 16:135–171, 1923.

14. Lee, I.-M., C.-C. Hsieh, and R. S. Paffenbarger, Jr. Exercise intensity and longevity in men: The Harvard Alumni Study. *JAMA.* 273(15):1179–1184, 1995.

15. Lusk, G. *The elements of the science of nutrition.* Saunders, Philadelphia, 1928.

16. Mitchell, J. H., W. C. Sproule, and C. B. Chapman. The physiological meaning of the maximal oxygen uptake test. *J. Clin. Invest.* 37:538–547, 1958.

17. Ornish, D. Can lifestyle changes reverse coronary artery disease? *World Rev. Nutr. Diet.* 72:38–48, 1993.

18. Paffenbarger, R. S., Jr., R. T. Hyde, A. L. Wing, I.-M. Lee, D. L. Jung, and J. B. Kampert. The association of changes in physical activity level and other lifestyle characteristics with mortality among men. *N. Eng. J. Med.* 328:538–545, 1993.

19. Raven, P. B., and W. G. Squires. What is science ? *Med. Sci. Sports Exerc.* 21(4):351–352, 1989.

20. Robergs, R. A. ACSM and exercise physiology: Past, present and future. *Profess. Exerc. Physiol.* 1(1): http://www.css.edu/users/tboone2/asep/pro1.htm.

21. Romijn, J. A., E. F. Coyle, S. Sidossis, X.-J. Zhang, and R. R. Wolfe. Relationship between fatty acid delivery and fatty acid oxidation during strenuous exercise. *J. Appl. Physiol.* 79(6):1939–1945, 1995.

22. Romijn, J. A., et al.. Regulation of endogenous fat and carbohydrate metabolism in relation to exercise intensity and duration. *Am. J. Physiol.* 265(8):E380–E391, 1993.

23. Sahlin, K., A. Katz, and S. Broberg. Tricarboxylic acid cycle intermediates in human muscle during prolonged exercise. *Am. J. Physiol.* 259(28):C834–C841, 1990.

24. Sherman, S. E., R. B. D'Agnostino, J. L. Cobb, and W. B. Kannel. Physical activity and mortality in women in the Framingham Heart Study. *Am. Heart J.* 128(5):879–884, 1994.

25. Taylor, H. L., E. R. Buskirk, and A. Henschel. Maximal oxygen intake as an objective measure of cardiorespiratory performance. *J. Appl. Physiol.* 8:73–80, 1955.

26. *Webster's Ninth New Collegiate Dictionary.* Merriam-Webster, Springfield, MA, 1984.

RECOMMENDED READING

Blair, S. N., K. W. Kohl, N. F. Gordon, and R. S. Paffenbarger Jr. How much physical activity is good for health? *Ann. Rev. Public Health.* 13:99–126, 1992.

Chapman, C. B., and J. H. Mitchell. The physiology of exercise. Scientific American. 212:88–96, 1965.

Costill, D. L. *Applied exercise physiology.* American College of Sports Medicine 40th anniversary lectures. American College of Sports Medicine, Indianapolis, 1994, pp. 69–80.

Lusk, G. *The elements of the science of nutrition.* Saunders, Philadelphia, 1928.

Robergs, R. A. ACSM and exercise physiology: past, present and future. *Profess. Exerc. Physiol.* 1(1): http://www.css.edu/users/tboone2/asep/pro1.htm.

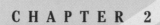

CHAPTER 2

Exercise: A Challenge of Homeostatic Control

earning how the body responds to exercise is essentially a study of control systems. We all know that we shiver when cold, or sweat when hot, and that responses exist to maintain an optimal body temperature. We are also aware that we eat when hungry, drink when thirsty, and sleep when tired. These behavioral and physical responses are not accidental, but are the result of intricate and often complicated biochemical control systems that exist within us. Exercise is a stress to the body that must be tolerated for continued activity. The stress of exercise is expressed in many body systems such as increased demands on the heart and lungs to maintain appropriate oxygen and carbon dioxide content in arterial blood; the regulation of muscle metabolism to provide rates of ATP (adenosine triphosphate) regeneration that meet the increased rates of ATP demand; functions of the heart, kidney, and cardiovascular system to optimize heat loss to the surroundings; functions of the heart, kidney, and peripheral vasculature in attempting to normalize blood pressure. If exercise is performed for too long, at a too high intensity, or in inappropriate environments, many of these body regulatory functions can fail, and exercise must be stopped. The purpose of this chapter is to explain the functioning of control systems and identify how exercise affects the major biological control systems of the body.

OBJECTIVES

After studying this chapter, you should be able to:

- Explain the differences between homeostasis and steady state.
- Define the components and functions of a biological control system.
- List several examples of biological control systems that function during exercise.
- Describe the concept of "negative feedback."
- Explain the concept of the "gain" of a control system.
- Describe how the correct function of control systems are crucial to normal body function and, in certain exercise situations, may preserve life.

KEY TERMS

homeostasis
steady state
biological control system
receptor

integrating control unit
effector mechanism

negative feedback
gain

Homeostasis

*T*he condition of bodily function when a constant or unchanging internal environment is maintained is called **homeostasis**. The homeostatic condition of the body is generally accepted to be at rest and unstressed and represents the state of the body in which it can most easily respond to a changing external environment. Despite these definitions, homeostasis is not a constant condition. There is a *dynamic balance* in bodily functions that combine to maintain homeostasis. For example, figure 2.1 illustrates the variation in systolic, mean and diastolic blood pressures obtained from every cardiac cycle during 4 min of supine rest. Neither measurement is constant, as each randomly fluctuates slightly above and below a mean value that we interpret as normal.

Homeostasis should not be interpreted as an ideal body condition. Later chapters of this text will explain how destructive a purely sedentary lifestyle is to human bodily function. In fact, exercise, a condition that can perturb homeostasis to large extremes, is gaining increased clinical recognition for its roles in disease prevention and rehabilitation. *The issues that are important about homeostasis are* (1) *how well the body can reduce the physiological consequences of applied stress and* (2) *the speed at which a homeostatic condition is once again attained.* Consequently, the student should view homeostasis as a reference, and focus interest on the processes of the body that are called upon when the body deviates from homeostatic function.

Steady State

In the study of exercise physiology, another common term used to describe seemingly constant conditions is **steady state.** Steady state during exercise is not homeostasis, but a condition where certain body functions have attained dynamic constancy at a new level. For example, during the transition from rest to low-intensity exercise the body is forced to increase oxygen transport and metabolism to fuel the contracting muscles. Thus, after a short period of time, the body has attained a steady state in oxygen consumption and the physiological processes that support this adaptation to the exercise. The adjustments in oxygen consumption and heart rate during a bout of low-intensity exercise are illustrated in figure 2.2. Each measure increased after the start of exercise, and then reached a steady state value. When concerned with prolonged continuous exercise, the ability to attain steady state for a given exercise intensity will determine the duration a person will be able to exercise. Thus, *when concerned with exercise, the condition of steady state has far more meaning than the condition of homeostasis.*

Control Systems of the Body

We have already expressed that the body has numerous control systems. A **biological control system** is a functioning unit that works to help maintain homeostasis. The components of a biological control system are a **receptor, integrating**

FIGURE 2.1

Tonometry is the continuous measurement of systemic blood pressure from a sensor placed over an artery. This method is noninvasive, provides blood pressure readings in intervals of less than 1 s, and is used routinely in hospitals to monitor blood pressure in patients during unconsciousness (e.g., surgery). In this figure, tonometry is used to show the variability in systolic, mean and diastolic blood pressures over time.

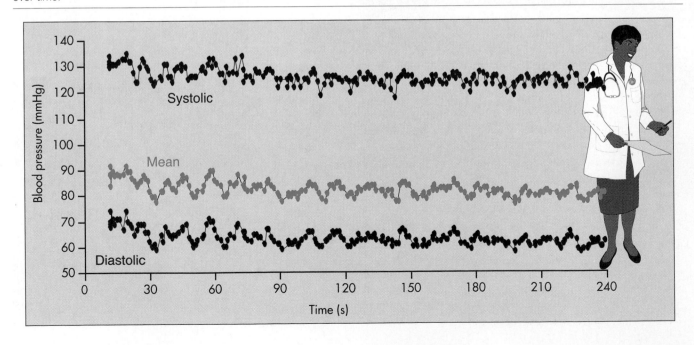

control unit, and an **effector mechanism.** Examples of biological control systems that function during exercise are illustrated in figure 2.3.

There are multiple sensory mechanisms that influence the body's control of blood pressure during exercise. Immediately as exercise begins, nerves from the brain and the contracting muscle(s) stimulate an increase in heart rate and blood flow around the body. These responses are necessary to support the muscles' needs for increased energy metabolism and waste removal, yet they have the potential to greatly increase blood pressure. To combat extreme exercise-induced increases in blood pressure, almost as abruptly as nerves stimulate an increased heart rate there are neural and chemical stimuli that decrease resistance to blood flow through the skin and contracting muscle (14). In fact, as illustrated in figure 2.4, at the start of exercise there are immediate decreases in both systolic and diastolic blood pressure that last several seconds and are followed by increases in systolic and mean arterial pressures (7, 11).

The receptors of blood pressure regulation during exercise are skeletal muscle, baroreceptors of the aortic and carotid arteries, and the atrium of the heart. The integrating control unit is located in the brain, and the effector mechanisms consist of nerves, hormones, and chemically related factors such as increased temperature, decreased pH, and the release of certain substances from muscle and/or the cell lining of the blood vessels within the contracting muscle that cause blood vessels to dilate (6, 13). As illustrated (fig. 2.4), these mechanisms provide a response that precedes the stimuli that they function to oppose, and is a good example of the speed at which biological control systems can function.

Another important biological control system integrates thermal and fluid balances. When we exercise, contracting muscles increase heat production. To maintain as normal a body temperature as possible, this heat must be directed to the surrounding environment. Most of the heat lost from the body during exercise is through the evaporation of sweat from our skin. Fluid lost as sweat during exercise can increase to a volume that exceeds 2 L/h if the environmental temperature is warm and/or humid, and exercise intensity is relatively high (8, 9). To maintain thermal balance, the body must therefore stress the regulation of fluid balance. Thus exercise can stress both thermal and fluid balance and, unless fluid balance can be maintained as best as possible, the body can experience large gains in heat storage, which in turn can cause tissue damage, organ failure, and even death.

The body has heat-sensitive receptors in peripheral tissues, as well as in the region of the brain responsible for integrating many sensory signals (hypothalamus). Increasing blood temperature sensed by the hypothalamus causes nerve stimulation that initiates an increase in sweating, redistributes more blood flow to the skin to assist in improved evaporative cooling of the body, and regulates the kidney to conserve fluid. As will be discussed in chapter 19, exercise in unusual environments adds to many of the stresses imposed on biological control systems within the body.

FIGURE 2.2

The increase in oxygen consumption (VO_2) and heart rate from rest to steady-state exercise. The steady-state condition is reflected by the near constant values for VO_2 and heart rate over time.

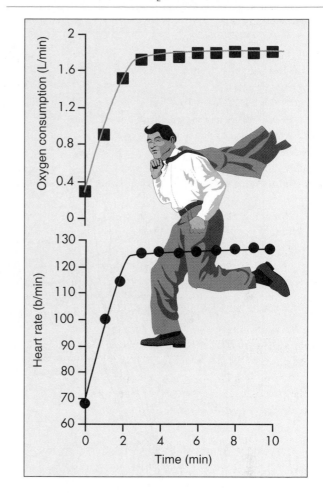

homeostasis the maintenance of a constant or unchanging internal environment

steady state a condition where certain bodily functions have attained dynamic constancy at a level different from homeostasis

biological control system a functioning unit of the body that functions to maintain homeostasis

receptor the component of a biological control system that senses a stimulus and relays information to the integrating control unit

integrating control unit the component that receives the sensory information from the receptor and redirects information to cause a response

effector mechanism the response resulting from receptor and integrating unit function

FIGURE 2.3

Examples of systems within the body that function as biological control systems during exercise stress. During exercise the heart and lungs increase their function in response to nerve stimulation. In addition, nerves are responsible for causing the muscle contraction of exercise. The skeletal system provides the framework of the body that enables movement. Bones also respond to exercise stress by becoming more tolerant of physical and load bearing stress.

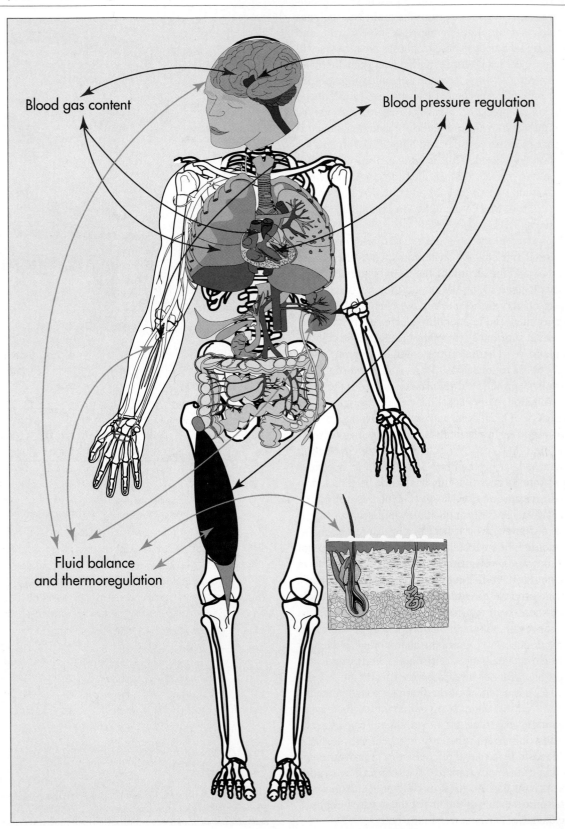

FIGURE 2.4

The immediate changes in systemic blood pressure in the transition from rest to exercise. Note the near-instantaneous decrease in both systolic and diastolic blood pressures after the start of exercise. Shortly after this, systolic pressure continues to increase, whereas diastolic pressure increases slightly and stabilizes at near-resting values.

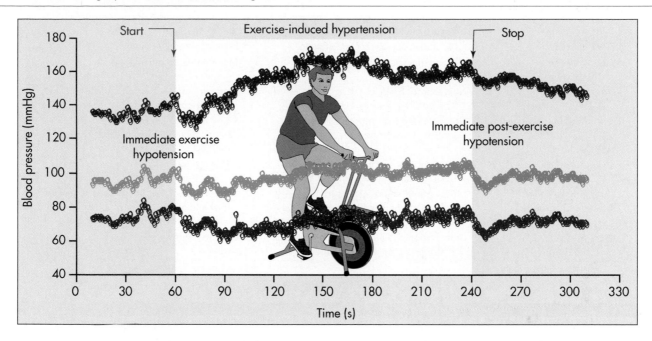

Table 2.1 lists the major control systems of the body, and their stimuli and effector responses that combine to regulate the body's acute response to exercise. These *control systems vary from intracellular biochemical functions to large multi-organ systems that work together to maintain normal bodily function as best as possible.* For example, the biochemical pathways of energy metabolism respond to increase the production of ATP (chemical energy) that is necessary to maintain the cellular ATP concentration that fuels muscle contraction and general cell function. Similarly, the lungs and heart function together to ensure that blood hemoglobin saturation with oxygen does not decrease during exercise despite what could be a 15-fold increase in oxygen consumption by the body. As you become more knowledgeable in exercise physiology it will become apparent that the body's physiological response to exercise can only be completely understood when one applies knowledge of how exercise can simultaneously influence multiple biological control systems.

Negative Feedback

From the examples provided of biological control systems, a consistent feature is that the response(s) to a stimulus that perturbs homeostasis causes a response that attempts to decrease the original stimulus and/or dampen the body's response to that stimulus. As these control system responses work in opposition to the initial stimulus response they are termed **negative feedback** responses.

The majority of the body's control response mechanisms operate via negative feedback. For example, blood pressure regulation during postural movement from a supine to a standing position can increase the occurrence of low blood pressure, or hypotension, because of a decreased flow of blood to the heart from the lower body (fig. 2.5). This condition is immediately sensed by specialized stretch receptors in the walls of the aorta and carotid arteries. Less blood flow to the heart decreases the volume of blood ejected by the heart, which decreases stretch on the arteries, which in turn decreases the rate of action potentials emanating from these receptors. This change is interpreted by the brain and results in a large neural and hormonal response that decreases the diameter of blood vessels in the lower limbs of the body, thus squeezing blood back to the heart and normalizing blood flow from the heart and blood pressure. The correction of blood pressure then increases the stretch on the receptors of the aorta and carotid arteries towards normal, increasing the signal output of the specialized stretch receptors. This was a negative feedback response as it reduced the initial signal that evoked the response. *Negative feedback systems therefore function to decrease the magnitude of the initial stimulus, resulting in the decreased need for further regulation.*

negative feedback responses of a biological control system that oppose the initial stimulus

TABLE 2.1

The major biological control systems of the body important during exercise

CONTROL SYSTEM EFFECT	STIMULI/EFFECTOR	FUNCTION
↑Energy metabolism	Chemical products of muscle contraction/cell organelles, enzymes	Maintain cellular ATP concentrations
↓Blood glucose	↑ Blood glucose/pancreas, ↑ insulin	Maintain blood glucose
↑Blood glucose	↓ Blood glucose/pancreas, ↑ glucagon	Maintain blood glucose
↑Lung ventilation	Nerves from brain, muscles, joints; ↑ blood CO_2/control of ventilation	Maintain normal oxygen and carbon dioxide content blood; maintain blood pH
↑Heart rate	Nerves from brain, muscles; hormones/control of heart rate	↑ Blood flow to provide oxygen for metabolism and remove wastes from metabolism
↑Sweat response	Nerves from spinal cord and brain; ↑ skin temp/ ↑ sweat gland function	↑ Blood flow to skin and ↑ sweat rate to ↑ heat transfer from body
↓Peripheral vascular resistance	Muscle metabolites, nerves from brain, ↑ muscle temp, ↑ muscle pH/blood vessel regulation	↑ Blood vessel dilation to ↓ resistance to flow and allow an ↑ in blood flow without a large ↑ in systemic blood pressure
↑Kidney water reabsorption	Dehydration, ↑ osmolality hypothalamus/ ↑ hormone regulation of kidney	Conserve body water

FIGURE 2.5

During the test of head-uptilt, hydrostatic forces retard blood flow back to the heart, which in turn transiently reduces the volume of blood pumped from the left side of the heart and systemic blood pressures. To protect the body from reduced blood pressure and low blood flow to the brain, neural and hormonal responses are triggered that increase resistance to flow in the peripheral blood vessels, which in turn normalizes or even increases systemic blood pressure above resting values. This response to head-uptilt may take only approximately 10 to 20 s to detect, as indicated in this illustration.

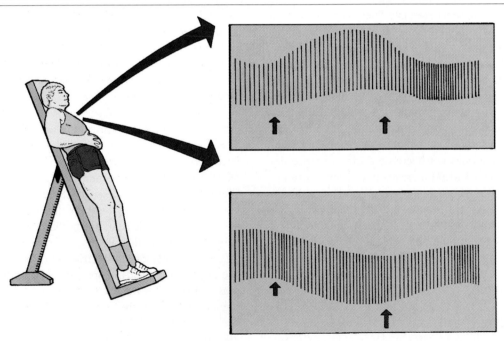

Positive feedback responses exist in the body, but are more rare. This should be obvious, as a positive feedback system would result in a biological response that exacerbates the original signal, which further stimulates the biological response. A good example of a positive feedback system is the T-cell network of the immune system. During infection, T cells of the body are stimulated to increase. During this process molecules are released that increase the formation of new T cells, causing an increasing rate of T-cell formation and improved immune function (15). However, as with all positive feedback systems, there must eventually be some means to "turn them off," which by definition involves negative feedback.

WEBSITE BOX

Chapter 2: Exercise: A Challenge of Homeostatic Control

The newest information regarding exercise physiology can be viewed at the following sites.*

arfa.org/index.htm
   Excellent site providing comprehensive information on many topics within exercise physiology.

http://www2.ncsu.edu/ncsu/cvm/people/autonomics/ PowerPoint slide show on homeostasis.

*Unless indicated, all URLs preceded by http://www.

Note: These URLs were valid at the time of publication, but could have changed or been deleted from Internet access since that time.

Gain of a Control System

Not all biological control systems are equal in their ability to prevent/dampen specific bodily functions. The precision by which a control system can prevent deviation from homeostasis is termed the **gain** of the system. For example, if the physiological measurement of concern is core body temperature, and 30 min of continuous steady-state exercise results in the expenditure of 291 kcal with only a 0.5°C increase in core temperature, an expression can be developed that compares body heat storage to heat production. As heat storage (specific heat) in the body has the relationship of 0.83 kcal/kg/°C, each 1°C increase in core temperature for a 70-kg person represents a heat storage of 58.1 kcal. Consequently,

2.1

$$\text{Gain} = \frac{\text{amount of correction needed}}{\text{amount of abnormality after correction}}$$

$$= \frac{\text{exercise heat production} - \text{resting heat production}}{\text{postexercise body heat storage} - \text{resting body heat storage}}$$

$$= \frac{(291 - 35)\ \text{kcal}}{(2,179 - 2,150)\ \text{kcal}}$$

$$= \frac{256\ \text{kcal}}{29\ \text{kcal}}$$

$$= 8.8$$

The calculated gain of approximately 9 for the above example means that the observed increase in body core temperature would have been 9 times greater if the control systems that exist to maintain body temperature were not functioning. Furthermore, control systems that have a more sensitive regulation and maintain "normal" or closer to "normal" conditions better have a larger gain.

The control systems of the body are not perfect. There are numerous examples of impaired body function resulting from exercise when one or a number of control systems fail. For example, deaths from hyperthermia (increased body temperature) during summer football training have occurred in the United States, as well as deaths from long-distance running during the summer heat in Australia. Similarly, life-threatening decreases in serum sodium concentrations (hy-ponatremia) during prolonged exercise have been reported in a few individuals because of incorrect regulation of body fluid and electrolytes (10).

Many clinical examples also exist for incorrectly functioning biological control systems. Individuals who suffer from high blood pressure (hypertension) may have this condition because of a failure in one of the many components involved in blood pressure regulation. Individuals who suffer from heart failure have impaired function because the muscles of their hearts cannot increase contraction force and velocity when stressed by an increased volume of blood returning to their hearts. Obviously, this seriously limits their abilities to exercise, and can eventually cause lung problems and additional life-threatening deterioration in organ function. Individuals who suffer from diabetes do so because they cannot produce insulin (type I) or have cells with reduced ability to be stimulated by insulin (type II), thereby preventing increased glucose use by cells. As a result glucose increases in concentration in the blood, causing damage to nerves and eventually risking loss of peripheral limbs and vision.

For many, but not all of clinical disease states, exercise can be beneficial in stimulating improved function of many components of biological control systems. Exercise training can improve glucose uptake by muscle in the type II diabetic (5). Exercise can decrease the resistance to blood flow in the peripheral tissues of the body, thereby assisting in the lowering of blood pressure in hypertensive individuals (3, 4). Exercise can also stimulate the body to retain more fluid in the blood, thereby providing more fluid for increased evaporative heat loss during future bouts of exercise (2). As discussed in chapter 1, the clinical importance of exercise and exercise training is increasing as we learn more about how the body responds to exercise stress, both *acutely* (during exercise) and *chronically* (long term). The role of exercise in improving health is becoming an important topic in the study of exercise physiology (see chapters 16 and 21) (1, 12) and is best understood by acquiring a thorough understanding of how the body functions as a multitude of interrelated biological control systems.

gain the theoretical amount of correction needed divided by the abnormality remaining after correction

SUMMARY

- The condition of bodily function where a constant or unchanging internal environment is maintained is called **homeostasis**. The homeostatic condition of the body is generally accepted to be at rest and unstressed and represents the state of the body in which it can most easily respond to a changing external environment.

- The issues that are important about homeostasis are (1) how well the body can reduce the physiological consequences of applied stress and (2) the speed at which a homeostatic condition is once again attained. Consequently, the student should view homeostasis as a reference and focus interest on the processes of the body that are called upon when the body deviates from homeostatic function.

- In the study of exercise physiology, another common term used to describe seemingly constant conditions is **steady state**. Steady state during exercise is not homeostasis, but a condition where certain body functions have attained dynamic constancy at a new level. When concerned with exercise, the condition of steady state has far more meaning than the condition of homeostasis.

- A **biological control system** is a functioning unit that works to help maintain homeostasis. The components of a biological control system are a **receptor**, an **integrating control unit**, and an **effector mechanism**.

- Examples of control systems of the human body that function during exercise are the regulation of (1) cellular ATP concentrations, (2) blood glucose concentrations, (3) blood oxygen content, (4) blood and tissue pH, (5) blood flow and blood pressure, (6) body temperature, and (7) body fluid/hydration.

- A constant feature of most biological control systems is that the response(s) to a stimulus that perturbs homeostasis causes a response that attempts to decrease the original stimulus and/or dampen the body's response to that stimulus. As these control system responses work in opposition to the initial stimulus response they are termed **negative feedback** responses.

- Not all biological control systems are equal in their ability to prevent/dampen specific bodily functions. The precision by which a control system can prevent deviation from homeostasis is termed the **gain** of the system. The gain of a control system equals the theoretical amount of correction needed divided by the abnormality remaining after correction. Control systems with large gain are more precise in regulating the parameter of concern.

STUDY QUESTIONS

1. Explain the differences between homeostasis and steady state.

2. Define a biological control system, and list the components of this system.

3. Do you know of any biological control systems that function during exercise? If so, list at least three and explain how they work.

4. Why do most biological control systems operate via negative feedback?

5. Explain what is meant by the term "gain" of a control system. Is a large or small gain desirable? Explain.

APPLICATIONS

1. Try to think of examples in clinical medicine where biological control systems are not working correctly. With each example, what are the consequences of this malfunction?

2. During the transition from rest to exercise, what are the biological control systems that immediately begin to function to enable us to eventually reach a steady state?

REFERENCES

1. Blair, S. N., K. W. Kohl, N. F. Gordon, and R. S. Paffenbarger, Jr. How much physical activity is good for health? *Ann. Rev. Public Health* 13:99–126, 1992.

2. Gillen, C. M., et al. Plasma volume expansion in humans after a single intense exercise protocol. *J. Appl. Physiol.* 71(5):1914–1920, 1991.

3. Harter, H. R, and A. P. Goldberg. Endurance exercise training: An effective therapeutic modality for hemodialysis patients. *Am. J. Clin. Nutr.* 33:1620-1628, 1980.

4. Hagberg, J. M., A. P. Goldberg, A. A. Ehsani, G. W. Heath, J. A. Delmez, and H. R. Harter. Exercise training improves blood hypertension in hemodialysis patients. *Am. J. Nephrol.* 3:209–212, 1983.

5. Lampman, R., and D. Schteingart. Effects of exercise training on glucose control, lipid metabolism, and insulin sensitivity in hypertriglycemic and non-insulin dependent diabetes mellitus. *Med. Sci. Sports Exerc.* 23(6):703–712, 1991.

6. Lerman, A., et al. Endothelin: A new cardiovascular regulatory peptide. *Mayo Clin. Proc.* 65:1441–1455, 1990.

7. Lightfoot, J. T. Can blood pressure be measured during exercise? A review. *Sports Med.* 12:290–301, 1991.

8. Noakes, T. D., B. A. Adams, K. H. Myburgh, C. Greeff, T. Lotz, and M. Nathan. The danger of an inadequate water intake during prolonged exercise. A novel concept revisited. *Eur. J. Appl. Physiol.* 57(2):210–219, 1988.

9. Noakes, T. D., et al. Metabolic rate, not percent dehydration, predicts rectal temperature in marathon runners. *Med. Sci. Sports Exerc.* 23(4):443–449, 1991.

10. Noakes, T. D. Hyponatremia during endurance running: A physiological and clinical interpretation. *Med. Sci. Sports Exerc.* 24(4):403–405, 1992.

11. O'Rourke, M. F. What is blood pressure? *Am. J. Hyperten.* 3:803–810, 1993.

12. Paffenbarger, R. S., Jr., R. T. Hyde, A. L. Wing, I.-M. Lee, D. L. Jung, and J.B. Kampert. The association of changes in physical activity level and other lifestyle characteristics with mortality among men. *N. Eng. J. Med.* 328:538–545, 1993.

13. Robergs, R. A., et al. Increased endothelin and creatine kinase after electrical stimulation of paraplegic muscle. *J. Appl. Physiol.* 75(6):2400–2405, 1993.

14. Rowell, L. B., and D. S. O'Leary. Reflex control of the circulation during exercise: Chemoreflexes and mechanoreflexes. *J. Appl. Physiol.* 69(2):407–418, 1990.

15. Shepherd, R. J., S. Rhind, and P. N. Shek. Exercise and the immune system: Natural killer cells, interleukins, and responses. *Sports Med.* 18(5):340–368, 1994.

RECOMMENDED READINGS

Blair, S. N., K. W. Kohl, N. F. Gordon, and R. S. Paffenbarger, Jr. How much physical activity is good for health? *Ann. Rev. Public Health* 13:99–126, 1992.

Noakes, T. D., K. H. Myburgh, J. du Plessis, L. Lang, M. Lambert, C. der Riet, and R. Schall. Metabolic rate, not percent dehydration, predicts rectal temperature in marathon runners. *Med. Sci. Sports Exerc.* 23(4):443–449, 1991.

O'Rourke, M. F. What is blood pressure? *Am. J. Hyperten.* 3:803–810, 1993.

Rowell, L. B., and D. S. O'Leary. Reflex control of the circulation during exercise: Chemoreflexes and mechanoreflexes. *J. Appl. Physiol.* 69(2):407–418, 1990.

Shepherd, R. J., S. Rhind, and P. N. Shek. Exercise and the immune system: Natural killer cells, interleukins, and responses. *Sports Med.* 18(5):340–368, 1994.

Lake Superior College Library

Metabolism

Exercise can be simply viewed as a condition that requires the repeated or sustained contraction of skeletal muscle. Continued muscle contraction requires that muscles provide, or be provided, a source of energy that can be used to fuel the contractions. This need stimulates certain reactions in skeletal muscle, and coincides with altered functions of the lungs, heart, and blood vessels, as well as other organs and tissues of the body (e.g.. liver, nervous system, glands and hormones, kidneys, skin, etc.). The altered functions of these tissues and organs either directly or indirectly support the energy requirements of muscle contraction. Because the focus of the cause of this energy need lies in skeletal muscle, an understanding of the changes in metabolism that occur when muscle function changes from rest to contraction is a tremendously important knowledge base of exercise physiology. Without this knowledge, it is difficult to appreciate the vast multiorgan and tissue responses to exercise, and why these responses occur at all. The purpose of this chapter is to introduce the study of cellular metabolism. The main reactions that occur in skeletal muscle will be outlined, and the importance of other organs and tissues that support skeletal muscle metabolism during exercise will be introduced.

OBJECTIVES

After studying this chapter, you should be able to:

- Explain why a fundamental understanding of bioenergetics helps the study of metabolism.
- Describe why ATP is an important molecule in metabolism.
- Describe the interrelationships between catabolism and anabolism.
- List and explain the reasons why enzymes are important in the regulation of metabolism.
- Explain the importance of creatine phosphate to skeletal muscle metabolism during intense exercise.
- Describe the function and products of glycolysis.
- Describe the function and products of the TCA cycle.
- Explain how oxygen is used and ATP is regenerated in mitochondrial respiration.
- Explain the rate at which ATP can be regenerated from the different reactions and pathways of catabolism during exercise.
- Provide examples of how the rapid recovery from intense exercise is important for sports performance.

KEY TERMS

chemical energy
bioenergetics
free energy
adenosine triphosphate (ATP)
metabolism
catabolism
anabolism
enzymes
phosphagen system
glycolytic metabolism
mitochondrial respiration

glucose
glycogen
triacylglycerols
fatty acids
amino acids
creatine phosphate (CrP)
glycogenolysis
glycolysis
lactate
redox potential
acetyl CoA
tricarboxylic acid cycle
electron transport chain (ETC)

oxidative phosphorylation
lipolysis
ß-oxidation
glycogen synthetase
transamination
transcription
ribosome
translation
gluconeogenesis

Exercise and Physical Activity Increase the Energy Needs of the Body

*I*magine yourself running a cross-country race, swimming a 400-m event, or sprinting down a football field dodging players of the opposing team. In each of these examples you could have moved from a standing posture to one of a fast pace. In doing this, the muscles used suddenly increase their demand for energy to fuel muscle contraction. Similarly, energy demands increase in organs that are used to support the exercise, such as the heart, lungs, glands, liver, and so forth. To tolerate this exercise, the body must have a means to rapidly "turn on" mechanisms that release energy, and have this regulation be suitable to allow the body to meet the energy demands so that certain stresses can be tolerated. For example, it would be devastating if the body's active muscles ran out of stored energy 30 s into a 5-min effort. Similarly, after the exercise the body must be able to use nutrients from ingested foods and liquid to restore body fluid and fuel reserves so that additional bouts of exercise can be completed.

The rapid recovery from exercise enables a person to repeat the exercise time and time again. The importance of being able to complete repeated exercise bouts in sports competition should be obvious, and examples of such events are soccer, American football, Australian football, rugby, tennis, cricket, track and field athletics, swimming, cycling, surfing. Similarly, we perform repeated bouts of exercise, or physical activity, in our daily lives. We climb stairs, walk at home and during school or work, run to catch a train or bus, and so on. Consequently, the need of our body to tolerate exercise is not just a sports need, but one of basic existence that allows us to complete activities of daily living.

The Rules that Govern How Cells Use Energy

The study of how cells use energy, and how this energy use is regulated is very complex. Most students complete 2 or 3 years of chemistry and biochemistry before a complete understanding of energy metabolism is acquired. As an undergraduate student you would benefit from the completion of an organic chemistry and introductory biochemistry class prior to your first exercise physiology class. However, not all undergraduate programs in exercise science require these prerequisites. Consequently, the contents of this chapter are written to provide an introductory explanation of cellular metabolism.

Energy Transfer

The body does not store energy in a form that is immediately available on demand, such as flipping a switch on a battery-powered flashlight, or the electric light switch on a wall, or turning a key to start the internal combustion engine. Rather, when body cells need energy, they must rapidly activate the breakdown of molecules and, in the process, release the energy stored in the bonds between atoms. The energy within chemical compounds is termed **chemical energy** (fig. 3.1). The two molecules that store chemical energy in human skeletal muscle cells are glycogen (containing glucose molecules) and triacylglycerols (containing fatty acid molecules) (see focus box 3.2).

How do cells release energy, and what regulates this release? The fact that we do not explode in a burst of energy when we exercise must mean that the energy release is gradual, and well controlled or regulated. The science that studies how energy is converted from one form to another in living things is called **bioenergetics** (1, 20). Bioenergetics is based on two very important laws.

1. *Energy cannot be created or destroyed, but can be changed from one form to another.*
2. *Energy transfer will always proceed in the direction of increased entropy, and the release of "free energy."*

The application of the laws of bioenergetics to metabolism is very important. When you look at a map, you cannot interpret the map without first reading the legend. Similarly, when you attempt to cook in a kitchen, you first need to follow a recipe. When applied to sports, you cannot play a

FIGURE 3.1

The release of chemical energy during reactions that "break down" molecules. The total chemical energy release during reactions is expressed in different forms, and can consist of heat, light, "free energy," and entropy.

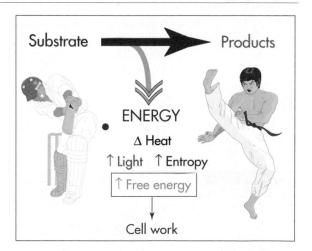

chemical energy energy stored in covalent and noncovalent chemical bonds within molecules

bioenergetics (bi'o-en-er-jet'iks) the study of energy transfer in chemical reactions within living tissue

game without first knowing the rules. This is where bioenergetics is important. Bioenergetics provides the laws by which metabolism functions. Thus, you cannot study metabolism without first knowing the laws of bioenergetics. If you have tried to study metabolism before, and failed or simply did not enjoy it, you probably were trying without an understanding of the laws of bioenergetics.

The first law indicates that energy is not destroyed when it is used or transferred from one form to another. For example, the energy released during a chemical reaction could produce usable energy, light energy, heat energy, and an unusable form of energy called entropy. Of these forms of energy, *only usable energy can be used by cells to produce work*. However, the heat released by reactions is important in increasing the rates of chemical reactions, and the maintenance of the body temperature of warm-blooded animals.

In many machines less than 25% of the energy used (input) is available to perform work. The ratio of energy input to output (work produced) is termed *efficiency*. As will be explained later in this chapter, the efficiency of the body's metabolic pathways can vary between 25 and 40%. Chapter 4 will reveal that the body is approximately 25 to 30% efficient in converting chemical energy into mechanical energy during exercise.

The second law of bioenergetics helps us understand why, or in which direction, a reaction is to proceed and therefore release chemical energy. Figure 3.1 indicates that when a chemical reaction occurs, energy is released in combinations of changes in heat, usable energy, entropy, and light. Usable energy is termed Gibbs **free energy** (ΔG, units = kcal/M), and it is this energy form that cells can harness to perform work. Entropy is a form of energy that cannot be used, and is defined by *increased randomness* or *disorder*. Based on the second law, all chemical reactions proceed in the direction that results in a release of free energy (denoted as a negative ΔG; $-\Delta G$), and are termed *exergonic* reactions. The more negative the ΔG, the more free energy that is released in the reaction. If ΔG is zero, the reaction is at *equilibrium*, and no net change in substrates, products or free energy transfer occurs.

ATP: The Cells's Way of Organizing Chemical Energy Exchange

Adenosine triphosphate (ATP) is a large molecule (fig. 3.2) that contains three phosphate (PO_3^-) groups. Inside a cell, the free energy released when one phosphate group is removed in a reaction approximates -14 kcal/M (26, 36). In other words, 14 kcal of energy is released for every 1 mole of ATP that is broken down to adenosine diphosphate (ADP) and a free phosphate (PO_3^-, or Pi) inside a cell. This is a lot of free energy, and can be used to power processes involved in cell work, such as muscle contraction, hormone secretion from glands, nerve conduction, and so forth. Do not confuse the value of -14 kcal/M with the standard ΔG ($\Delta G^{\circ\prime}$, for pH = 7, T = 25°C, initially 1 M of substrates and products) which is -7.3 kcal/M. I have used the conditions inside the cell because these are the ones that are important for cellular energy metabolism.

3.1   ATP ——> ADP + Pi $\Delta G = -14$ kcal/M

All chemical reactions can proceed in the opposite direction. This would mean that the energy to replace the phosphate on ADP and reform ATP would equal 14 kcal/M. Based on the second law of bioenergetics, this reaction is impossible because no reaction can occur that has a positive ΔG. However, chemical reactions in cells are designed so that reactions that require free energy are connected, or *coupled*, to reactions that release more free energy. Thus, the free energy release from one reaction can be used to "drive" a second coupled reaction.

3.2   ADP + Pi   ——> ATP $\Delta G = + 14$ kcal/M
3.3   CrP   ——> ATP + Cr $\Delta G = -14$ kcal/M
3.4   **CrP + ADP + H$^+$ ——> ATP + Cr $\Delta G = 0$ kcal/M**

ADP = adenosine diphosphate; ATP = adenosine triphosphate; Cr = creatine; CrP = creatine phosphate; H$^+$ = proton; Pi = inorganic phosphate.

FIGURE 3.2

The structure of adenosine triphosphate (ATP) and how it is formed from the phosphate addition to adenosine diphosphate (ADP).

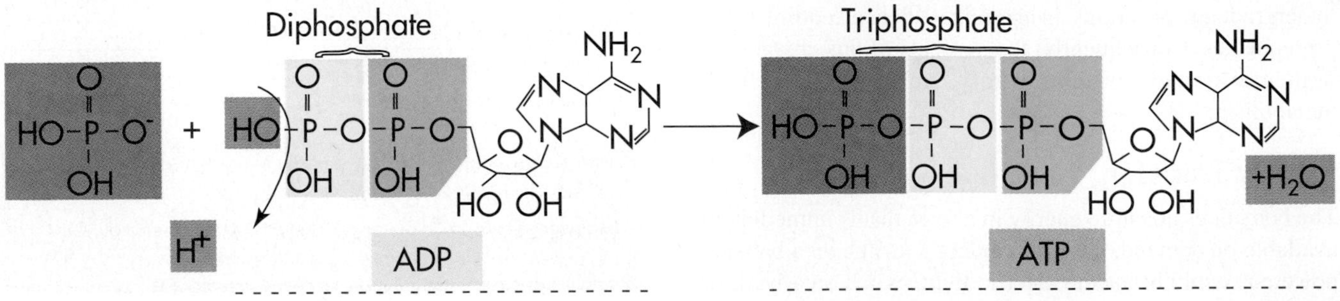

In the example equations above, creatine phosphate can release the free energy that is required to reform ATP. When the reactions are coupled the two free energy exchanges can be summed, resulting in a net free energy change that approximates zero, or can be at equilibrium for the resting concentrations of these molecules inside a cell. If the concentration of the substrates increases, then there will be a change in ΔG favoring the reaction to form ATP. Conversely, if the concentration of the products increase, then there will be a change in the direction of the reaction to favor the formation of CrP (in the reverse direction there is a $-\Delta G$). This is a consistent scenario in metabolism in cells. Reactions that require free energy are coupled to reactions that release free energy.

Figure 3.3 reveals that *in many instances reactions releasing free energy are coupled to the formation of ATP*. ATP formation can then be interpreted as a process that harnesses free energy. The free energy release from the breakdown of ATP is then used to "drive" chemical reactions that require free energy. ATP should therefore be viewed as an important molecule involved in the flow of free energy from reactions that release it to reactions that use it.

When the body has been given too much energy (from overeating!), cells do not increase their store of ATP. This is because cells just do not have sufficient space to accumulate ATP. During these conditions, the excess glucose molecules are used to form a storage molecule of glucose called *glyco-*

gen. In addition, in the liver and adipose tissue, glucose is broken down to two smaller 2-carbon-based molecules called acetyl CoA. The ATP formed from this conversion is used to combine acetyl CoA molecules to form fatty acids, which are stored in adipose tissue for later use when needed. Thus, both glycogen and fatty acids are energy-dense fuel stores that the body forms to have an available store of energy during times when the demand for energy during metabolism increases, like that during exercise, growth and repair, and times of illness or infection.

The Design of Cellular Metabolism

Figure 3.4 illustrates the relationships between the two main functions of **metabolism—catabolism** and **anabolism**. *Catabolism involves the breakdown of energy yielding nutrients, the release of free energy and electrons and their coupled transfer to intermediary molecules* (e.g., ATP), *and the formation of low-energy end products*. The intermediary molecules can be used in a controlled and regulated manner to provide free energy to make the reactions of anabolism exergonic. *Anabolism involves the covalent bonding of electrons, protons, and small molecules to produce larger molecules*. Thus, the free energy cost of building new and/or larger molecules occurs at the expense of the increased heat and entropy released from catabolism, as explained previously by the laws of bioenergetics.

Many of the catabolic and anabolic reactions of metabolism occur together. Greater stimulation for catabolism increases catabolism and reduces anabolism, and vice versa. Catabolism and anabolism therefore function in a *dynamic balance*, and the diversity of cell function is dependent upon the molecular balance and interactions between catabolism and anabolism.

Why Are Enzymes Important?

In a cell, the concentrations of molecules are extremely small. Thus, reactions would not proceed at a meaningful rate to support life if they were left on their own to react and form products. You have probably been taught that this is

---

FIGURE 3.3

Reactions that release free energy are coupled to ATP regeneration. Conversely, reactions that require free energy are coupled to ATP dephosphorylation.

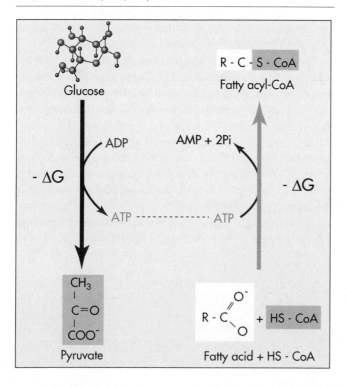

---

free energy the energy from a reaction that can be used to perform work

adenosine triphosphate (ATP) a large molecule that contains three phosphate (PO_3^-) groups

metabolism (me-tab'o-lizm) the sum of all reactions of the body

catabolism (ca-tab'o-lizm) the reactions of the body that decrease the size of molecules

anabolism (a-nab'o-lizm) the reactions of the body that increase the size of molecules

The relationships between anabolism and catabolism.

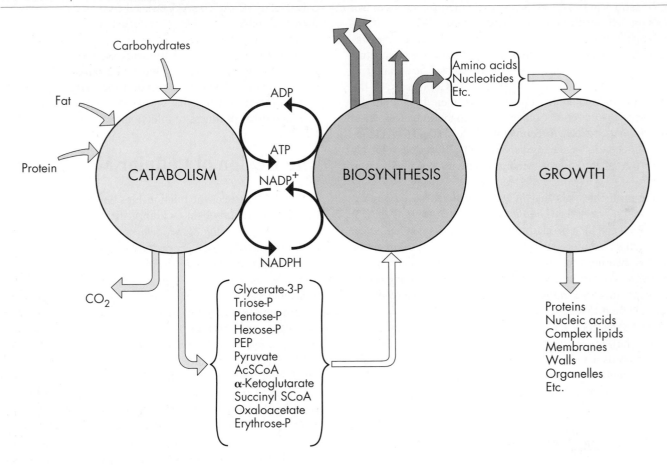

why **enzymes** are important. They function as a *biological catalyst*. They speed up chemical reactions without being involved in the reaction or altering the free energy release. This is correct, but it is by no means the only function of enzymes.

The enzymes in cells also provide the means to couple chemical reactions. For example, the enzyme creatine kinase catalyzes the reaction detailed in equation (3.4). If it were not for creatine kinase there would be no way to couple these two reactions and therefore no way to use ATP to reform creatine phosphate. The same would be true for any reaction that requires the free energy from the dephosphorylation of ATP to be used to drive otherwise positive ΔG reactions. The net result would be no anabolism, and the inability to sustain life.

Another important function of enzymes is that some of them can be regulated. This means that enzymes can be altered to either increase their effectiveness as catalysts, or decrease this effectiveness. The net result is that if cells can "turn on" (activate) or "turn off" (inhibit) enzymes, then this is a powerful way to determine which reactions, or pathways, can be functioning during given metabolic conditions. Enzymes that can be activated and inhibited are termed *allosteric enzymes*. The activation and inhibition of enzymes

results from the production of specific molecules during specific cell conditions that bind to the enzymes and either improve (activate) the ability of the enzyme to work, or impair (inhibit) this ability.

Despite the importance of enzyme regulation, not all enzymes can be regulated. Figure 3.5 indicates that most enzymes that are regulated are positioned at or near the beginning and end of metabolic pathways. If you think hard about this, it makes a lot of sense. Why have all enzymes regulated when a regulated enzyme at the start of a pathway can essentially be turned on or off to dictate whether the entire pathway is activated? In this way, fewer molecules need to be produced that alter enzyme activities, thereby simplifying the regulation of metabolism.

In summary therefore, enzymes are extremely important to cell function and metabolism because they

1. increase the rate of chemical reactions.
2. allow for the coupling of multiple chemical reactions, enabling the free energy release of one reaction to be used by another.
3. provide the means, by the regulation of the enzyme, of determining whether chemical reactions can proceed at a physiologically meaningful rate.

FIGURE 3.5

The regulation of enzymes that catalyze reactions early in pathways can redirect substrate to other connecting pathways. In this example, depending upon which enzymes are inhibited or activated, glucose entering a muscle cell can be directed to either glycogen synthesis, pentose phosphate formation, or catabolism in glycolysis.

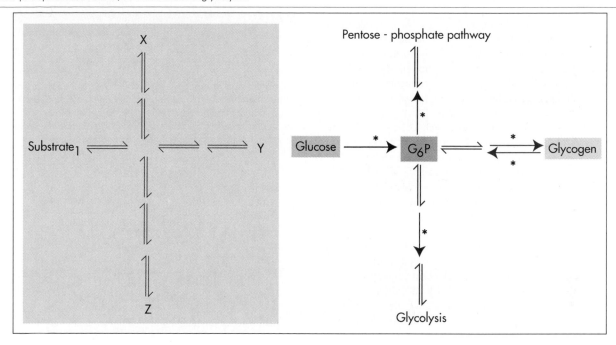

Catabolism in Skeletal Muscle

Overview

It is important to understand that all aspects of metabolism are occurring simultaneously, causing a dynamic balance that favors either net catabolism or anabolism, depending on the cell conditions. When studying metabolism it is difficult to appreciate this fact because most of the time you study one metabolic pathway at a time, and the connections between the pathways are not always emphasized. To prevent you from falling into this trap, it is best to superficially view what the major substrates are for catabolism, how these substrates are used in specific pathways, and how each pathway relates to each other. Once this "big picture" is appreciated, then it is time to focus in on the details.

Substrates and Pathways

The substrates used by cells in catabolism for the formation of ATP are carbohydrates, free fatty acids, and amino acids (focus box 3.1 and fig. 3.6). These molecules are catabolized during specific chemical pathways that release free energy, electrons, and protons (focus box 3.2). The metabolic pathways specific for each of carbohydrate, free fatty acids, and amino acids are glycolysis, ß-oxidation, and transamination, respectively. Carbon backbones from each substrate eventually enter into the tricarboxylic acid cycle (TCA cycle) of the mitochondria, where additional electrons and protons are removed, and the majority of carbon dioxide is produced. The electrons and protons harnessed from catabolism are used in

the electron transport chain of the mitochondria where the consumption of oxygen is coupled to the regeneration of ATP during the process of oxidative phosphorylation.

Both glycolysis and ß-oxidation therefore provide acetyl CoA, which can enter into the TCA cycle. Depending upon the carbon numbers of the amino acid side chains, amino acids can provide carbon molecules that can either enter into glycolysis, form acetyl CoA, or form molecules of the TCA cycle. The amine (NH_2) groups removed from amino acids are added to other carbon molecules (mainly pyruvate in skeletal muscle), removed from the cell, and circulated to the liver. In the liver the amine groups are processed to form urea, which is filtered from the blood by the kidney to be eventually removed from the body in urine.

The Reactions and Metabolic Pathways of Catabolism

Skeletal muscle can produce the ATP required to support muscle contraction from one or a combination of three metabolic reactions/pathways (fig. 3.7): (1) the transfer of the phosphate from creatine phosphate (CrP) to ADP to form ATP, (2) from glycolysis, and (3) from the use of oxygen in the mitochondria.

enzyme (en-zym) a protein molecule that functions as a biological catalyst

The Main Nutrients Involved in Energy Metabolism

The main nutrients of the body used in energy metabolism are carbohydrates, lipids, and amino acids (fig. 3.6). The nutrient most important to energy metabolism during moderate to intense exercise intensities is carbohydrate. There are many different types of carbohydrate molecules; however, **glucose** is the favored carbohydrate for metabolism in skeletal muscle, the liver, and adipose tissue. **Glycogen** consists of a protein core (glycogenin) from which chains of glucose molecules are attached (9, 20, 26). The glucose chains branch from themselves, resulting in a large structure with the ends of many glucose polymer chains exposed to the surrounding cellular medium. Glycogen molecules in skeletal muscle are visualized in electron microscopy as darkly stained circular structures dispersed throughout the cytosol, hence the term *glycogen granule* (9) (see Glycogenolysis).

There are many types of lipid molecules within cells. The main lipids of interest to energy metabolism are those that comprise **triacylglycerols.** A triacylglycerol consists of three **fatty acid** (FA) molecules attached to a carbohydrate backbone called *glycerol*. FA molecules that are bound to glycerol are termed *esterified* fatty acids, whereas FA free from glycerol are termed *nonesterified* fatty acids, or *free fatty acids* (FFA). The FFA molecule is catabolized in muscle during muscle contraction. Palmitate is a saturated FA consisting of 16 carbon atoms attached end to end to form a backbone from which hydrogen and oxygen molecules are also attached. *Palmitate is the predominant FA in the body* and is therefore used to represent the reactions and energy liberated from FFA catabolism (30, 35).

Amino acid molecules differ from carbohydrate and lipid molecules in that they contain nitrogen atoms. There are 20 amino acids within the body (35), and all have a structure comprising an acid (COOH), amine (NH_2), CH, and R-group (side chain) attached to a central carbon atom. *Amino acids differ by the structure of the R-group,* and can be classified by the *characteristics of the R-group,* or the *charge of the R-group.* Amino acids can be incorporated into catabolism by removing the amine group (*deamination*), and converting the remaining structure into a molecule of either the glycolytic or tricarboxylic acid (TCA) cycle pathways. Similarly, pyruvate produced from glycolysis can have an amine group added (*transamination*) from the deamination of another amino acid, producing alanine. Alanine then leaves the muscle and circulates to other tissues such as the liver.

During times of low-carbohydrate nutrition, when FFA catabolism is the predominant substrate, the liver can produce ketone bodies from acetyl CoA molecules. Ketone bodies comprise three different molecules: acetoacetate, ß-hydroxybutyrate, and acetone, with the main ketone body being acetoacetate. Once in the circulation, acetoacetate and β-hydroxybutyrate can enter into the circulation and be used by contracting muscle, the heart, and kidneys for substrate in catabolism.

FIGURE 3.6

The structures of key substrates involved in the pathways of metabolism. Glycogen consists of glucose molecules that are connected, and is a highly branched and structurally organized molecule. Fructose, like glucose, is another monosaccharide. Triacylglycerols comprise fatty acids and a glycerol molecule. Fatty acids can differ in carbon numbers and the degree of saturation. Amino acids are named for their amine group located on a central carbon atom, and differ in their side chain length, structure, and charge.

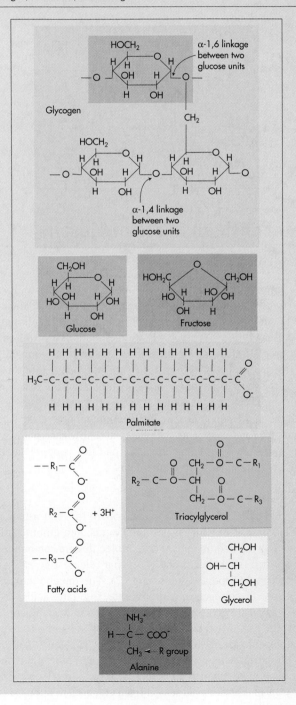

FIGURE 3.7

An overview of the reactions and pathways of catabolism in skeletal muscle.

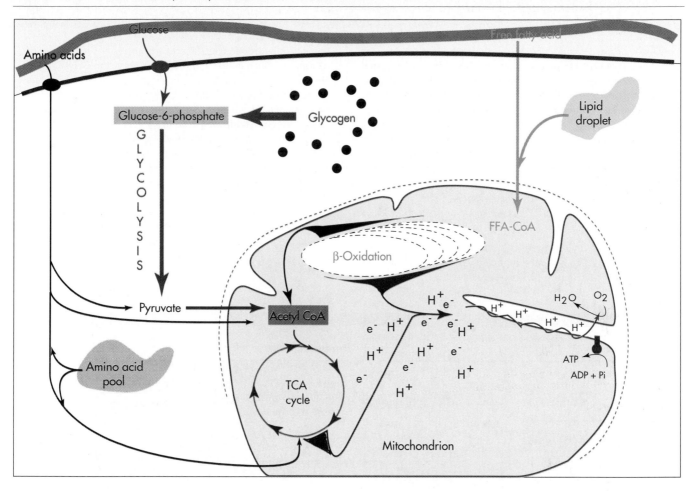

The production of ATP from CrP and glycolysis does not require the presence of oxygen, and has been referred to as *anaerobic metabolism.* Conversely, the ATP production from cellular respiration in mitochondria, which uses oxygen, has been termed *aerobic metabolism.* These terms are not entirely accurate for describing energy metabolism. Aerobic metabolism is not 100% aerobic because ATP from glycolysis is still produced even when all substrates are directed into the mitochondria. It is inappropriate to differentiate two extremes of energy metabolism when they can share a common central pathway (e.g., glycolysis in carbohydrate catabolism). Terms that are gaining increased acceptance for qualifying the source of ATP production are the **phosphagen system, glycolytic metabolism,** and **mitochondrial respiration,** respectively.

Phosphagen System

The **creatine phosphate (CrP)** reaction is the most rapid means to regenerate ATP, and is catalyzed by *creatine kinase.*

3.5
$$\text{CrP} + \text{ADP} + \text{H}^+ \xleftrightarrow{\text{Creatine kinase}} \text{ATP} + \text{Cr}$$

glucose (glu-kos) the form of sugar by which carbohydrate is metabolised in animals

glycogen (gli'ko-jen) a sugar polysaccharide that is the form of carbohydrate storage in animal tissues

triacylglycerol (tri-as'il-glis'er-ol) a lipid consisting of a glycerol backbone and three free fatty acid molecules, which is the principle form of fat storage in the body

fatty acids the lipid components of triacylglycerols, which are catabolized in tissues

amino acids amine (NH_2) containing molecules that are the primary components of proteins

phosphagen system the regeneration of ATP via creatine phosphate hydrolysis and ADP

glycolytic metabolism reactions of the glycolytic pathway

mitochondrial respiration reactions of the mitochondria which ultimately lead to the consumption of oxygen

creatine phosphate (CrP) a phosphorylated metabolite that releases a large amount of free energy during dephosphorylation

FOCUS BOX 3.2

Electrons, Protons, and Oxidation-Reduction Reactions

Electrons are negatively charged subatomic particles that circulate around the atom's nucleus. Electrons are essential for atoms to form covalent (electron-sharing) bonds. During many chemical reactions, electrons are either removed or added to molecules. Molecules that lose one or more electrons are *oxidized*, whereas molecules that gain electrons are *reduced*. Consequently, *oxidation involves the loss of electrons*, and *reduction involves the gaining of electrons*. As oxidation and reduction reactions occur together, they are often termed *oxidation-reduction* or *redox* reactions.

3.6 $A{:}e + B \longrightarrow A + B{:}e$

There are many examples of oxidation-reduction reactions in metabolism. The enzymes that catalyze these reactions are termed dehydrogenases. There are important examples of oxidation-reduction reactions in glycolysis, in which NAD^+ and NADH either receive or donate electrons, respectively. The same is true for the electron-carrier oxidation-reduction pair FAD^+ and FADH, which is used in mitochondrial respiration.

A proton is a hydrogen atom that has lost its electron. The symbol for the proton is H^+, and like electrons, protons are integral to the design of energy metabolism. The concentration of protons ($[H^+]$) in solution determines the acidity of the solution, and is represented numerically by the negative log of the $[H^+]$ ($pH = -\log[H^+]$). The movement of protons across the inner mitochondrial membrane during the electron transport chain is the driving force that eventually provides the free energy to phosphorylate ATP in the process of oxidative phosphorylation.

FIGURE 3.8

The creatine kinase and adenylate kinase reactions that cause rapid ATP regeneration in the vicinity of the contractile proteins.

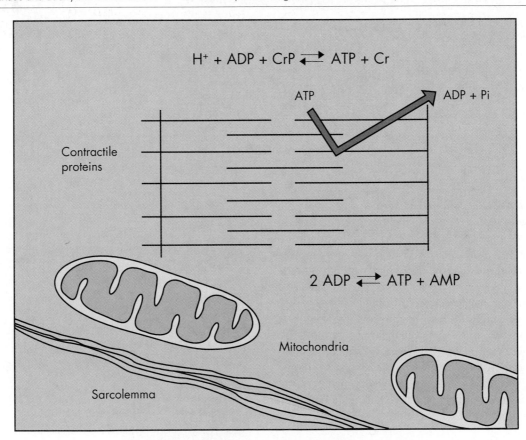

During muscle contraction when there are transient increases in ADP in the locations of the contractile filaments, the direction of the creatine kinase reaction favors ATP production (fig. 3.8). However, *the ATP production capacity of the creatine kinase reaction relies on a store of CrP*, which approximates 24 mmol/kg wet wt.

One additional enzyme-catalyzed reaction exists to regenerate ATP, and the enzyme involved is called *adenylate kinase.* The adenylate kinase reaction is similar to the creatine kinase reaction in that it is near equilibrium. This reaction also serves to produce the activator (AMP) of the allosteric enzymes phosphorylase (glycogenolysis) and phosphofructokinase (glycolysis), thus stimulating increased carbohydrate catabolism.

3.7
Adenylate kinase (myokinase)
$$ADP + ADP <-----> ATP + AMP$$

The importance of the phosphagen system is that it can regenerate ATP at the highest rate possible. During exercise that demands ATP production in excess of ATP supply from mitochondrial respiration or glycolysis, the creatine kinase reaction enables additional ATP to be produced to meet the ATP demand of muscle contraction. However, it can be calculated that the finite intramuscular store of CrP can be depleted during intense exercise in as little as 10 s. Table 3.1 lists activities that rely heavily on ATP regeneration from CrP hydrolysis, glycolysis, and oxidative phosphorylation.

Glycogenolysis

Muscle glycogen is a large molecule comprised of glucose units joined together by covalent bonds (focus box 3.1). Figure 3.9 is an electron micrograph of the subcellular organi-

zation of a skeletal muscle fiber. Glycogen can be seen as darkly stained granules distributed throughout the fiber (9).

The catabolism of glycogen is termed **glycogenolysis.** Glycogenolysis requires three enzymes for optimal function. However, the main enzyme is phosphorylase, which is allosteric and is responsible for releasing individual glucose

glycogenolysis (gli'-ko-jen-ol'i-sis) the removal of glucose units from glycogen, producing glucose 1-phosphate

FIGURE 3.9

An electron micrograph of skeletal muscle. The numerous small dark stained structures are glycogen granules (G).

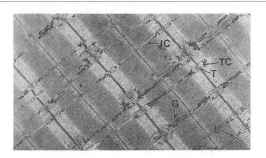

TABLE 3.1

Examples of activities that rely heavily on CrP, glycolysis, or mitochondrial respiration as the source for free energy to regenerate ATP in contracting skeletal muscle

| ACTIVITY | DEPENDENCE* | | APPROXIMATE DURATION | |
	PHOSPHAGEN	GLYCOLYTIC	MITOCHONDRIAL	(HOUR:MIN:SEC)
Kicking a football	High	Low	Low	0:0:05
Weight lifting (power)	High	Moderate	Low	0:0:05
Throwing events	High	Low	Low	0:0:10
Running up stairs	High	Low	Low	0:0:10
Pole vaulting	High	Moderate	Low	0:0:10
Jumping events	High	Low	Low	0:0:10
100–200-m run sprints	High	Moderate	Low	0:0:10–0:0:30
50–100-m swim sprints	High	Moderate	Low	0:0:10–0:0:30
Weight lifting (intervals)	High	Moderate	Low	0:0:30–0:2:00
400–800-m run sprints	High	High	Moderate	0:1:00–0:3:00
Wrestling	High	High	Moderate	0:0:30–0:5:00
200–400-m swim	High	High	Moderate	0:2:00–0:5:00
Hill running	High	High	Moderate	0:2:00–0:5:00
Ice hockey	High	High	Moderate	0:2:00–0:8:00
1500-m run	Moderate	Moderate	High	0:3:30–0:6:00
5,000–10,000-m run	Low	Low	High	0:12:00–0:30:00
Marathon run	Low	Low	High	2:0:00–4:0:00
Triathlons	Low	Low	High	2:0:00–5:0:00

*Relative to the maximal potential ATP supply from that energy system.

Note: No athletic/sports/exercise examples rely solely on one energy system.

residues from glycogen (6, 31). Phosphorylase activity is increased when an inorganic phosphate (Pi) is attached to the enzyme and when the intracellular concentration of calcium increases (such as occurs during muscle contraction). The phosphate attachment to phosphorylase occurs when the concentration of the intracellular second messenger cyclic AMP (cAMP) increases. cAMP is produced in response to epinephrine (a catecholamine hormone) binding to a specific receptor on the sarcolemma.

3.8
$$\text{Phosphorylase}$$
$$\text{Glycogen}_n + \text{Pi} \longrightarrow \text{glycogen}_{n-1} + \text{glucose-1-phosphate}$$

3.9
$$\text{Phosphoglucomutase}$$
$$\text{Glucose-1-phosphate} <\longrightarrow> \text{glucose-6-phosphate}$$

As indicated in equation (3.8), the presence of inorganic phosphate is also important for glycogenolysis. Muscle inorganic phosphate increases during conditions that rely more on creatine phosphate as a means to reform ATP. The net result of this is to also provide additional inorganic phosphate as substrate for glycogenolysis.

The importance of glycogenolysis is that it can *provide a rapid rate of production of glucose-6-phosphate*, which, as will be described below, is the first intermediate of glycolysis.

Glycolysis

Within skeletal muscle **glycolysis** begins either with the entry of glucose into the skeletal muscle fiber or from the eventual formation of glucose-6-phosphate (G6P) from glycogenolysis [equation (3.9)]. Glucose entry from the blood is facili-

---

FIGURE 3.10

The major contributor to G_6P formation is muscle glycogenolysis. However, low rates of glucose entry into skeletal muscle is facilitated by special transport proteins (GLUT proteins). $GLUT_1$ and $GLUT_4$ proteins are known to exist on the sarcolemma. $GLUT_4$ density on the sarcolemma is increased in response to insulin, and to exercise as explained in the text.

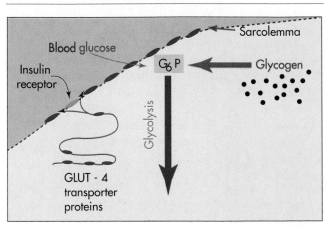

---

tated by glucose binding to specialized glucose transport proteins (GLUT proteins) located on the sarcolemma (fig. 3.10). *$GLUT_4$ is the major transporter in skeletal muscle,* and the number of $GLUT_4$ transporters can be increased in response to insulin and exercise (8, 10, 15). *The exercise stimulation of glucose transporters is additive and independent of the insulin response* (10, 13).

The enzyme hexokinase is bound to the outer mitochondrial membrane and/or the intracellular side of the sarcolemma (25, 26, 27), and catalyzes the conversion of glucose to G_6P coupled to the dephosphorylation of ATP. As G_6P concentrations are always very low in skeletal muscle cells, it is extremely difficult for G_6P to be converted to glucose in skeletal muscle. Thus, *conversion of glucose to G_6P in skeletal muscle retains glucose for either glycogen synthesis or glycolysis.*

G_6P is broken down sequentially by nine reactions that form the central carbohydrate metabolic pathway of glycolysis (fig. 3.11). *The important products of glycolysis are pyruvate, ATP, and NADH. Pyruvate is recognized as the final product of glycolysis,* and can be reduced to lactate in the cytosol, or be transported into the mitochondria and oxidized to acetyl CoA, which is further catabolized to form NADH and carbon dioxide (CO_2). *NADH is formed from NAD^+ by acquiring protons and electrons from specific chemical reactions.*

Lactate Production

Pyruvate can be reduced to **lactate** by the enzyme lactate dehydrogenase (LDH), as indicated in the equation below.

3.10
$$\text{Lactate dehydrogenase}$$
$$\text{Pyruvate} + \text{NADH} + \text{H}^+ <\longrightarrow> \text{lactate} + \text{NAD}^+$$

The ΔG of the LDH reaction is close to zero, and therefore is a near-equilibrium reaction (26). It is typically explained that this reaction first produces lactic acid, which then immediately releases a proton when produced at physiological pH, leaving lactate (fig. 3.12). However, growing evidence exists to indicate that the acidosis accompanying lactate production may be more complex than this, and is perhaps due more to the accumulation of $NADH + H^+$ and/or increased net ATP dephosphorylation (19). Therefore, it is more correct to say that *acidosis accompanies increased lactate production.*

A basal level of lactate production exists in skeletal muscle, resulting in a resting muscle lactate concentration of 1 mmol/kg wet wt. This resting concentration results from a balance between lactate production, metabolism within the same muscle fiber, and its removal from the cell for metabolism in other tissues (other skeletal muscle fibers, the heart, and the liver). The production of lactate under these steady-state conditions has been termed *aerobic glycolysis*; however, as glycolysis is totally anaerobic this term is misleading and should not be used.

Unless the free protons released during conditions of increased lactate production are buffered, increases in lac-

FIGURE 3.11

The reactions of glycolysis can be divided into two phases. Phase 1 involves the eventual catabolism of glucose into two three carbon molecules, and is ATP costly. The second phase of glycolysis produces ATP, reduces the coenzyme NAD$^+$, and eventually produces pyruvate.

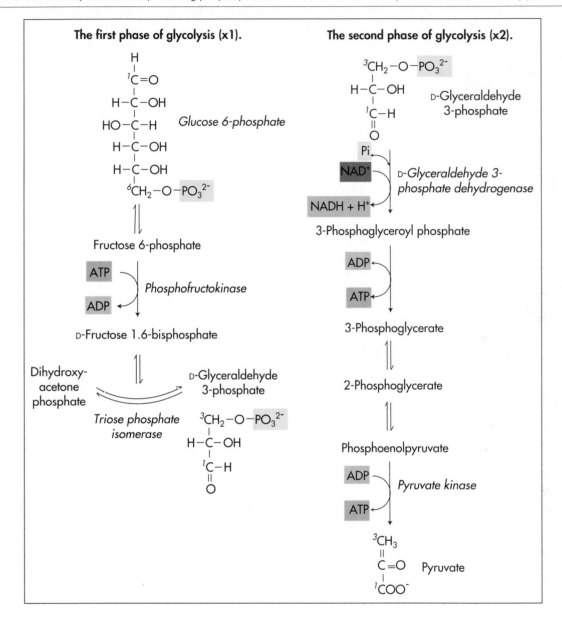

tate production coincide with decreases in cellular pH. For example, as exercise intensity increases, the rate of proton liberation eventually exceeds the buffering capacity of the cell, and pH decreases resulting in acidosis. Despite this occurance, *lactate production is not necessarily detrimental to muscle metabolism during exercise*. The production of lactate involves the reduction of pyruvate, and the electrons and protons required for this are provided by NADH + H$^+$. Lactate production therefore involves the oxidation of NADH, which regenerates NAD$^+$ for glycolysis. Lactate production therefore helps maintain the ratio between NAD$^+$ and NADH (termed the cytosolic **redox potential**), and supports continued glycolysis and a high rate of ATP regeneration during repeated

intense muscle contractions. Consequently, when you run fast, jump over fences, or perform any sustained high-intensity exercise, the production of lactate is necessary to enable glycolysis, and therefore a high rate of ATP production, to continue even when muscle creatine phosphate concentrations become low.

glycolysis (gli'-kol'i-sis) reactions involving the catabolism of glucose to pyruvate

lactate (lac'tate) product of the reduction of pyruvate

redox potential the ratio of NAD$^+$/NADH

FIGURE 3.12

The production of lactate in skeletal muscle. Lactate is the name for the deprotonated structure of lactic acid. During lactate production, pyruvate is reduced by the electrons from NADH, reforming NAD^+. Therefore, lactate production helps to maintain the cytosolic redox potential and provide the coenzyme NAD^+ for the glyceraldehyde 3-phosphate dehydrogenase reaction.

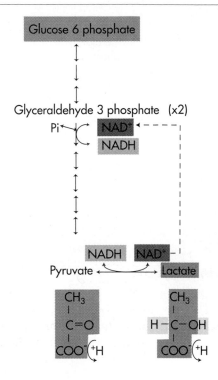

The metabolic conditions that cause an increase in lactate production are topics of research in exercise physiology and biochemistry. Despite evidence for lactate production during conditions of low or no oxygen (hypoxia) (19), lactate production can also occur in the presence of adequate oxygen (5, 17, 34). Consequently, lactate production should not be viewed as evidence of hypoxia (anaerobic conditions). *When the rate of pyruvate production exceeds the rate of pyruvate entry into the mitochondria, pyruvate will be converted to lactate.* This condition has been termed the *mass action* effect. Therefore, the production of lactate is not a detrimental occurrence. Because lactate and pyruvate can be removed from the muscle for metabolism in other tissues, lactate should be viewed as a substrate of metabolism.

Finally, it should be stressed that lactate production and accumulation in skeletal muscle does not directly cause fatigue and/or pain. Research has frequently measured blood or muscle lactate as an indication of muscle fatigue (5). However, lactate concentrations are used as an indirect reflection of acidosis. The production of lactate coincides with the release of a proton (H^+) and the potential for decreases in pH. It is the decrease in cellular and blood pH that accompany high rates of lactate production that has potential detriment to several enzymes of energy metabolism and muscle contraction. *The problem with lactate production is the accompanying acidosis and not the lactate molecule.*

Mitochondrial Respiration

During steady-state exercise conditions, the majority of pyruvate is not converted to lactate, but enters into the mitochondria to be further catabolized by a series of reactions that collectively yield carbon dioxide, release additional electrons and protons, consume oxygen, and produce large quantities of ATP.

Tricarboxylic Acid Cycle   During pyruvate entry into the mitochondria pyruvate is converted to **acetyl CoA** by a series of linked enzymes known collectively as pyruvate dehydrogenase.

Pyruvate dehydrogenase

3.11   Pyruvate + NAD^+ + CoA <————> acetyl CoA + NADH + H^+ + CO_2

The acetyl CoA formed from either carbohydrate or lipid catabolism can then enter into a catabolic pathway called the **tricarboxylic acid cycle** (TCA cycle) (fig. 3.13), which consists of nine reactions. *The combined products of the TCA cycle are carbon dioxide, ATP, NADH + H^+, and FADH.* All of the CO_2 produced in energy metabolism can be accounted for from the pyruvate dehydrogenase reaction and two reactions of the TCA cycle.

FIGURE 3.13

The intermediates and enzymes of the tricarboxylic acid cycle (TCA cycle). The products of the cycle are CO_2, NADH, FADH, and GTP. The TCA cycle is not a closed cycle, as intermediates can be used as substrates of other pathways of metabolism. Similarly, molecules (e.g., amino acids) can be converted to many of the TCA cycle intermediates and therefore integrated into catabolism.

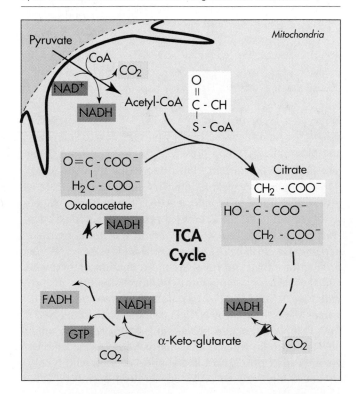

The reactions of the TCA cycle result in the production of three NADH, one FADH, one GTP, and two CO_2. The molecule GTP is guanine triphosphate, and is interconvertible with ATP so it is counted in the ATP tally of metabolism. *NADH + H^+* and *FADH + H^+ are the major products of the TCA cycle*, and harness electrons and protons for use in the electron transport chain. For every glucose molecule that is completely catabolized to CO_2 and water, the two pyruvate molecules that enter the mitochondria require two cycles of the TCA cycle (one cycle each).

Electron Transport Chain   The student should note that during all the catabolic pathways identified thus far, no mention has been made of oxygen, or of a large production of ATP. The biochemical use of oxygen occurs in the **electron transport chain (ETC)** (fig. 3.14). In the ETC, the proton and electrons acquired in NADH and FADH are utilized to add electrons to hydrogen atoms and oxygen to form water, and generate the free energy to add a phosphate to ADP to form ATP. The formation of water and ATP during the ETC is termed **oxidative phosphorylation.**

Electrons are transferred unidirectionally along the electron transport chain. The unidirectionality results from each electron acceptor of the chain having a progressively larger affinity for electrons. In biochemical terms, the measure of affinity for electrons is termed the *reduction potential*. NADH donates electrons and protons to the chain at the flavine mononucleotide (FMN) complex at the start of the chain. FADH donates electrons and protons at ubiquinone (coenzyme Q) further along the chain. The last electron receiver of the electron transport chain is molecular oxygen ($\frac{1}{2}O_2$), which has the largest reduction potential. Consequently, *the presence of oxygen inside the mitochondria essentially drives the electron transport chain, and all the reactions of the mitochondria*, which ultimately depend on the function of the chain to regenerate NAD^+ and FAD^+.

ATP production is coupled to the electron transport chain. As electrons are transferred down the chain, the protons are transported across the inner mitochondrial membrane, and accumulate in the intermembranous space (fig. 3.14). The unidirectional flow of protons develops a proton and pH gradient, which provides the potential for free energy to be harnessed from the controlled release of protons down the gradient. A special protein complex exists along the inner membrane that contains an ATP synthetase enzyme, and allows the flow of protons down the gradient across the inner membrane. According to the *chemiosmotic theory* of oxidative phosphorylation proposed by Peter Mitchell in 1961, the flow of protons down the gradient provides the free energy to phosphorylate ADP to ATP (14, 21). The electrons and protons provided to the chain by each NADH results in the production of three ATP. As FADH provides electrons and protons further along the chain than the flavin mononucleotide (FMN) prosthetic group of NADH-Q reductase, fewer protons can be transported across the membrane and only two ATP are produced for each FADH. Consequently, *the generally accepted ATP equivalents for NADH and FADH are 3 and 2, respectively*.

It is apparent that the production of ATP does not directly result from the reduction of oxygen and protons to form water. However, as previously explained, a stoichiometric relationship exists between the flux of protons across the inner membrane during the ETC and the production of ATP. This relationship indicates that these processes are somehow connected, or coupled, hence the combined name of *oxidative phosphorylation.*

Mitochondrial Membrane Shuttles   Several problems exist with oxidative phosphorylation occurring in mitochondria, which are enclosed by a double membrane. If the NADH produced from glycolysis is to be used as an electron and proton donor in the ETC, there must be a means to transfer this molecule and/or its electrons and protons into the mitochondria. In addition, there must be a means to transfer the ADP from the cytosol into the mitochondria, and the ATP produced in the mitochondria to the cytosol.

Cytosolic NADH does not enter into mitochondria. Instead, the electrons and protons of NADH are added to molecules that can be transported into the mitochondria, and these molecules are oxidized to release the electrons and protons to mitochondrial NAD^+. During cellular conditions when most of the pyruvate formed from glycolysis enters into the mitochondria, this shuttle mechanism is responsible for maintaining the cytosolic redox potential. There are two main methods of electron and proton transfer from the cytosol to mitochondria—the *glycerol-3-phosphate shuttle*, resulting in the formation of mitochondrial FADH + H^+, and the *malate-aspartate shuttle*, resulting in the formation of mitochondrial NADH + H^+.

The inner mitochondrial membrane also has an ATPase enzyme and a transport mechanism to transfer the terminal phosphate from mitochondrial ATP to a cytosolic ADP, regenerating ATP in the cytosol. In addition, an inner mitochondrial membrane–bound creatine kinase transfers a terminal phosphate from mitochondrial ATP to cytosolic creatine, regenerating creatine phosphate.

---

acetyl CoA molecule produced from carbohydrate and FFA catabolism that enters into the TCA cycle

tricarboxylic acid cycle mitochondrial reactions involving the addition of acetyl CoA to oxaloacetate, and the eventual release of carbon dioxide, electrons, and protons during the reformation of oxaloacetate

electron transport chain (ETC) the series of electron receivers located along the inner mitochondrial membrane that sequentially receive and transfer electrons to the final electron receiver—molecular oxygen

oxidative phosphorylation the production of ATP from the coupled transfer of electrons to the generation of a H^+ gradient between the two mitochondrial membranes

FIGURE 3.14

The location of the electron carrier molecules of the Electron Transport Chain across the inner mitochondrial membrane. Movement of electrons and protons occur in such a way that protons are transported to within the inter-membranous space, and generate a proton concentration (pH) gradient across both the inner and outer mitochondrial membranes. As explained in the text, the pH gradient is used to provide the free energy for ATP production during oxidative phosphorylation.

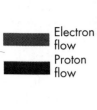

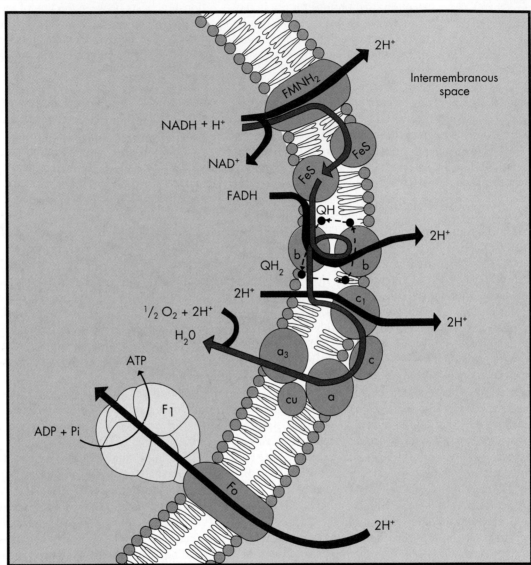

Lipolysis

Within skeletal muscle triacylglycerols are stored in lipid droplets that are easily visualized by electron microscopy (fig. 3.15). Lipid catabolism begins with the breakdown of triacylglycerols (**lipolysis**) (fig. 3.16). A special intracellular lipase enzyme (hormone-sensitive lipase) is activated by cAMP and sequentially releases free fatty acid molecules (FFAs) from the glycerol backbone of triacylglycerols (29, 30). Furthermore, another lipase enzyme, lipoprotein lipase, is attached to the endothelial lining of blood vessels and catabolizes triacylglycerols from blood lipoprotein molecules. The FFA molecules can then be catabolized by muscle, while the remaining glycerol molecule is circulated to the liver. However, glycerol removal by the liver, heart, and kid-

ney is a slow process; hence the use of glycerol as a marker for peripheral triacylglycerol catabolism (also termed FFA mobilization) and a nutrient that can increase the osmolality of body fluids and improve body hydration (see chapter 11).

Following intramuscular lipolysis, FFAs must be modified by the addition of a CoA to enable binding to carnitine and transport into the mitochondria where they are then catabolized in a metabolic pathway called **β-oxidation.** The β-oxidation pathway consists of four enzyme-catalyzed reactions that result in the removal of a 2-carbon end segment, producing acetyl CoA, NADH, FADH, and a FFA molecule that is two carbons shorter. The β-oxidation pathway can then continue, removing two carbon units with each cycle until only one acetyl CoA molecule is left.

FIGURE 3.15

A single lipid droplet can be seen in the central left region of this electron micrograph of myocardial muscle.

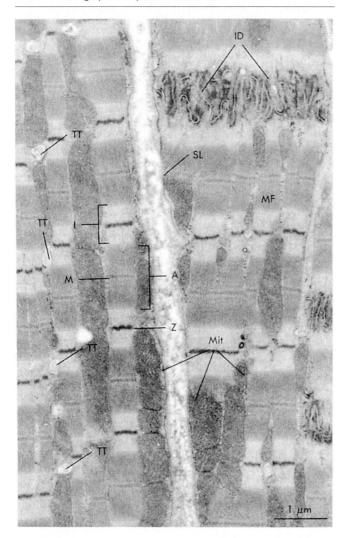

Does Lipid Burn in a Carbohydrate Flame within Skeletal Muscle? *In skeletal muscle, lipid does not burn in a carbohydrate flame.* This implies that molecules from carbohydrate metabolism can be produced and can enter the mitochondria and supplement TCA cycle intermediates. Unfortunately, many previous texts have indirectly promoted this adage by stating it without specific reference to a metabolically active tissue. Within skeletal muscle, lipid and carbohydrate metabolism share a common means of entry into the TCA cycle, acetyl CoA. As will be discussed in the section on glycogen synthesis, skeletal muscle does not have sufficient quantities of the enzymes to convert glycolytic intermediates (mainly pyruvate and phosphoenolpyruvate) into molecules that can be transported into the mitochondria to supplement TCA cycle intermediates. In fact, as indicated in the section on amino acid oxidation, a more accurate adage would be that *both muscle lipid and carbohydrate burn in an amino acid flame!*

Amino Acid Oxidation

Proteins can be catabolized to amino acids, and then have the nitrogenous amino group removed (deamination) with the carbon skeleton incorporated into the central pathways of carbohydrate and lipid metabolism. The exact location that the amino acid enters these pathways depends on the number of carbons in the molecule. The amine group from the process of deamination can be used to reform an amino acid (transamination) for storage in muscle, used in protein synthesis, or be released from the skeletal muscle fiber for uptake by the liver for conversion to urea and subsequent excretion in the urine.

Figure 3.17 presents the locations at which the carbon skeletons of each amino acid can enter into catabolism. The production of acetoacetyl CoA, a substrate of ketone body formation, can occur only in the liver and therefore doesn't apply to skeletal muscle metabolism. During prolonged exercise, when muscle glycogen and blood glucose concentrations are low, the incorporation of the carbon skeletons from amino acids into the TCA cycle is important for maintaining the concentrations of the intermediates, and therefore a high rate of mitochondrial respiration. The main amino acids oxidized in skeletal muscle are the branched chain amino acids isoleucine, leucine, and valine, as well as glutamine and glutamate (26).

The excessive deamination of amino acids is potentially harmful to cellular function. A by-product of deamination is ammonia (NH_3^-), which is released into the circulation and becomes toxic in high concentrations. During prolonged and intermittent intense exercise, when ammonia production increases, the accumulation of ammonia to small concentrations in plasma results in its inclusion in sweat and the odor of ammonia on the surface of the skin. Ammonia release from skeletal muscle is reduced by the transfer of the amine group from amino acids (mainly glutamate) to pyruvate to form alanine. Alanine is then released into the circulation where it can be taken up by the liver and metabolized (fig. 3.18).

The Tally of ATP Regeneration from Catabolism

We are now ready to sum the ATP produced from creatine phosphate, carbohydrate, lipid, and amino acid catabolism. Table 3.2 presents the sources of ATP during catabolism in skeletal muscle. Creatine phosphate provides one ATP per reaction, glycolysis provides three ATP from glycogen and two from glucose, one cycle of β-oxidation provides five ATP, one cycle of the TCA cycle provides 12 ATP, and the potential ATP yield from amino acid catabolism depends on the number of carbons in the molecule and therefore the

lipolysis (li-pol′i-sis) catabolism of triacylglycerol-releasing FFA and glycerol

β-oxidation the reactions of the oxidation of FFA molecules to acetyl CoA

FIGURE 3.16

The proposed roles of vascular and intracellular lipases in the mobilization of free fatty acids for muscle catabolism. *(a)* Mitochondrial catabolism of lipid requires the activation of cytosolic FFA molecules by the addition of CoA. *(b)* (next page) The activated acyl-CoA molecule can then be transported into the mitochondria by a special carnitine shuttle mechanism.

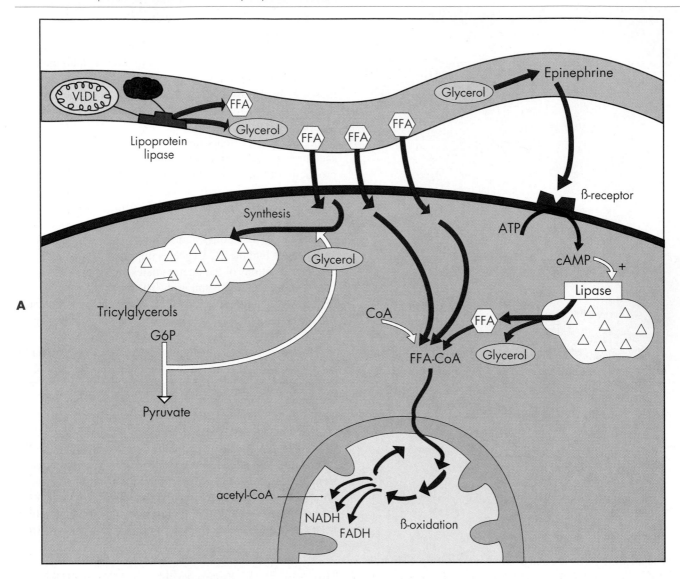

location of entry into the central catabolic pathways. The net ATP yield from the catabolism of glucose is therefore 2 or 3 if pyruvate is converted to lactate, and 36 when pyruvate is entered into mitochondrial respiration and the two cytosolic NADH enter the mitochondria via the glycerol-3-phosphate shuttle. The complete catabolism of palmitate provides 129 ATP, which accounts for the two ATP cost of FFA activation in the cytosol. Catabolism of valine and leucine to glutamine produces 16 molecules of ATP (26); however, as will be discussed in chapter 10, the rate of amino acid oxidation during exercise is low and increases to a maximum of only 15% of the ATP demand during prolonged (> 1 h) exercise.

Despite the comparatively larger ATP yield from palmitate compared to glucose, a comparison that equates acetyl CoA production proves interesting. Without including the ATP cost of free fatty acid activation, the ATP yield from two acetyl CoA molecules from palmitate amounts to 10, resulting from two NADH and two FADH from two cycles of β-oxidation. The ATP yield from the production of two acetyl CoA molecules from glucose equals 12 if the glycerol phosphate shuttle is operative, but equals 14 if the malate-aspartate shuttle is operative. As previously indicated, the metabolism of carbohydrate and lipid is identical after acetyl CoA formation. Based on this ATP tally, carbohydrate metabolism produces more ATP for a given number of acetyl CoA molecules. This requires less oxygen consumption for a given ATP production, and provides the biochemical explanation for *carbohydrate having a greater caloric equivalent for 1 L of oxygen consumed compared to lipid.* The practical

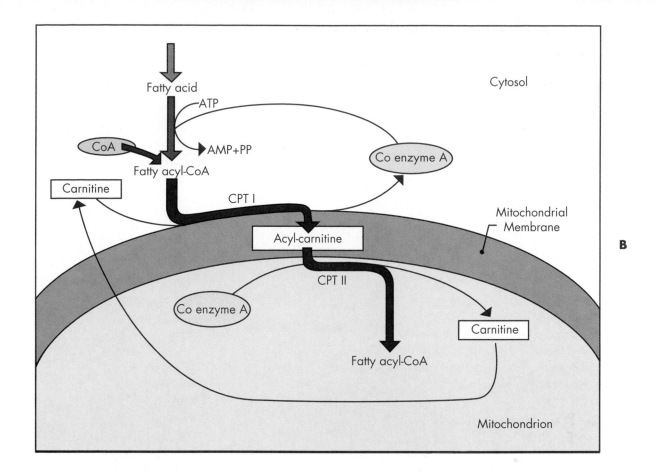

B

FIGURE 3.17

The entry points of amino acids into the main catatolic pathways of energy metabolism.

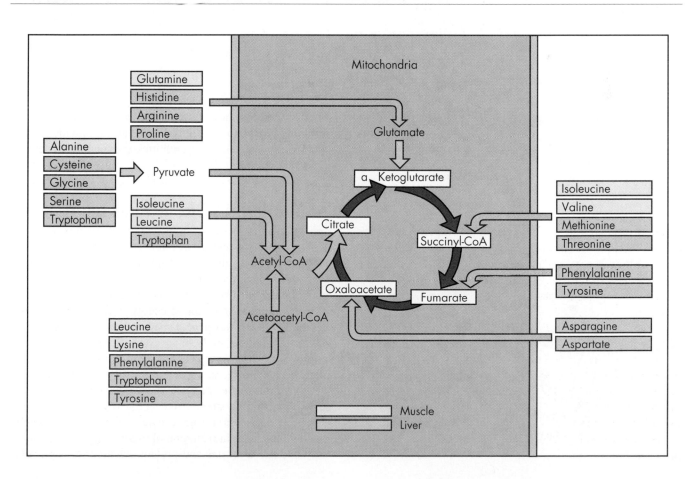

TABLE 3.2

The tally of ATP regeneration from the catabolism of creatine phosphate, carbohydrate, and lipid

REACTIONS		YIELD OF HIGH-ENERGY INTERMEDIATES			
		ATP	NADH	FADH	TOTAL ATP
Creatine Phosphate		1	0	0	1
Carbohydrate (Glucose)*					
Glycolysis					
Phosphorylation of glucose		−1			−1
Phosphorylation of fructose 6-phosphate		−1			−1
Dephosphorylation of 1,3, bisphosphoglycerate	(x2)	2			2
Oxidation of glyceraldehyde 3-phosphate†	(x2)		2		4
Dephosphorylation of phosphoenolpyruvate	(x2)	2			2
Mitochondrial (TCA cycle and ETC)					
Pyruvate oxidation to acetyl CoA	(x2)		2		6
Coupled phosphorylation of GTP from the oxidation of succinyl CoA	(x2)	2			2
Oxidation of isocitrate, α-ketoglutarate and malate	(x2)		6		18
Oxidation of succinate	(x2)			2	4
ATP tally					36
Free Fatty Acid (Palmitate, 16-Carbon)					
Cytosolic reactions					
Activation of the FFA		−2			−2
Mitochondrial (β-oxidation)					
Oxidation of acyl CoA	(x7)			7	14
Oxidation of 3-hydroxyacyl CoA	(x7)		7		21
Mitochondrial (TCA cycle and ETC)					
Acetyl CoA	(x8)	8	24	8	96
ATP tally					129

*The ATP cost of the first phase of glycolysis is 1 ATP if G_6P is produced from glycogen, which would result in either 37 or 39 ATP, depending on the NADH shuttle used.

†Assumes the glycero-phosphate shuttle is used.

FIGURE 3.18

The metabolic connections between the liver, adipose tissue and skeletal muscle. The exchange of lactate between skeletal muscle and the liver is termed the Cori Cycle. The exchange of alanine between skeletal muscle and the liver is termed the Alanine Cycle. The directionality and magnitude of flow of molecules between these tissues varies depending upon nutrient status and exercise intensity.

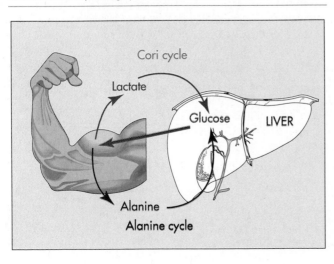

implications for the difference between carbohydrate and lipid in the oxygen requirement and carbon dioxide production for a given caloric expenditure are explained in detail in chapter 4.

Anabolism in Skeletal Muscle

An important concept in the application of exercise physiology to training for improved exercise performance is that the body needs a sufficient recovery to prepare itself for another bout of exercise. This recovery involves not only the removal of wastes or the restoration of energy stores, but also protein synthesis for the repair of damaged muscle and connective tissue. In addition, the cellular events that enable muscle to improve function to facilitate training improvements must also occur. Clearly, an appreciation of the metabolic events that occur during the recovery of exercise provides important knowledge for the exercise physiologist. Many of the reactions that occur during the recovery from exercise combine smaller molecules into larger molecules by the use of free energy and the electrons and protons released during catabo-

FIGURE 3.19

The reactions and metabolic conditions involved in muscle glycogen synthesis.

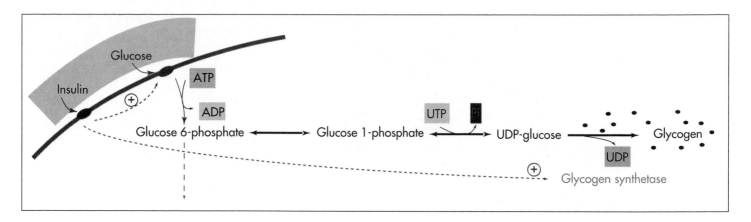

lism. The collective sum of these energy-requiring reactions are collectively referred to as *anabolism.*

Glycogen Synthesis

The enzyme responsible for catalyzing the addition of glucose residues to glycogen is called **glycogen synthetase.** However, the synthesis of glycogen is actually dependent on a series of reactions (fig. 3.19) involving the formation of G_6P, then glucose-1-phosphate (G_1P), then UDP-glucose, and finally the addition of the glucose to the glycogen molecule.

When glycogen synthetase is activated, glycogen synthesis will occur if there is a constant supply of substrate. *Substrate for glycogen synthesis in skeletal muscle can be blood glucose, or intramuscular G_6P.* A distinction is made between the two substrates, as G_6P is not only produced from the hexokinase reaction, but can accumulate in skeletal muscle during intense exercise, and be produced from the reversal of several of the reactions of glycolysis (3, 7, 23). During steady-state exercise, or intense exercise followed by an active recovery, there is minimal intramuscular metabolite accumulation, and substrate for glycogen synthesis is dependent on blood glucose as previously described.

After intense exercise, the increased accumulation of glycolytic intermediates may be diverted back to form G_6P (2, 22). However, although there are numerous findings from animal research that indicate the potential to reverse glycolysis in skeletal muscle, the data from human research are more contradictory (32). Despite this fact, muscle glycogen synthesis after intense exercise occurs at rates almost double that after steady-state exercises (32). These rates of synthesis, and the nutritional determinants of these rates are presented in chapter 11.

Glycogen synthesis is a very efficient storage of free energy. After G_6P formation, the only added energy expenditure is the two-ATP cost of the double phosphate cleavage from GTP during the formation of UDP-glucose. As previously explained, compared to glucose, glycogenolysis reduces the ATP cost of the first phase of glycolysis by one ATP. Therefore, *the net energy cost of forming glycogen is one ATP*. This is a small energy cost given that muscle glycogen is a more readily available substrate for glycolysis than blood glucose, and that if it were not for the muscle's store of glycogen there would not be a sufficient rate of substrate provision for glycolysis during intense exercise.

Triacylglycerol Synthesis

The presence of lipid (triacylglycerol) droplets within skeletal muscle has already been discussed. Because lipid is the predominant substrate catabolized during low to moderate intensities of exercise and at least 50% of this lipid comes from skeletal muscle (32, 33), the pathways that are responsible for these lipid stores deserve clarification.

Fatty acid synthesis does not occur at physiologically meaningful rates in skeletal muscle. The reason for this is the limited activity of the pentose phosphate pathway in skeletal muscle, which produces NADPH, the reducing coenzyme needed for several reactions in the pathway of fatty acid synthesis (35). Although malonyl CoA, the first molecule of fatty acid synthesis, has been shown to exist in skeletal muscle, the concentrations are too small to have metabolic significance (37).

The question therefore arises, Where do the free fatty acid (FFA) and glycerol molecules come from for muscle triacylglycerol synthesis? As illustrated in figure 3.20, the FFA molecules are taken from the blood. The synthesis of a triacylglycerol begins with the formation of glycerol-3-phosphate, which in skeletal muscle is predominantly formed from a glycolytic intermediate. Several enzymes

glycogen synthetase the enzyme catalyzing the addition of glucose residues from UDP-glucose to glycogen

FIGURE 3.20

Triacylglycerol synthesis within skeletal muscle. The synthesis of triacylglycerols is more involved than lipolysis, as several different enzymes are required to reduce glycerol-3-phosphate to phosphatidate and then eventually to a triacylglycerol.

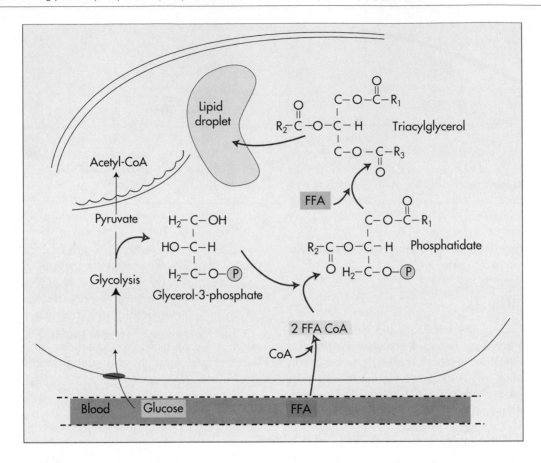

catalyze the addition of intramuscular FFA molecules (depending upon FFA length and saturation) to the glycerol-3-phosphate. The product formed after two FFA additions is called *phosphatidate*, and is a branch molecule in the synthesis of triacylglycerols and phospholipids. The third FFA acid molecule is added (by a lipase) after the phosphate is removed, forming a triacylglycerol. Limited research has been completed on muscle triacylglycerol synthesis, and the regulation of these reactions is unclear. This is unfortunate because muscle lipid is a major substrate for energy metabolism and therefore the biochemical regulation and mobilization of this energy store requires further understanding.

Amino Acid and Protein Synthesis

Many of the 20 amino acid molecules of the human body are produced from intermediates of glycolysis and the TCA cycle. Ten amino acids cannot be produced from metabolism and must be provided by the diet and are therefore termed *essential amino acids*. After the digestion and metabolism of protein into its constituent amino acids, the control of amino acid synthesis occurs via the regulated cellular metabolism of the amino acids glutamate and glutamine. Glutamate can be produced from adding an amine group to the TCA intermediate α-ketoglutamate. Amine groups can also be transferred from glutamate and glutamine, a process termed **transamination,** to carbon skeletons to form other amino acids. Not all amino acids are produced this way. Some have more involved pathways; others are produced from the modification of similarly structured amino acids. An important net result of protein synthesis in skeletal muscle is to increase the size of skeletal muscle by increasing the number of proteins used in muscle contraction (focus box 3.3).

Protein synthesis involves molecular events that involve communication between the nucleus and cytosol of a cell. An example of the stimulation of protein synthesis is provided in figure 3.22. Testosterone, a steroid hormone that increases protein synthesis in skeletal muscle, passes through the sarcolemma, binds to an intracellular transport protein, and is transported to the nucleus. Testosterone, as do other anabolic agents, stimulates the synthesis of a sequence of nucleotides that complement specific DNA sequences that code for the molecules necessary for skeletal muscle hypertrophy. In this process, termed **transcription,** a molecule similar to DNA is

FOCUS BOX 3.3

Researching Muscle Hypertrophy and Muscle Wasting

Muscular strength is proportional to the cross-sectional area of a muscle. Based on this fact, the need for increasing muscle size by hypertrophy, and perhaps by hyperplasia (see chapter 5), has stimulated numerous research questions. For example, there have been applied and clinical needs to understand the best ways to train for muscle hypertrophy, the time course of the hypertrophy response, and the time course of muscle wasting during detraining, immobilization, or from the result of various diseases (e.g., muscle wasting in individuals infected with HIV).

The capacity of human muscle to both increase and decrease in size is phenomenal. As will be discussed in later chapters of this text, complex interactions among genetics, exercise training, nutrition, endocrinology, and health combine to determine the degree of hypertrophy or wasting that results from a given condition. Until application of noninvasive methods for measuring muscle dimensions, such as the CAT (computed automated tomography) scan, or MRI (magnetic resonance imaging), indirect measures such as thigh girths have been used which are obviously less valid because of the unknown contribution of the skin and subcutaneous fat to the girth measurement.

MRI has been used effectively to document changes in muscle cross-sectional areas. Figure 3.21 presents the images of the thigh for two subjects. One subject has cycle trained for several years, while the other subject has not participated in regular exercise training of any sort due to HIV infection. Muscle cross-sectional areas are obtained by digitizing the circumference of the image on a computer screen and having a program mathematically calculate the area.

Muscle hypertrophy is not a rapid process. Several weeks of training are required to induce a detectable increase in muscle mass, and large increases in muscle cross-sectional area may take several months to years of committed training.

FIGURE 3.21

The images of the thigh obtained by MRI from *(a)* an individual who has muscle wasting induced by HIV infection, and *(b)* another individual trained in competitive cycling.

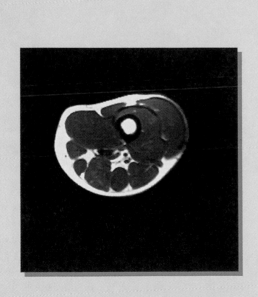

A

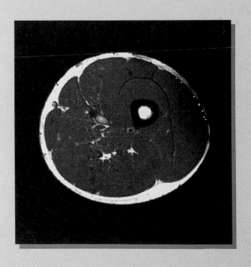

B

formed. This molecule is called *ribonucleic acid* and has nucleotide bases that complement those of the DNA. The transcribed RNA molecule is processed to produce a *messenger RNA* (mRNA), which is responsible for transferring the genetic code for specific molecules into the cytosol. Once in the cytosol, mRNA attaches to the organelle responsible for protein synthesis, the **ribosome.** *The ribosome provides the foundation from which the amino acids are connected*

transamination (trans-amin′a-shun) the removal of an amino group from one amino acid and its placement on a carbon chain that forms another amino acid

transcription (trans-krip′shun) the duplication of specific DNA regions in the form of RNA

ribosome (ri′bo-som) the cytosolic organelle involved in protein synthesis

FIGURE 3.22

Protein synthesis involves the formation of messenger RNA (mRNA) which then leaves the nucleus to attach to ribosome subunits in the cytosol. This event starts the process of joining amino acids into a protein molecule.

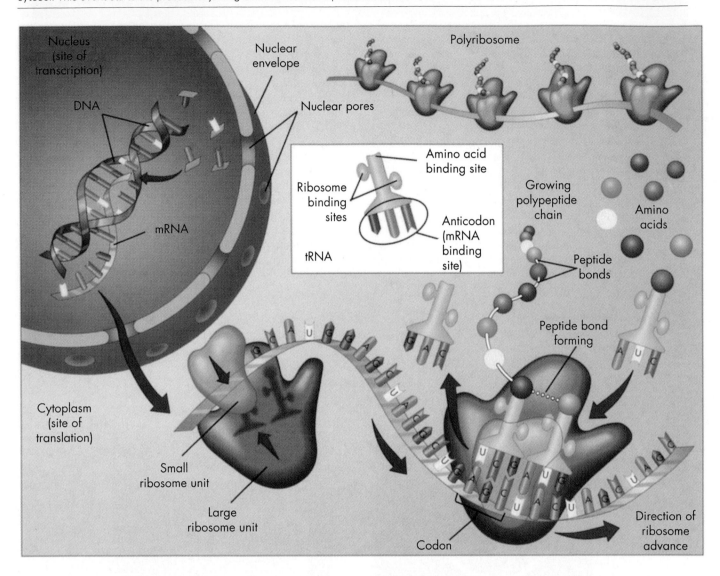

together by peptide bonds. Many ribosomes can work together to synthesize the protein coded by a mRNA molecule.

Amino acids are transported to the mRNA-ribosome structure by another special RNA molecule, called *transfer RNA* (tRNA). The tRNA molecule has a binding site (anticodon) for the RNA sequence that codes a specific amino acid (codon) and a binding site for the amino acid. Consequently, there is a specific tRNA molecule for each amino acid. In addition, specific enzymes exist that catalyze the binding of the tRNA to the mRNA, and the binding of the amino acid to the tRNA (12).

Protein molecules are synthesized by the interactions between the ribosomes, mRNA, and tRNA–amino acid molecules. As the ribosomes move along the mRNA molecule, the protein chain is elongated by the enzymatic addition of amino acids from the specific tRNA molecules, and this process is termed **translation.** Each tRNA–amino acid at-

tachment to the mRNA ribosome complex requires the dephosphorylation of one GTP. However, the GTP (equivalent to ATP) cost of each amino acid positioning on the ribosome mRNA complex is costly, as proteins can have more than several hundred amino acids that require a similarly numbered $(n - 1)$ ATP cost for synthesis.

The amino acid sequence of a protein is called the *primary structure,* and because many chains of proteins do not exist in a linear structure but twist into several types of formations (e.g., alpha helix of DNA), this three-dimensional arrangement is referred to as a *secondary structure.* Larger proteins can also form additional arrangements, where the secondary structure twists and turns, or changes structure, to form the *tertiary structure* (e.g., myoglobin). Finally, some proteins are so large that they consist of multiple units of a given tertiary structure (e.g., hemoglobin), and this arrangement is referred to as a *quaternary structure.*

The Contributions of the Liver and Adipose Tissue to Metabolism During Exercise

Exercise that is sustained for long periods of time places a severe energy stress on skeletal muscle and the liver. For example, the muscle store of glycogen may provide only sufficient carbohydrate to last close to 2 hours of continuous exercise. Clearly, added carbohydrate needs to be provided to skeletal muscle. More important, when liver glycogen stores become depleted blood glucose concentrations fall, causing impaired function of the central nervous system. To compensate for this, the liver must be able to produce new glucose from other molecules, and skeletal muscle must decrease its use of blood glucose (18). To assist in the preservation of blood glucose, skeletal muscle increases its reliance on its own store of FFA and amino acid molecules. Added FFA molecules are also circulated to muscle after they are released from adipose tissue.

Skeletal muscle also produces waste products, other than carbon dioxide, that must be removed. Molecules such as lactate, amino acids such as alanine and glutamate, and toxic waste products such as ammonia must be removed from skeletal muscle. These molecules can either serve as fuel sources to other tissues (lactate and alanine for the liver, lactate for the heart), or need to be processed and removed from the body (amino acid and ammonia conversion to urea for excretion as urine).

This basic description of metabolism during exercise reveals that *the liver and adipose tissue are important supportive organs/tissues to the metabolic needs of skeletal muscle.*

The Liver

The liver functions differently than skeletal muscle during and after exercise. Like skeletal muscle, the liver synthesizes glycogen, amino acids, triacylglycerols, and proteins. However, unlike skeletal muscle, the liver also produces glucose and FFAs, and regulates the production of various lipoprotein molecules that transport blood cholesterol, triacylglycerol, phospholipid, and protein structures to and from the extrahepatic (nonliver) tissues. The most important of these functions to exercise is the production of glucose from gluconeogenesis, and the synthesis of liver glycogen after exercise.

Gluconeogenesis

Gluconeogenesis refers to the production of glucose from noncarbohydrate precursors. The liver has enzymes that are not found, or are present in adequate quantities in skeletal muscle, that divert the two essentially irreversible reactions of glycolysis (7, 17, 24, 28). The gluconeogenic pathway is regulated by metabolites and hormones. During conditions of low blood glucose (< 3–4 mmol/L), glucagon is released

FIGURE 3.23

The production of glucose from non-carbohydrate precursors in the liver by the pathway of gluconeogenesis.

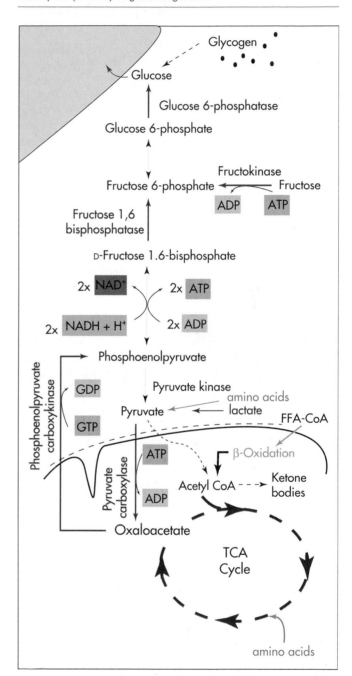

translation (trans-la'shun) the formation of amino acids from the enzymatic association between ribosomes, RNA, and tRNA

gluconeogenesis (glu'ko-ne-o-jen'e-sis) formation of glucose from noncarbohydrates, such as amino acids or alcohol

from the pancreas and inhibits pyruvate kinase activity, stimulates increased liver cAMP concentrations, and increases liver glycogenolysis. These conditions result in the increased production of G_6P (fig. 3.23). The low blood glucose concentration, minimal activity of glucokinase, and the presence of the enzyme G_6Pase allows for G_6P to be converted to glucose, with the release of glucose into the circulation.

Obviously, the pathway of gluconeogenesis is dependent on substrate. During prolonged exercise, liver glycogen stores can be depleted, causing a decreased ability to replenish blood glucose. During these conditions, skeletal muscle increases amino acid oxidation and the release of alanine. Alanine is then circulated to the liver as a substrate for gluconeogenesis (fig. 3.18). This process is known as the *alanine cycle*. Lactate is another substrate that is used by the liver in gluconeogensis (Cori cycle).

Glycogen Synthesis
In the liver, glucose is only a substrate for glycogen synthesis in the postabsorptive state after a high carbohydrate meal, when blood glucose concentrations are elevated enough for glucokinase activity to exceed rates of the reverse reaction catalyzed by G_6Pase. Research has shown that the main substrates for liver glycogen synthesis are lactate, fructose, alanine, glutamine, and glycerol (17, 18). This phenomenon has been termed the "glucose paradox," or the "indirect pathway" of glycogen synthesis (18).

Adipose Tissue

The main anabolic pathway of interest within adipose tissue is triacylglycerol synthesis. This pathway has been detailed in skeletal muscle metabolism. Nevertheless, the student should appreciate that adipose tissue is the main store of the body's triacylglycerols, and that excess carbohydrate or protein intake increases liver FFA synthesis, and it is the majority of this lipid that ends up in adipose tissue triacylglycerol stores.

WEBSITE BOX

Chapter 3: Metabolism

The newest information regarding exercise physiology can be viewed at the following sites.*

http://www.iol.paisley.ac.uk/courses/metabolism/metabolism_main.html
   Online tutorial on glycolysis, from University of Paisley, England.
http://biotech.chem.indiana.edu/glycolysis/glycohome.html
   Online tutorial on glycolysis.
http://mss.scbe.on.ca/DSRESPIR.htm
   List of links that provide complete coverage of topics within metabolic biochemistry.
http://prs.k12.nj.us/Schools/PHS/Science_Dept/APBiol/Glycolysis.html
   Lecture material on glycolysis.
http://intramet.ecu.edu/NUHM/CHOH/CARBO/
   Slide presentation of glycogen synthesis, from East Carolina University, Greenville, N.C.
http://disability.ucdavis.edu/Virtual_Library/Diaseas_Database/Glycogem_Storage_Diseases_Links.html
   Provides links of sites concerning glycogen storage diseases.
psu.edu/dept/cac/ets/archive/projects.1997/Nutrition/lipid/slisdes/index.html
   Slide show of lipid biochemistry.

http://www-classes.usc.edu/engr/ms/125/MDA125/cell/
   Lecture notes and slides on cell biology, including cellular biochemistry.
curtin.edu.au/curtin/dept/physio/pt/edres/exphys/e552_96/
   Index of brief reviews of exercise physiology content by students from Curtin University, Australia. Topics include nutrition, ergogenic aids, environmental physiology, training, and clinical applications.
neuro.wustl.edu/neuromuscular/pathol/diagrams/glycogen.htm
   Superb site providing the biochemistry of carbohydrate catabolism.
arfa.org/index.htm
   Excellent site providing comprehensive information on many topics within exercise physiology.
curtin.edu.au/curtin/dept/phyiol/pt/edres/exphys/ep552_96/Lactate/
   Lecture notes and reports on metabolism during exercise.

*Unless indicated, all URLs preceded by http://www.

Note: These URLs were valid at the time of publication, but could have changed or been deleted from Internet access since that time.

- The energy within chemical compounds is termed **chemical energy.** The science that studies how energy is converted in living things is called **bioenergetics.** Bioenergetics is based on two very important laws. (1) *Energy cannot be created or destroyed, but can be changed from one form to another.* (2) *Energy transfer will always proceed in the direction of increased entropy.*

- The usable energy (to complete work) released from chemical reactions is termed Gibbs **free energy** (ΔG). *Entropy* is a form of energy that cannot be used, and is defined by *increased randomness* or *disorder.* Based on the second law, all chemical reactions proceed in the direction that results in a release of free energy (denoted $-\Delta G$), and are termed *exergonic* reactions.

- **Adenosine triphosphate (ATP)** is a large molecule that contains three phosphate (PO_3^-) groups. Inside a cell, the free energy released when one phosphate group is removed in a reaction approximates -14 kcal/M. The free energy released from this reaction under standard conditions is 7.3 kcal/M.

- **Metabolism** can be defined as the sum of all chemical reactions in the body. **Catabolism** involves the breakdown of energy-yielding nutrients, the release of free energy and electrons, and their coupled transfer to intermediary molecules (e.g., ATP), and the formation of low-energy end products. **Anabolism** involves the covalent bonding of electrons, protons, and small molecules to produce larger molecules.

- **Enzymes** are protein molecules that function to increase the rates of chemical reactions. On the surface of an enzyme are specific binding sites for substrate(s), and depending upon the enzyme, other binding sites exist for molecules that either decrease or increase enzyme activity. Enzymes do not alter the free energy change of chemical reactions.

- Terms that are gaining increased acceptance in qualifying the source of ATP production are the **phosphagen system, glycolytic metabolism,** and **mitochondrial respiration,** respectively.

- The main nutrients of the body used in energy metabolism are *carbohydrates, lipids,* and *amino acids.* **Glucose** is the favored carbohydrate for metabolism in skeletal muscle, the liver, and adipose tissue. **Glycogen** consists of a protein core (glycogenin) from which chains of glucose molecules are attached. The main lipids of interest to energy metabolism are those that comprise **triacylglycerols.** A triacylglycerol consists of three **fatty acid** (FA) molecules attached to a carbohydrate backbone called *glycerol.* **Amino acid** molecules differ from carbohydrate and lipid molecules in that they contain nitrogen atoms. There are 20 amino acids within the body, and all have a structure comprising an acid (COOH), amine (NH_2), CH, and R-group (side chain) attached to a central carbon atom.

- **The creatine phosphate (CrP)** reaction is the most rapid means to regenerate ATP, and is catalyzed by *creatine kinase.* The phosphagen system is crucial to the muscles' abilities to tolerate increases in metabolic demand.

- The catabolism of glycogen is termed **glycogenolysis.** The importance of glycogenolysis is that it can *provide a rapid rate of production of glucose-6-phosphate* (G_6P), the first intermediate of glycolysis. Within skeletal muscle **glycolysis** begins with either G_6P or the entry of glucose into the skeletal muscle fiber. G_6P is broken down sequentially by nine reactions that form the central carbohydrate metabolic pathway of glycolysis. *The important products of glycolysis are pyruvate, ATP, and NADH.* The ratio of NAD^+ to NADH is called the **redox potential.**

- Pyruvate can be reduced to **lactate** by the enzyme *lactate dehydrogenase* (LDH). Lactate production and accumulation in skeletal muscle does not directly cause fatigue and/or pain. *The problem with lactate production is the accompanying acidosis and not the lactate molecule.*

- During pyruvate entry into the mitochondria, pyruvate is converted to **acetyl CoA** by a series of linked enzymes known collectively as pyruvate dehydrogenase. The acetyl CoA formed from either carbohydrate or lipid catabolism can then enter into a catabolic pathway called the **tricarboxylic acid cycle** (TCA cycle), which consists of nine reactions. *The combined products of the TCA cycle are carbon dioxide, ATP, NADH, and FADH.* All of the CO_2 produced in energy metabolism can be accounted for from pyruvate entry into the mitochondria and the TCA cycle.

- The biochemical use of oxygen occurs in the **electron transport chain (ETC).** *In the ETC, the proton and electrons acquired in NADH and FADH are utilized to add electrons to hydrogen atoms and oxygen to form water, and generate the free energy to add a phosphate to ADP to form ATP.* The formation of water and ATP during the ETC is termed **oxidative phosphorylation,** and our understanding of this process is based on the chemiosmotic theory.

- Within skeletal muscle, lipid catabolism begins with the breakdown of triacylglycerols (**lipolysis**). Following intramuscular lipolysis, FFAs must be modified by the addition of coenzyme-A for transport into the mitochondria where they are then catabolized in a metabolic pathway called **β-oxidation.** The β-oxidation pathway consists of four enzyme-catalyzed reactions that result in the removal of a 2-carbon end segment, producing acetyl CoA, NADH, FADH, and a FFA molecule that is two carbons shorter.

- The enzyme responsible for catalyzing the addition of glucose residues to glycogen is called **glycogen synthetase.** These enzymes, and others that affect their activity, are regulated by an epinephrine-cAMP mechanism, as well as

SUMMARY

intracellular metabolic conditions that favor synthetase activation during rest, low glycogen concentrations, and increased blood glucose and insulin concentrations.

■ After the digestion and metabolism of protein into its constituent amino acids, the control of amino acid synthesis occurs via the regulated cellular metabolism of the amino acids glutamate and glutamine. The transfer of amine groups from glutamate and glutamine (**transamination**) to carbon skeletons to form other amino acids is the main way amino acids are catabolized in skeletal muscle.

■ Protein synthesis involves molecular events that involve communication between the nucleus and cytosol of a cell. During **transcription,** a molecule similar to DNA is formed. This molecule is called *ribonucleic acid* and has nucleotide bases that complement those of the DNA. The transcribed RNA molecule is processed to produce a *messenger RNA* (mRNA), which is *responsible for transferring the genetic code for specific molecules into the cytosol.* Once in the cytosol, mRNA attaches to the organelle responsible for protein synthesis, the **ribosome.**

The ribosome provides the foundation from which the amino acids are connected by peptide bonds. Many ribosomes can work together to synthesize the protein coded by an mRNA molecule.

■ As the ribosomes move along the mRNA molecule, the protein chain is elongated by the enzymatic addition of amino acids from the specific tRNA molecules, and this process is termed **translation.** Each tRNA–amino acid attachment to the mRNA ribosome complex requires the dephosphorylation of one GTP.

■ The most important functions of the liver in exercise are the production of glucose from gluconeogenesis, and the synthesis of liver glycogen after exercise. **Gluconeogenesis** *refers to the production of glucose from noncarbohydrate precursors.* During prolonged exercise, liver glycogen stores can be depleted, causing a decreased ability to replenish blood glucose. During these conditions, skeletal muscle increases amino acid oxidation, and the release of alanine is circulated to the liver as a substrate for gluconeogenesis.

STUDY QUESTIONS

1. Define the terms energy, chemical energy, bioenergetics, entropy, exergonic, and metabolism.

2. What is ATP? Explain how ATP is used in coupled reactions in cellular metabolism.

3. Why do enzymes essentially regulate chemical reactions if they do not alter the thermodynamics of reactions?

4. Explain the multiple conditions that can alter enzyme activity.

5. How might the different rates of ATP regeneration from the catabolic reactions and pathways in skeletal muscle influence energy production during differing intensities of exercise?

6. What is the net ATP production from the different catabolic pathways of skeletal muscle?

7. Why are the concentrations of NAD^+ and NADH important to energy metabolism in the cytosol and mitochondria?

8. Why is lactate produced in skeletal muscle during exercise, and why it is wrong to view lactate as a detrimental molecule to muscle function?

9. Why is the capacity of skeletal muscle to synthesize glycogen important for the ability to perform exercise?

10. What are the differences between transcription and translation, and why are they important during protein synthesis?

APPLICATIONS

1. The second law of thermodynamics explains why concentrations of substrates and products can alter the directionality of chemical reactions. What problems would exist for cells if they solely relied on substrate and product concentrations for the regulation of the rate and directionality of chemical reactions?

2. Some individuals lack the enzyme phosphorylase (McArdle's disease). Phosphorylase is an allosteric enzyme. Based on what you know about allosteric enzymes, their importance to metabolism, and the catabo-

lism of carbohydrate, how would this condition alter the individuals' ability to tolerate exercise?

3. If allosteric enzymes are potentially more beneficial because of improved regulation, why aren't all enzymes of the body allosteric enzymes?

4. If more energy is stored in FFAs than in an equal amount of glycogen, why is glycogen the preferred fuel for contracting skeletal muscle?

5. Why would the majority of skeletal muscle protein synthesis have to occur during rest conditions?

REFERENCES

1. Atkinson, D. E. *Cellular energy metabolism and its regulation.* Academic Press, New York, 1977.

2. Bendall, J. R., and A. A. Taylor. The meyerhof quotient and the synthesis of glycogen from lactate in frog and rabbit muscle. *Biochem. J.* 118:887–893, 1970.

3. Bertorini, T. E., V. Shively, and B. Taylor. ATP degradation products after ischemic exercise: Hereditary lack of phosphorylase or carnitine palmityl transferase. *Neurology.* 35(9):1355–1357, 1985.

4. Carraro, F., S. Klein, J. I. Rosenblatt, and R. R. Wolfe. Effect of dichloroacetate on lactate concentration in exercising humans. *J. Appl. Physiol.* 66(2):91–97, 1989.

5. Chwalbinska-Moneta, J., R. A. Robergs, D. L. Costill, and W. J. Fink. Threshold for muscle lactate accumulation. *J. Appl. Physiol.* 66(6):2710–2716, 1989.

6. Chasiotis, D. Role of cyclic AMP and inorganic phosphate in the regulation of muscle glycogenolysis during exercise. *Med. Sci. Sports Exerc.* 20(6):545–550, 1988.

7. Crabtree, B., S. J. Higgins, and E. A. Newsholme. The activities of pyruvate carboxylase, phosphoenolpyruvate carboxykinase and fructose diphosphatase in muscles from vertebrates and invertebrates. *Biochem. J.* 130:391–396, 1972.

8. Douen, A.G., et al. Exercise induces recruitment of the "insulin responsive glucose transporter." *J. Biol. Chem.* 265(23):13,427–13,430, 1990.

9. Friden, J., J. Seger, and B. Ekblom. Topographical localization of muscle glycogen: An ultrahistochemical study in the human vastus lateralis. *Acta Physiol. Scand.* 135:381–391, 1989.

10. Fushiki, T., J. A. Wells, E. B. Tapscott, and G. L. Dohm. Changes in glucose transporters in muscle in response to exercise. *Am. J. Physiol.* 256(19):E580–E587, 1989.

11. Gollnick, P. D. Metabolic regulation in skeletal muscle: Influence of endurance training as exerted by mitochondrial protein concentration. *Acta Physiol. Scand.* 128(S556):53–66, 1986.

12. Grannar, D. K. Protein synthesis and the genetic code. In R. K. Murray, D. K. Granner, P. A. Mayes, and V. W. Rodwell (eds.), *Harper's biochemistry*, 22d ed. Appleton & Lange, Norwalk, CT, 1990, pp. 395–407.

13. Henrikson, E. J., R. E. Bourey, K. J. Rodnick, L. Koranyi, A. Permutt, and J. O. Holloszy. Glucose transporter protein content and glucose transport capacity in rat skeletal muscle. *Am. J. Physiol.* 259(22):E593–E598, 1990.

14. Hinkle, P. C., and R. E. McCarry. How cells make ATP. *Scientific American* 238(5):104–123, 1978.

15. Houmard, J. A., et al. Elevated skeletal muscle glucose transporter levels in exercise-trained middle-aged men. *Am. J. Physiol.* 261(24):E437–E443, 1991.

16. Hurley, B. F., P. M. Nemeth, W. H. Martin III, J. M. Hagberg, G. P. Dalsky, and J. O. Holloszy. Muscle triglyceride utilization during exercise: Effect of training. *J. Appl. Physiol.* 60(2):562–567, 1982.

17. Johnson, J. L., and G. J. Bagby. Gluconeogenic pathway in liver and muscle glycogen synthesis after exercise. *J. Appl. Physiol.* 64(4):1591–1599, 1988.

18. Katz, J., and J. D. McGarry. The glucose paradox. Is glucose a substrate for liver metabolism? *J. Clin. Invest.* 74:1901–1909, 1984.

19. Katz, A., and K. Sahlin. Regulation of lactic acid production during exercise. *J. Appl. Physiol.* 65(2):509–518, 1988.

20. Lehninger, A. L. *Principles of biochemistry.* Worth, New York City, 1993.

21. Mayes, P. A. Biologic oxidation. In R. K. Murray, D. K. Granner, P. A. Mayes, and V. W. Rodwell (eds.), *Harper's biochemistry.* 22d ed. Appleton & Lange, Norwalk, CT, 1990, pp. 105–111.

22. McLane, J. A., and J. O. Holloszy. Glycogen synthesis from lactate in three types of skeletal muscle. *J. Biol. Chem.* 254(14):6548–6553, 1979.

23. Munger, R., E. Temler, D. Jallut, E. Haesler, and J. Felber. Correlations of glycogen synthase and phosphorylase activites with glycogen concentration in human muscle biopsies: Evidence for a double-feedback mechanism regulating glycogen synthesis and breakdown. *Metabolism* 42(1):36–43, 1993.

24. Newgard, C. B., L. J. Hirsch, D. W. Foster, and J. D. McGarry. Studies on the mechanism by which exogenous glucose is converted into liver glycogen in the rat. *J. Biol. Chem.* 258(13):8046–8052, 1983.

25. Newsholme, E. A., and B. Crabtree. Flux generating and regulatory steps in metabolic control. *Trends in Biochem. Sci.* 6:53–55, 1981.

26. Newsholme, E. A., and E. R. Leech. *Biochemistry for the medical sciences.* Wiley, Chichester, 1983.

27. Newsholme, E. A., B. Crabtree, and M. Parry-Billings. The energetic cost of regulation: An analysis based on the principles of metabolic-control-logic. In J. M. Kinney, and H. N. Tucker (eds.), *Energy metabolism: Tissue determinants and cellular corollaries.* Raven Press, New York, 1991, pp. 467–498.

28. Opie, L. H., and E. A. Newsholme. The activities of fructose 1,6-diphosphatase, phosphofructokinase and phosphoenolpyruvate carboxykinase in white muscle and red muscle. *Biochem. J.* 103:391–399, 1967.

29. Oscai, L. B. Type L hormone-sensitive lipase hydrolyzes endogenous triacylglycerols in muscle in exercised rats. *Med. Sci. Sports Exerc.* 15(4):336–339, 1983.

30. Oscai, L. B., and W. K. Palmer. Cellular control of triacylglycerol metabolism. *Exerc. Sport Sciences Rev.* 11:1–23, 1983.

31. Ren, J. M., and E. Hultman. Regulation of phosphorylase activity in human skeletal muscle. *J. Appl. Physiol.* 69(3):919–923, 1990.

32. Robergs, R. A. Nutritional and exercise determinants of postexercise muscle glycogen synthesis. *Int. J. Sports Nutrition* 1:307–337, 1991.

33. Romjin, J. A., E. F. Coyle, L. S. Sidossis, X. J. Zhang, and R. R. Wolfe. Relationship between fatty acid delivery and fatty acid oxidation during strenuous exercise. *J. Appl. Physiol.* 79(6):1939–1945, 1995.

34. Stanley, W. C., E. W. Gertz, J. A. Wisneski, D. J. Morris, R. A. Neese, and G. A. Brooks. Systematic lactate kinetics during graded exercise in man. *Am. J. Appl. Physiol.* 249(12):E595–E602, 1985.

REFERENCES

35. Stryer, L. *Biochemistry*. Freeman, New York, 1991.

36. Veech, R. L., J. W. Randolph Lawson, N. W. Cornell, and H. A. Krebs. Cytosolic phosphorylation potential. *J. Biol. Chem.* 254(14):6538–6547, 1979.

37. Yan, Z., M. K. Spencer, P. J. Bechtel, and A. Katz. Regulation of glycogen synthase in human muscle during isometric contraction and recovery. *Acta Physiol. Scand.* 147:77–83, 1993.

RECOMMENDED READINGS

Friden, J., J. Seger, and B. Ekblom. Topographical localization of muscle glycogen: An ultrahistochemical study in the human vastus lateralis. *Acta Physiol. Scand.* 135:381–391, 1989.

Houmard, J. A., P. C. Egan, P. D. Neufer, J. E. Friedman, W. S. Wheeler, R. G. Israel, and G. L. Dohm. Elevated skeletal muscle glucose transporter levels in exercise-trained middle-aged men. *Am. J. Physiol.* 261(24):E437–E443, 1991.

Hurley, B. F., P. M. Nemeth, W. H. Martin III, J. M. Hagberg, G. P. Dalsky, and J. O. Holloszy. Muscle triglyceride utilization during exercise: Effect of training. *J. Appl. Physiol.* 60(2):562–567, 1982.

Oscai, L. B., and W. K. Palmer. Cellular control of triacylglycerol metabolism. *Exerc. Sport Sciences Rev.* 11:1–23, 1983.

Robergs, R. A. Nutritional and exercise determinants of post-exercise muscle glycogen synthesis. *Int. J. Sports Nutrition* 1:307–337, 1991.

Romjin, J. A., E. F. Coyle, L. S. Sidossis, X. J. Zhang, and R. R. Wolfe. Relationship between fatty acid delivery and fatty acid oxidation during strenuous exercise. *J. Appl. Physiol.* 79(6):1939–1945, 1995.

CHAPTER 4

Ergometry and Calorimetry

hen we exercise, our bodies use chemical energy derived from catabolism to cause muscle contraction. During this process we use energy and therefore expend calories and generate mechanical power and work. To better understand the processes of power, work, and energy expenditure during exercise, scientists have developed methods that can quantify these capacities. For example, the introduction of the stationary cycle enabled the quantification of work and power output during cycle exercise. Similarly, the development of equipment and techniques allowing the measurement of *oxygen consumption* provided an indirect means to quantify the metabolic intensity of steady-state exercise and to calculate changes in energy expenditure with changes in exercise intensity. When controlling exercise intensity, metabolic responses can be compared between differing individuals (male vs. female, young vs. old, etc.), or for the same individual exposed to differing circumstances (e.g., pretraining to posttraining, low vs. high altitude, etc.). The purpose of this chapter is to explain the methods available for quantifying exercise intensity for various modes of exercise and to present the methods used to measure or indirectly calculate the energy expenditure of the body. The importance of the concepts of energy, work, and power during exercise to the science of exercise physiology cannot be overemphasized.

OBJECTIVES

After studying this chapter, you should be able to:

- Define ergometry and provide examples of its application to exercise.
- Calculate work and power for bench step, cycle, and treadmill ergometry examples.
- Use conversion factors to equate units of work, energy, and power.
- Explain the differences between direct and indirect calorimetry.
- Calculate oxygen consumption, carbon dioxide production, and energy expenditure for given exercise data examples.
- List the caloric equivalents (per unit weight and also relative to oxygen consumption) for pure fat and pure carbohydrate catabolism.
- State the assumptions and limitations of the nonprotein RER values used in indirect calorimetry.
- Identify modern methods available for indirect calorimetry data measurement and computation during exercise.
- Explain the importance of indirect calorimetry to the calculation of oxygen consumption, and how this measure is important in the study and research of exercise physiology.

KEY TERMS

ergometry	calorimeter	Haldane
ergometer	respiratory	transformation
work	quotient (RQ)	economy
power	respiratory	efficiency
calorimetry	exchange ratio (RER)	

Ergometry

*T*he science of **ergometry** concerns the measurement of work. Work (*W*) is accomplished during the application of force against gravity (*F*) over a distance (*D*), and hence is expressed as follows;

4.1
$$W = F \times D$$

Like the science of thermodynamics, ergometry was originally applied to mechanical systems. However, as the body is based on lever systems which produce mechanical work during dynamic muscle contraction, ergometry also has application to human movement. A device which can be used to measure work is called an **ergometer**.

One of the earliest ergometers was a bench step (fig. 4.1*a*). To measure work and power, a subject steps up and down on a bench, thus raising the body weight against gravity. When stepping a bench of a known height at a constant rate the amount of positive work performed is equal to:

Force = body weight = 70 kg

Distance = step height × rate × time = 0.25 m/step × 30 steps/min × 30 min

4.2   = 225 m

Work = 70 kg × 225 m

      = 15,750 kgm

Power = work / time (min)

      = 15,750 kgm / 30

      = 525 kgm/min

Appendix C provides conversions between different scientific units. The internationally recognized unit of work is the joule (J), and the recognized unit for power is J/s (or J/min) (18, 30). These units are extremely small, so they are often expressed in increments of 1000 units of energy (kJ). Unfortunately, the scientific literature in many countries uses alternative units, and energy is still often expressed as kilocalories (kcals) and power is expressed as watts (W). This is especially true for the United States. An understanding of the relationships between kcal and kJ and W and kJ/min is advantageous for the understanding of research findings from internationally circulated journals.

Using the scientific conversions of appendix C (1 W = 6.118 kgm/min = 0.060 kJ /min, 1 kgm = 0.0023 kcal, and 1 kcal = 4.1868 kJ), the bench stepping exercise involved an average power output of 85.8 W (5.1480 kJ /min), and a total mechanical energy generation of 36.23 kcals or 151.66 kJ. This energy value is not the biological energy expended for this activity, but the energy derived from the mechanical work produced. As the body is not 100% efficient in converting chemical energy to mechanical energy, *the biological energy expenditure by the body during exercise is always greater than the mechanical energy cost*. The concept of efficiency will be explained, and values calculated, in a later section of this chapter.

The distinction between work and power is important during exercise. Almost any individual can perform a given amount of work if given enough time. However, not all individuals can perform a similar quantity of work in a given time interval. Consequently, exercise intensity is quantified in units of power, which enables comparisons to be made within and between individuals. Individuals that can sustain high-power outputs during prolonged exercise without becoming fatigued have high *cardiorespiratory endurance* fitness. Conversely, individuals that can generate high maximal power values during very short bursts of exercise have high *muscle power*, and would be suited to sprint and other intense short-term exercises.

Cycle Ergometry

The development of the cycle ergometer enabled the calculation of work and power during cycle exercise. A modern example of a cycle ergometer and the principles it uses to quantify work and power is illustrated in Figure 4.1*b*.

On a cycle ergometer, the application of friction via a belt around the front flywheel is quantified by the force required to move a pendulum attached to the belt. The distance moved by the pendulum is calibrated, and generally labeled in 0.5 kg units on a scale fixed behind the pendulum. A person pedaling the bike will spin the front flywheel, and the product of the distance transversed by the circumference of the flywheel and the frictional force applied to the belt is equal to work, expressed as kilogram meters (kgm). Bikes can differ in the circumferential distance transversed with one crank revolution. The Body Guard™ and Monark™ ergometers transverse 6 m per crank revolution, and the Tunturi™ transverses 3 m per crank revolution.

For a Monark ergometer, **work** and **power** can be calculated as follows:

4.3   Work = cadence (rpm) × load (kg) × 6 (m) × duration (min)

For example, a person riding at 60 rpm against a 2 kg load for 30 min will perform work equal to:

Work (kgm) = 60 × 2 × 6 × 30

          = 21,600

ergometry (er-**gom**′e-**tree**) the science of the measurement of work and power

ergometer (er-**gom**′e-**ter**) a device used to measure work

work the product of an applied force exerted over a known distance against gravity

power the application of force relative to time

FIGURE 4.1

Illustrations of common ergometers used during exercise. *(a)* The bench step. *(b)* The cycle ergometer. During cycle ergometry, resistance is usually applied via a friction belt surrounding the front flywheel. This friction system is calibrated, with the frictional resistance, or load, measured in kilograms. *(c)* The constant load cycle ergometer. Electrical resistance is applied to a copper flywheel, and the resistance is automatically adjusted with increases or decreases in cadence to maintain a constant power output. *(d)* The treadmill. The movement of the treadmill belt at given velocities is used to generate known walking or running speeds. Walking or running up hill can also be mimicked by increasing the inclination of the treadmill. *(e)* An arm egometer, which is also based on the principles used in cycle ergometry.

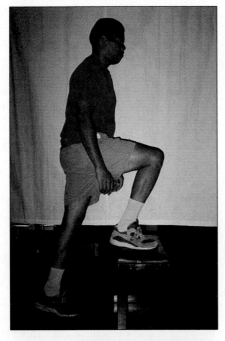

A

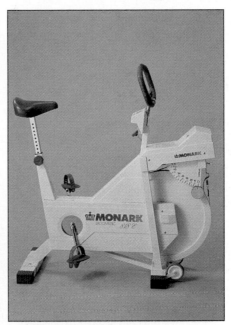

B

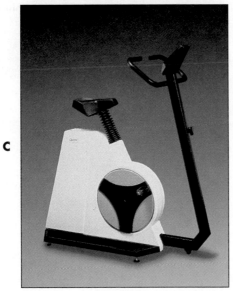

C

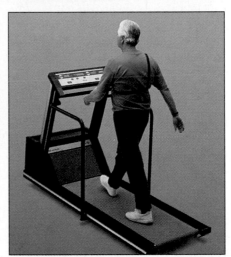

D

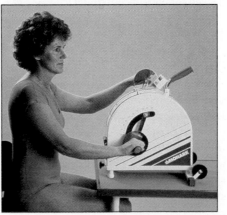

E

When expressing power relative to work performed in a minute (kgm per min, kgm/min), the above example computes to:

$$
\begin{aligned}
\text{Power (kgm/min)} &= 21{,}600 / 30 \\
&= 720 \\
\text{Power (W)} &= 720 / 6.118 \\
&= 118 \\
\text{Power (kJ/min)} &= 118 \times 0.060 \\
&= 7.08
\end{aligned}
$$

There are many different types of cycle ergometers in use in research and fitness facilities. A popular cycle ergometer used in well-equipped research laboratories is the constant load ergometer (fig. 4.1c). The constant load ergometer has an electronic resistance mechanism that applies resistance to a flywheel that varies with cadence. The ability to apply variable resistance enables the subject to vary cadence within a range specified by the bike manufacturer. Consequently, unlike the traditional cycle ergometer, a given power output (usually set as watts) is maintained automatically by the bike across a wide range of cadence. This is advantageous in a research setting, because less time and effort by the researchers is required to ensure the correct cadence for a given exercise intensity, which decreases the likelihood of experimental error.

Another type of cycle ergometer is the isokinetic ergometer (fig. 4.1d). This cycle provides the user with the option to set a given cadence, and then measures the force applied to the crankshafts during cycling. These forces are used to calculate both power and work. With the advances in computer and video technology, the isokinetic ergometer is becoming popular in many fitness facilities because of additional options like videotape integration, competitive racing programs, and specific terrain imitating circuits. Similar ergometers also exist for rowing (fig. 4.2).

Each of the constant load and isokinetic ergometers are not without fault. The traditional cycle ergometer can be calibrated manually, but the constant load or isokinetic ergometers need to be either returned to the manufacturer for recalibration or provided with an expensive calibration device. Each ergometer should be routinely checked for correct calibration.

Treadmill Ergometry

Compared to cycling, it is more difficult to apply principles of ergometry to treadmill running or walking (17). Level walking or running does not directly involve a translation of force against gravity. Although the body's center of gravity is moved vertically during a stride, this height is hard to quantify, differs between individuals, and is therefore hard to control. The easiest solution to this problem is to have the subject walk or run on a treadmill set at an incline, or suspend a weight over a pulley behind the treadmill (fig. 4.3). The larger the angle, the steeper is the grade, and a vertical distance (against gravity) can be calculated from the application of simple trigonometry (fig. 4.3a). The accepted unit of treadmill grade is % grade, and represents the relative expression of the vertical distance divided by the horizontal distance during treadmill walking or running. The conversions between % grade and angle (°) for various % grades are presented in table 4.1.

Swimming Ergometry

Of all the popular exercise modes, swimming has proved the most difficult to apply the principles of ergometry. The main

FIGURE 4.2

Students collecting expired air in a Douglas bag from a subject exercising on a rowing ergometer.

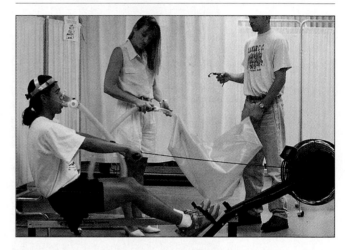

TABLE 4.1

Conversions between angle and % grade of a treadmill

% GRADE	TANGENT Θ	Θ (DEGREES)
1	0.01	0.57
2	0.02	1.15
3	0.03	1.72
4	0.04	2.29
5	0.05	2.86
6	0.06	3.43
7	0.07	4.00
8	0.08	4.57
9	0.09	5.14
10	0.10	5.70
12	0.12	6.28
14	0.14	7.97
16	0.16	9.09
18	0.18	10.20
20	0.20	11.31

FIGURE 4.3

(a) The inclination of a treadmill is measured as a percent grade (% grade), which is defined as the vertical rise per 100 units of horizontal translation. It is easily calculated as the tangent of the angle multiplied by 100. However, in reality, measuring the angle is not easy or accurate. Consequently, measuring the vertical height (rise) of a triangle (y) and dividing it by the horizontal length of the triangle (x) will yield the grade expressed as a fraction. The inverse tangent of this value is the angle. *(b)* Suspension of a weight from the subject provides a force exerted against gravity, thus allowing the calculation of work during treadmill exercise. *(c)* Instead of a weight, subjects can also be connected to a strain gauge positioned at the rear of a special low resistance free-spinning treadmill. During walking or running, the subject's attempts at forward movement spins the treadmill belt and force is exerted by the body on the strain gauge.

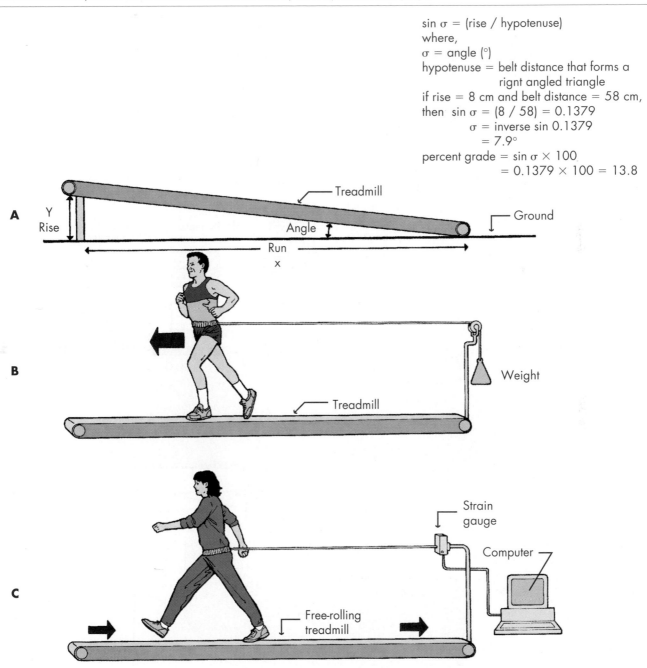

$\sin \sigma = (\text{rise} / \text{hypotenuse})$
where,
$\sigma = \text{angle } (°)$
$\text{hypotenuse} = \text{belt distance that forms a}$
$\qquad\qquad\qquad \text{rignt angled triangle}$
if rise $= 8$ cm and belt distance $= 58$ cm,
then $\sin \sigma = (8 / 58) = 0.1379$
$\qquad \sigma = \text{inverse } \sin 0.1379$
$\qquad\quad = 7.9°$
percent grade $= \sin \sigma \times 100$
$\qquad\qquad\qquad = 0.1379 \times 100 = 13.8$

method to gauge and increment exercise intensity during swimming is based on a simple pulley and suspended weight system (fig. 4.4*a*). Maintaining the suspended weight in the same position requires effort that can be expressed as a force (weight against gravity), exerted continuously over time. Al-

though there is no true distance component and therefore calculations of power and work cannot be performed, this method enables researchers to perform tests with increments of intensity, similar to the principles of a treadmill or cycle ergometer incremental exercise test.

FIGURE 4.4

Methods used to quantify exercise intensity, or measure power and velocity, during swimming. *(a)* The suspended weight method. *(b)* The use of an isokinetic system enables the measurement of power developed by the swimmer in the water. Connecting the wire device suitable for velocity measurement will provide information of changes in speed. *(c)* The swimming flume.

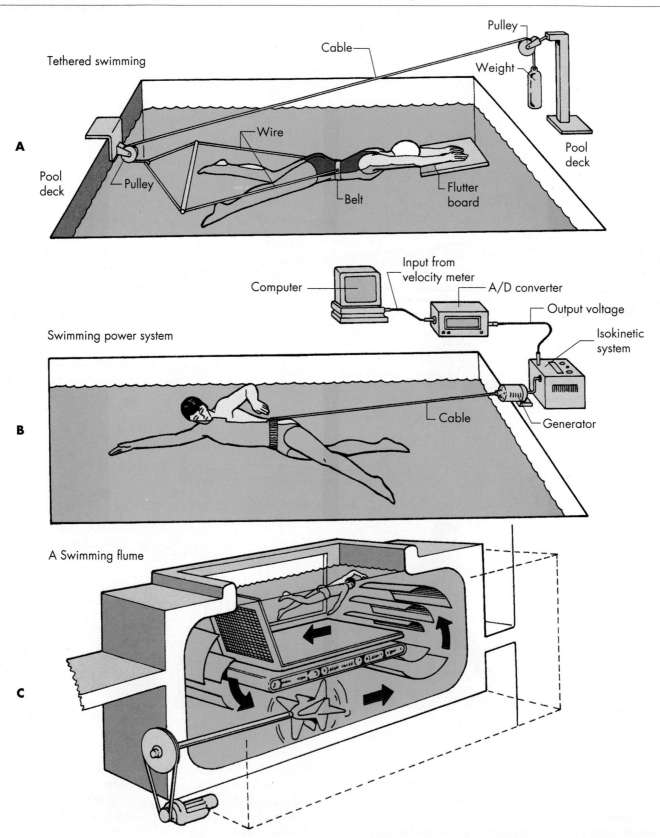

Another swimming method more suitable for ergometry is the swimming power test developed by David Costill (8) (fig. 4.4*b*). A belt is placed around the waist of a swimmer and to the belt is attached a wire, which in turn is connected to a modified isokinetic device. The swimmer then swims as hard as possible. The isokinetic device maintains a constant velocity and the strain exerted on the wire is measured as a force. This test provides data of maximal power generation during swimming, and has been used to correlate swimming power and performance in competitive swimmers, as well as monitor the effects of training programs and skill coaching for in-water power development. Similar systems have been developed for assessing velocity changes during the varied propulsive phases of the different strokes (9, 10).

Swimming research can also be conducted with a flume (fig. 4.4*c*). A swimming flume is a small swimming pool, fitted with electronically controlled water circulation devices that generate known water velocities within the pool. A swimmer must swim against the water velocity to maintain her or his position in the flume, thereby swimming at a known speed. Indirect calorimetry procedures can be performed with the swimmer in the water and swimming at various velocities. Research of this description has determined the variation in energy cost of different swimming strokes, and differences between individuals with differing swimming techniques for a given stroke (11). Obviously swimming flumes and the ability to measure the effectiveness of different stroke technique changes are important for the improvement in swimming technique for both the elite and recreational swimmer. For these and other reasons, a swimming flume exists at the International Center for Aquatics Research, located at the U.S. Olympic Training Center in Colorado Springs, and a flume also exists at the Institute for Exercise and Environmental Medicine in Dallas. Many European countries also have swimming flumes that are used for advances in the swimming techniques of their elite athletes.

Calorimetry

Many chemical reactions occur to support our body's basic needs for function and survival. The sum of all these reactions is referred to as *metabolism*. Recalling the first law of thermodynamics from chapter 2, energy is neither created nor destroyed, but simply changes form. The forms and products of changes in energy that concern our bodies are heat, light, chemical energy and work, mechanical work, and entropy. It is difficult to measure and quantify changes in entropy, light, and the chemical energy of the body. However, mechanical work can be measured as previously described in the section on ergometry and, as will be explained, changes in heat are suited to measurement and the calculation of energy expenditure in both animals and humans.

Another important meaning of the first law of thermodynamics is that energy release from the combustion of chemicals is a constant. The quantity of heat release, free energy, and entropy from the breakdown of glucose to water and carbon dioxide is the same regardless of how the breakdown occurs. For example, the catabolism of glucose will yield 648 kcal/mol (3.72 kcal/g) of energy if the catabolism occurs via the numerous reactions of the body, or if the glucose molecule was combusted in a flame (16, 19). For palmitate, the body's predominant free fatty acid molecule, the heat release from its complete catabolism or combustion amounts to 2340 kcal/mol (9.3 kcal/g) (16, 19). As heat is a major biproduct of the chemical reactions in the body, *the heat production from reactions is proportional to the number or rate of the reactions*. Similarly, the measurement of the heat generated by the body would be a reflection of the rate of body metabolism.

The science that quantifies the heat release from metabolism is termed **calorimetry** (fig. 4.5). Calorimetric methods that involve the direct measurement of heat dissipation from the body are termed *direct calorimetry* (4, 23). When heat dissipation is calculated from other measurements, these methods are termed *indirect calorimetry*. Indirect calorimetry can also be subdivided into *open-* and *closed-circuit* systems. Closed-circuit indirect calorimetry involves the recirculation of inhaled and exhaled air, thus necessitating the removal of carbon dioxide and the replenishment of oxygen. Open-circuit indirect calorimetry can involve the inhalation of atmospheric air and the sampling and measurement of exhaled air for respiratory gas analysis. Other forms of indirect open-circuit calorimetry exist, such as measuring total carbon and nitrogen exchange and measuring the exchange of labeled water within the body (29).

Calorimetry Has a Long History

Calorimetry is an old science that dates back to the eighteenth century. However, it was not until the formulation of

---

FIGURE 4.5

The divisions of calorimetry.

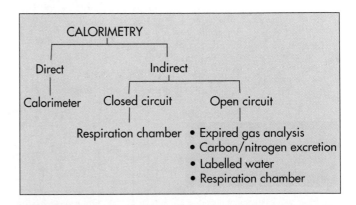

calorimetry (kal′o-ri-met′ri) the measurement of body metabolism from heat release from the body

the first law of thermodynamics in 1842 that scientists focused more directly on quantifying the total heat release from metabolism. As early as 1849 the first closed-circuit respirometer was built and used in animal research to measure the changes in oxygen consumption and carbon dioxide production resulting from different diets (22).

In 1860 Bischoff and Voit completed calculations on the caloric and respiratory gas exchange involved in the combustion of certain foods and pure nutrients. The **calorimeter** used to combust food was called a bomb calorimeter. Bomb calorimetry was an important advancement to understanding the energy value of foods. A typical bomb calorimeter is illustrated in figure 4.6. When a food source was ignited in an oxygen-rich environment, the heat release was measured via the increase in temperature of circulating water, and measurements of oxygen consumption and carbon dioxide were also made. Consequently, if a given quantity of pure carbohydrate, fat, or protein is combusted, given amounts of oxygen consumption, carbon dioxide production, and heat re-

lease can be measured. These values are listed in table 4.2. Researchers knew that the products of carbohydrate and fat catabolism were similar for the body and combustion; however, for nitrogen catabolism the products of metabolism were different from combustion. Catabolism of protein in the body yielded carbon dioxide, water, urea, nitrogen waste in feces, and additional carbon compounds in urine and feces (e.g., creatinine). Consequently, the excreted nitrogen and carbon compounds accompanying protein metabolism represented a loss in potential heat release, which needed to be subtracted from known bomb calorimetry caloric equivalents for protein.

Rubner determined the caloric value of protein combustion in a bomb calorimeter, measured the energy release of dried urine and feces, and calculated the difference in energy release from protein between bomb calorimetry and metabolism. In 1901, Rubner published caloric equivalent values for different types of carbohydrate, fat, and protein molecules that are metabolized in the body (table 4.2) (22).

FIGURE 4.6

A typical bomb calorimeter. The calorimeter consists of a heavy insulated metal shell, a capsule for the sample to be combusted, a water bath pressurized with at least 20 atmospheres of oxygen, a thermometer to measure water temperature, and an electric fuse to ignite the food sample. The number of calories used to combust the food is determined by the increase in water temperature. Analyzing the air for decreases in oxygen and increases in carbon dioxide, enable calculations of oxygen consumption and carbon dioxide production.

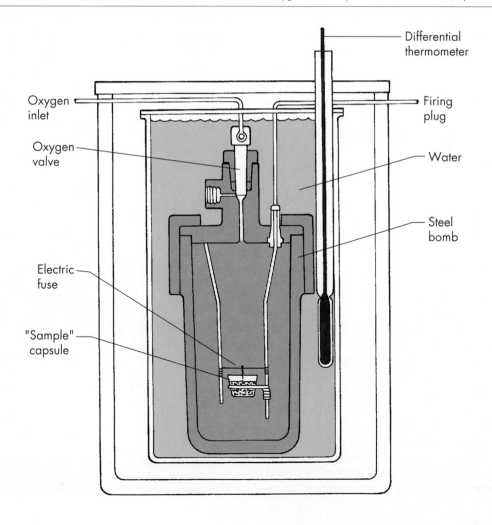

TABLE 4.2

The heat release[†] and caloric equivalents for oxygen[†] for the main macronutrients of catabolism

FOOD	RUBNER'S kcal/g	kcal/g BOMB CALORIMETER	kcal/g* BODY	RQ	kcal/L O_2
Mixed carbohydrate	4.1	4.1	4.0	1.0	5.05
Glycogen		4.2		1.0	5.05
Glucose		3.7		1.0	4.98
Fructose		3.7		1.0	5.00
Glycerol		4.3		0.86	5.06
Mixed fat	9.3	9.3	8.9	0.70	4.73
Palmitate (C 16:0)		9.3		0.70	4.65
Stearate (C 18:0)		9.5		0.69	4.65
Triacylglycerol (C 18:0)		9.6		0.70	4.67
Medium chain length triacylglycerols		8.4		0.74	4.69
Mixed protein	4.1	5.7	4.3	0.81	4.46
Alanine		4.4		0.83	4.62
Aspartate		2.69		1.17	4.60
Glutamate		3.58		1.0	4.58
Isoleucine		6.89		0.73	4.64
Alcohol		7.1	7.0	0.82	4.86
Mixed diet				0.84	4.83

*The lower values for the caloric release during combustion in the body compared to the bomb calorimeter are due to relative inefficiencies of digestion. The respective adjustments for carbohydrate, fat, and protein for the inefficiency of digestion are –2%, –5%, and –25% (–8% digestion and –17% loss in urine) (13).

[†]Data are compiled from Lusk (22), Livesey and Elia (19), Bursztein et al. (4), and Fox et al. (14).

Assuming percentage contributions of these molecules to total metabolism, Rubner deduced that the appropriate average values to use for each of carbohydrate, fat, and protein were 4.1, 9.3, and 4.1 kcal/g, respectively. Rubner's findings were replicated in human subjects by Atwater and Benedict in 1904 with a more sophisticated closed-circuit respiration calorimeter (1, 22) (fig. 4.7). It is ironic that Atwater, an American, has received historical recognition for these values when the pioneering original work was published by Rubner, a German, before the experiments of Atwater and Benedict had begun!

Lusk (22) removed the caloric release, oxygen consumption and carbon dioxide production due to basal protein catabolism from total body metabolism. The remainder of oxygen consumption, carbon dioxide production and heat release was then attributable to carbohydrate and fat metabolism (table 4.3). As carbohydrate and lipid catabolism differs in oxygen consumption and carbon dioxide production, the ratio of the volume of carbon dioxide production and oxygen consumption [**respiratory quotient (RQ)**] was used to indicate the predominance of carbohydrate or fat as the substrate for catabolism. Because of the subtraction of protein from this data set, it is often referred to as *nonprotein* data.

As early as 1866, Pettenkofer and Voit demonstrated that moderate amounts of exercise did not increase protein me-

tabolism, and therefore that increased energy was provided by the metabolism of carbohydrate and fat (22). These findings were supported by more elaborate research by Atwater in 1904 (1). However, research had also been completed that contradicted these findings. Campbell and Webster (5) reported that a man who expended 100,000 kgm of work on a cycle ergometer increased urinary nitrogen from 8.01 g/day to 10.25 g/day. Additional research involving more intense and shorter duration exercise also indicated an increase in protein catabolism (22). Ironically, the implications of these early findings were shadowed by the many studies in humans and animals that verified the predominance of carbohydrate and fat catabolism during exercise (22). As will be explained in chapter 6, the topic of an increase in protein catabolism during exercise was reevaluated in the 1970s, and through the use of more sophisticated techniques proved that prolonged exercise can increase protein catabolism. Nevertheless, the nonprotein RQ and caloric equivalents are still

calorimeter (kal′o-rim′eter) an instrument that measures heat release from the body

respiratory quotient the ratio of carbon dioxide production to oxygen consumption during metabolism

FIGURE 4.7

An illustration of the Atwater-Benedict respiration calorimeter, which was developed during the early 1900s. The walls of the chamber are insulated. Direct calorimetry measurements were made from the chamber from the simple measurement of the change in temperature of water as it was circulated though the chamber. Indirect calorimetry measurements were made from the circulation of air through the chamber, requiring oxygen replenishment to replace that used, and the removal of the carbon dioxide produced by soda lime. Carbon dioxide production was then measured chemically by the change in the weight and composition of the soda lime per unit time.

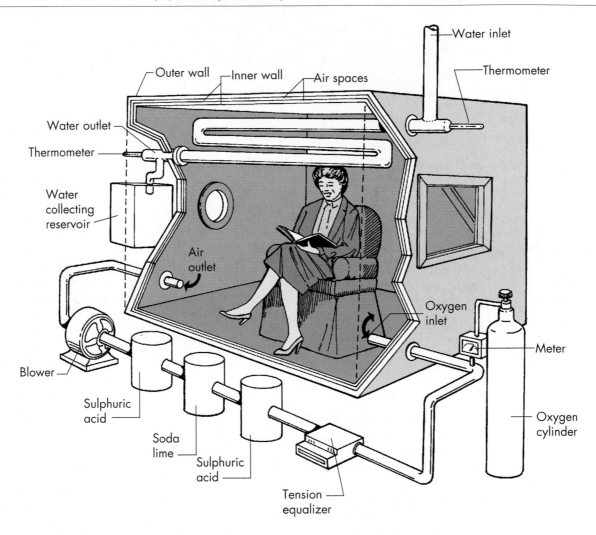

used today for computing caloric expenditure during many, but not all, rest and exercise conditions.

The validation of indirect (using oxygen consumption and carbon dioxide production [respiration]) methods of calorimetry enabled application of indirect open-circuit gas analysis calorimetry to varied metabolic conditions. Researchers measured basal energy requirements under different environmental conditions and established the relationships among metabolic rate and body temperature, body surface area, and the intensity of exercise (5, 6, 21, 22). Interestingly, research done as early as 1910 demonstrated the superiority of carbohydrate as the main dietary component to fuel the muscles during exercise (22).

The recent history of calorimetry witnessed the development of more sophisticated instrumentation and alternative methods of both direct and indirect calorimetry. For indirect

calorimetry, expired gas collection bags (Douglas bags), portable gas collection and analysis units, improved electronic gas volume and gas analyzer instrumentation, and computerization of data collection have enabled greater use of this technique during varied conditions (fig. 4.8*a, b,* and *c,* respectively). Direct calorimeters are currently used in many metabolic and nutrition divisions of hospitals to research metabolic abnormalities in patients, and the validation of alternative indirect methods such as doubly labeled body water have enabled research of long-term metabolism without the expense and confinement of large direct calorimeters. Nevertheless, the science of direct and indirect calorimetry still relies on the classic work by researchers such as Rubner, Voit, and Atwater. This fact is testament to the quality of work completed by these pioneering researchers when the equipment and techniques they used

TABLE 4.3

The caloric equivalents for the range of nonprotein respiratory quotient (RQ) values; caloric values from each of carbohydrate and fat are also listed for each RQ value

RQ	kcal/L O_2	% CHO*	kcal/L O_2 CHO	% FAT	kcal/L O_2 FAT
1.00	5.047	100.00	5.047	0.0	0.000
0.99	5.035	96.80	4.874	3.18	0.160
0.98	5.022	93.60	4.701	6.37	0.230
0.97	5.010	90.40	4.529	9.58	0.480
0.96	4.998	87.20	4.358	12.80	0.640
0.95	4.985	84.00	4.187	16.00	0.798
0.94	4.973	80.70	4.013	19.30	0.960
0.93	4.961	77.40	3.840	22.60	1.121
0.92	4.948	74.10	3.666	25.90	1.281
0.91	4.936	70.80	3.495	29.20	1.441
0.90	4.924	67.50	3.324	32.50	1.600
0.89	4.911	64.20	3.153	35.80	1.758
0.88	4.899	60.80	2.979	39.20	1.920
0.87	4.887	57.50	2.810	42.50	2.077
0.86	4.875	54.10	2.637	45.90	2.238
0.85	4.862	50.70	2.465	49.30	2.397
0.84	4.850	47.20	2.289	52.80	2.561
0.83	4.838	43.80	2.119	56.20	2.719
0.82	4.825	40.30	1.944	59.70	2.880
0.81	4.813	36.90	1.776	63.10	3.037
0.80	4.801	33.40	1.603	66.60	3.197
0.79	4.788	29.90	1.432	70.10	3.356
0.78	4.776	26.30	1.256	73.70	3.520
0.77	4.764	22.30	1.062	77.20	3.678
0.76	4.751	19.20	0.912	80.80	3.839
0.75	4.739	15.60	0.739	84.40	4.000
0.74	4.727	12.00	0.567	88.00	4.160
0.73	4.714	8.40	0.396	91.60	4.318
0.72	4.702	4.76	0.224	95.20	4.476
0.71	4.690	1.10	0.052	98.90	4.638
0.707	4.686	0.0	0.000	100.00	4.686

*To convert kcal to kJ, multiple by 4.186.

Source: Based on data from Lusk (22).

were more labor intensive, tedious, and open to more potential error than that of today's scientific equipment and methodology.

Direct Calorimetry

The previous description of the historical development of calorimetry revealed that the direct calorimeter was the first tool used to measure caloric expenditure in animals and humans. As can be appreciated by the previous discussion, direct calorimeters are expensive pieces of equipment. In ad-

dition, they are more suited to measuring basal metabolic demands than those of exercise for several reasons:

1. Exercise performed in a direct calorimeter causes added heat production from friction developed by the ergometer and the subject.
2. During exercise the body stores heat as evidenced by the rise in core temperature.
3. The method is not suited to providing data in small time intervals, which is necessary to measure the rapidity of the changes in metabolic rate during changes in exercise intensity.

Today direct calorimetry is used to study basal metabolic rate, daily energy expenditure, and the influence of altered environmental or physiological conditions on these parameters. For example, use of direct calorimeters that are large enough to allow people to live inside for several days have been used to determine the factors that influence basal and daily metabolic rate (2).

Indirect Calorimetry

The fact that a known amount of oxygen is required to combust gram equivalents of carbohydrate, fat, and protein is extremely important. If one could measure oxygen consumption, and have a means to quantify the proportion of carbohydrate, fat, or protein used during metabolism, one could then simply calculate heat release (caloric expenditure). The most common procedure used to do this is referred to as *indirect gas analysis calorimetry*. Indirect gas analysis calorimetry can be performed via an open- or closed-circuit system.

Open-Circuit Indirect Calorimetry
Although the mathematical calculations of open-circuit indirect calorimetry have remained unchanged since the respiration calorimetry work of Rubner and Atwater, the equipment that was originally used differs considerably from the computerized systems that exist today. The principles, equations, and assumptions of indirect calorimetry are presented in focus box 4.1.

When concerned with exercise, the predominant application of indirect calorimetry is for the measurement of oxygen consumption, and therefore an assessment of the metabolic intensity of exercise. Also, the ratio between carbon dioxide production and oxygen consumption is used to indicate the contribution of fat and carbohydrate substrates to energy production. However, as will be discussed in the section on energy production, there are several factors that can invalidate the accurate use of indirect calorimetric calculations for determining the contribution of fat and carbohydrate to energy production.

Respiratory Quotient and the Respiratory Exchange Ratio
The ratio between carbon dioxide production and oxygen consumption is traditionally called the *respiratory quotient*

FIGURE 4.8

Common methods used to collect and sample expired gases during indirect gas analysis calorimetry. *(a)* The use of a Douglas bags, gas analyzers, and a gas flow meter to obtain measurements required in calorimetry. The air collected in the Douglas bag is saturated with water vapor and at room temperature. A small volume of this collected air is pumped through gas analyzers to determine the fraction of oxygen and carbon dioxide. The volume of collected air is then measured via a flow meter. The expired volume must be converted to standard conditions before being used in the calculations of Box 6.1 (see Appendix B). *(b)* A simple, portable, time averaged system for indirect calorimetry. Expired gas flow is measured via a pneumotach, expired air is sampled from a mixing bag and pumped to oxygen and carbon dioxide electronic analyzers, and data is acquired, processed, and calculations completed by a computer. *(c)* An advanced breath-by-breath system. Rapidly responding analyzers and powerful computerization enable calculations to be made every breath.

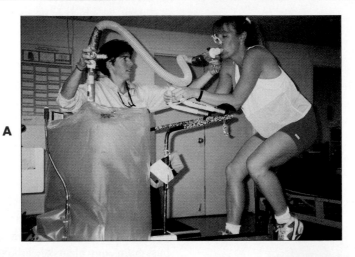

A

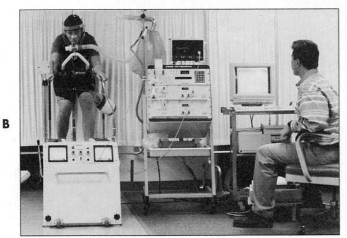

B

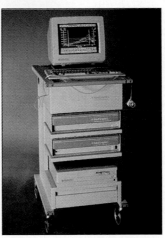

C

(RQ). This measure is calculated the same as the **respiratory exchange ratio (RER)**; however, the conditions of production of carbon dioxide differ. The RQ is used to indicate cellular respiration, and therefore the VO_2 and VCO_2 resulting from the catabolism of food. The RER is used when VO_2 and VCO_2 are measured from ventilated air resulting from external respiration at the lung. When sampling air from the lung, the ratio of VCO_2/VO_2 can be modified by increased exhalation of CO_2 that is unrelated to the cellular production of CO_2 from the catabolic pathways of carbohydrate, fat, or protein. *When gas volumes are calculated or measured that relate solely to cellular respiration, the term RQ should be used. When gas volumes are measured that can be influenced by additional sources of CO_2 production,*

the term RER should be used. These rules will be adhered to in this text.

4.4 $$RER = VCO_2 / VO_2$$

The energy released from catabolism for every liter of oxygen consumed at different nonprotein RQ values is listed in table 4.3. The RQ values theoretically reflect carbohydrate and lipid catabolism, with an RQ value of 1.0 reflecting pure carbohydrate catabolism, and an RQ value of 0.71 reflecting pure lipid catabolism.

The RQ is important because when carbon dioxide production is occurring only from cellular metabolism, and assuming that no change in protein (amino acid) catabolism

FOCUS BOX 4.1

The Principles, Equations, and Assumptions of Indirect Gas Analysis Calorimetry

The Principles

The fundamental principle of indirect calorimetry is that the volume of oxygen consumed by the body equals the difference between the volumes of inspired and expired oxygen.

4.5
$$VO_2 = V_IO_2 - V_EO_2$$

Each of the variables V_IO_2 and V_EO_2 can be further partitioned, with equation (4.5) expressed differently as,

4.6
$$VO_2 = (V_IF_IO_2) - (V_EF_EO_2)$$

where F_IO_2 = fraction of oxygen in inspired air

F_EO_2 = fraction of oxygen in expired air

To solve for the dilemma of needing to measure both inspired and expired volumes of air, and because nitrogen is physiologically inert and, therefore, on average inspired nitrogen must equal expired nitrogen, use equation (4.6) to solve for V_I.

4.7
$$V_IN_2 = V_EN_2$$

4.8
$$\text{and } V_IF_IN_2 = V_EF_EN_2$$

4.9
$$\text{thus,} V_I = (V_EF_EN_2) / F_IN_2$$

4.10
$$V_I = V_E (F_EN_2 / F_IN_2)$$

The gas fractions in atmospheric air are as follows:

GAS	FRACTION
Oxygen	0.2093
Nitrogen	0.7903
Carbon dioxide	0.0003
Argon and helium, etc.	0.0001
Total	**1.0000**

If one neglects the rare gas component of air, the F_EN_2 can be rewritten as $[1 - (F_ECO_2 + F_EO_2)]$, and equation (4.10) can be rewritten as,

4.11
$$V_I = V_E \times \frac{[1 - (F_ECO_2 + F_EO_2)]}{0.7903}$$

Equating V_I and V_E by assuming that inspired nitrogen equals expired nitrogen is called the **Haldane transformation** (20). Although data also exist to refute its accuracy (9, 15), replicated studies have been performed that have documented the similarity of inspired and expired nitrogen volumes (20, 26, 28). Consequently, the Haldane transformation, and resulting indirect calorimetry equations for calculating oxygen consumption, carbon dioxide production, and energy expenditure are widely accepted by educators and scientists.

Incorporating equation (4.11) into equation (4.6) provides the final equation to calculate oxygen consumption:

4.12
$$VO_2 = (V_E \times \frac{[1 - (F_ECO_2 + F_EO_2)]}{0.7903} \times F_IO_2) - (V_E \times F_EO_2)$$

Carbon Dioxide Production

Carbon dioxide production is equal to the carbon dioxide expired minus the carbon dioxide inspired:

4.13
$$VCO_2 = (V_EF_ECO_2) - (V_IF_ICO_2)$$

Solving for this equation is relatively easy compared to calculating oxygen consumption. Assuming that oxygen consumption is calculated first, V_I is then already calculated, and all that is needed is to incorporate V_I, V_E (measured), F_ICO_2 (0.0003), and F_ECO_2 (measured) into equation (4.13). Because of the small value for F_ICO_2, a ventilation even as large as 150 L/min would yield only a value of 0.045 L/min for inspired carbon dioxide. Consequently, seemingly accurate values can be obtained by simply equating VCO_2 and $V_EF_ECO_2$. Nevertheless, it is recommended that the student complete the calculation with equation (4.13) to uphold the principle of the measurement.

occurs during exercise, the RQ value can be used to accurately reflect the proportion of fat and carbohydrate catabolized for energy during exercise. The caloric equivalent for a given RQ can then be used to calculate energy expenditure during exercise.

For many metabolic and exercise conditions, the RER is often assumed to be equal to the RQ, and is then used to calculate contributions of either fat and carbohydrate to catabolism and caloric expenditure. However, the assumption of equality between RQ and RER cannot be made under certain conditions. These conditions and their interpretations are:

1. *Metabolic acidosis:* Within the cell the production of carbon dioxide cannot exceed the consumption of oxygen, and the maximal value of 1.0 for VCO_2/VO_2 occurs from

Haldane transformation the use of equal inspired and expired nitrogen volumes to solve for either inspired or expired ventilatory volumes

respiratory exchange ratio the ratio of carbon dioxide production to oxygen consumption, as measured from expired gas analysis indirect calorimetry

the metabolism of pure carbohydrate. During metabolic conditions that increase acid production (intense exercise, ketosis, etc.), the added carbon dioxide produced from the buffering of acid in the body increases VCO_2 independently of oxygen consumption (VO_2), and therefore RER values can exceed 1.0. Consequently, during exercise the RER value can also be used as an indirect measure of exercise intensity. During exercise, if the RER increases to above 1.0, it can be concluded that acid production is increasing (presumably associated with increased lactate production). If the RER continues to increase above 1.0 during exercise, then fatigue will be eminent unless the exercise intensity is decreased.

Basal conditions of acidosis, such as during ketosis, would raise the RER and cause an incorrect assumption of an increased contribution of carbohydrate to catabolism.

2. *Non-steady-state conditions:* When a person has increased his or her exercise intensity, it takes time for the VO_2 to increase to a level that accounts for the ATP produced during metabolism. During these times, the ATP is produced from alternative sources, namely from creatine phosphate hydrolysis and glycolysis. Calculating VO_2 during non-steady-state conditions would give a lower metabolic intensity than if the person was at steady state. In addition, a higher RER may be calculated, and together these values would yield incorrect calculations of energy expenditure and the contribution of fat and carbohydrate to steady-state catabolism. If the exercise intensity is not too high, between three to five min are required for the attainment of steady state.

3. *Hyperventilation:* Excessive exhalation will increase the volume of carbon dioxide exhaled from the lung. If this phenomenon occurred without similar increases in VO_2, a higher VCO_2 would result from indirect gas analysis calorimetry, yielding an inflated RER value.

4. *Excess postexercise VO_2:* After exercise, VO_2 declines but remains above preexercise values for several minutes, whereas VCO_2 decreases rapidly. Consequently, the RER may decline below resting values for several minutes.

5. *Prolonged exercise:* The longer the exercise duration, the greater the contribution of amino acid catabolism to energy metabolism. For durations of exercise exceeding 90 min, especially when muscle and liver glycogen stores become low, estimations of fat and carbohydrate contributions to metabolism using the nonprotein RER data become more and more inaccurate. During these conditions, researchers typically measure or estimate the amino acid oxidation and correct the nonprotein RER data (25).

The aforementioned circumstances that can alter RER values must be understood when performing research or interpreting exercise responses. These circumstances could cause error in calculations of the contribution of food stuffs to catabolism, as will be explained in the calculations of energy expenditure.

Energy Expenditure The calculation of energy expenditure using the nonprotein data of Lusk (table 4.3) is a simple process, involving the multiplication of oxygen consumption (L/min), time (min), and the caloric equivalent for the respective RER of the exercise (kcal/L O_2).

4.14 $$kcal = VO_2 \text{ (L/min)} \times RER \text{ caloric equivalent (kcal/L)} \times time \text{ (min)}$$

For example, when performing exercise for 30 min requiring a VO_2 of 1.5 L/min, with an average RER of 0.9, caloric expenditure can be calculated as,

$$kcal = 1.5 \times 4.924 \times 30$$
$$= 221.6$$

Based on Table 4.3, the contribution of fat and carbohydrate to the energy expenditure can be calculated. For example, from the previous calculation of VO_2, RER, and kcal,

% kcal from fat $= [(1 - RQ)/(1 - 0.7)] \times 100$

% kcal from carbohydrate (CHO) $= 100 - (\% \text{ kcal from fat})$

With a reported RQ $= 0.9$, 33.3% of the kcal are derived from fat and 66.7% of the kcals are derived from carbohydrates:

kcals from fat $= 0.33 \times (221.6 \text{ kcal}/30 \text{ min})$
$= 2.46 \text{ kcal/min}$

kcals from CHO $= 0.667 \times (221.6 \text{ kcal}/30 \text{ min})$
$= 4.93 \text{ kcal/min}$

Assume caloric densities of 4 kcal/g for CHO and 9 kcal/g for fat:

Fat usage $= (2.46 \text{ kcal/min}) / (9 \text{ kcal/g})$
$= 0.27 \text{ g fat/min}$

CHO usage $= (4.93 \text{ kcal/min}) / (4 \text{ kcal/g})$
$= 1.23 \text{ g CHO/min}$

If dietary, disease, or exercise conditions exist that are accompanied by increased protein catabolism, calculations of energy expenditure using the nonprotein RER data of Lusk may be inaccurate. However, even as early as the 1920s it was understood that the error inherent in increased protein catabolism was negligible. For example, a 10% increase in urinary nitrogen with an RER of 0.9 would lower the caloric equivalent for oxygen from 4.925 to 4.90 kcal/L O_2, resulting in a 1% error in caloric expenditure for a VO_2 of 2.0 L/min. Recent nutrition research by Livesey and Elia (19) has supported this fact.

However, although the errors are negligible when computing caloric expenditure during conditions of increased protein catabolism, approximating contributions of fat or carbohydrate to energy expenditure can have errors as large as $\pm 60\%$ under these conditions (19). Metabolic conditions that would increase protein catabolism are starvation, diabetes mellitus, prolonged exercise during restricted carbohydrate nutrition, and excess protein ingestion.

Table 4.2 presents known heat release and caloric equivalents for the combustion of certain carbohydrates, fats, and amino acids. The caloric release during food combustion has high variability within and between food categories, and high variability also exists for the measures of RQ and kcal/L O_2. The lower values for the caloric release during combustion in the body compared to the bomb calorimeter are due to relative inefficiencies of digestion. The respective adjustments for carbohydrate, fat, and protein for the inefficiency of digestion are –2%, –5%, and –25% (–8% digestion and –17% loss in urine) (13).

Systems Used in Indirect Calorimetry

Within the last 20 years the sophistication of the equipment used in indirect calorimetry has increased remarkably. Today, data is obtained, processed, and calculated within seconds, enabling the monitoring of changes during very small time intervals. Ventilation measurement is now performed by advanced electronics less than one-tenth the size of the original volume meters, and the response time of the electronic analyzers for oxygen and carbon dioxide are now as short as 100 ms. When these improvements are combined with computer software and hardware advances that enable the handling of computer bits of information at high rates, the automation of indirect calorimetry data collection is now a common feature of many advanced research and clinical exercise testing laboratories.

Time-Averaged and Breath-by-Breath Calculations of Oxygen Consumption Today's computerized sophistication with indirect calorimetry has enabled the production of several different systems (15). The basic designs of computerized indirect calorimetry systems are illustrated in figure 4.9. For the time-averaged system (fig. 4.9*a*), the subject breathes room air through a volume measuring device; expired air flows into a mixing chamber. Air from the mixing chamber is continuously pumped to and through separate oxygen and carbon dioxide analyzers. Electrical signals from the volume measurement and gas analyzers are diverted to a computer where they are first converted from electrical current (analog) to digital signal via an analog-to-digital (A-D) converter. For example, for ventilation and gas fraction measurement, electronic accessory equipment is connected to the equipment so that a change in the measurement condition of the instrument exerts a proportional change in electrical voltage output. This voltage change is converted to computer language by the A-D converter (4, 27).

Time-average systems are able to calculate indirect calorimetry values such as VO_2, VCO_2, RER, caloric expenditure, and other respiratory parameters in intervals of time restricted by software and hardware capacities. For example, if the ventilation meter and gas analyzers have slow re-

sponse times, and the computer processor has small memory and slow processing speed, data may be calculated in intervals of 15 or 30 s.

Indirect calorimetry systems exist that have rapidly responding analyzers and advanced computerization that enable the calculation of parameters with every breath. These systems are appropriately called breath-by-breath systems (fig. 4.9*b*). The circuitry of a breath-by-breath system is a little different from that of time-averaged systems. Expired air is sampled close to the mouth, avoiding the need for a mixing chamber, and ventilation is measured by sophisticated devices such as a pneumotach or a low-mass impeller, rather than the traditional volume meter.

Economy and Efficiency of Human Movement

The words economy and efficiency are often used synonymously when describing exercise conditions. This is incorrect because these terms pertain to very different conditions of the body. **Economy** of movement refers to *the energy cost of that movement* (3, 12). **Efficiency** of movement refers to *the mechanical energy produced during the movement relative to the metabolic energy used to cause the movement.*

Economy of movement is best exemplified during running, and in this context has been termed *running economy* (12, 24). Another term used to describe this energy demand is *submaximal oxygen consumption* (3). Figure 4.10 presents data for two different individuals running on a treadmill. Subject A has better running economy; for a given running speed subject A consumes less oxygen relative to body weight than subject B. Researchers have explained differences in running economy by different running techniques (biomechanics) (24).

The concept of efficiency, and some difficulties inherent in calculating efficiency, are best illustrated using subjects A and B of figure 4.10 as an example. These two runners have differing submaximal oxygen consumptions (differing economy), and the increase in VO_2 for a given intensity is also different between the two individuals. To compute the efficiency of movement for an individual, the change in energy output during ergometry is expressed relative to the change in the chemical energy used during the movement. In this instance, subject B requires a smaller increase in VO_2 for a given increase in intensity. If all else is equal (i.e., mechanics), this would mean that subject B is more efficient.

4.15   Efficiency = Δ energy generation / Δ energy of metabolism

economy the concept pertaining to the oxygen consumption required to perform a given task

efficiency when applied to exercise, the ratio (expressed as percentage) between the mechanical energy produced during exercise to the energy cost of the exercise

FIGURE 4.9

Schematics of time averaged and breath-by-breath indirect calorimetry systems. *(a)* A typical time averaged system. Ventilation is measured on the inspired side via a large capacity low resistance flow meter. Expired air is directed to a mixing chamber, from which air is pumped to electronic oxygen and carbon dioxide analyzers. The flow meter and analyzers are electronically connected to an analog to digital (A-D) converter, and digital signals are received by a computer which runs software enabling the calculations of indirect calorimetry to be made, and printed or displayed on a screen. *(b)* The breath-by-breath system is configured differently. Expired air samples are obtained from tubing connected to the mouthpiece, and are pumped to rapidly responding analyzers. Expired air flow rate is measured by a pneumotach, or a low resistance impeller, with the exhaust air returned to the room. Electronic connections to a powerful high capacity computer enables calculations to be performed, and the display of data on the screen in tabular or graphical form while the test is conducted.

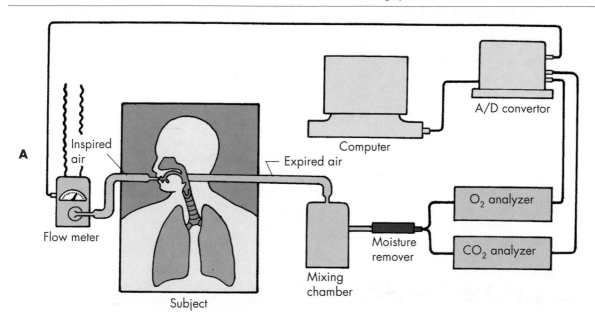

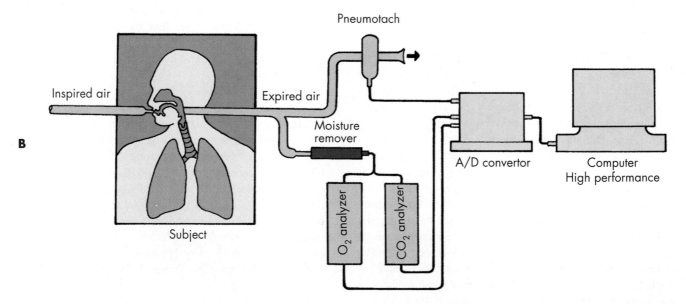

However, this definition poses problems when trying to compute efficiency of running. As previously described, the calculation of mechanical work during level treadmill walking or running requires a modification in how the treadmill is used. Suitable modifications are running or walking up a grade and measuring the horizontal force applied by the subject to a strain gauge or the vertical force from a suspended weight attached to the subject. Unless either of these modifi-

cations are accomplished, the term "efficiency" has little meaning to level running, walking, or cross-country skiing.

For a change in exercise intensity during cycle ergometry from 100 to 250 W, a subject increases energy generation each minute from 1.4333 kcal to 3.5832 kcal. If the subject's steady-state VO_2 during the two cycle intensities was 1.6 L/min and 3.1 L/min, respectively, with an RER of 0.83, then efficiency can be calculated as,

Efficiency = Δ mechanical energy production / Δ metabolic
              energy cost

4.16

= 3.5832 − 1.4333 kcal/min / 14.9978 − 7.7408 kcal

= 2.1499 kcal/min / 7.2570 kcal/min

= 8.9995 kJ/min / 30.3778 kJ/min

= 0.2962

= 29.62%

Generally, efficiency during exercise is very similar between individuals because of the constant efficiency of our metabolic pathways. For example, the standard free energy change of glycolysis is equal to –47.0 kcal/mol glucose, and the production of two ATP in muscle from glucose during glycolysis, for standard conditions, is equal to –14.6 kcal/mol glucose. The ratio of the two is equal to 0.361, or 36%. This value is slightly higher than the normal range of total body efficiency during exercise of 25 to 30% (13)

FIGURE 4.10

The change in oxygen consumption (VO_2) for two subjects when running at different velocities on a level treadmill.

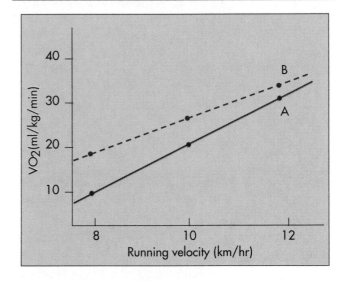

WEBSITE BOX

Chapter 4: Ergonometry and Calorimetry

The newest information regarding exercise physiology can be viewed at the following sites.*

af.mil/news/may1996/n19960520_960473.html
    Brooks Airforce Base descriptions of how they use cycle ergometry in fitness testing.
lode.nl/medical/indexprod.html
    Ergometer products from Lode medical instruments, The Netherlands.
http://131.84.1.31/news/Jul1998/n19980702_980979.html
    Article on how the U.S. Air Force uses a cycle ergometry protocol to assess cardiorespiratory fitness.

vertimax.com/
    Commercial site that presents a novel method for quantifying muscle jumping power, and training for an explosive vertical jump.
nau.edu/~hp/proj/rah/courses/exs337/outlines/ergo/.html
    Lecture notes on ergometry from Northern Arizona University.

_____

*Unless indicated, all URLs preceded by http://www.

Note: These URLs were valid at the time of publication, but could have changed or been deleted from Internet access since that time.

SUMMARY

▪ The science of **ergometry** concerns the measurement of work. A device that can be used to measure work is called an **ergometer**. Examples of ergometers used for exercise and research are the bench step, cycle, treadmill, and rowing apparatus.

▪ Ergometry enables the calculation of **work**, **power**, and external energy production during exercise. The general components of these calculations are a resistance or load, a distance the load is moved against gravity and over time, and the duration (repetition) of the movement. The preferred unit to express energy is the kJ, which equals 4.1868 kcal. Power is expressed as kJ/min, where 1 kJ/min equals 16.667 W.

▪ The direct measurement of heat dissipation is termed direct **calorimetry**. When heat dissipation is calculated from other measurements, these methods are termed indirect calorimetry. Indirect calorimetry can also be subdivided into open- and closed-circuit systems.

▪ The direct **calorimeter** was the first tool used to measure caloric expenditure in animals and humans. With the validation of indirect calorimetry, and therefore less expensive methods of calorimetry, attention turned away from direct methods.

▪ The most common method of indirect calorimetry involves the collection and measurement of expired gas, allowing the computation of oxygen consumption (VO_2)

SUMMARY

and carbon dioxide production (VCO_2). The ratio of VCO_2 to VO_2 is termed the **respiratory quotient (RQ),** and when measured under conditions of ventilatory gas exchange is termed the **respiratory exchange ratio (RER)**. These calculations are based on the **Haldane transformation** which is derived from the fact that nitrogen is physiologically inert.

▪ The following conditions will alter VCO_2 disproportionately to VO_2 and invalidate use of RER values for use in

energy expenditure calculations: metabolic acidosis, non-steady-state exercise conditions, hyperventilation, excess postexercise VO_2, and prolonged exercise in excess of 90 min during low-carbohydrate conditions.

▪ **Economy** of movement refers to the energy cost of that movement. **Efficiency** of movement refers to the mechanical energy production of the movement relative to the metabolic energy used to cause the movement and approximates 30% during exercise.

STUDY QUESTIONS

1. Define the terms ergometry, economy, efficiency, and calorimetry.

2. Calculate work and power for the following exercise examples:

   a. A 75 kg person bench stepping a 15-cm bench, 15 times per minute, for 30 min.

   b. A person riding a cycle ergometer with a 6-m-per-revolution flywheel, for 45 min, at a load setting of 1.5 kg and a cadence of 80 rpm.

   c. A person riding the aforementioned cycle ergometer for 2 min at a load of 5.0 kg at 95 rpm.

   d. In examples b and c above, which example would be more likely to be maintained at a metabolic steady state? Why?

3. What are the difficulties of applying principles of

ergometry to treadmill walking or running and swimming?

4. What are the differences between direct and indirect calorimetry?

5. What are the differences between open- and closed-circuit indirect calorimetry?

6. Calculate each of $V_E STPD$, $V_I STPD$, VO_2, VCO_2, RER, and energy expenditure for the examples provided in appendix D.

7. What is the difference between the respiratory quotient (RQ) and the respiratory exchange ratio (RER)?

8. Under what conditions does the RER not equal the RQ?

9. What are the components of a modern computerized system for indirect gas analysis calorimetry?

APPLICATIONS

1. The absolute oxygen consumption of the body during exercise, combined with exercise duration, are the two most important determinants of energy expenditure. A friend wants you to explain the best way he or she can "burn" as many calories from fat as possible during exercise. Applying the first law of bioenergetics from chapter 2, what would you tell him or her?

2. Why is the inspired volume of air not always equal to the expired volume of air?

3. Which of the following are examples of scientific ergometers, and why: stationary cycle, treadmill, stair stepper, versi-climber, aerobic rider? How would the researchers determine the oxygen cost of exercising at different intensities on the equipment that cannot provide calculations of work and power?

REFERENCES

1. Atwater, W. O. Coefficients of digestibility and availability of the nutrients of food. *Proc. Am. Physiol. Soc.* 1:30, 1904.

2. Bisdee, J. T., W. P. T. James, and M. A. Shaw. Changes in energy expenditure during the menstrual cycle. *Brit. J. Nutr.* 61:187–199, 1989.

3. Bransford, D. R., and E. T. Howley. Oxygen cost of running in trained and untrained men and women. *Med. Sci. Sports Exerc.* 9:41–44, 1977.

4. Bursztein, S., D. H. Elwyn, J. Askanazi, and J. M. Kinney. *Energy metabolism, indirect calorimetry, and nutrition.* Williams and Wilkins, Baltimore, 1989.

5. Campbell, J. A., and T. A. Webster. Day and night urine during complete rest, laboratory routine, light muscular work and oxygen administration. *Biochem. J.* 15:660–664, 1921.

6. Campbell, J. A., D. Hargood-Ash, and L. Hill. Effect of cooling power of the atmosphere on body metabolism. *J. Physiol. Lond.* 52:259–264, 1922.

7. Cissik, J., and R. Johnson. Myth of nitrogen equality in respiration: Its history and implications. *Aerospace Med.* 43:755–758, 1972.

8. Costill, D. L., F. Rayfield, J. Kirwan, and R. Thomas. A computer based system for the measurement of force and power during front crawl swimming. *J. Swim. Res.* 2(1):16–19, 1986.

9. Costill, D. L., G. Lee, and L. J. D'Aquisto. Video-assisted analysis of swimming technique. *J. Swim. Res.* 3(2):5–9, 1987.

10. D'Aquisto, L. J., D. L. Costill, G. M. Gehlsen, W. Young, and G. Lee. Breaststroke economy, skill, and performance: Study of breaststroke mechanics using a computer based "velocity-video" system. *J. Swim. Res.* 4(2):9–13, 1988.

11. deGroot, G. Fundamental mechanics applied to swimming: Technique and propelling efficiency. In B.E. Ungerechts, and K. Reischle (eds.), *Swimming Science V, International Series on Sport Sciences* 18:17–30, 1986.

12. Daniels, J. T. A physiologist's view of running economy. *Med. Sci. Sports Exerc.* 17(3):332–338, 1985.

13. Fox, E. L., and R. Bowers. Steady-state equality of respiratory gaseous N_2 in resting man. *J. Appl. Physiol.* 35(1):143–144, 1973.

14. Fox, E. L., R. W. Bowers, and M. L. Foss. *The physiological basis for exercise and sport*, 5th ed. Brown & Benchmark, Madison, 1993.

15. Jones, N. L. Evaluation of a microprocessor-controlled exercise testing system. *J. Appl. Physiol.* 57:1312–1318, 1984.

16. Kleiber, M. *The fire of life: an introduction to animal energetics*. Robert E. Kreiger Publishing, Huntington, 1975.

17. Lakomy, H. K. A. An ergometer for measuring the power generated during sprinting. (Abstract) *J. Physiol. Lond.* 354:33P, 1984.

18. Lippert, H., and H. P. Lehmann. *SI units in medicine. An introduction to the international system of units with conversion tables and normal ranges*. Urban & Schwarzenberg, Baltimore, 1978.

19. Livesey, G., and M. Elia. Estimation of energy expenditure, net carbohydrate utilization, and net fat oxidation and synthesis by indirect calorimetry: evaluation of errors with special reference to the detailed composition of fuels. *Am J. Clin. Nutr.* 47:608–628, 1988.

20. Luft, U., L. Myhre, and J. Loeppky. Validity of Haldane calculation for estimating respiratory gas exchange. *J. Appl. Physiol.* 35(4):546–551, 1973.

21. Lusk, G., and E. F. DuBois. On the constancy of the basal metabolism. *J. Physiol. Lond.* 54:213–216, 1924.

22. Lusk, G. *The elements of the science of nutrition*, 4th ed. Saunders, Philadelphia, 1928.

23. McLean, J. A., and G. Tobin. *Animal and human calorimetry*. Cambridge University Press, New York, 1987.

24. Morgan, D. W., P. E. Martin, G. S. Krahenbuhl, and F. D. Baldini. Variability in running economy and mechanics among trained male runners. *Med. Sci. Sports Exerc.* 23(3):378–383, 1991.

25. Romjin, J. A., et al., Regulation of endogenous fat and carbohydrate metabolism in relation to exercise intensity and duration. *Am. J. Physiol.* 265(28):E380–E391, 1993.

26. Wagner, J., S. Horvath, T. Dahms, and S. Reed. Validation of open-circuit method for the determination of oxygen consumption. *J. Appl. Physiol.* 34(6):859–863, 1973.

27. Weissman, C., M. C. Damask, J. Askanazi, S. H. Rosenbaum, and J. M. Kinney. Evaluation of a non-invasive method for the measurement of metabolic rate in humans. *Clin. Sci.* 69:135–141, 1985.

28. Wilmore, J., and D. L. Costill. Adequacy of the Haldane transformation in the computation of exercise VO_2 in man. *J. Appl. Physiol.* 35(1):85–89, 1973.

29. Wong, W. W., W. J. Cochran, W. J. Klish, E. O'Brien Smith, L .S. Lee, and P. D. Klein. In vivo isotope-fractionation factors and the measurement of deuterium- and oxygen-18-dilution spaces from plasma, urine, saliva, respiratory water, and carbon dioxide. *Am. J. Clin. Nutr.* 47:1–6, 1988.

30. Young, D. S. Implementation of SI units for clinical laboratory data. Style specifications and conversion tables. *Annal. Intern. Med.* 106:114–120, 1987.

RECOMMENDED READINGS

Bursztein, S., D. H. Elwyn, J. Askanazi, and J. M. Kinney. *Energy metabolism, indirect calorimetry, and nutrition*. Williams and Wilkins, Baltimore, 1989.

Daniels, J. T. A physiologist's view of running economy. *Med. Sci. Sports Exerc.* 17(3):332–338, 1985.

Livesey, G., and M. Elia. Estimation of energy expenditure, net carbohydrate utilization, and net fat oxidation and synthesis by indirect calorimetry: evaluation of errors with special reference to the detailed composition of fuels. *Am J. Clin. Nutr.* 47:608–628, 1988.

Lusk, G. *The elements of the science of nutrition*, 4th ed. W.B. Saunders, Philadelphia, 1928.

McLean, J. A., and G. Tobin. *Animal and human calorimetry*. Cambridge University Press, New York, 1987.

2

oxygen

$Q = SV \times HR$

$HRmax = 220 - age$

RQ

fatigue RER

stress

mmHg

VO_2max

Systemic Responses to Exercise

Neuromuscular Function and Adaptations to Exercise

hen we move our body, or body parts, we require very complex functions of nerves and skeletal muscle to be performed in fractions of a second. For repeated muscle contractions, these events are repeated for several seconds, minutes, and even hours depending upon the duration of exercise or physical activity. In addition, some contractions need to be weak and finely controlled (e.g., handwriting), whereas others are required to be as forceful as possible (e.g., throwing the shot put). Some movements that we perform do not require us to think about them, such as the muscle contractions required in talking, breathing, and some actions that protect us when we fall (using our arms for improved balance or protection). Other movements that we voluntarily perform require conscious effort, such as throwing a ball, kicking a football, or jumping a fence. Clearly, our brain must organize nerve and skeletal muscle function differently depending on the type of movements required. The purpose of this chapter is to identify the important interactions that exist between nerves and skeletal muscle, explain the process of skeletal muscle contraction, document the different neural and muscle metabolic properties of the human neuromuscular system, and identify the acute and chronic adaptations of neuromuscular structure and function that result from exercise.

OBJECTIVES

After studying this chapter, you should be able to:

- Explain how nerves and skeletal muscle combine to control muscle contraction.
- Explain the molecular events that occur during the contraction of skeletal muscle.
- Define and explain the function of motor units and muscle fiber types.
- List the neural, contractile, and metabolic differences among motor units.
- Draw the different curves of muscle torque and power for changes in contraction velocity.
- Explain the multiple functions of the muscle spindle.
- Describe the potential changes in muscle fiber type proportions after endurance, strength, or power training.
- Explain the definitions of the terms; hypertrophy, hyperplasia, atrophy.

KEY TERMS

nerves	myofibrils	electromyography (EMG)
action potential	sarcomere	muscle biopsy
axon	myosin	fiber type
synapse	actin	muscle spindle
neurotransmitter	tropomyosin	alpha-gamma coactivation
receptors	troponin	resistance exercise
motor cortex	motor unit	hypertrophy
neuromuscular junction	concentric	hyperplasia
fibers	eccentric	atrophy
sarcolemma	isometric	
	isokinetic	

The Nervous System

he nervous system of the body provides the means to have rapid communication between the brain and the different tissues and organs of the body. **Nerves** are special cells that function to conduct a rapid change in the charge across a membrane (**action potential**) along a long thin component of the cell (**axon**). The nerve axon extends the nerve from one part of the body to another, thereby conducting the action potential to a specific location (fig. 5.1). Where a nerve connects to another nerve, or the target tissue, is called a **synapse**. At the synapse, a special chemical (**neurotransmitter**) is released that results in the transmission of the action potential to the connecting tissue. This process is facilitated by the presence of specific proteins (**receptors**) on the connecting-tissue (postsynaptic) membrane that bind the neurotransmitter and regenerate the action potential (table 5.1). When the action potential reaches the target tissue, the binding of the neurotransmitter to the specific receptor of the postsynaptic membrane instigates a cell/tissue response that is very specific to the receptor. For example, such events can cause the contraction of skeletal muscle, relaxation of certain smooth muscle, release of certain hormones, acceleration of heart rate, or alteration in function of enzymes within specific metabolically active tissues. These events can occur in as little as 5 msec, which is a clear example of the speed of neural communication within the body.

The nervous system can be divided into functional and anatomic divisions. The functional divisions of the nervous system can be divided into involuntary and voluntary control divisions. The voluntary, or *somatic* nervous system, is best exemplified by the nerves that innervate skeletal muscle. We have voluntary control over whether to use or not use these nerves, giving us voluntary control over our movement. The involuntary, or *autonomic* nervous system, is composed of two divisions that our body uses to regulate cellular, tissue, and organ functions—sympathetic and parasympathetic. These subdivisions exist because of differences in anatomy and *neurotransmitter* release, *and not necessarily function.* For example, the parasympathetic nerves all leave the central nervous system (CNS) at the lower brain level, whereas the nerves of the sympathetic division leave the spinal cord at levels that generally reflect the anatomical location of the organs and tissues they innervate. In addition, all parasympathetic nerves release the neurotransmitter acetylcholine on their target tissues, whereas sympathetic nerves mostly release norepinephrine (table 5.1). Depending on the type of receptor on the target cell membrane, the cellular response to parasympathetic and sympathetic innervation may differ, or may be similar; such as blood vessel vasoconstriction or vasodilation.

The parasympathetic division works in combination with the sympathetic division to control such things as heart rate and heart muscle (myocardium) contraction velocity, the contraction of the smooth muscle surrounding certain blood vessels, the bladder, and sweat glands, and the release of hormones from certain glands. The importance of the autonomic nervous system will be discussed and exemplified in later chapters of the book concerning muscle metabolism (chapter 6), cardiovascular functions (chapter 7), and hormone functions (chapter 9).

Anatomically, the nervous system comprises the central and peripheral systems (fig. 5.2) where the CNS comprises the brain and spinal cord. The peripheral nervous system comprises sensory nerves, nerves from the parasympathetic and sympathetic divisions of the autonomic nervous system, and motor nerves. Within the peripheral nervous system, nerves that leave the CNS and direct action potentials to peripheral tissue are termed *efferent* nerves, and nerves that originate in specialized sensory structures (receptors) in peripheral tissues that direct action potentials to the CNS are termed *afferent* nerves.

Nerve-Muscle Interactions

When you move your body, your first awareness of the results of this action comes when you feel or see your muscles contract and your limbs move. However, the movement is really the end result of a sequence of neural and muscular events. Complex neural events take place before your skeletal muscles contract, and to learn and understand why muscles contract, attention should be directed to the functions of the central nervous system that initiate muscle contraction.

Initiating Movement

The neural events that eventually cause muscle contraction begin in several locations in the brain, with the involvement of each location dependent on the complexity of movement. If you think hard about what is needed from the brain to orchestrate movement, you come to the conclusion that movement is a remarkable feat of life. Multiple muscles must be

---

nerves the cells of the nervous systems that conduct action potentials

action potential the rapid change in the membrane potential of excitable cells that is conducted along an excitable membrane

axon (ak'son) the long component of a nerve that conducts the action potential from one location to another within the body

synapse (sin'aps) the junction between two nerves

neurotransmitter (nu'ro-trans-mit'er) a chemical released at a synapse in response to the depolarization of the presynaptic membrane

receptors (re-sep'tors) proteins located within a membrane that are able to bind another molecule (typically a hormone or neurotransmitter)

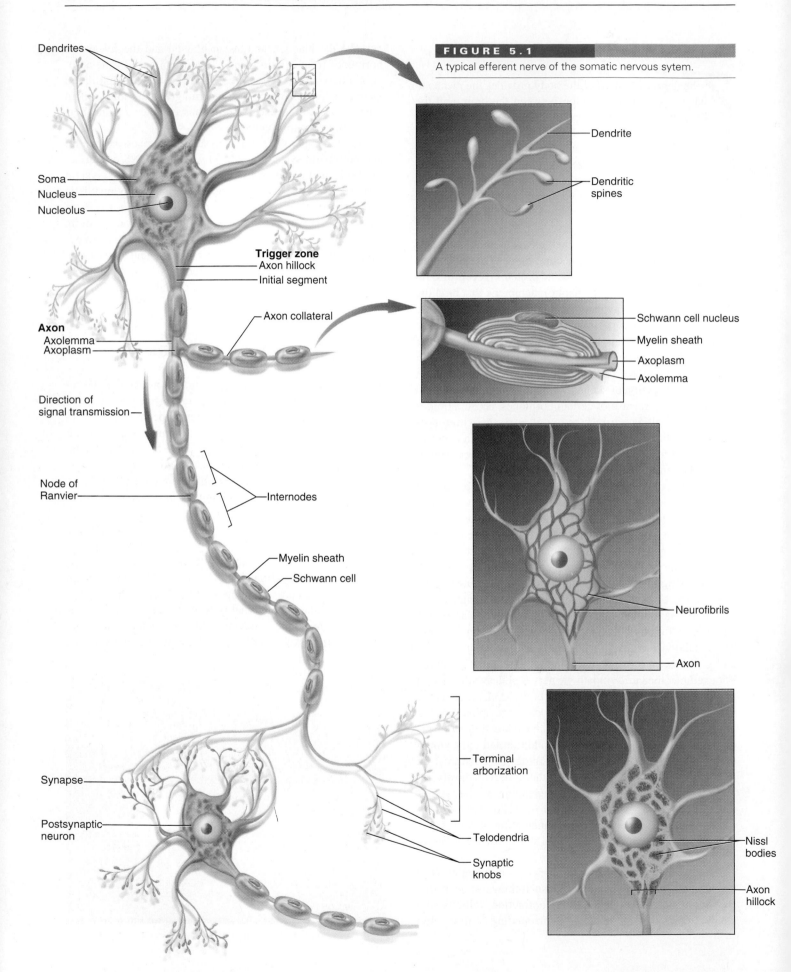

FIGURE 5.1

A typical efferent nerve of the somatic nervous sytem.

TABLE 5.1

Examples of the fast-acting* neurotransmitters of the nervous system, the main regions of the nervous system in which they occur, and examples of their importance during exercise

NEUROTRANSMITTER	LOCATIONS	FUNCTIONS DURING EXERCISE
Acetylcholine	Motor cortex, basal ganglia, Aα motor nerves, some nerves of the autonomic nervous system	↑ Muscle contraction,↑ sweating
Norepinephrine	Brainstem, hypothalamus, most post ganglionic nerves of the sympathetic nervous system	↑ Heart rate, cardiovascular regulation, blood glucose regulation, ↑ muscle metabolism
Epinephrine	Adrenal medulla	↑ Heart rate, cardiovascular regulation, blood glucose regulation, ↑ muscle metabolism
Dopamine	Basal ganglia	Motor coordination
Serotonin	Brainstem, spinal cord, hypothalamus	↑ Perceptions of fatigue
γ-aminobutyric acid (GABA)	Brainstem, spinal cord, cerebellum, cortex	Motor coordination

* The nervous system also uses slow-acting neurotransmitters, or neuropeptides, that are synthesized in the soma of a nerve and not in the presynaptic region of the nerve.

FIGURE 5.2

The anatomical (structural) and functional divisions of the nervous system.

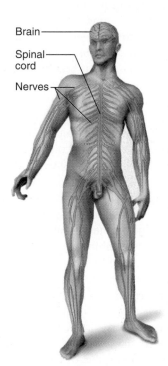

stimulated to contract, and some relax, in a well-timed sequence, with added control over the magnitude and speed of muscle force development. For the 100-m sprint runner, bouts of muscle contraction and opposing muscle relaxation are occurring several times per second. For the gymnast, rapid muscle contractions are also required, but with an overall emphasis on grace, and biomechanical and aesthetic perfection. How is it possible for the human body to accomplish such tasks?

In a localized region of the outer layers of the brain (cortex), anterior to the main convoluted fold (gyrus) of the brain, is a region called the **motor cortex** (fig. 5.3).

motor cortex the cortex region of the precentral gyrus responsible for the origin of the neural processing that instigates most contraction of skeletal muscle

FIGURE 5.3

The anatomical and functional association between the neuromuscular components involved in body movement. The basal ganglia are several nuclei within the mid and lower brain that receive nerves from the motor cortex, and primarily return nerves back to the cortex. Skilled movements, and movements requiring cognitive input such as throwing, kicking, shoveling, and writing require the presence of the basal ganglia. The main nucleus of the basal ganglia, the caudate nucleus, receives input from numerous regions of the brain and combines these inputs to "inform" the motor cortex of appropriate movement patterns, or the appropriate speed at which movement patterns should occur. The red nucleus is responsible for assisting the motor cortex in causing refined movement of the distal muscles of the body, such as the forearms, and lower leg. The red nucleus has a spatial arrangement similar to the motor cortex.

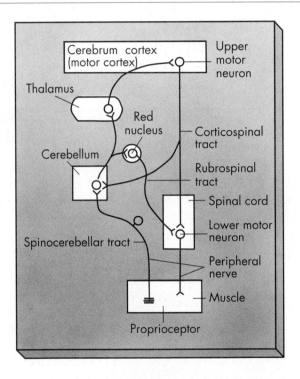

This cortical matter is responsible for developing neural patterns that eventually cause muscle contraction. The three-dimensional area of the motor cortex is divided into regions that are specific to different muscles of the body. The greater the number of motor units of the muscle, and the more intricate the neural control over a given muscle's contraction, the greater the area of the cortex that is assigned to that muscle. Thus, muscles that we use to cause intricate movement patterns, such as the forearm and hand for writing, typing, painting, or the muscles of the face for expression and talking, all have a relatively large area of the motor cortex. Not surprisingly, more than 50% of the motor cortex concerns the muscles of the hands and face (35).

The nerves that leave the motor cortex group together at the level of the lower brain and pass down the spinal cord in the *corticospinal tract* (or pyramidal tract). The nerves of the corticospinal tract cross in the medulla, so that the right side of the motor cortex controls movement on the left side of the body, and vice versa. This is best seen in patients suffering from stroke, as a stroke on the left side of the brain affects movment of the right side of the body, and vice versa.

Before nerve action potentials leave the brain and pass along the spinal cord, many patterns are modified in other sections of the brain. This modification is essential for refinement, correction, and sudden changes that are required in the movement. Why have a system that requires a change to be made in the motor cortex, when adjustments can occur faster, with less mental effort, somewhere else? One of the main locations of the refinement of movement patterns is called the cerebellum. In addition, the cerebellum is also important for the preparation of future motor patterns, and for storing correct movement sequences (35). For example, after considerable training of particular movment, more of the details of the movement can be retrieved from the cerebellum, leaving less need of the motor cortex. This is akin to requiring less conscious effort to do a particular task. In sports, this would mean that a person is able to concentrate on other aspects of performance, such as tactics, teamwork, or the ability to anticipate future events. These are the neurological facts behind the saying, "practice makes perfect."

As illustrated in figure 5.3, all the components of the motor control regions of the brain operate together in a complex manner that results in the controlled and precisely orchestrated series of action potentials that are propagated to the appropriate Aα motor nerves of the spinal cord. Nerves are classified by their axon diameter, degree of myelination, and conduction velocity. The motor nerve has the largest diameter and highest conduction velocity, and the letters "Aα" indicate this. *Many nerves innervate the soma of an Aα motor nerve*, as efferent nerves from the different components of the motor control system of the brain can synapse either directly or indirectly on the Aα nerve. In addition, afferent nerves function to invoke inhibition or excitation of the Aα motor nerve, thus providing important refinement at the level of the spinal cord.

The distribution of Aα motor nerves down the spinal cord is somewhat organized into a *segmental distribution*, where the Aα motor nerves leave the spinal cord at a vertebral level that reflects the anatomical position of the skeletal muscle (13). For example, the Aα motor nerves from the motor units of the muscles of the shoulder girdle, abdominal muscles, and muscles from the upper and lower leg leave the spinal cord at various levels of the cervical, thoracic, and sacral vertebrae, respectively.

Instigating Movement

The stimulation of the Aα motor nerves results in the propagation of action potentials to the skeletal muscle fibers of the muscles required to contract during the given

FIGURE 5.4

Electron micrographs of neuromuscular junctions. *(a)* A scanning electron micrograph of a motor nerve axon and its neuromuscular junction. The neuromuscular junction is an enlarged end region of the nerve axon that extends in many directions across the surface of the muscle fiber. *(b)* When the axon and neural components of the neuromuscular junction are removed, invaginations can be seen in the muscle fiber, within which are further clefts and folds.

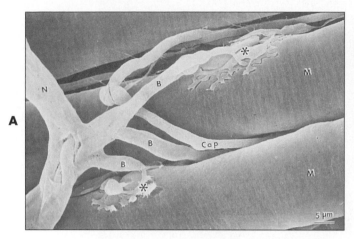

A

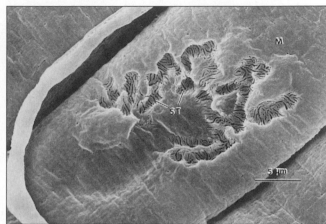

B

fibers of the muscles required to contract during the given movement. The divergence of the Aα motor nerve results in the formation of many junctions between the nerve and skeletal muscle fibers. These junctions are special synapses, and as such are referred to as *neuromuscular junctions*.

The Neuromuscular Junction

As for the synapse, the function of the **neuromuscular junction** is to transmit the action potential across a synaptic cleft. Unlike the synapse, the postsynaptic membrane is not a nerve but the *sarcolemma* of a skeletal muscle fiber.

Electron micrographs of tissue preparations containing neuromuscular junctions are presented in figure 5.4*a* and *b*. Some muscle fibers have more than one neuromuscular junction, each neuromuscular junction is an enlarged structure that extends over an area far greater than the cross-sectional area of the Aα motor nerve axon, and an extensive invagination exists in the skeletal muscle fiber under the neural extensions of the junction.

An enlarged simplified illustration of the cross section of a neuromuscular junction is presented in figure 5.5. The postsynaptic region of the sarcolemma, sometimes termed the *motor endplate*, is not only a large invagination, but within it exist numerous other invaginations that serve to increase the cross-sectional area exposed to the release of acetylcholine. As with the postsynaptic membrane of a nerve synapse, the region of the sarcolemma at the neuromuscular junction contains special Na$^+$ channels that open when bound by acetylcholine. The sarcolemma is then depolarized, and an action potential spreads across the sarcolemma and down special tubules that eventually leads to the molecular events of muscle contraction.

Skeletal Muscle Contraction

Skeletal muscle is one of three types of muscle in the human body: *skeletal muscle*, *cardiac muscle*, and *smooth muscle*. The individual cells in each muscle type are referred to as muscle **fibers**, and the specialized excitable cell membrane of skeletal muscle fibers is called the **sarcolemma**. Skeletal muscle, as with all the types of muscle, can receive an action potential, and can conduct the action potential across and within muscle fibers. This property is termed *excitability*. In addition, skeletal muscle can respond to action potentials by contracting (*contractility*), and then return to its precontraction length because of the property of *elasticity*.

Skeletal muscle functions to contract and either cause body movement or the stability of body posture. Skeletal muscle contraction must be able to be performed with a decrease or increase in muscle length. In performing these functions, *skeletal muscle is required to contract and generate tension throughout the length of the muscle*. Depending on the muscle and movement, skeletal muscle must also be able to develop a wide range of tensions, with the ability to alter tension in small increments. These general requirements necessitate a structure with enormous capacity in change in length, and be structurally and functionally

---

neuromuscular junction the connection between a branch of an alpha motor nerve and a skeletal muscle fiber

fibers muscle cells

sarcolemma (sar'ko-lem'ah) the cell membrane of a muscle fiber

FIGURE 5.5

An illustration of the cross-section of a neuromuscular junction. The intracellular structures and membrane channels that are involved in neuromuscular transmission of the action potential are included, as are the membrane features of the post-synaptic membrane.

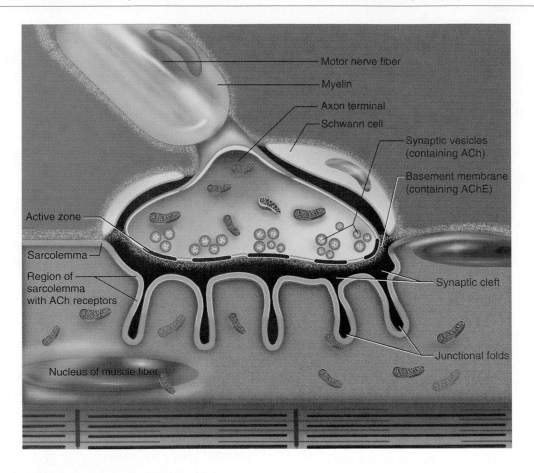

FIGURE 5.6

A transverse section of human skeletal muscle, illustrating the striated appearance of skeletal muscle fibers.

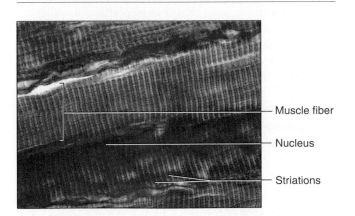

organized to contract and generate both minutely small and extremely large forces.

Structure

When viewed in transverse section (fig. 5.6), the striated appearance of skeletal muscle fibers results from the organized arrangement of proteins. The main proteins of skeletal muscle are myosin, actin, tropomyosin, and troponin: *myosin and actin are involved in the process of muscle contraction; troponin and tropomyosin are involved in the regulation of muscle contraction.*

Striated muscle proteins are organized into subcellular structures called **myofibrils**, which extend along the length of the muscle fiber. The myofibrils are aligned beside each other resulting in a similar three-dimensional pattern of the contractile proteins within the entire fiber. Within a myofibril, the contractile proteins are arranged in units called **sar-**

FIGURE 5.7

The organization of the contractile proteins in skeletal muscle as viewed through an electron microscope.

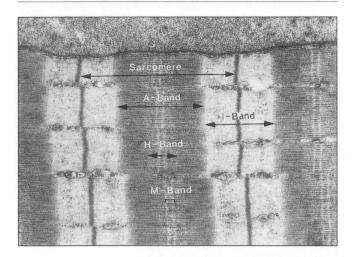

comeres (fig. 5.7). The sarcomere is bordered by proteins that form the Z-lines. F-actin molecules extend from each Z-line toward the middle of the sarcomere. The myosin molecules do not extend to each Z-line, and are maintained in the central region of the sarcomere by proteins that form the M-line (81). When viewed three dimensionally, each myosin molecule is associated with six different F-actin molecules in a hexagonal structure.

The different visual regions of the sarcomere have been named. The darkly stained region indicating the region of myosin is termed the A-band. Located centrally within the A-band is a less darkly stained region where no actin is associated with the myosin, termed the H-band. On either side of the Z-lines are unstained (clear) regions comprised solely of actin molecules, termed the I-band.

The contractile proteins of the myofibrils differ in structure and function (fig. 5.8). **Myosin**, the largest of the proteins, is a two-stranded helical structure, and consists of two forms of myosin (light and heavy). In vivo the two heavy chains contain a hinged region, a linear end region, and two globular heads (S_1 units) at one end. The S_1 units contain the enzyme myosin ATPase. The activity of myosin ATPase is believed to be influenced by the myosin light chains (50, 82, 83), although the details of this interaction remain unclear.

Actin is a globular protein (G-actin), however, in vivo it aggregates to form a two-stranded helical structure (F-actin). Associated with the F-actin is a rod-shaped molecule called **tropomyosin**, which exists as multiple strands, each of which associates with six or seven G-actin molecules along the length of the F-actin (8, 43, 44). At the end of each tropomyosin molecule is bound a **troponin** molecule, which is involved in the regulation of skeletal muscle contraction.

Contraction and Regulation

For one muscle, hundreds of separate $A\alpha$ nerves may be stimulated, and for a given $A\alpha$ motor nerve, divergence of the main axon into hundreds of branches results in the innervation of hundreds of muscle fibers. The muscle fibers and the $A\alpha$ motor nerve that innervates them comprise what is called a **motor unit** (fig. 5.9). When stimulated, a motor unit responds by contracting maximally. Therefore, *the motor unit is the functional unit of muscle contraction.* Contraction of a skeletal muscle results from the combined contraction of many motor units.

The electrochemical and molecular sequence of events during muscle contraction are listed in sequential order in table 5.2 and illustrated in figure 5.10. When an action potential is transmitted to and propogated along the sarcolemma, the depolarization is internalized within the fiber by the *t-tubule* network. When the wave of depolarization reaches the junction of the t-tubule and sarcoplasmic reticulum (*triad*), calcium is released from the *sarcoplasmic reticulum* (SR) and increases the concentration of free calcium within the fiber.

The binding of the calcium ions to the troponin molecules induces a conformational shift in the actin-troponin-tropomyosin association. This shift in three-dimensional molecular structure exposes a site which enables the noncovalent association of actin and the S_1 units of myosin. The position of the myosin S_1 units prior to calcium release from the SR is often illustrated as a vertical structure, and represents the "favorable" or "less strained" position of the S_1 unit.

The binding of the S_1 units to actin enables the release of the ADP (adenosine diphosphate) and Pi (inorganic phosphate) molecules, which strengthens the actin-myosin complex (58). During this event, the S_1 units return to their "less strained" or "favored" position causing shortening of the sarcomere. The myosin and actin association is broken by the binding of ATP (adenosine triphosphate) to the

myofibril (mi′o-fi′bril) the longitudinal anatomical unit within skeletal and cardiac muscle fibers that contains the contractile proteins

sarcomere (sar′ko-mere) the smallest contractile unit of skeletal muscle, consisting of the contractile proteins between two Z-lines

myosin (mi′o-sin) the largest of the contractile proteins of skeletal muscle

actin (ac′tin) a contractile protein of skeletal muscle

tropomyosin (tro′po-my′osin) a contractile protein of striated muscle

troponin (tro′po′nin) the regulatory calcium binding contractile protein of striated muscle

motor unit an alpha motor nerve and the muscle fibers that it innervates

FIGURE 5.8

The molecular structure of the contractile proteins of skeletal and cardiac muscle. Filamentous actin (F-actin) is comprised of separate units of G-actin. Troponin and tropomyosin are located along the F-actin filament. Myosin is a more complex molecule than actin. Myosin can be enzymatically cleaved at two sites. The long tail is termed light meromyosin (LMM), and the remaining hinge and two-head structure is termed heavy meromyosin (HMM). HMM can be further divided into two S_1 units, with each S_1 unit having two light chains. One of the light chains from each S_1 head is a regulatory light chain. The enzyme myosin ATPase is also located on each S_1 unit.

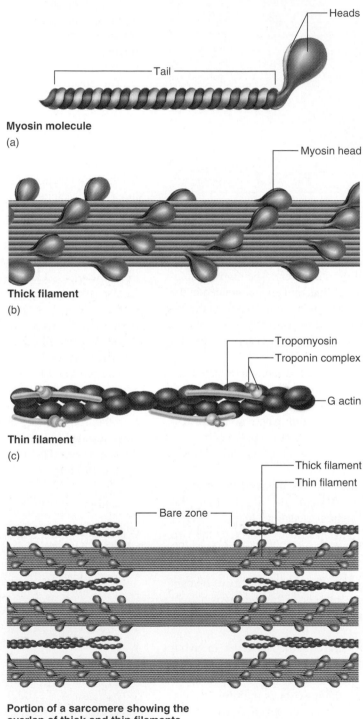

FIGURE 5.9

The motor nerve and muscle fiber components of the motor unit.

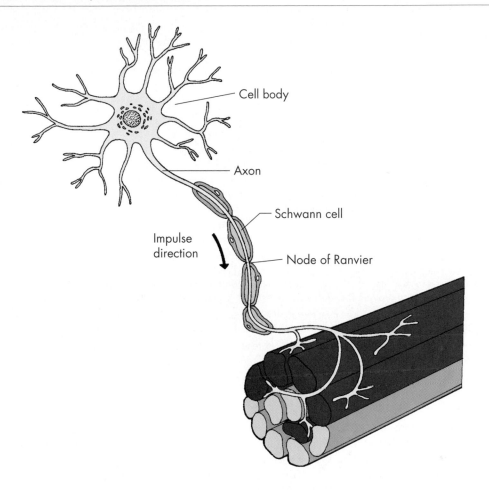

myosin S_1 heads and the release of the ADP. The hydrolysis of ATP then provides the free energy to move the S_1 units of myosin to their strained position. The presence of ADP and Pi on the S_1 units retains the S_1 units in this position until calcium ions bind to troponin. Consequently, if free calcium is still present within the myofibrillar apparatus and calcium remains bound to troponin, as soon as the S_1 units are returned to their strained position the contraction process will occur once again. The continued cycling of the S_1 units, which *requires the presence of calcium and the continual production and hydrolysis of ATP*, is termed *contraction cycling*. Contraction cycling accounts for the ability of skeletal muscle to generate force despite no (isometric) or minimal changes in length, and for the ATP and metabolic demands of these contractions. The summation of contraction cycling and sarcomere shortening within a myofibril, muscle fiber, and motor unit, and among multiple motor units, results in the shortening of muscle during dynamic muscle contraction.

Function

Types of Contractions   Skeletal muscle can contract in a variety of ways. Contractions causing a change in muscle length are called *isotonic* contractions. When the muscle length shortens, the isotonic contraction is referred to as a **concentric** contraction. When the muscle length increases during contraction, the isotonic contraction is referred to as **eccentric** (fig. 5.11). However, by definition a contraction involves muscle shortening. For this reason many researchers now refer to an eccentric contraction as an eccentric action. Nevertheless, because the American College

concentric (kon-sen'trik) in reference to skeletal muscle contraction; a contraction involving the shortening of muscle

eccentric (e-sen'trik) in reference to skeletal muscle contraction; a contraction involving the lengthening of muscle

---

TABLE 5.2

The sequence of events during contraction in striated muscle

When striated muscle is relaxed, ADP and Pi are bound to the S_1 unit of myosin, the myosin head is in the vertical "strained" position, there is a low intracellular calcium concentration, and therefore negligible actin-myosin binding and contraction.

1. The depolarization is received at the sarcolemma and is propagated down the t-tubule network to the sarcoplasmic reticulum (SR).

2. Depolarization of the SR in the region of the triad initiates the release of calcium from the SR and an increase in intracellular calcium.

3. Increased intracellular calcium increases calcium binding to troponin.

4. The troponin-calcium complex causes a structural change in the position of troponin and tropomyosin on the F-actin polymer, enabling actin to bind to the S_1 units of myosin.

5. Actin-myosin binding enables the S_1 units to immediately move to their "less strained" or "favorable" position, thus causing the movement of the attached actin toward the central region of the sarcomere. During this process, ADP and Pi are released from each S_1 unit. This constitutes muscle contraction.

6. Because actin is connected to the Z-lines, actin movement results in the shortening of each sarcomere within the fibers of the stimulated motor unit, resulting in muscle contraction.

7. Provided ATP is continually replenished at the myosin-actin sites of the sarcomere, ATP molecules once again bind to the myosin S_1 units, which causes the release of each S_1 unit from actin. During the release of actin and myosin, ATP is hydrolyzed to ADP and Pi and the S_1 units change conformation to a vertical "strained" position. The ATP hydrolysis is believed to provide the free energy needed to move the S_1 units to the "strained" position.

8. If the increased intracellular calcium concentration is maintained (because of continued neural stimulation), the myosin S_1 units will continue the cyclical attachment and detachment to actin, termed *contraction cycling*.

9. Relaxation occurs when the action potentials are not received by the neurmuscular junction and calcium is actively "pumped" back into the SR.

---

of Sports Medicine recommends that the word "contraction" be retained because of the broad acceptance and application of its nonspecific meaning (62), it will be used in this text. Eccentric muscle contractions can generate greater force than concentric contractions (82), with the difference due to combined effects of gravity assistance (when performed with gravity), stored elastic energy, and the passive tension of the contractile proteins and musculotendinous junctions (focus box 5.1). Muscle contractions causing no change in muscle length are called **isometric** contractions.

A third type of contraction (muscle action) is **isokinetic**. Isokinetic contractions are a special type of concentric contraction, where the velocity of muscle shortening remains constant (hence the term *isokinetic*). These contractions require specialized and expensive equipment that instantaneously modifies resistance in proportion to the force generated at specific joint angles (refer to fig. 1.6). The result of this is to provide maximal resistance when musculoskeletal mechanics allow maximal force production and vice versa (fig. 5.12).

Length-Tension Relationship For a given muscle, the force of a maximal concentric contraction depends on the length of the muscle (8). When a muscle is removed from the body, with one end connected to a micrometer and the other end connected to a force transducer, stimulation of

the muscle will cause contraction without shortening (isometric) and the development of tension on the force transducer (fig. 5.13a). By stimulating the muscle and recording the resulting forces for various muscle lengths, the data can be graphed as a length-tension curve (fig. 5.13b). However, because simply stretching the muscle generates *passive tension*, this passive component must be subtracted from the *total tension* measured, resulting in the *active tension*. Muscle length influences tension development because excessive stretch and inadequate length decrease actin and myosin interaction (fig. 5.13c). These facts have direct application to exercise because warm-up and flexibility preparation prior to an event optimize the length-tension relationship of skeletal muscle, allow increased force production and power generation, and can improve performance.

Force-Velocity and Power-Velocity Relationships Skeletal muscle tension development is also known to vary with the velocity of the shortening. Greatest tension development occurs at zero-shortening velocity (isometric) contractions. The force developed during maximal isometric contractions is referred to as the *maximal voluntary contraction* (MVC) force. As contraction velocity increases, peak tension development decreases (fig. 5.15). The force-velocity curve can differ among muscles with training/detraining, and among individuals who differ in fiber type proportions. The skeletal

FIGURE 5.10

The sequence of events during skeletal and cardiac muscle contraction. The depolarization of the sarcolemma is propagated down the t-tubules and causes calcium release from the SR *(a)*. As long as calcium is not pumped back into the SR, the sequence of events from A to E continues, and represents contraction cycling. *(b)* The binding of calcium to troponin causes the conformational alteration of actin-tropomyosin interaction, exposing the actin-myosin S_1 unit binding sites. *(c)* Binding of actin and the S_1 units of myosin causes the translation of the actin and myosin, causing contraction. *(d)* The regeneration of ATP from metabolism enables a new ATP molecule to bind to the S_1 unit, which causes the deattatchment of actin and the S_1 units of myosin. *(e)* The S_1 units of myosin return to the vertical or "strained" position, powered by the free energy of ATP dephosphorylation.

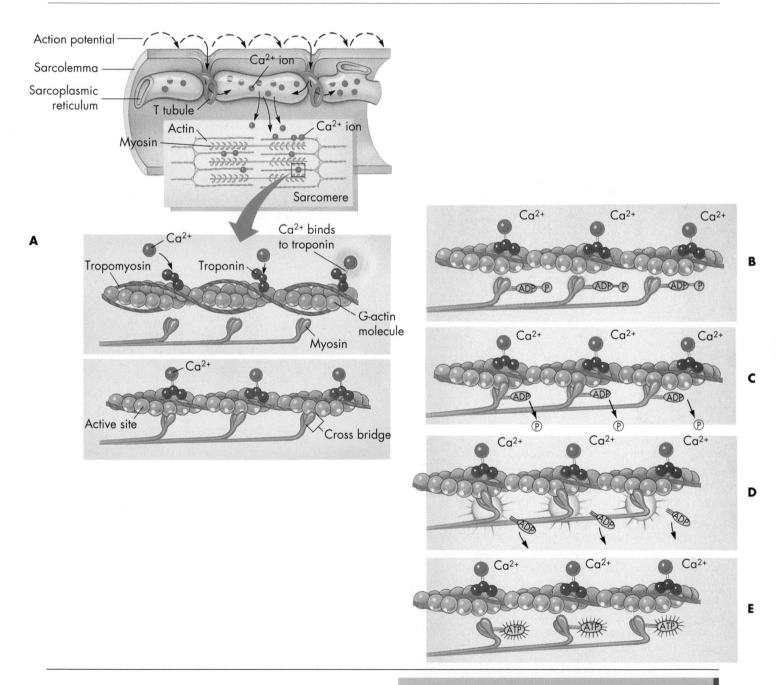

isometric (i-so-met'rik) in reference to skeletal muscle contraction; a contraction involving no change in the length of muscle

isokinetic (i-so-ki-net'ik) in reference to skeletal muscle contraction; a contraction involving a constant velocity

FIGURE 5.11

The different types of skeletal muscle contraction. Concentric contractions occur with a rapid increase in *external force* application. However, because of the influence of joint angle on force development, *contractile tension* varies during a full joint range of motion contraction. During eccentric contractions the *external force* profile is similar to that of concentric contractions; however, muscle tension development is greatest when the force of gravity is perpendicular to the lever arm. Greater forces can be developed during eccentric contractions than for concentric contractions.

FIGURE 5.12

Isokinetic contractions performed with maximal effort produce a variable force. The data presented are for maximal isokinetic knee flexion and extension, and show force curves during the range of motion during flexion and extension. Force production is less for the start and end of a contraction, where musculoskeletal mechanics (joint angles) limit force generation. Training muscle for strength and power using isokinetic equipment has received support for its ability to maximize resistance at optimal joint angles, and for the ability to set specific contraction velocities. However, the isolation of specific muscles and muscle groups decreases the suitability of this training to actions that involve multiple muscle groups (adapted from Thorstensson A., G. Grimby and J. Karlsson. Force-velocity relations and fiber composition in human knee extensor muscles. *J. Appl. Physiol.* 40(1):12-16, 1976).

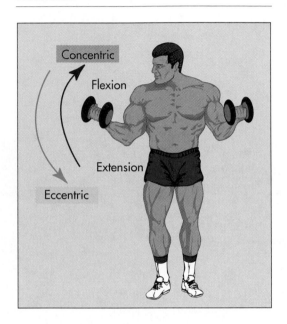

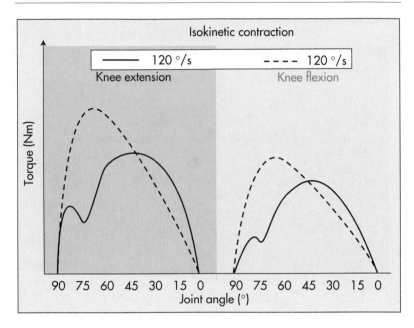

muscle force-power curve reveals that an optimal velocity exists for developing power.

During repeated maximal effort contractions, muscle fatigues. Fatigue is illustrated as a decay in force generation with subsequent contractions (fig. 5.13). Interestingly, muscles with greater force generation capabilities, or muscles trained to increase strength, exhibit more rapid decrements in muscle force. Conversely, muscles trained for long-term endurance have small maximal force capabilities and less force decrement during fatigue.

Summation and Tetanus   The skeletal muscle twitch response is extremely long (150 to 250 ms) compared to the action potential (< 5 ms). As previously explained, skeletal muscle contraction results from the combined contraction of many motor units. The long contraction time and short stimulation time provide opportunity for additional neural stimulation prior to the complete relaxation of the muscle or motor unit. In these circumstances, the force of the total muscle or motor unit twitch can increase with in-

creased stimulation frequency, and is called *summation*. As stimulation frequency increases, twitch tension also increases until a smooth maximal tension is reached, which is called *tetanus*. Tetanus is not a normal occurrence during voluntary muscle contraction, but exemplifies the ability of skeletal muscle to respond to high-frequency stimulation. Furthermore, during abnormal muscle function, such as during cramp, the resulting response is similar to tetanus and can often exceed the maximal voluntary contraction force.

Resting Muscle Tone   At rest a small amount of muscle motor unit contraction occurs to maintain firmness or *tone* of skeletal muscle. The resting muscle tone is known to be caused by neural stimulation because neurally isolated muscles are flaccid. In addition, when afferent nerves from muscle are cut, thereby preventing feedback from muscles to the central nervous system, muscle tone is lost (8). This fact illustrates that resting muscle tone is caused by afferent nerve feedback from muscle to the spinal cord, which then stimu-

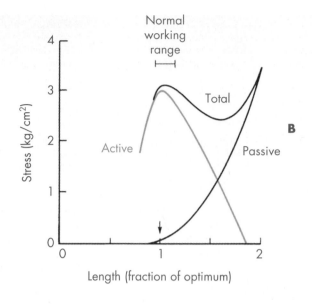

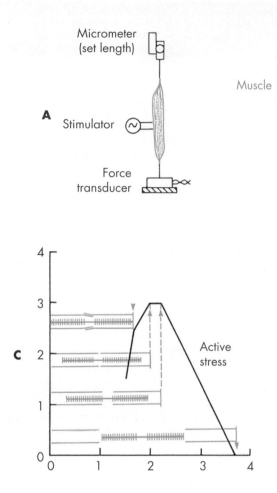

FIGURE 5.13

(a) Invitro research of muscle contraction has produced curves illustrating the relationship between muscle length and tension development *(b)*. Active tension is the tension remaining after the passive tension component is removed, and reflects the molecular interaction between actin and myosin *(c)*.

lates efferent fibers that innervate a small number of skeletal muscle motor units (8).

Identifying Motor Units and Muscle Fiber Types

Research of neuromuscular function was first conducted using samples from animals. The earliest animal models used to research nerve function and muscle contraction were the triceps surae and gastrocnemius muscles of the cat (10, 11, 12, 36, 38). This research identified that differences existed in the morphology and function among the nerves of certain motor units, and that the metabolic and contractile characteristics of muscle fibers innervated by different nerves were also different. The complete classification of a motor unit requires data of nerve and muscle morphology and physiology, and differences in these characteristics have resulted in a motor unit classification based on nerve recruitment order and conduction velocity, muscle contraction velocity and force, and muscle fiber metabolic capacities (table 5.3). Motor units exist in human

muscle that are fast-twitch and slow-twitch. Within the fast-twitch category are two subdivisions that differ in oxidative capacity.

Nerve and Recruitment Characteristics

The attainment of a threshold membrane potential of the soma of the nerve occurs more rapidly in an SO (slow-twitch oxidative) motor unit than in either the FOG (fast-twitch oxidative glycolic) or FG (fast-twitch glycolic) motor unit, resulting in a recruitment order of motor units. *SO motor units are recruited first during incremental exercise, followed by a progressive increase in FOG and FG motor unit recruitment as exercise intensity increases.* This pattern of recruitment has been termed the *size principle*, and causes SO motor units to be recruited predominantly during low to moderate exercise intensities, and each of SO, FOG, and FG motor units to be recruited during exercise requiring intense contractions against high resistance or fast muscle contractions (27, 38, 39, 40, 67). *During contractions of increased velocity the size principal is still retained*, however, the difference in recruitment order among the different types of motor units is less pronounced (27).

FOCUS BOX 5.1

Eccentric Contraction–Induced Skeletal Muscle Injury

When exercise is performed that involves eccentric muscle contractions, especially when the exercise duration or intensity are unaccustomed, microscopic muscle damage occurs. This damage is associated with the development of elevated serum creatine kinase activity, swelling, soreness, and restricted range of motion during the ensuing 48 h (14, 18, 21, 41). Originally, this condition was termed delayed onset muscle soreness (DOMS), however, research conducted since the early 1980s has indicated that the muscle damage that accompanies DOMS can be quite severe, induces an immune response, increases calcium release from muscle, which in turn can activate many protein-degrading enzymes and exacerbate the microtrauma to skeletal muscle. The biochemical events that accompany these responses probably induce the inflammation and soreness. In short, delayed onset muscle soreness is a nondescript term for the condition, and the term *exercise-induced muscle damage* is becoming more accepted.

Figure 5.14 presents an electron micrograph of damaged skeletal muscle. The disruption of the Z-lines is termed Z-line streaming, and probably results from damage to proteins that stabilize the actin and myosin molecules to the Z-line proteins. After approximately 12 h, infiltration of the damaged muscle region by macrophages and lymphocytes occurs, resulting in the destruction of the damaged region of muscle. It is theorized that chemicals released from the immune response induce both the swelling and

pain symptoms, and that the influx of calcium into the damaged cells may activate enzymes that degrade protein and further accentuate the muscle damage.

Clarkson and Tremblay (18) have documented that recovery from even a single bout of exposure to eccentric muscle contractions protects the muscle from the same damage during a second bout of eccentric muscle contractions. This rapid adaptability to eccentric contractions is remarkable; however, the cellular events and changes that this tolerance is attributable to are unknown.

FIGURE 5.14

Microscopic skeletal muscle damage resulting from eccentric exercise. The disruption of the Z-line has caused this damage to be termed "Z-line streaming."

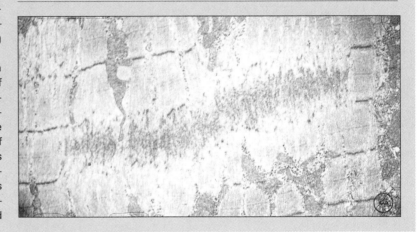

Apart from the soma and recruitment order, the Aα motor nerves of different motor units also differ in size, conduction velocity, and stimulation characteristics (fig. 5.16). The area dimensions of the soma and cross-sectional area of the axon of the Aα motor nerve is larger in the FG motor unit than in the SO motor unit (13, 40, 66). In addition the Aα motor nerve has a higher conduction velocity in the FG motor unit than in the SO motor unit, and SO motor units are stimulated in a more consistent manner compared to the rapid and intermittent manner of the FG motor units (40). However, because of considerable overlap among motor units for these characteristics Burke (13) has commented that motor units cannot be classified based on nerve characteristics alone.

The contribution of human motor unit recruitment to muscle function has been indirectly studied using **electromyography (EMG).** The signal obtained from EMG is proportional to electrical activity, which in turn is proportional to the number of muscle fibers and therefore the num-

ber of motor units stimulated to contract (6). EMG has revealed the increase in electrical activity that occurs when muscle contractions develop increased tension, and the different electrical activity and recruitment for concentric, eccentric, and isokinetic muscle contractions (focus box 5.2).

Muscle Characteristics

The muscle fibers of a motor unit have biochemical and contractile capacities that influence how the motor unit is suited to different exercise intensities and durations.

Contractile Force and Velocity

The contractile force of muscle within the different motor units increases in a progression from SO, to FOG, to FG motor units (fig. 5.16), whereas the duration of the contraction decreases in the progression from SO, to FOG, to FG motor units. The force of contraction of a motor unit is determined

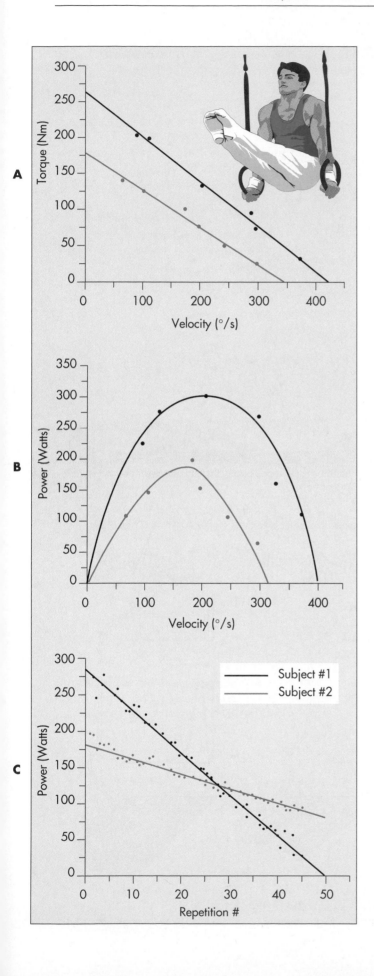

FIGURE 5.15

(a) The relationship between muscle contraction force and contraction velocity. Data is shown from two subjects that have different maximal force capabilities of the quadriceps. Subject 1 is an untrained individual, and subject 2 is a national competitive triathlete. Even though subject 2 was endurance trained for prolonged exercise, subject 1 had greater maximal force. *(b)* The relationship between muscle power and contraction velocity of the quadriceps for the same two subjects. Subject 1 had greater power, with both subjects having the optimal power-velocity relationship at velocities between 150 and 200°/s. *(c)* The decrease in power during multiple contractions of skeletal muscle in the same two subjects. Subject 2 had far greater endurance (less decrease in power).

by the size of the muscle fibers within a motor unit, and by the number of muscle fibers within a motor unit. FT (fast-twitch) motor units generally contain more muscle fibers than ST (slow-twitch) motor units.

Contractile velocity of motor units is determined by the conduction velocity of the Aα motor nerves and the type of myosin proteins and myosin ATPase enzyme within the muscle fibers. The myosin heavy and light chains and ATPase enzyme are known to result from separate genes, and their expression is therefore determined by gene translation, which is believed to be differentiated within the first year of life (13). Different structures of the myosin light chains are known to be present in FT compared to ST muscle fibers, as are different structures of the enzyme myosin ATPase. These differences result in faster contraction times in FT compared to ST motor units; however, the contribution from other determinants to contractile velocity, such as neuromuscular transmission, t-tubule and sarcoplasmic reticulum density, and calcium pump characterstics are unknown (67).

Muscle Fiber Biochemical and Enzymatic Capacities

Skeletal muscle fibers from SO motor units have a high oxidative capacity. In other words, they possess relatively high concentrations of myoglobin, high mitochondrial membrane density and, therefore, relatively high concentrations of the enzymes of the TCA (tricarboxylic acid) cycle, β-oxidation, and electron transport chain. The added myoglobin and mitochondria of SO muscle compared to FG muscle are the reasons for the "red" appearance and "white" appearance of the respective muscle types. Muscle fibers from FOG motor units have moderate concentrations of these molecules and enzymes, with muscle from FG motor units having the lowest concentrations. However, the differentiation of muscle fibers based on metabolic capacities is by far less sensitive than that of histochemical staining based in the different pH stability of myosin ATPase, and has been interpreted as evidence of a

electromyography (EMG) (e-lek'tro-mi'og-ra'fi) study of neuromuscular electrical activity at rest and during muscle contraction

TABLE 5.3

The classification nomenclature of mammalian skeletal muscle motor units

CLASSIFICATION METHOD	NOMENCLATURE			
Visual	Red		White	
Contractile velocity [Hennemen and Mendell (40)]	Slow-twitch		Fast-twitch	
Contractile velocity and metabolism [Brooke and Kaiser (9)]	I Slow-twitch	IIab Fast-twitch intermediate	IIa Fast-twitch fatigue resistant	IIb Fast-twitch fatigable
Contractile velocity and metabolism [Burke et al. (11, 13)]	S Slow-twitch	F(int) Fast-twitch intermediate	FR Fast-twitch fatigue resistant	FF Fast-twitch fatigable
Contractile velocity and metabolism [Peter et al. (59)]	Slow-twitch oxidative (SO)		Fast-twitch oxidative gly-colytic (FOG)	Fast-twitch glycolytic (FG)

Source: Adapted from Burke (13), Peter (59).

A more complex classification, resulting in additional subdivisions can be found in Pette and Straron (60).

FIGURE 5.16

The different neural, stimulatory, contractile, and metabolic differences among the three main types of motor units of human skeletal muscle. SO = slow-twitch oxidative, FOG = fast-twitch oxidative glycolytic, FG = fast-twitch glycolytic.

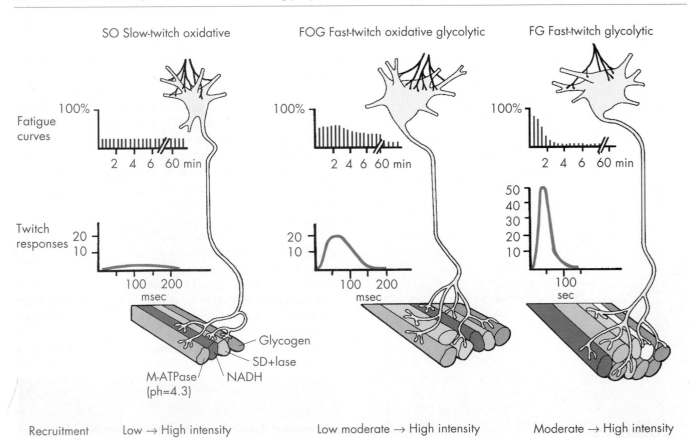

FOCUS BOX 5.2

Electromyography: Measuring Neuromuscular Electrical Activity During Muscle Contraction

What is Electromyography?

Electromyography (EMG) is the study of muscle function from the detection of electrical activity emanating from the depolarization of nerves and muscle membranes that accompany contraction (6). The electrical activity is detected by the placement of one or more electrodes over the contracting muscle(s) of interest. The type of electrodes can be either needle or surface: needle electrodes are inserted into a muscle belly or a specific nerve, and surface electrodes are placed on the skin over the muscle(s) of interest (fig. 5.17).

The EMG Signal

The observed unprocessed signal is the composite of all neural and muscle membrane depolarization, and as such consists of signals from Aα motor nerves of the recruited motor units, muscle receptors, and afferent nerves. Understandably, the EMG signal can be very complex! The raw signal can be processed by adding the squared deviations from the baseline signal, and this signal processing when expressed relative to the duration of the signal is referred to as *integrated EMG*. Another method of analysis is to record the frequency of individual spikes in the EMG signal. Increased frequency of EMG signals indicates increased conduction velocities (and/or increased FT recruitment), whereas a decrease in frequency represents muscle fatigue (6). In addition, the ability of skeletal muscle to increase force application after exercise training despite no increase in EMG signal has been used to indicate a neural component to training adaptation, such as an increased synchronization of motor unit firing (28, 56).

EMG Evidence of Motor Unit Recruitment

The use of the EMG to detect changes in motor unit recruitment has been based on an increase in signal amplitude and an increase in integrated EMG signal (fig. 5.18). Both parameters increase in an exponential manner as the muscle contraction force increases.

FIGURE 5.18

The increase in integrated EMG signal with increases in the strength of muscle contraction.

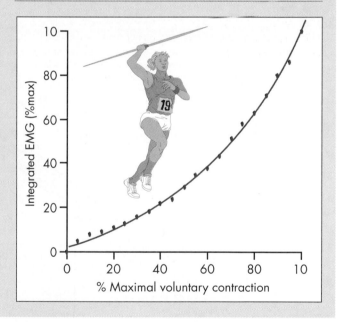

FIGURE 5.17

Photograph of an EMG with surface electrodes attached to a subject.

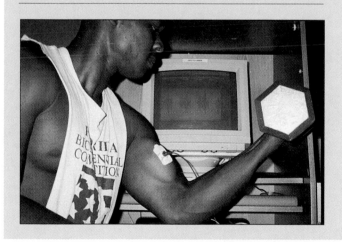

---

metabolic continuum that exists within and between muscle fibers of different motor units (see focus box 5.3) (9, 12, 13, 32, 66, 67).

These metabolic differences make SO motor units more suited to prolonged exercise, and allow muscle catabolism of lipid and carbohydrate via mitochondrial respiration. Conversely, the low mitochondrial density of the skeletal muscle fibers from FG motor units makes these muscle fibers reliant on glycolytic catabolism, and therefore the production of lactate and the development of acidosis (25, 31). Muscle

fibers from SO motor units are therefore termed *fatigue resistant*, whereas muscle fibers from FG motor units are *fatigable*.

Researchers have documented the metabolic differences among muscle fibers from different motor units by several methods. An increasingly common but laborious technique is to isolate individual muscle fibers from a biopsy sample, determine their fiber type by an enzymatic assay, pool the fibers into different fiber type populations, and then assay the muscle samples for the activity of additional enzymes of

FOCUS BOX 5.3

Applications of Muscle Biopsy to Exercise Physiology

The Muscle Biopsy Procedure

Human muscle biopsy is an invasive procedure that removes a small piece of muscle tissue from the human body. It is performed by first injecting a local anaesthetic into the skin and underlying connective tissue where the biopsy is to be performed. Once the anaesthetic has taken effect, a small incision (usually 1 cm long) is made through the skin and down through the fascia sheath covering the muscle. The biopsy needle (fig. 5.19) is then forced into the opening. When in place, the center plunge and guillotine is raised and, to increase the size of the biopsy sample, suction is generated within the needle to force muscle into the window of the needle (26). The guillotine is then forcefully lowered, cutting the muscle. The needle is then withdrawn, with the muscle specimen inside.

How Are Muscle Biopsy Specimens Processed and Analyzed?

When the muscle specimen is removed from the needle, it can be processed in several ways. For biochemical assay, the muscle specimen is frozen in liquid nitrogen as rapidly as possible. Some researchers place the needle, with the muscle inside, immediately into liquid nitrogen to prevent the added delay in removing the muscle from the needle! If the specimen is to be used for histological preparations, the rapidity of freezing is less important (see below).

Freeze Drying vs. Wet Weight

When frozen, the muscle specimen can either be stored as is, or have the water content of the tissue removed by vacuum sublimation (freeze drying). If the muscle is left frozen in its raw form, it contains a large amount of water, which dilutes the concentration of metabolites. Conversely, freeze drying enables the water to be removed, increasing the concentration of metabolites, and thereby improving the ability to detect metabolites by enzymatic assays. The drawback to freeze drying is that metabolites are not in their true in vivo concentration; however, dividing metabolite concentrations expressed relative to muscle dry weight (e.g., mmol/kg dry wt) by 4.11 will give a concentration close to wet weight values (depending upon the change in tissue hydration).

FIGURE 5.19

An illustration of the biopsy needle, identifying the inner guillotine, window for muscle sampling, and attached suction device. The needle can come in several different sizes, with the size of the standard needle approximating the diameter and length of a lead pencil.

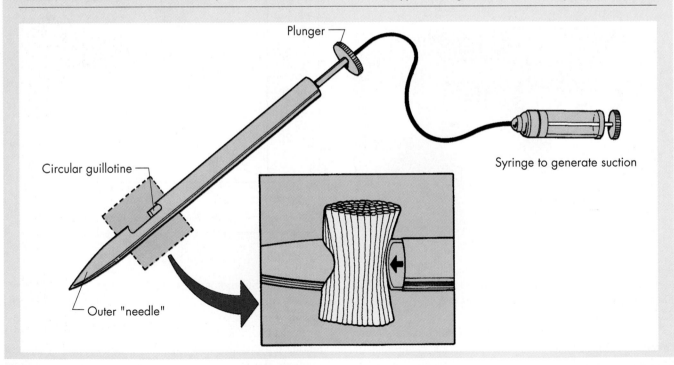

Plunger

Syringe to generate suction

Circular guillotine

Outer "needle"

Enzymatic Biochemistry

Muscle metabolites and enzyme activities are most frequently determined by first homogenizing the muscle in a solution containing buffers and electrolytes. For the assay of metabolites, a sample of this homogenate is then added to test tubes containing appropriate enzymes, substrates, and enzyme activators to induce reactions that will eventually increase the concentration of a suitable end product that can be measured via an indirect technique (usually NADH, which can be measured by spectrophotometry or fluorometry).

Histology

For histological preparation, the muscle specimen needs to be cleaned of excess blood and connective tissue, and then mounted within a special paste on a small platform (usually cork). The mounted specimen is then frozen slowly in an organic solvent (e.g., isopentane) to prevent damage to the specimen that occurs during rapid freezing, and is then stored in liquid nitrogen for later histological preparation.

Microscopically thin slices of frozen tissue are obtained in a *cryostat*. Serial sections of the tissue are then placed in solutions containing chemicals that specifically favor a given reaction, or selectively denature enzymes in given muscle fiber types. For example, the periodic acid-Schiff stain produces a pink color, with the color intensity being proportional to muscle carbohydrate (glycogen) (fig. 5.20b).

The myosin ATPase stain, if it involves a preincubation of the sections in an acid medium of pH = 4.3, denatures the myosin ATPase enzyme in fast-twitch muscle fibers and allows the following incubation and reactions to deposit cobalt in the slow-twitch fibers whose myosin ATPase is still active. This stains slow-twitch fibers black, and leaves fast-twitch fibers unstained (white) when viewed by light microscopy. A preincubation in a solution of pH = 10.3 will denature the myosin ATPase from slow-twitch muscle fibers, thus allowing subsequent incubations to stain the fast-twitch muscle fibers which have active myosin ATPase. Consequently, when preincubated at pH = 10.2, fast-twitch fibers stain black and slow-twitch fibers remain unstained. If the preincubation is at a moderately low pH (pH = 4.6), some muscle fibers that are classified as fast-twitch by either of the 4.3 or 10.3 preincubation procedures retain some myosin ATPase activity (fig. 5.20a). These fibers reveal a slight stain from the incubation and reactions that follow, and have been classified as fast-twitch oxidative (IIa or FOG) fibers.

FIGURE 5.20

Sections of skeletal muscle stained for *(a)* myosin ATPase activity after a preincubation pH of 4.6, and *(b)* carbohydrate content by the periodic acid Schiff (PAS) stain. The PAS stain section is from a post-exercise condition. The difference in stain intensity (glycogen content) for the muscle fibers is evident. For the ATPase stain section, there are multiple shades of staining for many fast-twitch fibers. Note, these are not serial sections.

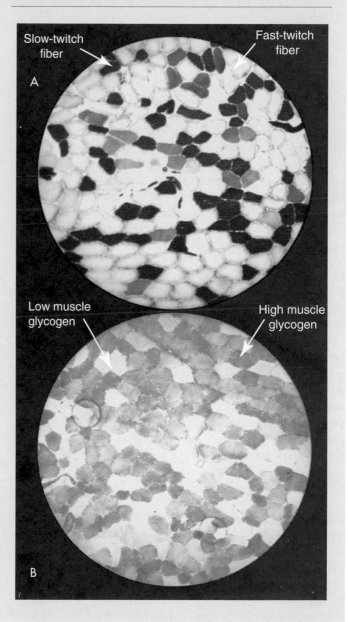

either glycolysis, β-oxidation, the TCA cycle, or the electron transport chain (16, 46). Researchers can also analyze whole muscle biopsy samples, and based on additional myosin AT-Pase fiber typing, compare enzyme activities among samples that have differing percentages of ST and FT muscle fibers. Another method is to histochemically assay sections of muscle biopsy samples for specific enyzme activities.

Based on single-fiber research, muscle fibers from the different motor units have distinctive enzymatic capacities that are best discriminated by the activity of mitochondrial enzymes, or by ratios of activities from enzymes of glycolytic versus mitochondrial pathways (60). When using histochemical methods to detect differences in the quantity of NADH in muscle fibers, SO fibers stain darkest and a progressive decrease in stain intensity occurs for the FOG and FG fibers.

Muscle Glycogen Stores   Muscle glycogen stores have been reported to be higher in FT than ST muscle fibers prior to exercise (47, 63, 69, 78, 79, 80). However, because of the recruitment order of motor units and the bias to ST muscle metabolism that would exist in daily locomotion requirements, this finding may be due to an activity-related lowering of muscle glycogen in ST muscle fibers rather than a difference in glycogen storage. This interpretation is understandable given the predominance of carbohydrate catabolism in skeletal muscle during both intense prolonged exercise and short-term intense exercise.

Capillary Density

Research on the density of capillaries in rodent skeletal muscle has revealed that within a muscle of homogenous fiber type, a greater capillary density is evident in slow-twitch compared to fast-twitch muscle. Because human muscle is heterogenous in fiber type, a similar investigation cannot be completed. Nevertheless, Anderson (3) studied the capillary density of human muscle relative to the area occupied by either of the fiber types. Greatest capillary density occurred around SO muscle fibers, and there was no difference in capillary density between FG and FOG muscle fibers. Consequently, even in human muscle with a heterogenous distribution of fiber types there appear to be *more capillaries surrounding SO muscle fibers*.

Fiber Type Proportions

The differences in biochemical capacities and myosin AT-Pase pH stability among the muscle fibers of differing motor units has enabled histochemical methods to become those predominantly used to determine motor unit proportions in human **muscle biopsy** samples (focus box 5.3) from skeletal muscle. However, as the myosin ATPase histochemical procedure involves only the muscle fiber component of the motor unit, the term **fiber type** has often replaced the more correct expressions SO, FOG, and FG *motor unit* proportions. This is unfortunate, as evidence exists to indicate that mus-

cle fibers have a greater potential for diversity than do the neural components of the entire motor unit. For example, at least eight different muscle fiber types based on the myosin ATPase stain have been shown (32) and, as will be discussed in later sections of this chapter, exercise training can alter the genetic function of skeletal muscle fibers resulting in the transcription of myosin light chains that typically occur in other fiber type subcategories (60). Consequently, changes in fiber type proportions may not reflect actual motor unit changes, and it remains unclear whether fiber type changes are more important than nerve changes for the function of motor units during exercise.

Sensory Functions

During rest and exercise conditions, neural functions of our body are continually operating to provide feedback to the CNS of the conditions experienced by our internal organs and peripheral tissues. The neural information is derived from specialized *sensory receptors* that convert a biochemical (e.g., reactions altered by light in retina of the eye), physical (e.g., temperature), or mechanical (joint movement) stimulus into an action potential that is propagated to the CNS. The main sensory receptors that function during exercise are listed in table 5.4. Of these, the receptors of importance to neuromuscular function are the muscle spindle, golgi tendon organ, and joint receptors.

General Function of Sensory Receptors

The function of receptors and their afferent nerves is to "inform" the CNS of changes in local conditions. To do this effectively, there must be a means to (1) detect these changes and (2) relay neural information of the magnitude of these changes.

The Receptor Potential   A given receptor has a specialized structure that enables a specific sensory stimulus (modality) to alter the membrane potential. The depolarization of the receptor membrane is called a *receptor potential*. As with the postsynaptic membrane, or the soma of a nerve, if the receptor potential exceeds a *threshold* value an action potential is generated and propagated toward the CNS.

The magnitude of the stimulus to a receptor is relayed to the CNS by the rate of action potentials leaving the receptor. *The greater the stimulus strength, the larger the receptor potential and, if above threshold, the greater the rate of action potentials leaving the receptor.*

The Muscle Spindle   During exercise, where many muscles are contracting during very complex movements, it is easy to overlook the complex interactions that must exist between nerves and muscle. In fact, the contraction of skeletal muscle is only one of several neuromuscular interactions during movement. During muscle contraction and the movement of the body, there is continual feedback by affferent nerves that

TABLE 5.4

The sensory receptors of the body most pertinent to exercise

RECEPTOR	FUNCTION DURING EXERCISE
Mechanoreceptors	
Muscle spindle	Smooth muscle contractions; kinesthesis
Golgi tendon organ	Prevention of muscle injury
Pacinian corpuscles	Pressure sensation
Joint receptors	↑ Ventilation rate
Free nerve endings	↑ Blood pressure and heart rate
Cochlea	Sound
Vestibular apparatus	Equilibrium and balance
Baroreceptors	Blood pressure and blood volume regulation
Atrial stretch receptors	Blood pressure and blood volume regulation
Thermoreceptors	
Cold receptors	Thermoregulation
Warm receptors	Thermoregulation
Electromagnetic receptors	
Rod and cone cells	Vision
Chemoreceptors	
Aortic and carotid bodies	Blood O_2 and CO_2 concentrations, ventilatory regulation
Osmoreceptors	Blood osmolality, fluid balance, kidney function, and blood volume regulation
CNS blood CO_2 sensors	Ventilatory regulation, blood acid-base regulation
Glucose receptors	Blood glucose regulation, carbohydrate metabolism

Source: Adapted from Guyton (35).

originate in receptors within skeletal muscle. The main skeletal muscle receptor of interest is the **muscle spindle**, which continually *allows neural information to be relayed back to the CNS of muscle stretch, muscle length, and the rate of change in muscle length*. These functions are a result of the anatomical arrangement between afferent and efferent nerves and the components of the muscle spindle (fig. 5.21).

The muscle spindle contains specialized muscle fibers, which are collectively termed *intrafusal fibers*. These fibers run parallel to the normal skeletal muscle fibers, which for the sake of clarity are termed *extrafusal fibers*. There are two types of intrafusal fibers, which are termed *nuclear bag* and *nuclear chain* fibers, and the typical spindle has several of each type, with the chain fiber being more numerous (12, 27, 35, 42).

The nuclear bag and chain fibers get their names from their anatomical appearances. Nuclear bag fibers are the larger of the two, and have multiple nuclei clustered centrally within the fiber. Nuclear chain fibers also have multiple nuclei, yet because of their smaller diameter the nuclei

are aligned in a single line, resembling a chain in the central region of the fiber. The intrafusal fibers also differ with regard to efferent and afferent nerve connections. The bag fiber has a Ia afferent nerve that encapsulates the central nuclear region. The multiple encapsulation of the Ia nerve around the bag fiber is termed an *annulospiral ending* (actually the origin or receptor of the afferent nerve). The chain fibers also have annulospiral Ia afferent nerve connections and, in addition, have group II afferent connections (flower spray endings) located distally and proximally to the central region of the fiber. The Ia afferent nerves have a greater conduction velocity than the group II afferents and therefore relay information faster to the CNS. Both the bag and chain fibers have γ efferent nerves innervating the distal and proximal ends of each fiber where the contractile proteins are located.

Functions of the Spindle   The muscle spindle is sensitive to static stretch, dynamic stretch, and to changes in muscle length, as described below.

Static Stretch   During static stretch the central regions of the bag and chain fibers are forcefully elongated and cause receptor potentials in the annulospiral and flower spray endings of the type Ia afferents of the bag and chain fibers and type II afferent nerves of the chain fibers. These action potentials are propagated back to the spinal cord, where they synapse directly to a type Aα motor nerve. This nerve innervates the stretched muscle, causing a contraction of the fibers innervated by the motor nerve. This stretch response is termed the *static stretch reflex* because it is performed at the spinal cord level without the involvement of the higher-level centers of the CNS. The static stretch reflex is maintained for as long as the muscle is stretched.

Dynamic Stretch   The neuromuscular response to dynamic stretch is slightly different from the static stretch reflex. A sudden stretch of a skeletal muscle induces a receptor potential solely in the type Ia annulospiral endings from the bag and chain fibers. The ensuing reflex is rapid, causing a forceful contraction of the stretched muscle, and is completed in a fraction of a second.

Changes in Muscle Length   During muscle contraction and relaxation there is a repeated increase and decrease in the length of the extrafusal fibers. If the muscle spindle is to remain effective in responding to changes in muscle length, at differing initial lengths, the spindle must also change length

muscle biopsy the procedure of removing a sample of skeletal muscle from an individual

fiber type a categorization of muscle fibers based on their enzymatic and metabolic characteristics

muscle spindle the sensory receptor within skeletal muscle that is sensitive to static and dynamic changes in muscle length

FIGURE 5.21

The skeletal muscle spindle. The muscle spindle is located parallel to the extrafusal fibers of a muscle. The spindle consists of several smaller, and relatively more specialized, intrafusal fibers which are encapsulated in a connective tissue sheath. As explained in the text, the differentiation between afferent and efferent nerve association in the intrafusal fibers is integral to the multiple functions of the spindle.

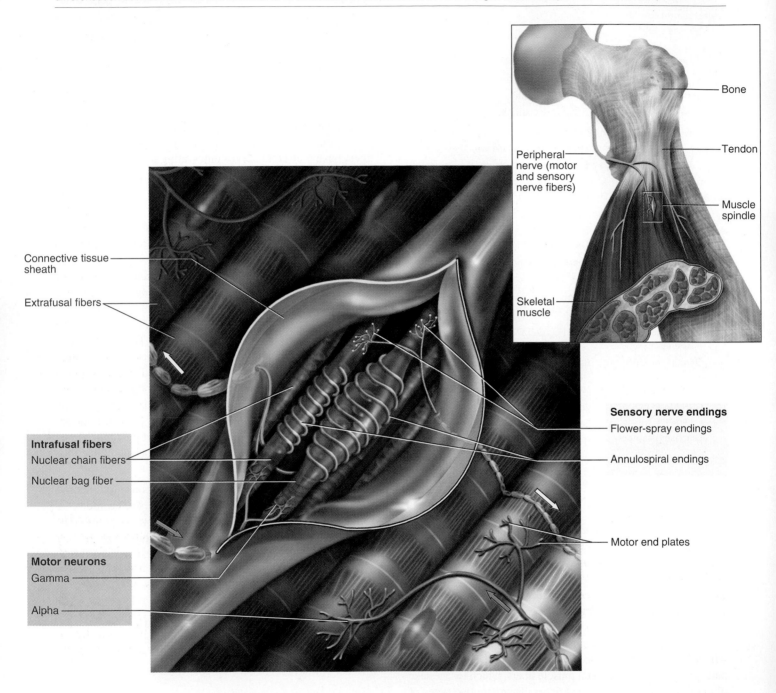

in concert with the extrafusal fibers. This does happen, and represents a very important additional function of the γ efferent nerves. When Aα nerves are stimulated, γ nerves are also stimulated so that the change in length of the intrafusal fibers matches that of the extrafusal fibers. This process is called **alpha-gamma coactivation**, and allows the spindle to be at near-optimal sensitivity regardless of the changing length of the extrafusal muscle fibers. Alpha-gamma coacti-

vation enables continual afferent feedback from the contracting muscle that informs the CNS of muscle length almost continually during a contraction. This dynamic sense has been termed *kinesthesis*, whereas the term *proprioception* is used to describe the general state of body awareness in the resting state. Our abilities of proprioception and kinesthesis are used in daily activities, as well as in exercise and athletic performance.

Other Muscle Receptors

As well as the muscle spindle, other receptors exist that connect to afferent nerves and the CNS. As the name implies, the *Golgi tendon organs* are located in the tendons of skeletal muscle. They are receptive to tension generated in the tendon during excessively strong muscle contractions, and action potentials are directed to the spinal cord by type Ib afferent nerves, where they synapse on an inhibitory interneuron, which then inhibits the respective Aα motor nerve(s).

Research has documented the existence of other muscle afferents that are probably either special mechanoreceptors or receptors sensitive to metabolites from metabolism, or both. Muscle contraction is known to elicit increases in cardiovascular parameters, such as heart rate and blood pressure, and to increase ventilation. These afferent nerves are believed to be type III and IV nerves, and therefore have a slower conduction velocity compared to the Ia and Ib nerves of the spindle and golgi tendon organ (35). These added receptors provide evidence for the role of nerves in orchestrating extremely rapid multisystemic responses to muscle contraction, and therefore partially account for how the body can rapidly adapt to exercise stress.

Neuromuscular Adaptations to Exercise

The Metabolic Contribution of Muscle Fiber Types during Exercise

The dissimilar metabolic capacities of muscle fibers from different motor units, combined with the recruitment transition of slow- to fast-twitch motor units during increases in exercise intensity, emphasize the need to interpret metabolic changes during and following exercise relative to the specific contributions from specific types of muscle fibers. Because of these facts, the following sections are structured to present research on specific contributions of fiber type to muscle metabolism relative to the intensity of exercise and specific metabolic pathways.

Steady-State Exercise and Intense Exercise

Glycogenolysis   During exercise at intensities that can be sustained for periods of time in excess of 30 min, research using serial muscle sections stained by the Periodic Acid Schiff (PAS) and myosin ATPase methods has revealed greater use of glycogen from SO compared to FG and FOG muscle fibers (30, 49, 69, 78). After 60 min of cycling at 43% VO_{2max}, muscle biopsy specimens sectioned and stained by the PAS procedure revealed that SO muscle fibers contributed 80% of the change in muscle glycogen, with the remainder due to FOG fiber recruitment. The FOG contribution to glycogen breakdown increased at 61% VO_{2max},

and at 91% VO_{2max} glycogen breakdown continued to occur in SO and FOG fibers, and also in FG fibers (78). In similar research of muscle glycogen changes during an active recovery at 40% VO_{2max}, muscle glycogen increased in FOG and FG muscle fibers, which were presumably not recruited during the low-intensity exercise (57). Collectively, this evidence is used to indirectly indicate preferential recruitment of SO motor units during low-intensity long-duration exercise.

The previous evidence does not mean that fast-twitch motor units are never recruited during low-intensity exercies. As muscle glycogen is depleted from SO muscle fibers and exercise is continued, FOG and FG motor units are recruited to allow for continued activity (78). However, the level of motor skill often diminishes during these conditions because the larger number of muscle fibers of the FOG and FG motor units decreases refinement in the gradations of contractile strength. In addition, as will be explained in chapter 6, decreases in muscle glycogen are associated with decreases in liver glycogen and blood glucose, which are conditions that invoke additional metabolic adaptations that decrease the ability to maintain relatively high steady-state exercise intensities.

Muscle Lactate Acccumulation   As will be discussed in chapter 6, during prolonged steady-state exercise, where slow-twitch motor unit recruitment predominates, minimal lactate is produced (45). However, as exercise intensity increases above the lactate threshold (see chapter 6) lactate production increases. Part of the cause for increased lactate production is the recruitment of fast-twitch glycolytic motor units (46).

Weight Lifting Exercises

Minimal research of fiber type specific glycogen depletion has occurred during weight lifting or **resistance exercise.** Nevertheless, data indicate that glycogenolysis occurs simultaneously and equally in slow- and fast-twitch fibers during maximal single-leg isokinetic leg extension exercise at 180°/s (7). This result is to be expected for such moderate-speed muscle contraction because of the involvement of all three motor unit types. However, animal research has shown that rapid muscle contraction can preferentially recruit fast-twitch motor units. Whether this is true for human voluntary exercise remains unclear.

---

alpha-gamma coactivation the interaction between alpha and gamma motor nerves and type I and II afferent nerves of skeletal muscle and muscle spindles that results in smooth and controlled dynamic muscle contractions

resistance exercise muscle contractions performed against a resistance, typically in the form of external loads like that used in weight lifting

Fiber Type Determinants of Exercise Performance

The metabolic and contractile differences between slow- and fast-twitch motor units can not only alter metabolic responses to exercise, but also influence exercise performance. For elite athletes, where muscle metabolic capacities are highly developed, motor unit proportions can set genetically based limitations to the magnitude of training adaptations.

Long-Term Endurance Exercise

A summary of research on human muscle fiber type proportions in elite athletes from different activities is presented in figure 5.22. Based on this compilation of cross-sectional data, the elite athletes who are involved in long-term activities, such as distance running, cycling, or swimming have predominantly SO muscle fibers in the muscles that contribute most to their respective exercise. Conversely, the proportion of FG and FOG muscle fibers predominate in athletes who have excelled in activities more reliant on muscle strength and power. These data are derived from genetically favored individuals and *should not be interpreted as evidence for muscle fiber type changes that are specific to the intensity and duration of exercise training* (see section, Training Adaptations).

Experimental evidence exists to provide a mechanistic association between fiber type proportions and exercise performance. For example, a high ST proportion in muscle causes a high mitochondrial capacity, a high capacity for oxygen consumption (45), a high lactate threshold (see chapter 6), and superior distance running and cycling performance (20, 45).

Short-Term Intense Exercise

A high FT proportion in muscle is accompanied by the continued ability to generate power at increasing contraction velocities (34, 77), and superior performance in explosive activities (19, 22, 34). It has often been accepted that such a bias toward FT proportions would favor all types of intense exercise; however, research exists to question this. Colliander and colleagues (19) investigated performance during three bouts of intense single-leg knee extensions performed at 180°/s, with each bout separated by 1 min of recovery. Individuals with high FT fiber type proportions generated greater *torque* than those with predominantly ST proportions during the first bout of contractions; however, torque was no different between groups for bouts two and three.

FIGURE 5.22

The proportions of ST and FT muscle fibers in elite athletes from different events. The more long term the activity, the greater is the proportion of ST muscle fibers in select muscles of the athletes.

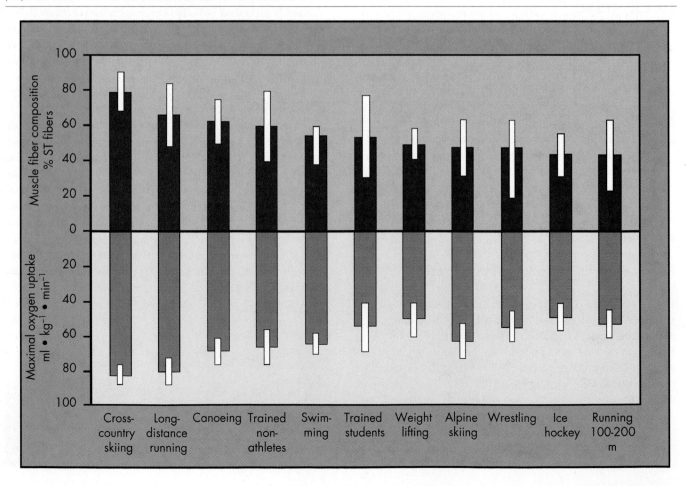

Individuals with greater ST fiber type proportions in their vastus lateralis had greater metabolic recovery between bouts. The results indicated that when multiple bouts of intense exercise are to be performed, ST muscle fibers are important for allowing recovery between bouts. Conversely, individuals with greater FT fiber proportions will probably perform better during single bouts of intense exercise, or if they are provided more recovery between successive bouts of intense exercise.

Weight Lifting Exercise

Research using isokinetic exercise equipment has provided added evidence for potential for varied fiber type proportions to influence strength and endurance exercise performance (34, 77). In this research design, muscle fiber type proportions determined from myosin ATPase staining for individuals are compared to the abilities of these individuals to contract their muscles to generate torque at different velocities of contraction. Figure 5.23 indicates that individuals with high FT fiber type proportions in the vastus lateralis can generate greater torque at contraction velocities between 90 and 300°/s (34). These results are similar for trained males and females (42). Interestingly, at low contraction velocities and isometric contractions, where force generation is greatest (see chapter 3), there is no difference in force generation between individuals with high ST or high FT fiber type proportions (34). These results suggest that individuals involved in powerful single-contraction events would benefit by having a

greater FT fiber type proportion in their active muscles. Conversely, for pure stength development, the fiber type proportion is less influential in determining performance.

Training Adaptations

The following sections will focus on how exercise training affects the additional characteristics of muscle fibers that are important in distinguishing their classification as SO, FOG, and FG fiber types. These characteristics are central nervous system activation and neuromuscular function, fiber size and number, myosin ATPase and myosin isozyme content, and capillary density. Specific comment and reference to different exercise intensities will be provided in each section.

Fiber Size and Number

The increase in size, or more specifically the cross-sectional area, of muscle fibers is termed **hypertrophy.** In endurance-trained individuals, the size of the SO muscle fibers can be larger than either of the FOG or FG muscle fibers (29), with considerable variation in size within a fiber type in the same muscle (15). These findings indicate some degree of selective hypertrophy of muscle fibers from different motor units, and is presumably a result of an increased mitochondrial and membranous mass and increased muscle filaments within the fibers.

During more intense exercise, such as sprinting or weight lifting, muscle hypertrophy is greater than for endurance activities (17, 23). The fiber type hypertrophy is not as selective as for endurance exercise, because all motor unit types are recruited in these activities (53).

Animal research has indicated the potential for muscle fibers to split and form new fibers during intense training (4). Although there are various animal models, those involving voluntary exercise, and therefore most similar to human exercise, have repeatedly reported increases in muscle fiber numbers from 5 to 15% after long-term resistance training (> 10 weeks) (33, 73). The increase in the number of muscle fibers is termed **hyperplasia**. It is unclear whether hyperplasia occurs from the splitting of existing fibers or the generation of new fibers.

Although there is no experimental evidence for hyperplasia in human muscle following training for long-term muscular endurance, Antonio and Gonyea (4) have very meticulously detailed the large body of indirect evidence for hyperplasia. When entire muscles have been obtained postmortem, comparison between left and right tibialis anterior muscles from previously healthy men revealed a 10%

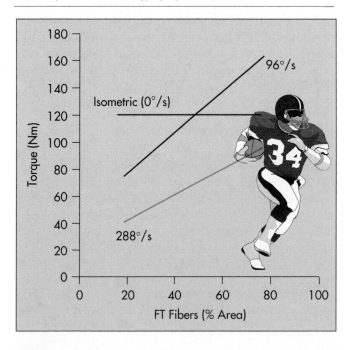

FIGURE 5.23

The difference in torque generation at different contraction velocities for individuals with different FT and ST muscle fiber type proportions. Individuals having higher FT muscle fiber proportions can generate greater torque at higher contraction velocities. However, maximal torque generation during isometric contractions is not dependent on fiber type proportions.

hypertrophy (hi-per'tro-fi) the increase in size of skeletal muscle due to the increased size of individual muscle fibers

hyperplasia (hi'per-pla'zi-ah) the increase in muscle fiber number in skeletal muscle

difference in fiber numbers (68). Research that has compared muscle fiber areas between hypertrophied trained athletes and sedentary controls has revealed no difference in fiber areas, yet large differences in muscle size (2, 48, 70, 74, 75, 76). However, a similar body of research exists that has shown the muscle fiber hypertrophy can account for differences in muscle cross-sectional area between trained and untrained individuals (36, 54, 61, 68).

The generally accepted interpretation of these findings is that *muscle fiber hypertrophy accounts for the largest increases in muscle cross-sectional area*, with a small contribution that may occur from hyperplasia.

Central Nervous System Activation, Neuromuscular Function, and Muscular Strength

Generally speaking, maximal force development during muscle contractions (muscular strength) is proportional to the cross-sectional area of skeletal muscle. Consequently, training that increases muscle mass will increase muscular strength. However, research indicates that muscular strength is not just dependent on muscle mass, as the neural components of motor unit recruitment are also important. For example, during the initial weeks of a strength-training program, muscular strength increases, yet there is no evidence of muscle hypertrophy. Results from research using isokinetic training and electromyography have indicated that such strength gains without changes in muscle size are because of alterations in motor unit recruitment (15, 22). The motor unit recruitment alterations involve an increase in the number of motor units recruited and the stimulation of these motor units in a manner that increases the number of motor units that are stimulated at the same time (more synchronous) (15, 22, 77).

The neural component of muscular strength is important because it explains why some individuals can generate large contractile forces without large muscles and, as previously explained, accounts for the initial strength gains during resistance training. Furthermore, the training findings indicate that the central nervous system can be trained to improve function (motor unit recruitment).

Research has also addressed the best way to train to optimize muscle strength gains. Greatest strength gains result from training using concentric and eccentric muscle actions (24, 37). It remains unclear why an eccentric component is needed to optimize muscular strength during concentric contractions. However, is has been theorized that the microscopic damage to skeletal muscle that occurs during the eccentric phases might further increase the cellular stimulus for muscular hypertrophy.

Myosin ATPase and Myosin Structures

Animal research has clearly documented the importance of neural activation and muscle contraction as determinants of the altered expression of myosin and myosin ATPase in skeletal muscle fiber types. Both nerve cross reinnervation and artificial electrical stimulation of motor nerves have been shown to reverse the metabolic and contractile profiles of muscle fibers (64). Connecting muscle fibers to an opposite motor nerve, or stimulating a nerve in the opposite frequency and intensity converts the muscle fibers to reflect the muscle normally innervated by the nerve and stimulation profile (64). However, these interventions are extreme and not reflective of voluntary activation of human motor units in patterns that reflect low-intensity or high-intensity muscle contractions.

In humans, exercise training for improvement in long-term muscular endurance, strength, or power lifting causes changes in the genetic expression of myosin ATPase, certain structural components of the myosin molecule (heavy and light chains), and the contractile function of myosin in select populations of muscle fibers (1). These changes result in altered contractile function that favor the specific demand of training. However, in human voluntary exercise training, these changes do not alter the basic proportions of slow- and fast-twitch muscle fibers. Rather, the relative proportions of the FG and FOG fiber types change so that endurance training increases the proportion of FT fibers that stain as FOG fibers (decreased FG fibers), whereas pure strength training may either increase (71) or decrease (1, 5, 54, 55) the proportion of muscle fibers that stain as FG fibers (decreased FOG).

Capillary Density

Exercise training for long-term muscular endurance also increases the number of capillaries per cross-sectional area of muscle. As previously mentioned, Anderson (3) documented a selective increase in capillary density around SO muscle fibers in human muscle samples that have a heterogenous distribution of fiber types. Exercise training for long-term endurance further increases capillary density, thus providing more potential for blood flow to and from the contracting muscle fibers. As these new capillaries cannot be totally associated with only SO muscle fibers, this adaptation also provides a more oxygen-rich microenvironment to certain FG and FOG fibers, thus further supporting the potential for increased capacities for mitochondrial respiration in these fibers.

Disuse Atrophy

During detraining, muscle mitochondrial metabolic capacities are lost at a fast rate and those of glycolysis remain unchanged or increase slightly (51, 52). However, alterations in fiber type proportions require more severe disuse, like forced bed rest and immobilization of a limb (e.g., limb casts) (52), or deinnervation (e.g., spinal cord injury) (53) (focus box 5.4). Generally, there is a shift in fiber type from SO to FOG to FG; however, the shift is not consistent in all muscles that are affected by the intervention (64, 65, 72). Increased activity can reverse this **atrophy** response, even by artificial electrical stimulation of the immoblized muscle(s) (55).

Making Paralyzed Muscle Contract Again

Individuals who suffer injury causing a complete break of their spinal cord experience many symptoms of impaired neuromuscular, cardiac, and pulmonary function. When concerned with skeletal muscle, the muscles that are now *deinnervated* from the injury experience severe wasting. Such wasting is aesthetically unappealing to the individual. Furthermore, a large loss of muscle, if retrained and used to assist in exercise, could increase the trainability of such individuals. The result of this would be to decrease the risk for developing risk factors for coronary artery disease, resulting in improved health and quality of life.

Research has been conducted within the last decade that has evaluated the results of artificial electrical stimulation on the paralyzed muscle of individuals with spinal cord injury (SCI).

Artificial Electrical Stimulation

Artificial electrical stimulation (AES) of skeletal muscle involves the placement of surface or needle electrodes on/in muscles of interest, and the stimulation of these muscles with a small electric current at predetermined intervals. This stimulation results in the synchronous contraction of all motor unit types, with the number of motor units recruited dependent on the strength (voltage) of the stimulation.

Researchers from Wayne State University in Detroit, Michigan, have further developed AES to enable individuals with complete spinal cord injury to perform cycle ergometry or walking by providing computer-controlled AES to several muscles. For example, correctly programmed AES to the quadraceps, hamstrings, and gluteal muscles can result in movement of the lower legs similar to voluntary cycling. Such use of AES has been termed computerized functional electrical stimulation (CFES) (fig. 5.24), and has enabled many individuals with complete spinal cord injury to once again experience the movement pattern of riding a bike.

Human Paralyzed Muscle Training by Electrical Stimulation

Denervated muscle eventually experiences a decrease in fiber number, and when histologically prepared have unusually large fiber cross-sectional areas with inconsistent myosin ATPase staining. Paralyzed muscle also experiences an increase in fast-twitch fiber type expression (55). Collectively, these alterations decrease the contractile function and endurance of the muscle, as indicated by the minimal endurance and strength capabilities of paralyzed muscle when initially exposed to artificial electrical stimulation (47).

AES and CFES have been shown to increase the endurance capacity of paralyzed muscle (47). When AES is used as a means of exercise training, there is an increase in slow-twitch muscle fiber type expression toward normal values, and associated increases in mitochondrial enzyme activity

(55). In addition, if multiple muscles are stimulated and therefore the muscle mass stimulated is large, there is a considerable production of lactate that can raise systemic blood lactate concentrations above 4 mmol/L even for extremely low exercise intensities (47).

Initial application of artificial electrical stimulation to paralyzed muscle causes eventual muscle fatigue and contractile failure within as little as 1 min, with the fatigue probably due to neuromuscular or intramuscular electrochemical impairment. However, when an individual with SCI is trained by CFES, muscle endurance increases dramatically, as does the person's ability to increase his or her peak heart rate and VO_2 during exercise (47).

FIGURE 5.24

An individual with spinal cord injury receiving computerized functional electrical stimulation (CFES) that enables her to perform cycle ergometry.

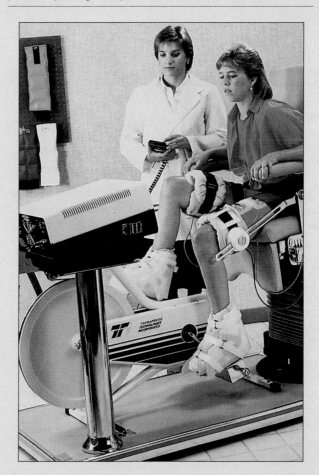

atrophy (a-tro'fi) the degeneration of muscle, often resulting in a decrease in size and functional capacities

WEBSITE BOX

Chapter 5: Neuromuscular Function and Adaptations to Exercise

The newest information regarding exercise physiology can be viewed at the following sites.*

yorku.ca/faculty/academic/ecaf/home/
Website of the neuromuscular physiology lab of York University, Canada.

http://savell-j.tamu.edu/muscontract.html
Events involved in the contraction of skeletal muscle.

http://ortho84-13.ucsd.edu/MusIntro/struct.html
Description of basic skeletal muscle structure and function.

http://ortho84-13.ucsd.edu/MusIntro/Jump.html
All you need to know about many topics on skeletal muscle structure, contraction, fiber types, metabolism, etc.

http://weber.u.washington.edu/~rlc/fes/
Introduction and explanation of functional electrical stimulation.

ptcentral.com/muscles/
The Hosford Muscle Tables: index site of information of the origin, insertion, action, blood supply, and innervation of every human skeletal muscle.

http://haiti.stanford.edu/~thu/MuscleHut.html#top
Detailed site from Stanford University detailing everything you need to know about skeletal, cardiac, and smooth muscle—anatomy, fiber types, etc.

http://education.vetmed.vt.edu/Education/curriculum/
VM8054/Labs/Lab10/Examples.exspindl.htm
Awesome histolotical color himage of a muscle spindle between skeletal muscle fibers. A detailed discussion of the spindle is also provided.

nwmissouri.edu/~0100064/KINCH6/sld001.htm
Powerpoint slide (14 slides) presentation of the biomechanical aspects of neuromuscular function.

http://anatomy.adam.com/mhc/top/003416.htm
Detailed site containing information of the numerous medical applications of the biopsy technique.

-----

*Unless indicated, all URLs preceded by http://www.

Note: These URLs were valid at the time of publication, but could have changed or been deleted from Internet access since that time.

SUMMARY

■ **Nerves**, like all excitable tissues, can generate a rapid change in their membrane potential, called an **action potential.** Action potentials are conducted along the **axon** of a nerve, and are transmitted from one nerve to another, or from a nerve to a target tissue/organ via a **synapse.**

■ Almost all the synapses of the body function by releasing a chemical substance from the *presynaptic membrane* that diffuses across the space between nerves, or *synaptic cleft*, where the chemical binds to special **receptors** on the *postsynaptic membrane*. Such chemicals are called **neurotransmitters.** All synapses function unidirectionally.

■ All the components of the motor control regions of the brain operate together in a complex manner that results in the controlled and precisely orchestrated series of action potentials that are propagated from the **motor cortex** or other regions to the appropriate Aα motor nerves of the spinal cord. The distribution of Aα motor nerves down the spinal cord is somewhat organized into a *segmental distribution*. The Aα motor nerves leave the spinal cord at a vertebral level that reflects the anatomical position of the skeletal muscle.

■ As for the synapse, the function of the **neuromuscular junction** is to transmit the action potential across a synaptic cleft. Unlike the synapse, the postsynaptic membrane is not a nerve but the sarcolemma of a skeletal muscle fiber.

■ The individual cells in each muscle type are referred to as muscle **fibers,** and the specialized excitable cell membrane of skeletal muscle fibers is called the **sarcolemma.** Striated muscle proteins are organized into subcellular structures called **myofibrils,** which extend along the length of the muscle fiber. The myofibrils are aligned beside each other resulting in a similar three-dimensional pattern of the contractile proteins within the entire fiber. Within a myofibril, the contractile proteins are arranged in units called **sarcomeres.**

■ The contractile proteins of the myofibrils differ in structure and function. **Myosin** is the largest of the proteins, is a two-stranded helical structure, and consists of two forms of myosin (light and heavy). In vivo the two heavy chains contain a hinged region, a linear end region, and two globular heads (S_1 *units*) at one end. The S_1 units contain the enzyme myosin ATPase. The activity of myosin ATPase is believed to be influenced by the myosin light chains. **Actin** is a globular protein (G-actin); however, in vivo it aggregates to form a two-stranded helical structure (F-actin). Associated with the F-actin is a rod-shaped molecule called **tropomyosin,** which exists as multiple strands, each of which associates with six or seven G-actin molecules along the length of the F-actin. At the end of each tropomyosin molecule is bound a **troponin** molecule, which is involved in the regulation of skeletal muscle contraction.

■ The muscle fibers and the Aα motor nerve that innervates them comprise what is called a **motor unit.** When stimulated, a motor unit responds by contracting maximally. Therefore, *the motor unit is the functional unit of muscle contraction.* Contraction of a skeletal muscle results from the combined contraction of many motor units.

■ Skeletal muscle can contract in a variety of ways. Contractions causing a change in muscle length are called *isotonic* contractions. When the muscle length shortens, the isotonic contraction is referred to as a **concentric** contraction. When the muscle length increases during contraction, the isotonic contraction is referred to as **eccentric.** Muscle contractions causing no change in muscle length are called **isometric** contractions. **Isokinetic** contractions are a special type of concentric contraction, where the velocity of muscle shortening remains constant (hence the term *isokinetic*).

■ The long contraction time and short stimulation time of skeletal muscle motor units provide opportunity for additional neural stimulation prior to the complete relaxation of the muscle or motor unit. In these circumstances, the force of the total muscle or motor unit twitch can increase with increased stimulation frequency and is called *summation.* As stimulation frequency increases, twitch tension also increases until a smooth maximal tension is reached, which is called *tetanus.*

■ The earlier attainment of a threshold membrane potential of the soma of the nerve of an SO motor unit than of either an FOG or FG motor unit results in a recruitment order of motor units. *SO motor units are recruited first during incremental exercise, followed by a progressive increase in FOG and FG motor unit recruitment as exercise intensity increases.* This pattern of recruitment has been termed the *size principle,* and causes SO motor units to be recruited predominantly during low to moderate exercise intensities, and SO, FOG, and FG motor units to be recruited during exercise requiring intense contractions against high resistance or fast muscle contractions.

■ **Electromyography (EMG)** is the study of muscle function from the detection of electrical activity eminating from the depolarization of nerves and muscle membranes that accompany contraction. The electrical activity is detected by the placement of one or more electrodes over the contracting muscle(s) of interest.

■ The contractile force of muscle within the different motor units increases in a progression from SO, to FOG, to FG motor units, and the duration of the contraction decreases in the progression from SO, to FOG, to FG motor units. Contractile velocity of motor units is determined by the conduction velocity of the Aα motor nerves and the type of myosin proteins and mysoin ATPase enzyme within the muscle fibers.

■ Skeletal muscle fibers from SO motor units have a high oxidative capacity. In other words, they possess relatively high concentrations of myoglobin, high mitochondrial membrane density and therefore relatively high concentrations of the enzymes of the TCA cycle, β-oxidation, and electron transport chain. The added myoglobin and mitochondria of SO muscle compared to FG muscle are the reasons for the "red" appearance and "white" appearance of the respective muscle types. Muscle fibers from FOG motor units have moderate concentrations of these molecules and enzymes, with muscle from FG motor units having the lowest concentrations.

■ The differences in biochemical capacities and myosin ATPase pH stability among the muscle fibers of differing motor units has enabled histochemical methods to become predominantly used to determine motor unit proportions in human **muscle biopsy** samples from skeletal muscle. However, as the myosin ATPase histochemical procedure involves only the muscle fiber component of the motor unit, the term **fiber type** has often replaced the more correct expressions SO, FOG, and FG motor unit proportions.

■ The main skeletal muscle receptor is the **muscle spindle,** which continually *allows neural information to be relayed back to the CNS of muscle stretch, muscle length, and the rate of change in muscle length.* These functions are a result of the anatomical arrangement between afferent and efferent nerves and the components of the muscle spindle. When Aα nerves are stimulated, γ nerves are also stimulated so that the change in length of the intrafusal fibers matches that of the extrafusal fibers. This process is called **alpha-gamma coactivation,** and allows the spindle to be at near-optimal sensitivity regardless of the changing length of the extrafusal muscle fibers.

■ During exercise at intensities that can be sustained for periods of time in excess of 30 min, there is greater use of glycogen from SO compared to FG and FOG muscle fibers. As muscle glycogen is depleted from SO muscle fibers and exercise is continued, FOG and FG motor units are recruited to allow for continued activity. During low-intensity exercise, where slow-twitch motor unit recruitment predominates, minimal lactate is produced.

■ Minimal research of fiber type specific glycogen depletion has occurred during weight lifting or **resistance exercise.** Nevertheless, data indicate that glycogenolysis occurs simultaneously and equally in slow- and fast-twitch fibers during maximal single-leg isokinetic leg extension exercise at 180°/s.

■ The increase in size, or more specifically the cross-sectional area, of muscle fibers is termed **hypertrophy.** The increase in the number of muscle fibers is termed **hyperplasia.** It is unclear whether hyperplasia occurs from

SUMMARY

the splitting of existing fibers or the generation of new fibers. *Muscle fiber hypertrophy accounts for the largest increases in muscle cross-sectional area*, with a small contribution that may occur from hyperplasia. Disuse of skeletal muscle causes a decrease, or **atrophy**, of muscle.

▪ In humans, exercise training for improvement in long-term muscular endurance, strength or power lifting results

in altered contractile function that favors the specific demands of training. However, in human voluntary exercise training, *these changes do not alter the basic proportions of slow- and fast-twitch muscle fibers*. Rather, endurance training increases the proportion of FT muscle that stains as FOG fibers, whereas strength/power training increases the proportion of muscle fibers that stain as FG fibers.

STUDY QUESTIONS

1. How can the nervous system be divided based on both structure and function?

2. Detail and sequence the molecular events of skeletal and cardiac muscle contraction.

3. Explain the differences among concentric, eccentric, and isokinetic muscle contractions.

4. How does the velocity of skeletal muscle contraction affect force and power development?

5. What are the functions of the muscle spindle?

6. What is a motor unit, how many different types are there, and how do they differ within and between different muscles of the body?

7. What is a fiber type, and how are they determined in research?

8. What is electromyography, and how has it been used in exercise-related research?

9. Can extremes in fiber type proportions influence an individual's potential for success in given types of exercise or sports competition? Explain.

10. What are the changes in muscle fiber type proportions that one should expect from training for either endurance or muscular power?

11. When muscles increase in cross-sectional area after resistance training, is the increase due to hypertrophy or hyperplasia?

12. What muscle fiber changes occur during severe disuse, like that of immobilization of a limb or deinnervation?

APPLICATIONS

1. During episodes of skeletal muscle cramp, relief is often promoted by immediate massage and the stretching of the muscle. Propose explanations for why these immediate treatment modalities might be effective.

2. Why do electrolyte imbalances in blood (Na^+, K^+, Ca^{++}) impair the ability of muscle to respond appropriately to neural stimulation?

3. What type of resistance (weight) training should athletes perform to induce the greatest adaptations in skeletal muscle, and thereby provide more optimal benefits to performance? Why?

4. How might the preferential decrease in muscle glycogen from SO muscle fibers influence performance during exercise lasting in excess of 2 hours?

REFERENCES

1. Abernethy, P. J., J. Jurimae, P. A. Logan, A. W. Taylor, and R. E. Thayer. Acute and chronic response of skeletal muscle to resistance exercise. *Sports Medicine* 17(1):22–38, 1994.

2. Alway, S. E., W. H. Grumbt, J. Stray-Gundersen, and W. J. Gonyea. Effects of resistance training on elbow flexors of highly competitive bodybuilders. *J. Appl. Physiol.* 72(4):1512–1521, 1992.

3. Anderson, P. Capillary density in skeletal muscle of man. *Acta Physiol. Scand.* 95:203–205, 1975.

4. Antonio, J. A., and W. J. Gonyea. Skeletal muscle fiber hyperplasia. *Med. Sci. Sports Exerc.* 25(12):1333–1345, 1993.

5. Baldwin, K. M., G. H. Klinkerfuss, R. L. Terjung, P. A. Mole, and J. O. Holloszy. Respiratory capacity of white, red, and intermediate muscle: Adaptive response to exercise. *Am. J. Physiol.* 222:373–378, 1972.

6. Basmajian, J. V., and C. J. DeLuca. *Muscles alive: Their functions revealed by electromyography,* 5th ed. Williams & Wilkins, Baltimore, 1985.

7. Bell, D. G., and I. Jacobs. Muscle fiber-specific glycogen utilization in strength-trained males and females. *Med. Sci. Sports Exerc.* 21(6):649–654, 1989.

8. Berne, R. M., and M. N. Levy. *Physiology*, 3rd ed. Mosby-Year Book, St. Louis, 1993.

9. Brooke, M. H., and K. Kaiser. Three "myosin adenosine triphosphatase" systems: The nature of their pH lability and sulfhydryl dependence. *J. Histochem. Cytochem.* 18:670–672, 1970.

10. Burke, R. E. Firing patterns of gastrocnemius motor units in the decerebrate cat. *J. Physiol.* 196:631–654, 1968.

11. Burke, R. E., D. N. Levine, P. Tsairis, and F. E. Zajac. Physiological types and histochemical profiles in motor units of the cat gastrocnemius. *J. Physiol. London* 234:723–748, 1973.

12. Burke, R. E., and V. R. Edgerton. Motor unit properties and selective involvement in movement. *Exerc. Sport Sci. Rev.* 3:31–81, 1975.

13. Burke, R. E. Motor units: Anatomy, physiology and functional organization. In V. B. Brooks (ed.), *Handbook of physiology: The nervous system*, Sect. 1, Vol. 11. The American Physiological Society, Bethesda, MD, 1981, pp. 345–422.

14. Byrnes, W. C., P. M. Clarkson, J. Spencer White, S. S. Hsieh, P. N. Frykman, and R. J. Maughan. Delayed onset muscle soreness following repeated bouts of downhill running. *J. Appl. Physiol.* 59:710–715, 1985.

15. Caiozzo, V. J., J. J. Perrine, and V. R. Edgerton. Training-induced alterations of the in vivo force-velocity relationship of human muscle. *J. Appl. Physiol.* 51(3):750–754, 1981.

16. Chi, M. M.-Y., et al. Effects of detraining on enzymes of energy metabolism in individual human muscle fibers. *Am. J. Physiol.* 244:C276–C287, 1983.

17. Clarke, D. H. Adaptations in strength and muscular endurance resulting from exercise. *Exerc. Sports Sci. Rev.* 1:73–102, 1973.

18. Clarkson, P. M., and I. Tremblay. Exercise-induced muscle damage, repair and adaptation in humans. *J. Appl. Physiol.* 65(1):1–6, 1988.

19. Collainder, E. B., G. A. Dudley, and P. A. Tesch. Skeletal muscle fiber composition and performance during repeated bouts of maximal, concentric contractions. *Eur. J. Appl. Physiol.* 58:81–86, 1988.

20. Costill, D. L., W. J. Fink, and M. L. Pollock. Muscle fiber composition and enzyme activities of elite distance runners. *Med. Sci. Sports Exerc.* 8(2):96–100, 1976.

21. Costill, D. L., D. D. Pascoe, W. J. Fink, R. A. Robergs, and S. I. Barr. Muscle glycogen resynthesis after eccentric exercise. *J. Appl. Physiol.* 69:46–50, 1990.

22. Coyle, E. F., et al. Specificity of power improvements through slow and fast isokinetic training. *J. Appl. Physiol.* 51(6):1437–1442, 1981.

23. Dons, B., K. Bollerup, F. Bonde-Peterses, and S. Hancke. The effect of weight lifting exercise related to muscle fiber composition and muscle cross-sectional area in humans. *Eur. J. Appl. Physiol.* 40:95–106, 1979.

24. Dudley, G. A., P. A. Tesch, B. J. Miller, and P. Buchanan. Importance of eccentric actions in performance adaptations to resistance training. *Aviation Space Environ. Med.* 62:543–550, 1991.

25. Essen, B., E. Jansson, J. Henriksson, A. W. Taylor, and B. Saltin. Metabolic characteristics of fiber types in human skeletal muscle. *Acta Physiol. Scand.* 95:153–165, 1975.

26. Evans, W. J., S. J. Phinney, and V. R. Young. Suction applied to muscle biopsy maximizes sample size. *Med. Sci. Sports Exerc.* 14:101–102, 1982.

27. Freund, H. J. Motor unit and muscle activity in voluntary motor control. *Physiol. Rev.* 63:387–436, 1983.

28. Garfinkel, S., and E. Cafarelli. Relative changes in maximal force, EMG, and muscle cross-sectional area after isometric training. *Med. Sci. Sports Exerc.* 24(11):1220–1227, 1992.

29. Gollnick, P. D., R. B. Armstrong, C. W. Saubert, K. Piehl, and B. Saltin. Enzyme activity and fiber composition in skeletal muscle of untrained and trained men. *J. Appl. Physiol.* 33(3):312–319, 1972.

30. Gollnick, P. D., K. Piehl, and B. Saltin. Selective glycogen depletion pattern in human skeletal muscle fibers after exercise of varying intensity and at varying pedal rates. *J. Physiol.* 241:45–57, 1974.

31. Gollnick, P. D., M. Reidy, J. J. Quintinskie, and L. A. Bertocci. Differences in metabolic potential of skeletal muscle fibers and their significance for metabolic control. *J. Exp. Biol.* 115:91–199, 1985.

32. Gollnick, P. D., and R. D. Hodgson. The identification of fiber types in human skeletal muscle: A continual dilemma. *Exercise. Sport Sciences Reviews.* 14:81–104, 1986.

33. Gonyea, W. J., D. G. Sale, F. B. Gonyca, and A. Mikesky. Exercise-induced increases in muscle fiber number. *Eur. J. Appl. Physiol.* 55:137–141, 1986.

34. Gregor, R. J., V. R. Edgerton, J. J. Perrine, D. S. Campion, and C. DeBus. Torque-velocity relationships and muscle fiber composition in elite female athletes. *J. Appl. Physiol.* 47(2):388–392, 1979.

35. Guyton, A. C. *Textbook of medical physiology,* 8th ed. Saunders, Philadelphia, 1991, chap. 8, pp. 87–95.

36. Haggmark, T., E. Jansson, and B. Svane. Cross-sectional area of the thigh muscle in man measured by computed tomography. *Scn. J. Clin. Lab. Invest.* 38:355–360, 1978.

37. Hather, B. M., P. A. Tesch, P. Buchanan, and G. A. Dudley. Influence of eccentric actions on skeletal muscle adaptations to resistance training. *Acta Physiol. Scand.* 143:177–185, 1991.

38. Henneman, E., G. Somjen, and D. O. Carpenter. Functional significance of cell size in spinal motor neurons. *J. Neurophysiol.* 28:560–580, 1965.

39. Henneman, E., G. Somjen, and D. O. Carpenter. Excitability and inhibitability of motor neurons of different sizes. *J. Neurophysiol.* 28:599–620, 1965.

40. Henneman, E., and L. M. Mendell. Functional organization of motorneurone pool and its inputs. In V. B. Brooks (ed.), *Handbook of physiology: The nervous system:* Sec. 1, Vol. 11. The American Physiological Society, Bethesda, MD, 1981, pp. 345–422.

41. Hortobagyi, T., and T. Denaham. Variability in creatine kinase: Methodological, exercise, and clinically related factors. *Int. J. Sports Med.* 10:69–80, 1989.

42. Hunt, C. C. Mammalian muscle spindle: Peripheral mechanisms. *Physiol. Rev.* 70(3):643–662, 1991.

REFERENCES

43. Huxley, H. E. Molecular basis of contraction in cross-striated muscle. In G. H. Bourke (ed.), *The structure and function of muscle:* Vol. 1, Part 1. Academic Press, New York, 1972, pp. 302–388.

44. Ishikawa, H., H. Sawada, and E. Yamada. Surface and internal morphology of skeletal muscle. In L. D. Peachey, R. H. Adrian, and S. R. Geiger (eds.), *Handbook of physiology: Sec. 10, Skeletal Muscle.* American Physiological Society, Bethesda, MD, 1983, pp. 1–22.

45. Ivy, J. L., R. T. Withers, P. J. Van Handel, D. H. Elger, and D. L. Costill. Muscle respiratory capacity and fiber type as determinants of the lactate threshold. *J. Appl. Physiol.* 48(3):523–527, 1980.

46. Ivy, J. L., M.M.-Y Chi, C. S. Hintz, W. M. Sherman, R. P. Hellendall, and O. H. Lowry. Progressive metabolite changes in individual human muscle fibers with increasing work rates. *Am. J. Physiol.* 252(21):C630–C639, 1987.

47. Kraus, J., et al. Cardiorespiratory effects of computerized functional electrical stimulation (CFES) and hybrid training in individuals with spinal cord injury. *Med. Sci. Sports Exerc.* 25(9):1054–1061, 1993.

48. Larsson, L., and P. A. Tesch. Motor unit fiber density in extremely hypertrophied skeletal muscles in man. *Eur. J. Appl. Physiol.* 55:130–136, 1986.

49. Lesmes, G. R., D. W. Benham, D. L. Costill, and W. J. Fink. Glycogen utilization in fast- and slow-twitch muscle fibers during maximal isokinetic exercise. *Ann. Sports Med.* 1:105–108, 1983.

50. Lowey, S., and D. Risby. Light chains from fast and slow muscle myosins. *Nature* 234:81–85, 1971.

51. MacDougall, J. D., G. R. Ward, D. G. Sale, and J. R. Sutton. Biochemical adaptation of human skeletal muscle to heavy resistance training and immobilization. *J. Appl. Physiol.* 43:700–703, 1977.

52. MacDougall, J. D., E. C. B. Elder, D. G. Sale, J. R. Moroz, and J. R. Sutton. Effects of strength training and immobilization on human muscle fibers. *Eur. J. Appl. Physiol.* 43:25–34, 1980.

53. MacDougall, J. D., D. G. Sale, E. C. B. Elder, and J. R. Sutton. Muscle ultrastructural characteristics of elite power lifters and body builders. *Eur. J. Appl. Physiol.* 48:117–126, 1982.

54. MacDougall, J. D., D. G. Sale, S. E. Elway, and J. R. Sutton. Muscle fiber number in biceps brachia in body builders and control subjects. *J. Appl. Physiol.* 57:1399–1403, 1984.

55. Martin, T. P., R. B. Stein, P. H. Hoeppner, and D. C. Reid. Influence of electrical stimulation on the morphological and metabolic properties of paralyzed muscle. *J. Appl. Physiol.* 72(4):1401–1406, 1992.

56. Narici, M., G. Roi, L. Landoni, M. Minetti, and P. Cerretelli. Changes in force, cross-sectional area, and neural activation during strength training and detraining of the human quadriceps. *Eur. J. Appl. Physiol.* 59:310–319, 1989.

57. Nordheim, K., and N. K. Vollestad. Glycogen and lactate metabolism during low-intensity exercise in man. *Acta Physiol. Scand.* 139:475–484, 1990.

58. Pate, E., and R. Cooke. A model of crossbridge action: The effects of ATP, ADP, and Pi. *J. Muscle Res. Cell Motility* 10:181–196, 1989.

59. Peter, J. B., R. J. Barnard, V. R. Edgerton, C. A. Gillespie, and K. E. Stempel. Metabolic profiles of three types of skeletal muscle in guinea pigs and rabbits. *Biochemistry* 11:2627–2633, 1972.

60. Pette, D., and R. S. Staron. Cellular and molecular diversities of mammalian skeletal muscle fibers. *Rev. Physiol. Biochem. Pharmacol.* 116:2–76, 1990.

61. Prince, F. P., R. S. Hikida, and F. C. Hagerman. Human muscle fiber types in power lifters, distance runners and untrained subjects. *Pflugers Archives* 363:19–26, 1976.

62. Raven, P. B. Editorial. *Med. Sci. Sports Exerc.* 23(7):777–778, 1991.

63. Robergs, R. A., et al. Muscle glycogenolysis during differing intensities of weight-resistance exercise. *J. Appl. Physiol.* 70(4):1700–1706, 1991.

64. Roy, R. R., K. M. Baldwin, and V. R. Edgerton. The plasticity of skeletal muscle: Effects of neuromuscular activity. *Exercise and Sport Sciences Reviews* 19:269–312, 1991.

65. Sale, D. G. Influence of exercise and training on motor unit activation. *Exerc. Sport Sci. Rev.* 15:95–151, 1987.

66. Saltin, B., J. Henriksson, E. Nygaard, and P. Anderson. Fiber types and metabolic potentials of skeletal muscles in sedentary man and endurance runners. *Annals New York Acad. of Sci.* 301:3–29, 1977.

67. Saltin, B., and P. D. Gollnick. Skeletal muscle adaptability: Significance for metabolism and performance. In *Handbook of physiology: Sec. 10, Skeletal muscle.* American Physiological Society, Bethesda, MD, 1983, pp. 555–631.

68. Schantz, P., E. Randall Fox, P. Norgen, and A. Tyden. The relationship between muscle fiber area and the muscle cross-sectional area of the thigh in subjects with large differences in thigh girth. *Acta Physiol. Scand.* 113:537–539, 1981.

69. Secher, N. H., and N. E. Jenssen. Glycogen depletion patterns in type I, IIA, and IIB muscle fibers during maximal voluntary static and dynamic exercise. *Acta Physiol. Scand.* (Suppl. 440):174–181, 1976.

70. Sjostrom, M., J. Lexell, A. Eriksson, and C. C. Taylor. Evidence of fiber hyperplasia in human skeletal muscles from healthy young men? *Eur. J. Appl. Physiol.* 62:301–304, 1992.

71. Staron, R. S., E. S. Malicky, M. J. Leonardi, J. E. Falkel, F. C. Hagerman, and G. A. Dudley. Muscle hypertrophy and fast fiber type conversions in heavy resistance-trained women. *Eur. J. Appl. Physiol.* 60:71–79, 1990.

72. Stephens, J. A., and T. P. Usherwood. The mechanical properties of human motor units with special reference to their fatigabililty and recruitment threshold. *Brain Research* 125:91–97, 1977.

73. Tamaki, T., S. Uchiyama, and S. Nakano. A weight-lifting exercise model for inducing hypertrophy in the hindlimb muscles of rats. *Med. Sci. Sports Exerc.* 24:881–886, 1992.

74. Tesch, P. A., A. Thorsson, and P. Kaiser. Muscle capillary supply and fiber type characteristics in weight and power lifters. *J. Appl. Physiol.* 56(1):35–38, 1984.

75. Tesch, P. A., and L. Larsson. Muscle hypertrophy in body builders. *Eur. J. Appl. Physiol.* 49:301–306, 1984.

76. Tesch, P. A., A. Thorsson, and P. Kaiser. Muscle capillary supply and fiber type characteristics in weight and power lifters. *J. Appl. Physiol.* 56(1):35–38, 1984.

77. Thorstensson, A., G. Grimby, and J. Karlsson. Force-velocity relations and fiber composition in human knee extensor muscles. *J. Appl. Physiol.* 40(1):12–16, 1976.

78. Vollestad, N. K., O. Vaage, and L. Hermansen. Muscle glycogen depletion pattern in type I and subgroups of type II fibers during prolonged severe exercise. *Acta Physiol. Scand.* 122:433–440, 1984.

79. Vollestad, N. K., and P. C. S. Blom. Effect of varying exercise intensity on glycogen depletion in human muscle fibers. *Acta Physiol. Scand.* 125:395–405, 1985.

80. Vollestad, N. K., P. C. S. Blom, and O. Gronnerod. Resynthesis of glycogen in different muscle fiber types after prolonged exhaustive exercise in man. *Acta Physiol. Scand.* 137:15–21, 1989.

81. Wang, K. Sarcomere-associate cytoskeletal lattices in striated muscle. In J.W. Shay (ed.), *Cell muscle motility:* Vol. 6. Plenum, New York, 1985, pp. 315–369.

82. Westing, S. H., and Y. Segar. Eccentric and concentric torque-velocity characteristics, torque output comparisons and gravity effect torque corrections for quadriceps and hamstring muscles in females. *Int. J. Sports Med.* 10:175–180, 1989.

83. Young, O. A. A possible role for myosin light chain 1 slow of bovine muscle. *J. Muscle Res. Cell Motility* 10:403–412, 1989.

RECOMMENDED READINGS

Antonio, J. A., and W. J. Gonyea. Skeletal muscle fiber hyperplasia. *Med. Sci. Sports Exerc.* 25(12):1333–1345, 1993.

Clarkson, P. M., and I. Tremblay. Exercise-induced muscle damage, repair and adaptation in humans. *J. Appl. Physiol.* 65(1):1–6, 1988.

Coyle, E. F., et al. Specificity of power improvements through slow and fast isokinetic training. *J. Appl. Physiol.* 51(6):1437–1442, 1981.

Gollnick, P. D., and R. D. Hodgson. The identification of fiber types in human skeletal muscle: A continual dilemma. *Exec. Sport Sci. Rev.* 14:81–104, 1986.

Gollnick, P. D., M. Reidy, J. J. Quintinskie, and L. A. Bertocci. Differences in metabolic potential of skeletal muscle fibers and their significance for metabolic control. *J. Exp. Biol.* 115:91–199, 1985.

Hortobagyi, T., and T. Denaham. Variability in creatine kinase: Methodological, exercise, and clinically related factors. *Int. J. Sports Med.* 10:69–80, 1989.

Hunt, C. C. Mammalian muscle spindle: Peripheral mechanisms. *Physiol. Rev.* 70(3):643–662, 1991.

Kraus, J., et al. Cardiorespiratory effects of computerized functional electrical stimulation (CFES) and hybrid training in individuals with spinal cord injury. *Med. Sci. Sports Exerc.* 25(9):1054–1061, 1993.

Martin, T. P., R. B. Stein, P. H. Hoeppner, and D. C. Reid. Influence of electrical stimulation on the morphological and metabolic properties of paralyzed muscle. *J. Appl. Physiol.* 72(4):1401–1406, 1992.

Peter, J. B., R. J. Barnard, V. R. Edgerton, C. A. Gillespie, and K. E. Stempel. Metabolic profiles of three types of skeletal muscle in guinea pigs and rabbits. *Biochemistry* 11:2627–2633, 1972.

Thorstensson, A., G. Grimby, and J. Karlsson. Force-velocity relations and fiber composition in human knee extensor muscles. *J. Appl. Physiol.* 40(1):12–16, 1976.

Vollestad, N. K., O. Vaage, and L. Hermansen. Muscle glycogen depletion pattern in type I and subgroups of type II fibers during prolonged severe exercise. *Acta Physiol. Scand.* 122:433–440, 1984.

CHAPTER 6

Metabolic Adaptations to Exercise

uring the muscle contractions that accompany exercise or physical activity, ATP (adenosine triphosphate) must be replaced at a rate that is as close as possible to the rate of ATP hydrolysis. If this does not occur, muscle ATP will decline, skeletal muscle fatigue will develop, and exercise will have to stop or be performed at a lower intensity. The need to replenish muscle ATP during muscle contraction reveals the importance of the chemical reactions that exist to regenerate ATP, as was discussed in chapter 3. Exercise is therefore useful to research how skeletal muscle metabolism is regulated so that muscle fibers can tolerate transitions from rest to exercise; a change that can increase the demand for ATP regeneration more than 100-fold. The immediate changes, or *acute adaptations,* that occur in muscle biochemistry during muscle contraction are classic examples of the responsiveness of skeletal muscle to metabolic stress. Furthermore, skeletal muscle that is routinely exposed to exercise stress can develop changes that are retained for more prolonged periods of time, or *chronic adaptations.* Chronic adaptations typically function to decrease the stress associated with exercise. The purpose of this chapter is to present information that reveals the acute changes that occur in muscle metabolism to meet the muscles' needs to increase the regeneration of ATP, and the chronic adaptations that improve the muscles' abilities to regenerate ATP during exercise. In addition, important concepts used in the study of the metabolic response to exercise will be identified.

OBJECTIVES

After studying this chapter, you should be able to:

- Describe the metabolic implications of a range of exercise intensities when expressed relative to VO_{2max} or the lactate threshold.
- Identify how incremental, steady-state, and intense exercise affect the multiple catabolic pathways of energy metabolism: creatine phosphate, glycolysis, mitcohondrial respiration.
- Describe how to measure VO_{2max}, and how exercise can be quantified relative to VO_{2max}.
- Identify the factors that may cause a muscle and blood lactate threshold during incremental exercise.
- Describe the metabolic events that occur during the recovery from different exercise intensities.
- Explain how skeletal muscle metabolism adapts chronically to repeated exposures to short term and long-term endurance exercise.
- Explain how chronic muscle metabolic adaptations are specific to the type of metabolic pathway stressed during exercise, and to a lesser extent the type of exercise performed.

KEY TERMS

acute adaptations	lactate threshold (LT)	chronic adaptations
incremental exercise	acidosis	buffering capacity
maximal oxygen consumption (VO_{2max})	redox potential	
	oxygen deficit	
phosphorus magnetic resonance spectroscopy (^{31}P MRS)	anaerobic capacity	
	excess postexercise oxygen consumption (EPOC)	

Acute Adaptations

*T*he reactions involved in increasing muscle metabolism during exercise, and altering muscle metabolism in the recovery from exercise, are termed **acute adaptations**. During exercise, catabolic reactions within skeletal muscle are stimulated to release the free energy required to regenerate the ATP used to fuel muscle contraction. Figure 6.1 expresses the connection between exercise duration (intensity) and the predominance of a certain catabolic pathway. Figure 6.1 applies to maximal exercise performed to fatigue, such that if fatigue occurs at 30 s, most of the ATP would be regenerated from creatine phosphate hydrolysis. Exercise causing fatigue after 2 min would mainly rely on ATP from glycolysis, whereas exercise performed in excess of 3 min would rely more on ATP from mitochondrial respiration. The illustration should not be interpreted to indicate that creatine phosphate is used only in the first 30 s of exercise, that glycolysis then follows, with mitochondrial respiration being important only after 3 min. As will be discussed in this chapter, creatine phosphate has important biochemical functions even during long-duration exercise, and *muscle glycogenolysis, glycolysis and mitochondrial respiration are stimulated almost immediately when muscle contraction begins.*

During the recovery after exercise, both catabolic and anabolic reactions occur to replenish the energy stores used during exercise, and to recover from such things as acidosis, muscle damage, and local disturbances in fluid and electrolyte balances. The processes that occur in skeletal muscle in the recovery from exercise are also examples of acute adaptations to exercise.

Because of the importance of exercise intensity and duration to the skeletal muscle metabolic response to exercise, and whether the condition is exercise or recovery, information of how skeletal muscle adapts to exercise will be organized in sections concerning the type of adaptation, the nature of the exercise, and the type of recovery from exercise.

Adaptations During Exercise

Incremental Exercise

Incremental exercise involves the increase in exercise intensity over time. Other names for this type of exercise are "progressive" or "graded." Incremental exercise protocols can be either continuous, where successive increases in intensity occur without rest periods, or intermittent, where a rest period is provided between increments. In addition, incremental protocols can be maximal, requiring the subject to exercise against increasing intensities until volitional fatigue, or submaximal, when exercise is terminated at a predetermined intensity prior to volitional fatigue. Incremental exercise protocols can also vary in the duration of each specific intensity (stage), and the magnitude of the increment. In addition, protocols exist that continuously increase intensity over time (speed and/or grade on a

> **acute adaptations** changes in body structure and function during or immediately following exercise stress
>
> **incremental exercise** exercise performed at intensities that progressively increase over time

---

FIGURE 6.1

The relationships between exercise duration during exhaustive exercise and the contribution of the creatine phosphate, glycolytic, and mitochondrial respiration pathways of ATP regeneration.

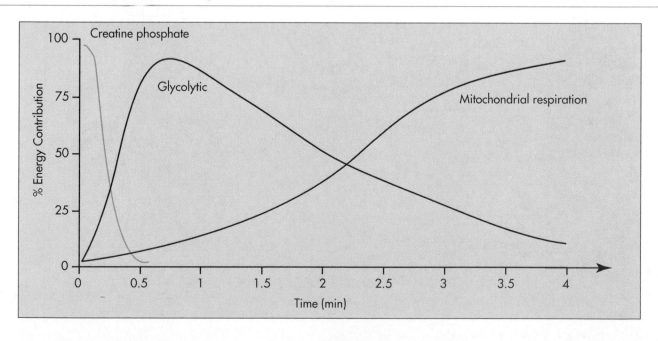

treadmill, and resistance on a cycle ergometer), and these are termed *ramp protocols*.

Maximal Oxygen Consumption   Maximal oxygen consumption (VO_{2max}) is the maximal rate at which the body can consume oxygen during exercise. Traditionally, VO_{2max} is verified when it coincides with a plateau in VO_2 despite further increases in intensity, an RER (respiratory exchange ratio) that exceeds 1.1 (30, 54, 60), and a maximal heart rate within ± 10 b/min from predicted (220 – age) (60). A true VO_{2max} is most likely to be attained in healthy, moderately to highly endurance-trained individuals, and when using a protocol duration between 8 to 12 min (19, 60, 100). Students should read the excellent review by Howley and associates (60) on the experimental criteria needed for accurately measuring VO_{2max}. As exercise intensities are often expressed relative to VO_{2max}, this measure must be understood prior to discussing energy metabolism during both steady-state and intense exercise conditions.

Figure 6.2 presents the change in VO_2 during two different protocols (ramp and 50W increment, 3-min stage) for the same individual using breath-by-breath indirect calorimetry. The ramp protocol increased VO_2 in a smooth linear manner to the plateau at VO_{2max}; however, during the initial stages, the 3-min stage protocol induced a "staircase" effect in the increase in VO_2. This effect makes it difficult to plot and interpret changes in metabolism over time during incremental protocols; however, it provides close to steady-state VO_2 values for the lower exercise intensities, which may be useful for computing economy. Given that the duration of a test of VO_{2max} should be between 8 to 12 min, and should progressively increase intensity, there is merit in devising protocols that are specific to given individuals. In this way, there is more certainty that the protocol will cause a person to attain VO_{2max} rather than a submaximal peak VO_2 response.

Units of Expression of VO_{2max} VO_{2max} values can be expressed as an absolute volume of oxygen per unit time (L/min), or relative to body mass (mL/kg/min). Typically, the absolute expression is used for exercise modes where body weight is externally supported (e.g., cycling), and the relative expression is used for exercise modes where body weight is

---

FIGURE 6.2

During incremental exercise, VO_2 increases in a manner that is dependent on the type of protocol used. The triangles show the linear increase in VO_2 during cycle ergometry using a ramp protocol (see text). During a 50 W incremental protocol, with 3-min stage durations, VO_2 increases to near-steady-state values at each stage during the early part of the test, revealing a "staircase" effect as shown with the squares. During the last half of the test, the intensity increment and absolute intensity are too great for a steady state to be attained, and VO_2 increases more linearly to VO_{2max}.

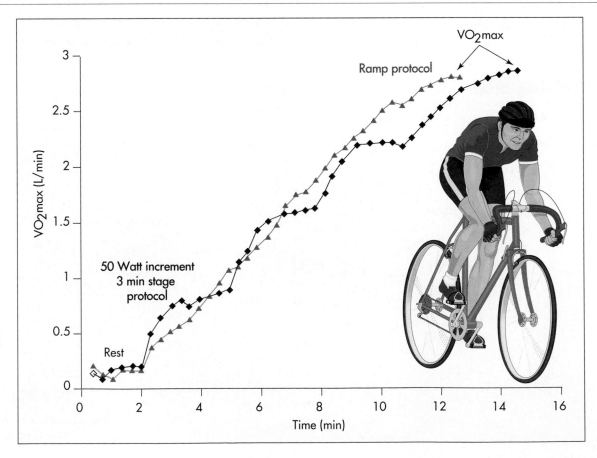

supported by the individual and therefore contributes to the intensity of the exercise (e.g., running). However, there is considerable evidence that a better relative expression of VO_{2max} is to adjust body mass to the power of 0.75, rather than absolute body mass (124). This recommendation is based on the fact that the variation in VO_2 for a given exercise intensity is in direct proportion not to body mass but to body mass$^{0.75}$. However, this expression of submaximal VO_2 or VO_{2max} is not yet widely used in research, clinical, or fitness assessment applications of exercise physiology.

For comparing VO_{2max} values between genders, the relative expression of VO_{2max} should use lean body mass (LBM – kg) rather than body mass (kg) (125), because of the lower LBM of women compared to men of equal total body mass.

Individual Variation in VO_{2max} VO_{2max} values are dispersed between extremely low capacities, like those of chronically ill individuals (< 20 mL/kg/min), and the capacities of well-trained and elite endurance athletes (> 80 mL/kg/min) (fig. 6.3). The factors that combine to influence VO_{2max} are a high proportion of slow-twitch motor units, high central and peripheral cardiovascular capacities, and the quality and duration of training. Having more slow-twitch muscle fibers increases the oxidative capacity of the muscle (66). As discussed in chapter 5, muscle motor unit proportions are genetically determined and, therefore, a person's abilities to respond to endurance training and increase VO_{2max} have genetic constraints.

VO_{2max} During Different Exercise Modes VO_{2max} is known to differ depending upon the type of exercise and the type and extent of training performed by the individual. Figure 6.4 provides a comparison between VO_{2max} obtained from a treadmill run protocol and that obtained from step-test, cycle ergometry, arm ergometry, and swimming incremental protocols. Generally, VO_{2max} is greatest during running and stepping and lowest during arm ergometry. The reason for these differences is believed to be due to muscle mass, as a larger muscle mass is exercised during running, and a relatively small muscle mass is exercised during arm ergometry (30). However, when comparing cycling and treadmill running, VO_{2max} values have been shown to be greatest in the trained exercise mode, with cycling VO_{2max} equal to or greater than treadmill VO_{2max} in well-trained cyclists (35).

> **maximal oxygen consumption (VO_{2max})** the maximal rate of oxygen consumption by the body

---

FIGURE 6.3

The variation in VO_{2max} for individuals that range in functional capacity from the chronically ill, to elite cross-country skiers. These differences are not totally explained by training, as the genetic determinants of VO_{2max} include motor unit and central cardiovascular capacities that provide a foundation of genetic potential that will determine the magnitude of training improvement.

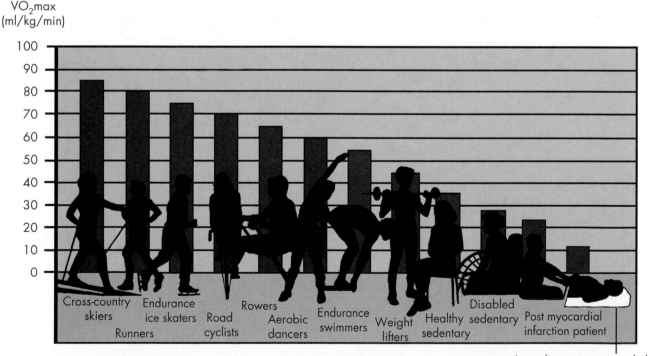

VO_2max (ml/kg/min)

FIGURE 6.4

A comparison between VO_{2max} obtained for a given individual during different exercise modes. The VO_{2max} values are expressed relative to treadmill run VO_{2max}, which represents the zero value of the *y*-axis. The changes for relatively untrained individuals is provided, with values for individuals highly trained in one exercise mode also provided.

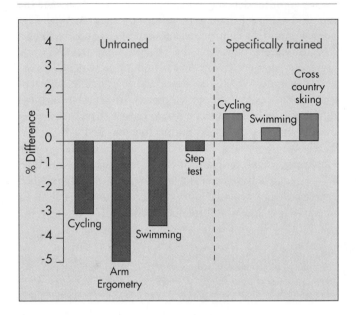

Despite the association between increasing VO_{2max} and the size of the muscle mass exercised, the actual relationship is not linear but an "inverted U" (∩) (fig. 6.5). Adding increased work by the upper-body to lower-body exercise will eventually result in a decrease in VO_{2max} because of cardiovascular limitations to "maximal" muscle blood flow (see chapter 7).

Is There a Controversy over the Measurement and Use of VO2max?

There has been recent interest in whether the traditional interpretations of a plateau in VO_2 during incremental exercise is valid (9, 94–96, 108). Since the initial work on the VO_{2max} concept by Hill and Lupton in 1923 (56), it has been generally accepted that the plateau in VO_2 during incremental exercise to volitional exhaustion represents the inability of the body's cardiovascular system to provide sufficient oxygen to the working muscles (see chapter 7). This assumption has resulted in the interpretation of VO_{2max} to represent the body's maximal cardiorespiratory capacity, or "maximal aerobic power."

The main criticism of the VO_{2max} concept is that a true plateau in VO_2 during incremental exercise has only been shown in 30 to 50% of tests conducted on healthy subjects (85). This incidence decreases dramatically when testing individuals who are sedentary, diseased, or disabled (108). Noakes (94–96) has argued that VO_{2max} must not really be a true maximal value, but the end result of not central limitations to oxygen delivery, but limitations in oxygen use by the contracting muscles. Bassett and Howley (9) have argued against this notion.

FIGURE 6.5

VO_{2max} initially increases with an increase in the muscle mass exercised. However, after an optimal muscle mass, further increases in the exercised muscle mass cause decreases in VO_{2max}, as explained in the text.

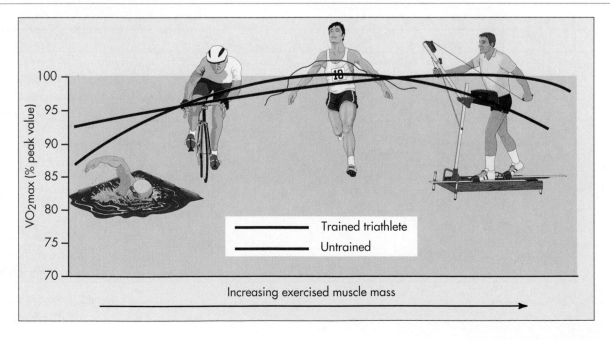

Robergs (108) responded to the debate on the validity of VO_{2max} by providing another review of the topic, and revealed that the VO_{2max} concept is valid, but that it is difficult to accurately measure in all individuals. Just because a cardiovascular limitation to VO_2 may not occur in all individuals does not mean that it does not exist. Clearly, in individuals that will have difficulty in exercising to true volitional fatigue caused by cardiovascular limitations to oxygen consumption, the expression VO_{2max} should be replaced with VO_{2peak} (108). If the two main criteria for the attainment of a VO_{2max} are not met (plateau and RER > 1.1), then the term VO_{2peak} should be used. Once again, the individuals who are more likely to attain a VO_{2peak} rather than VO_{2max} are:

- Prepubescent children
- Sedentary individuals (including the elderly)
- Individuals with acute illness (cold, flu, exercise-induced bronchoconstriction, asthma, etc.)
- Individuals with disease (cardiovascular diseases, muscle diseases, etc.)

FIGURE 6.6

The radiofrequency data received from the surface coil during ³¹P MRS of the forearm. *(a)* The raw radiofrequency signal from rest, referred to as a free induction decay (FID). *(b)* After FID has been Fourier Transformed it is converted to a spectrum revealing the intensity of signal of separate ₃₁P-containing molecules, and the signal frequency difference between each molecule.

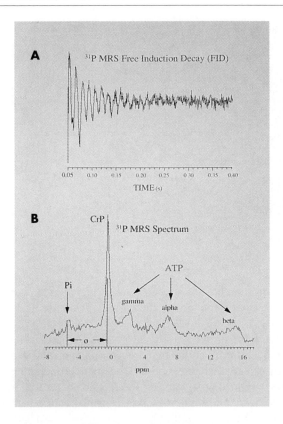

For a complete and interesting review of the more advanced issues of this topic, students should read the publications of Bassett and Howley (9), Noakes (94–96), and Robergs (108).

% VO₂ₘₐₓ: A Relative Measure of Exercise Intensity   The measurement of VO_{2max}, or VO_{2peak}, is not only an important measure in itself, but also serves as a value for the relative expression of exercise intensity. As the increase in VO_2 is a linear function of exercise intensity, exercise intensities below VO_{2max} can be expressed as a percent of VO_{2max} (% VO_{2max}), thus *allowing metabolic responses at the same relative intensity to be compared between individuals who may have very different VO_{2max} values*. In addition, the linear relationship between intensity and VO_2 enables synonymous use of the expression %VO_{2max} and % workload at VO_{2max}.

Exercise intensities can also be performed above that attained at VO_{2max}; however, such intensities have been incorrectly termed "supramaximal," which has caused some confusion because a supramaximal load would theoretically be one that could not be performed! This fact should not cause confusion because the intensity at VO_{2max} is attained after 8 to 12 min of continuous exercise culminating in the maximal rate of oxygen consumption. An individual can tolerate far higher exercise intensities, but because these intensities are associated with an overreliance on glycolysis, development of acidosis, depletion of creatine phosphate, and the development of additional cellular and neural conditions associated with muscle fatigue, exercise sessions are much shorter in duration. As will be discussed and presented in almost every chapter of this book, the expression of exercise intensities relative to VO_{2max} (or VO_{2peak}), or the % workload at VO_{2max} are common features of exercise-related research.

Metabolic Adaptations to Exercise

Creatine Phosphate   The previous description and graphic representation of a maximal exercise test indicated the development of metabolic acidosis, as evidenced by an RER exceeding unity, and the fact that the test is terminated by volitional fatigue! Obviously, muscle creatine phosphate stores must be used to supplement ATP regeneration from mitochondrial respiration during the later stages of the test, and research using ³¹P MRS (focus box 6.1) has shown an increasing reliance on creatine phosphate above intensities corresponding to 60% of the maximal incremental workload (1, 24, 129, 140).

Glycogenolysis and Glycolysis   The information in figure 6.1, and the previously described changes in muscle CrP (creatine phosphate) during incremental exercise, indicate that increased glycogenolysis and glycolysis must also occur with an increase in intensity. Furthermore, at intensities in excess of 60% VO_{2max}, lactate production also increases, and coincides with increases in muscle acidosis (focus box 6.2). Research has measured increased glycogenolysis and glycolysis during incremental exercise indirectly via measuring changes in blood or muscle lactate. Blood and muscle

FOCUS BOX 6.1

Research Using Phosphorus Magnetic Resonance Spectroscopy (^{31}P MRS)

Phosphorus magnetic resonance spectroscopy (^{31}P MRS) is a method that is being used increasingly to study muscle metabolism during exercise. The method is based on the principle of *magnetic resonance*, which concerns the characteristic and predictable behavior of certain atomic nuclei when placed in a magnetic field. For example, when placed in a magnetic field, atoms that have a negative number of electrons exhibit a characteristic spinning (or precession). When radiofrequency electromagnetic energy is applied to the atoms, the nuclei are forced to precess differently. When the energy is removed, the nuclei return to their original precession and give off radiofrequency electromagnetic energy. This energy is recorded, and its intensity is proportional to the concentration of atoms in the specimen studied (human tissue). Furthermore, the frequency of the energy released is specific to each atom and is slightly modified by neighboring atoms. Thus the signal released from the phosphate of CrP is slightly different from the signals of the phosphates from ATP and inorganic phosphate (Pi), but very different from the signals from the protons (^{1}H^{+}) of water, lipid, lactate, creatine, and so on.

The electromagnetic energy released from the phosphate molecules of wrist flexor muscles of the forearm is presented in figure 6.6*a*. When this signal is processed (fig. 6.6*b*) by signal frequencies (called Fourier transformation), peaks that represent CrP, Pi, and ATP are revealed. Cellular pH is indirectly calculated from the frequency difference between the Pi and CrP peaks. During increasing acidity, protons attach to the Pi causing a change in the frequency of its signal, and result in the Pi peak moving closer to the CrP peak. ADP is too low in concentration to be detected by ^{31}P MRS, but can be calculated from the data of CrP, Pi, ATP, and pH. During moderate to intense exercise, the CrP peak decreases, the Pi peak increases, the ATP peaks remain unchanged, and the Pi peak moves closer to the CrP indicating increasing *acidosis.*

The use of ^{1}H MR imaging (MRI) to detect differences in the anatomical structure of the body is based on the different signal intensities of different tissues (fig. 6.7). For example, lipid appears bright on an image from MRI as it has a more dense proton content than muscle, cartilage, or tendon.

There is increasing application of MR to study muscle metabolism during exercise and muscle hypertrophy in response to different types of training. Knowledge of these techniques will help you learn more from current research in exercise physiology and the related biological sciences.

FIGURE 6.7

Images of the thigh from *(a)* an individual with AIDS wasting of skeletal muscle, and *(b)* an endurance-trained individual. The difference in proton density of the different tissues of the leg (fat, muscle, bone, muscle fascia) provide anatomical differentiation.

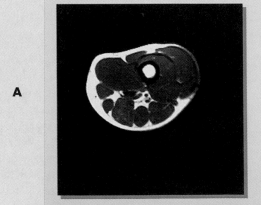
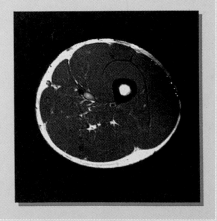

A   B

lactate concentrations increase abruptly at a certain exercise intensity, which has been termed the **lactate threshold (LT).**

Lactate Thresholds   The lactate threshold has mainly been researched during cycle ergometry and treadmill running. When increased lactate concentrations are measured from blood during incremental exercise, the measurement is termed the *blood lactate threshold*. When lactate concentrations are measured in muscle during incremental exercise, the measurement is termed the *muscle lactate threshold* (23, 44, 71).

Figure 6.8 presents a typical graph of blood lactate concentrations from venous blood during incremental exercise. In this example, at an exercise intensity approximating 60% of the workload at VO_{2max}, blood lactate concentrations begin to increase abruptly. As indicated in figure 6.8, the in-

FOCUS BOX 6.2

Lactic Acid, Lactate, and Acidosis

Lactic Acid vs. Lactate

Lactic acid is a carboxylic acid compound, and is termed a *strong acid*. The strength of an acid is quantified by the ability of an acid to release a hydrogen ion (or proton, H^+), into solution. For lactic acid, this proton comes from the carboxylic acid group (-COOH). The pH of a solution that causes half the acid molecules to lose the proton (deprotonated) is termed the *pK*. The stronger the acid, the lower is the pK. The pK of lactic acid is approximately 3.7. The intracellular pH of skeletal muscle approximates 7.0. During intense exercise, muscle cellular pH may fall to between 6.4 and 6.0 (2, 24, 83, 140). Consequently, muscle lactic acid is nearly completely deprotonated during rest and exercise conditions. When an acid is deprotonated it has a negative charge, and to even the charge it binds to a positively charged ion (sodium or potassium) and is referred to as an acid salt (in this case, CH_3-CHOH-COO$^-$Na$^+$). As the molecule is no longer an acid, the suffix "ate" is added to the end of the molecule name. Thus, inside the body (in vivo), there is really no such thing as lactic acid, but only its deprotonated form called *lactate*. Other examples of acid salts pertinent to energy metabolism are pyruvate, citrate, palmitate, and so on.

Lactate Production and Acidosis

If pyruvate and lactate are deprotonated acid salts, then how does **acidosis** develop during the production of lactate? As presented in chapter 3, the production of lactate is a reaction catalyzed by lactate dehydrogenase, and involves the reduction of pyruvate to lactate. The electrons and protons of this reaction are provided by NADH + H^+. Early research on this topic assumed that the protons that are released during lactate production came from lactic acid. However, an additional cause of the acidosis may be the decrease in redox potential (NAD+/NADH) that coincides with increased lactate production, resulting in an accumulation of NADH + H^+. Similarly, the breakdown of ATP to ADP releases a proton (95). Regardless of the direct mechanism, given that increasing NADH$^+$ H$^+$ in the cytosol can increase lactate production, the accumulation of lactate in blood and muscle is associated with a decrease in pH.

The apparent similarity between acidosis and lactate accumulation enables the measurement of blood or muscle lactate as useful indirect indicators of acidosis (23). Unfortunately, too many people assume that because it is the lactate that is measured, it is lactate that is detrimental to muscle function during exercise. *The problem with increased lactate production is not lactate, but the associated acidosis.*

---

crease in blood lactate is more clearly resolved when expressing blood lactate as logarithmic values (10). This particular intensity can be expressed as a VO_2, Watts (if cycling), or running speed (if treadmill running). Research indicates that *the intensity at the lactate threshold represents the maximal intensity at which steady-state exercise can be maintained* (79, 133). Consequently, studies that have correlated running velocity at the lactate threshold to long-distance running have reported correlations exceeding 0.9 for running distances from 5 km to the marathon (46 km) (79). The higher the intensity at the lactate threshold, the higher the intensity that can be sustained in endurance exercise.

We know that a similar lactate threshold occurs in muscle. As early as 1972, data existed that demonstrated that during low-intensity exercise muscle lactate remained close to rest concentrations (1 mmol/kg wet wt), and after a given intensity, muscle lactate then increased abruptly (71). Despite these early findings, more recent research has indicated that muscle lactate production may increase linearly with exercise intensity (44). However, these findings have not been reproduced, whereas those of a threshold increase in muscle lactate accumulation have (23).

What may cause a muscle and blood lactate threshold? There are several proposed explanations for the lactate threshold:

- The decreased removal of lactate from the circulation
- An increased recruitment of fast-twitch glycolytic motor units
- An imbalance between the rate of glycolysis and mitochondrial respiration
- A decreased redox potential (increased NADH relative to NAD^+)
- Muscle hypoxia (lowered muscle oxygen content, or anaerobiosis)
- Ischemia (lowered blood flow to skeletal muscle)

Decreased removal of lactate Research using radioactive isotopes has demonstrated that lactate production increases even during low-intensity exercise, and that as exercise

---

phosphorus magnetic resonance spectroscopy (^{31}P MRS) the detection of differing frequency sound waves from precessing objects in a magnetic field, and the processing of these signals allowing the graphic illustration and quantification of the different signals and their respective intensities

lactate threshold (LT) the term used to denote the intensity of exercise when there is an abrupt increase in lactate accumulation in blood or muscle

acidosis (as'i-do'sis) the decrease in pH (increase in free hydrogen ion concentration)

FIGURE 6.8

The change in blood lactate concentrations during an incremental exercise test. *(a)* The detection of the lactate threshold by converting lactate to log values. The lactate threshold represents the intensity at which the two regression lines intersect. *(b)* The identification of the lactate threshold from visual detection of the abrupt increase in blood lactate.

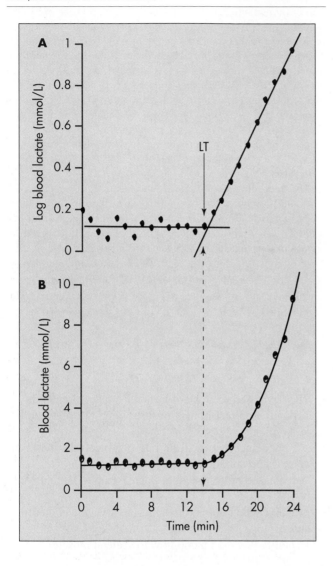

intensity increases beyond a certain point the removal of lactate from the circulation does not increase at the same rate (122). However, these data do not provide a mechanism for the further increase in lactate production during incremental exercise.

Increased fast-twitch glycolytic motor unit recruitment   The delayed recruitment of fast-twitch glycolytic (FG) motor units during incremental exercise will influence lactate production. Muscle fibers from FG motor units have a high glycolytic capacity and a low oxidative capacity. Therefore, recruiting FG motor units will bias metabolism away from mitochondrial respiration to glycolysis. The inevitable result will be an increase in lactate production.

The fiber type proportion determinants of the lactate threshold have also been revealed from comparing the intensity of the lactate threshold to the proportion of slow-twitch fiber types in muscle, and to muscle oxidative capacity (66). The oxidative potential of the muscle, and therefore the genetic and training determinants of this capacity are important determinants of the exercise intensity at the lactate threshold.

Mass action   The argument that lactate production increases because of a greater rate of glycolysis than mitochondrial respiration has been termed the *mass action* effect. Because of the large potential increases in glycogenolysis and glycolysis during exercise, pyruvate can be produced at high rates which may exceed the ability for all pyruvate molecules to enter into the mitochondria and be converted to acetyl CoA. Under these conditions, pyruvate will be converted to lactate.

Decreased cytosolic redox   The lactate dehydrogenase reaction converts pyruvate to lactate and vice versa. Apart from pyruvate, an important substrate for this reaction is NADH + H$^+$, which provides the electrons and protons necessary to reduce pyruvate to lactate. Consequently, the production of lactate also regenerates NAD$^+$, which is a coenzyme for the glyceraldehyde-3-phosphate dehydrogenase reaction of phase 2 of glycolysis. Lactate production can be viewed as a result of a decreased capacity for exchange of NAD$^+$ and NADH between the mitochondria and cytosol, as would occur when mitochondrial NADH increases. To help maintain NAD$^+$ in the cytosol, pyruvate needs to be converted to lactate. The ratio between NAD$^+$/NADH is termed the **redox potential**.

Is there an anaerobic threshold?   The name "anaerobic threshold" was first reported in 1964 by Wasserman and McIlroy (133). At that time the sudden increase in blood lactate was interpreted to indicate increased lactate production, which in turn was interpreted to indicate an inadequate supply of oxygen within the contracting skeletal muscle. The concept of an anaerobic threshold was based on experimental research that documented increased lactate production during conditions of low blood oxygen partial pressures (*hypoxia*), or low blood flow conditions (*ischemia*). At that time Wasserman and McIlroy thought that it was logical for increased lactate production during incremental exercise to be interpreted as evidence for a lack of oxygen in the contracting muscles. However, there was no experimental evidence for the development of hypoxia within muscle during incremental exercise, and because of methodological constraints, even today we are still unable to measure intracellular partial pressures of oxygen.

Despite our inability to measure intracellular pressures of oxygen, several indirect measures may indicate reduced cellular oxygen content. Each of these measures is based on the fact that if there is a lack of oxygen in muscle, then the rate of electron transport would be slowed, which would slow the rate of the TCA (tricarboxylic acid) cycle. These events would increase the concentration of NADH in both the mitochondria and cytosol, and decrease the concentration of NAD^+. Consequently, the $NAD^+/NADH$ (redox potential), would be a reflection of the oxygen availability in muscle. As most of the NAD^+ and NADH are found in the mitochondria (75, 77, 112, 113), a total muscle measure of $NAD^+/NADH$ is interpreted to reflect the mitochondrial redox potential.

The lactate threshold has also been estimated from gas exchange parameters determined from indirect gas analysis calorimetry, with the name *ventilatory threshold* used to reflect the measure's dependence on ventilation. Because the ventilatory threshold involves acute ventilatory responses to incremental exercise, it will be explained in chapter 7.

All of the previous explanations of the lactate threshold may be involved in determining when blood or muscle lactate may increase abruptly. A lack of oxygen will cause each of the mitochondrial redox, cytosolic redox, and mass action scenarios to develop. The increase in fast-twitch motor unit recruitment will exacerbate each of the aforementioned conditions. The actual mechanism(s) causing the lactate threshold remains an interesting and challenging research topic, but one must remember that the applied importance of the lactate threshold to endurance performance, that of the maximal steady-state exercise intensity, is not at question.

Other lactate thresholds The blood lactate response to exercise has also been evaluated using prolonged steady-state intensities (12, 50, 84). Researchers have subjects exercise for between 10 to 20 min at a given intensity, and measure blood lactate at repeated intervals. The test is then repeated at different increased exercise intensities. The exercise intensity that corresponds to the highest blood lactate concentration that exists before a continual increase occurs has been termed the *onset of blood lactate accumulation* (OBLA) (50, 84), or the maximal lactate steady-state (MLSS) workload (12). Mader and Heck (84) have shown that OBLA occurs at blood lactate concentrations approximating 4 mmol/L; however, recent research indicates that the blood lactate concentration at OBLA varies among different exercise modes within the range of 3.1 to 6.6 mmol/L (12).

Steady-State Exercise

As explained in chapter 2, steady-state exercise is attained when almost all the ATP demand from muscle contraction is met by oxidative phosphorylation. As such, during steady-state exercise oxygen consumption has reached a plateau and there is no development of metabolic acidosis. The metabolic issues of interest involve how steady state is attained, how each of glycogenolysis, glycolysis, lipolysis, β-oxidation, and amino acid oxidation contribute substrate to mitochondrial respiration, and how the contribution of these substrates may change with different steady-state exercise intensities and durations.

Oxygen Kinetics During Transitions to Increased Exercise Intensity The increase in VO_2 that accompanies an increase in exercise intensity is immediate, but takes time to reach a steady-state condition. For low to moderate intensities, small increases in intensity result in an exponential increase in VO_2 until steady state is reached. The time to reach steady state requires approximately 3 min (46, 47, 55, 62, 136); however, there is variation in this time depending upon the magnitude of the increment and the fitness of the individual (47, 55). The larger the increment the longer the time to steady state, although individuals with high cardiorespiratory endurance have a shorter time to steady state (fig. 6.9). The oxygen cost of recovering from the use of these immediate sources of ATP regeneration occurs during the steady-state exercise, and also during the recovery from the exercise (see section on EPOC).

Because of the time delay in attaining steady-state VO_2, ATP must be regenerated by creatine phosphate hydrolysis and glycolysis to enable continued muscle contraction. The energy provided by creatine phosphate and glycolysis that supplements mitochondrial respiration is called the **oxygen deficit**. As endurance training can decrease the time to steady state, it also decreases the oxygen deficit (47, 55). Performing a warm-up can also decrease the oxygen deficit. Presumably, a warm-up increases the body's ability to respond to exercise by increasing blood flow, muscle temperature, and stimulation to mitochondrial respiration (105).

The Drift in VO₂ During Prolonged Exercise Although exercise at a submaximal intensity will result in a steady-state VO_2 after approximately 3 min, prolonged exercise at a given submaximal intensity will cause a slight increase in VO_2, known as *oxygen drift*. Westerlind and colleagues (135) demonstrated that the oxygen drift was significantly greater (approximately 18 to 22 mL/kg/min) during 30 min of downhill running at 40% VO_{2max} compared to level running at the same intensity, where no drift was reported. However, in studies that evaluated VO_2 for longer periods of time, and at higher submaximal steady-state exercise intensities (> 60% VO_{2max}), an upward drift in VO_2 has been reported (26, 46). It seems that a combination of increased muscle temperature and circulating catecholamine hormones contribute to the oxygen drift during level running. It appears that the larger oxygen drift during downhill running is not due to muscle damage but to greater increases in muscle temperature during negative work (135).

Carbohydrate and Lipid Catabolism The metabolic data obtained from indirect calorimetry for steady-state exercise at different intensities are graphed in figure 6.10. The increasing

---

redox potential the ratio between NAD^+ and NADH concetrations ($NAD^+/NADH$)

oxygen deficit the difference between oxygen consumption and the oxygen demand of exercise during non-steady-state exercise conditions

FIGURE 6.9

The change in VO$_2$ during the transition from rest to submaximal exercise revealing *(a)* the exponential increase in VO$_2$ and the detection of the time to steady state. The distinction between the integrated differences of measured VO$_2$ and the steady-state VO$_2$ represents the oxygen deficit. For a given increment in exercise intensity, the oxygen deficit will be less in an individual trained for long-term endurance. *(b)* The oxygen deficit increases for larger increments in exercise intensity.

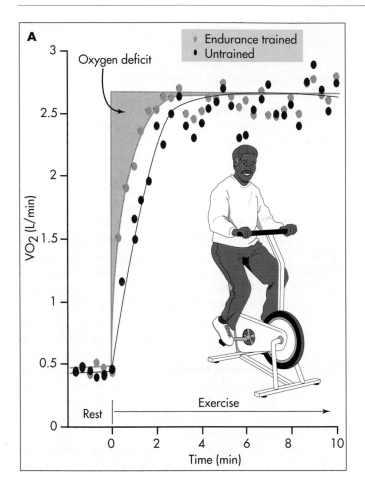

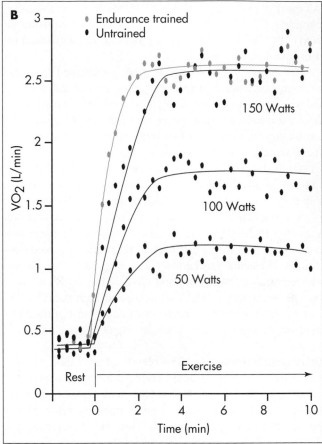

VO$_2$, VCO$_2$, and RER for increases in exercise intensity indicate that VO$_2$ increases linearly with an increase in intensity, VCO$_2$ initially increases linearly but at a slightly larger rate and then increases more abruptly, and RER increases linearly. The difference between the VO$_2$ and VCO$_2$ response is explained by RER. An increase in RER indicates an increasing reliance on carbohydrate catabolism, which involves an increase in CO$_2$ production. For example, at rest, when lipid catabolism predominates, RER approximates 0.7 and indicates that VCO$_2$ is less than VO$_2$. During exercise the increase in RER toward unity indicates an increase in VCO$_2$ relative to VO$_2$. Consequently, exercise performed at a low intensity, when RER is close to 0.7, involves lipid as the predominant substrate.

Not all steady-state exercise will rely predominantly on lipid as a fuel. O'Brien and associates (91) mimicked the marathon run inside a laboratory using a treadmill and demonstrated that RER averaged 0.99 for fast runners (< 165-min duration at 73.3% VO$_{2max}$). Interestingly, both muscle glycogen and blood glucose were substrates for mus-

cle catabolism. The muscle, liver, and blood stores of carbohydrate are therefore of importance to more intense steady-state exercise, and RER values close to 1.0 occur at exercise intensities close to the LT.

Where does the lipid come from that fuels muscle contraction during low-intensity steady-state exercise? Traditionally, lipid catabolism was thought to involve the mobilization of free fatty acids (FFA) from triglycerides stored in plasma lipoproteins or adipose tissue. These free fatty acids were assumed to enter into muscle fibers from the capillary circulation and be used in β-oxidation. These interpretations were based on animal and human research that revealed that free fatty acid uptake into skeletal muscle increased in proportion to the concentration of free fatty acids in blood (27, 101, 104). However, several studies have been conducted that indicate circulating free fatty acids are not the only or major source of lipid during muscle lipid catabolism. Carlson and colleagues (20) documented that more than 60% of lipid used during submaximal exercise comes from lipid stores within the contracting skeletal muscle. In addition, Hurley and associates

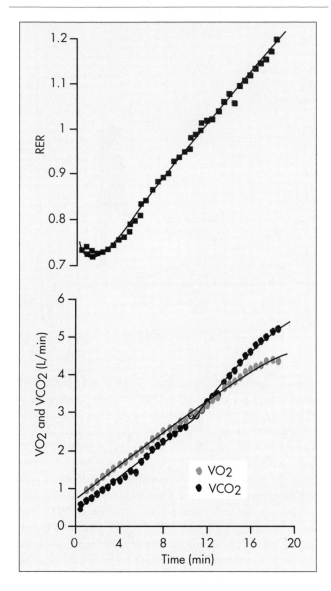

FIGURE 6.10

The change in VO$_2$, VCO$_2$, and RER during an incremental exercise test.

(65) demonstrated that after endurance training, when lipid catabolism increases for a given exercise intensity, circulating FFA and glycerol concentrations decrease, and the use of muscle triglycerides increase. More recently, Romjin and colleagues (109, 110) reported that circulating FFA are the predominant source during low-intensity exercise, but that muscle lipid catabolism increases during moderate-intensity exercise. These data indicate that the role of blood and muscle lipid as the source of fat catabolism during exercise is influenced by exercise intensity, and that for endurance-trained individuals, the main source of lipid for metabolism is not blood or adipose tissue, but intramuscular stores of lipid.

The rate of muscle glycogenolysis during steady-state and intense exercise is dependent on exercise intensity (41). Figure 6.11 presents the decrease in muscle glycogen concentrations for different relative exercise intensities. The lower the exercise intensity, the longer the duration to muscle glycogen depletion. For the near-maximal steady-state intensities (60 to 80% VO$_{2max}$), muscle glycogen stores would become low for durations in excess of 2 h. As muscle glycogen concentrations become low there is a decrease in continued glycogenolysis and glycolysis, the concentrations of the TCA cycle intermediates decrease (114), there is an increased reliance on lipid catabolism (42), the rate of mitochondrial respiration decreases, blood glucose concentrations decrease, and an individual's perception of effort increases (fig. 6.12a, b, and c). Low muscle glycogen concentrations are therefore associated with decreases in exercise performance, and a metabolic shift away from carbohydrate catabolism. As will be explained in chapter 11, it is during these metabolic conditions that carbohydrate supplementation during exercise is beneficial.

Amino Acid and Ketone Body Catabolism   The depletion of muscle glycogen during prolonged exercise requires that additional substrates be used to fuel muscle contraction. The main additional source of carbohydrate is blood glucose, which is released from the liver. However, like skeletal muscle, the liver has a finite store of glycogen. As liver glycogen stores become low, the liver is forced to produce glucose from sources other than glycogen. Consequently, liver gluconeogenesis increases, with the molecules lactate and amino acids as the main substrates. Similarly, in skeletal muscle the TCA cycle intermediates must be supplemented if mitochondrial respiration is to be maintained at a relatively high rate. The main additional substrates for supplementing muscle TCA cycle intermediates are muscle and blood amino acids.

The indirect evidence for an increase in amino acid oxidation during long-term steady-state exercise is the increase in blood and muscle ammonia (NH$_3^+$) (82). Ammonia is formed from the deamination of amino acids that are oxidized in the catabolic pathways, and from the conversion of AMP (adenosine monophosphate) to IMP (inosine monophosphate). Amino acid catabolism increases during long-term exercise, and may contribute as much as 10% of the energy expenditure. The catabolized amino acids come from muscle proteins, intramuscular amino acid stores, and the amination of molecules within the liver or muscle to form nonessential amino acids that are used by other tissues (e.g., alanine). Therefore, amino acid catabolism during exercise is important for three reasons:

- For free energy during exercise to fuel muscle contraction
- To increase concentrations of TCA cycle intermediates, and therefore support carbohydrate and lipid catabolism
- To serve as gluconeogenic precursors for the liver

Prolonged exercise during low muscle and liver carbohydrate conditions also increases the production of ketone bodies in the liver. The ketone bodies are then released and are used by more active tissues (skeletal muscle, heart, kidney) as a form of carbohydrate. The main ketone body from the liver, β-hydroxybutarate (β-HB) is released from the liver

FIGURE 6.11

The change in muscle glycogen during different intensities of exercise. For intense exercise, muscle glycogen does not decrease in a linear manner, but reveals an exponential decrease.

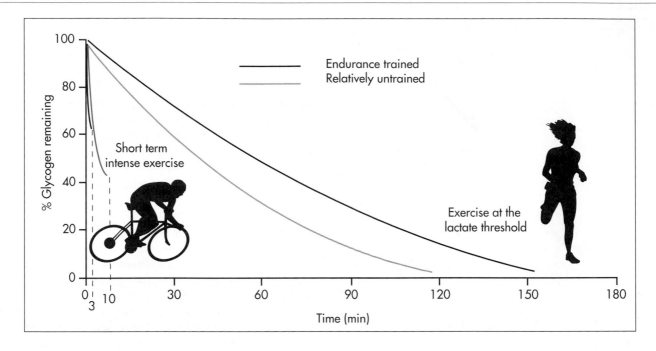

during exercise (or starvation) and circulated to the active skeletal muscle where it is taken up, converted to two acetyl CoA molecules, and utilized in mitochondrial respiration. Interestingly, in severe cases of ketosis, such as diabetes, the increased blood concentration of β-HB can induce acidosis. However, it is unclear whether the increased acid production by β-HB during prolonged exercise contributes to the increased perceptions of fatigue.

Intense Exercise

Intense exercise can be defined as any intensity that exceeds an individual's capabilities to maintain a steady-state condition. Intense exercise can be performed in many ways, with common examples being the intense powerful exercises of sprint running, cycling, swimming, skating, and skiing, and the more strength-dependent exercise of weight lifting. During intense exercise ATP regeneration from mitochondrial respiration must be supplemented by creatine phosphate hydrolysis, and by glycolysis causing increased production of lactate and the associated development of acidosis. The extent and rate of change in creatine phosphate stores, glycolytic rate, and the development of metabolic acidosis have been heavily researched topics of muscle function during intense exercise.

Mitochondrial Respiration   The easiest way to assess increases in mitochondrial respiration is to measure increases in oxygen consumption. Generally, exercise physiologists do this by measuring total body changes in VO_2 during exercise using the procedures of indirect gas analysis calorimetry outlined in chapter 4.

During intense exercise, the increase in mitochondrial respiration occurs very quickly. For example, during 30 s of maximal cycling, the contribution of ATP from mitochondrial respiration to muscle contraction is estimated to be between 25 to 40% (86, 88, 89). Figure 6.13 presents the different curves obtained from the breath-by-breath measurement of VO_2 when changing from unloaded cycling to different absolute exercise intensities for 5 min. The larger the intensity, the more rapid is the increase in VO_2. However, as these curves reveal a gradual increase in VO_2 over time, the greater the exercise intensity, the larger is the oxygen deficit, and therefore the greater is the reliance on creatine phosphate and glycolysis for ATP regeneration.

Creatine Phosphate   Figure 6.14 illustrates results from muscle biopsy research that measured the decrease in muscle creatine phosphate at different intervals of a 100-m sprint (57). The resting muscle creatine phosphate store was 22 mmol/kg wet wt, which decreased during a warm-up to 11 mmol/kg wet wt. During the sprinting, the decrease in creatine phosphate was largest during the first 40 m, and then decreased in small decrements in each remaining 20-m segment. Interestingly, speed increased in an exponential decay to 60 m, and then gradually and consistently decreased to 100 m. Although muscle biopsy research can be applied to field settings, such as the one described, the time delay in having the subjects stop exercising, be positioned for the biopsy, have the biopsy performed, and then the muscle sample frozen can be as long as 20 s, during which time considerable creatine phosphate may be reformed.

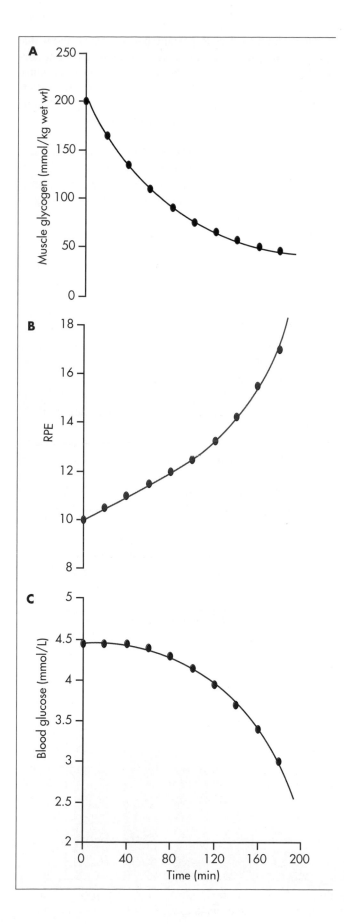

FIGURE 6.12

The change in (a) muscle glycogen, (b) ratings of perceived exertion (RPE), and (c) blood glucose during prolonged submaximal exercise. The association among decreases in glycogen, blood glucose, and RPE may indicate the role of hypoglycemia in the mechanism of fatigue during prolonged exercise.

Research has also demonstrated that creatine phosphate content is higher in fast-twitch than slow-twitch muscle fibers, and that there is a greater decrease in creatine phosphate from fast-twitch muscle during intense exercise (128). During intense exercise to fatigue, ^{31}P MRS has revealed that muscle ATP concentrations decrease only slightly, muscle CrP is almost completely depleted, inorganic phosphate increases mirror the decreases is CrP, ADP (adenosine diphosphate) increases, and cellular pH lowers from 7.0 to approximately 6.1 (6, 13, 90). The concentrations of ADP in skeletal muscle are too small to detect by ^{31}P MRS, but can be calculated by using the creatine phosphate, ATP and inorganic phosphate concentrations, and muscle pH conditions.

Glycogenolysis   Figure 6.11 illustrated the change in muscle glycogen over time for exercise performed at different intensities. The larger the exercise intensity, the greater was the decrease in muscle glycogen for a given time interval.

Is Intense Exercise Performance Impaired When Muscle Glycogen Is Low?   It appears that muscle glycogen concentrations as low as 50 mmol/kg wet wt do not impair muscle contraction during intense exercise (13). However, researchers have not answered this question when muscle glycogen concentrations were very low (< 20 mmol/kg wet wt). Obviously, muscle glycogen is important for intense exercise, but generally the short time to fatigue, and the progressively decreasing rates of glycogenolysis during intense exercise decreases the need for large preexercise muscle glycogen stores.

Glycolysis   AMP concentrations increase in skeletal muscle during intense exercise. AMP is an activator of phosphorylase, the important allosteric enzyme that increases the rate of glycogenolysis and therefore glucose-6-phosphate (G6P) production, and phosphofructokinase (PFK), the allosteric enzyme that converts fructose-6-phosphate to fructose-1,6-bisphosphate. The remaining reactions of glycolysis are either close to equilibrium, or highly exergonic, so that increasing G6P production and activation of PFK essentially activates the entire glycolytic pathway.

Alanine Production   The release of amino acids from skeletal muscle increases during intense exercise (134, 137, 139). Based on radioactive labeling research, it has been deduced that the primary source of the alanine is the amination of pyruvate formed from glycolysis, and that the capacity for alanine formation was greater in more oxidative muscle fibers than in pure fast-twitch fibers (137, 139).

FIGURE 6.13

The increase in VO₂ determined by breath-by-breath indirect gas analysis calorimetry during an increment from rest to a steady-state intensity, and during large increments from rest to non-steady-state intensities. The rate of change in the VO₂ response to the non-steady-state conditions were larger than that for steady state. However, minor differences exist among the rates of VO₂ increase during the three non-steady-state intensites. Obviously, the oxygen deficit is large for increments in intensity to non-steady-state conditions.

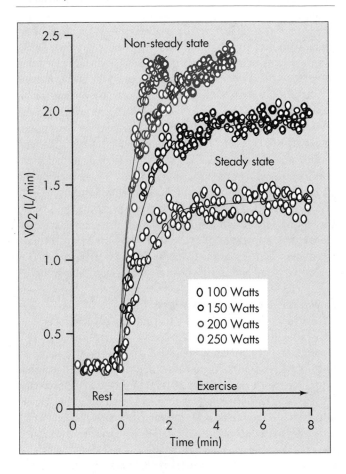

These findings are important because they show that amino acid involvement in energy metabolism is not confined to prolonged exercise during low carbohydrate nutrition states. In addition, the removal of pyruvate from muscle as alanine prevents further increases in acidosis by providing a pathway for pyruvate other than lactate formation.

Lactate Production and Acidosis   Both muscle and blood acidosis are characteristics of high-intensity exercise. As explained in focus box 6.2, the production of lactic acid from the oxidation of pyruvate occurs at a pH that, even during intense exercise (pH = 6.1 to 7.0), greatly exceeds the pK of lactic acid (pH = 3.7). Consequently, the protons that increase during metabolic conditions that increase lactate production are free to either bind to other proteins, be buffered by the intracellular phosphate buffer system, or leave the muscle cell to be buffered by blood bicarbonate, plasma proteins, or hemoglobin (see Buffering Capacity in Chronic Adaptations section).

Muscle biopsy research has measured muscle pH as low as 6.4 (63, 98, 120); however, ³¹P MRS has measured muscle pH as low as 6.1 (6, 13, 21, 83, 129), which represents an eightfold increase in muscle [H⁺] compared to rest. Blood pH does not vary across the range evident in muscle. During intense exercise to volitional fatigue, venous blood pH has been reported to decrease to 7.15, which represents almost a doubling of [H⁺] above the normal resting blood pH of 7.4. In arterial blood, pH changes are not as large and may decrease to 7.24 (78, 104). As will be explained in chapter 8, the blood and lungs combine to be a very powerful buffer of acidosis.

Can Muscle Acidosis Impair Muscle Energy Metabolism?   As enzyme function can be negatively affected by acidosis, research has evaluated whether increased muscle acidosis can

FIGURE 6.14

The decrease in muscle creatine phosphate and increase in blood lactate during different segments of the 100-m sprint.

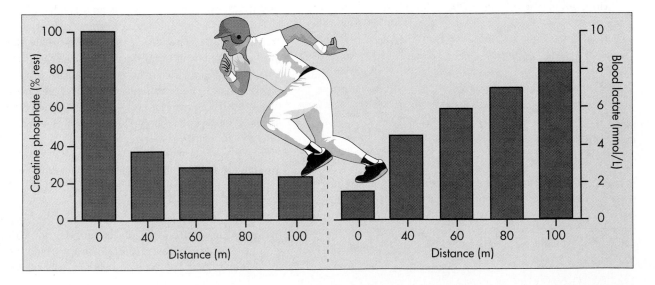

FIGURE 6.15

The changing contribution to ATP regeneration from creatine phosphate, glycolysis, and mitochondrial respiration during intense exercise of increasing duration.

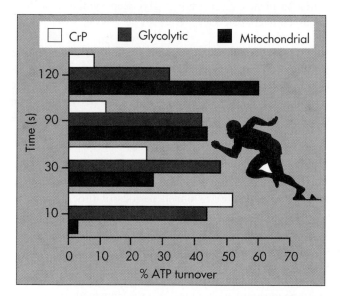

have a measurable effect on the glycolytic rate. As previously stated, the main regulatory enzyme of glycolysis is PFK, and in vitro research has indicated that it can be inhibited by low pH (104). Researchers indirectly assess pH inhibition of PFK by measuring the concentrations of fructose-6-phosphate (F6P) and fructose-1,6-bisphosphate (F1,6P). An increase in the ratio of F6P/F1,6P indicates that there is a rate limitation at the PFK reaction, which has been interpreted to be due to in vivo pH inhibition of PFK (22, 118–120). A decreasing cellular pH can also affect other enzymes, such as the ATPases that are associated with muscle contraction, calcium pumps, and the Na^+/K^+ pump, but the magnitude of pH inhibition of these enzymes in vivo has not been determined.

What Is the Anaerobic Capacity of Skeletal Muscle?   This is an important question because the measurement of an individual's **anaerobic capacity** would provide a value that could reflect an individual's suitability for intense exercise. Researchers have attempted to calculate the energy released from anaerobic pathways during intense muscle contraction (6, 45, 88, 89, 118, 119). Figure 6.15 presents the contribution to ATP production from each of creatine phosphate, glycolysis, and mitochondrial respiration at different time intervals during intense exercise. As with muscle glycogenolysis, the rate of creatine phosphate hydrolysis exhibits an exponential decay. However, glycolysis can provide a high rate of ATP regeneration for as long as 2 min. Despite this fact, muscle fatigue increases over this time frame, and can reduce muscle tension to values less than 50% of the initial force application in less than 1 min.

Medbo and associates (88, 89) have published several articles on how accumulating the oxygen deficit during exercise

can be used as a measure of the capacity of the anaerobic sources of ATP regeneration for a given bout of intense exercise. When calculating the ATP provision from accumulated muscle lactate and decreases in creatine phosphate, and comparing this to the ATP provision calculated from accumulating the oxygen deficit, the correlation obtained was 0.94. Although some controversy exists on the validity of the *accumulated oxygen deficit* (6, 45), these findings may have potential to better evaluate the capacity to perform intense exercise.

Adaptations During the Recovery After Exercise

Muscle recovery occurs after exercise, and is characterized by the continued removal of waste products and by-products of metabolism (lactate, H^+, CO_2), and the restoration of endogenous substrates used during exercise (creatine phosphate, glycogen, lipid). Depending upon the exercise duration and intensity, and the conditions of the recovery (active vs. passive, nutrition), these processes may take from minutes to several days. Because the long-term recovery of energy substrates in muscle is mainly determined by exercise nutrition, a detailed discussion of the exercise and nutritional determinants of postexercise muscle glycogen resynthesis will be presented in chapter 11. The remainder of the material pertinent to understanding muscle recovery after exercise will be organized by the intensity of exercise, metabolic pathways, and, when appropriate, whether the recovery is passive or active.

Steady-State Exercise

As previously explained, during steady-state exercise muscle metabolism is predominantly dependent upon a combination of fat and carbohydrate catabolism. Creatine phosphate stores are not being taxed, and glycolysis is occurring at a rate that does not induce metabolic acidosis. Therefore, recovery primarily concerns the effects of the intensity of exercise and the type of recovery on mitochondrial respiration and the restoration of endogenous stores of glycogen and triacylglycerols.

Mitochondrial Respiration   During a passive recovery from exercise, the body's VO_2 decreases in an exponential manner, with an initial fast component followed by a slow component (fig. 6.16). Consequently, the body has an elevated VO_2 after exercise. It was originally proposed that the elevated VO_2 after exercise was an *oxygen debt*, which existed to pay back the *oxygen deficit* incurred during exercise (38). This interpretation was based on the oxygen cost of replenishing creatine phosphate and for the oxidation of lactate to glycogen, glucose, or TCA cycle intermediates. However,

anaerobic capacity the maximal amount of ATP able to be regenerated from creatine phosphate hyrolysis and glycolysis during intense exercise

FIGURE 6.16

The continued elevation of VO_2 above basal levels (EPOC) during the recovery from exercise.

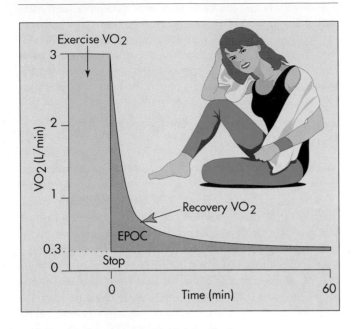

we now know that several factors contribute to the retained elevation in VO_2 after exercise:

1. Replenishment of creatine phosphate and the metabolism of lactate
2. Muscle glycogen and protein metabolism
3. Reoxygenation of venous blood
4. Increased body temperature
5. Increased heart rate
6. Increased ventilation rate
7. Increased circulating concentrations of catecholamine hormones and their effect on increasing cellular metabolism

Each of the aforementioned factors would increase metabolic rate, and therefore increase VO_2. Researchers have abbreviated the **excess postexercise oxygen consumption** as EPOC (3, 4, 39, 43).

The intensity and duration of exercise will determine the relative contribution of each factor to the size of EPOC, and to the magnitude of EPOC itself. For example, 20, 40, and 80 min of cycling at 70% VO_{2max} retained a 12-h EPOC that amounted to 24, 33, and 69 kcal, respectively (3). Conversely, studies that required lower intensities of exercise (35 to 55% VO_{2max}) demonstrated an EPOC that lasted less than 1 h (14, 97).

Reproducible values for the maximal EPOC range between 15 and 21 L O_2, and when assuming a caloric equivalent of 4.74 kcal/L O_2, this amounts to an added expenditure of between 70 and 100 kcal. Findings of larger values for EPOC have been reported for cycle ergometry and less-endurance-trained individuals (85). However, it is unclear how endurance training status, time of day, and exercise mode combine to influence EPOC.

Glycogen Synthesis   The ability of exercised skeletal muscle to resynthesize glycogen after steady-state exercise is dependent on diet, the presence of muscle damage, and whether the recovery is active or passive. The dietary contribution to postexercise muscle glycogen synthesis will be discussed in chapter 11.

Passive Recovery   During steady-state exercise muscle glycogen can be decreased to low levels if exercise is performed for long enough. During the recovery, if adequate carbohydrate is ingested (0.7 g CHO/kg body wt/h), the maximal rate of synthesis approximates 7 to 10 mmol/kg wet wt/h, with minimal synthesis occurring without carbohydrate ingestion (106).

This rate of glycogen resynthesis may be lowered if the exercise bout induced muscle damage, as is common when running downhill for extended periods of time, especially when unaccustomed to downhill running (28, 33, 106). However, the impaired muscle glycogen synthesis accompanying muscle damage is not apparent until after 12 h of recovery (28, 33). It is believed that glycogen synthesis is lowered during muscle damage because of the infiltration of macrophages and leukocytes into the damaged region. Because white blood cells rely solely on blood glucose as a substrate for catabolism, the white blood cells compete with the exercised muscle for blood glucose, resulting in decreased glucose availability to muscle. It is because of the simple competition for glucose that raising the carbohydrate content of the diet, and further increasing the blood glucose response to the ingested food, can increase muscle glycogen synthesis toward normal rates (106).

Active Recovery   During an active recovery, a metabolic load is still placed on the muscles, and the resynthesis of glycogen is impaired (16, 17). Consequently, muscle glycogen concentrations continue to decrease. For low-intensity exercise during an active recovery, muscle glycogen use continues in slow-twitch muscle, but glycogen may be synthesized in the inactive fast-twitch muscle (132).

Triacylglycerol Synthesis   Previous descriptions of lipid metabolism in skeletal muscle have indicated the limited knowledge we have of the regulation, rates, and timing of triacylglycerol lipolysis during exercise. The same is true for muscle triacylglycerol synthesis after exercise and the source of free fatty acids used to fuel muscle metabolism during the recovery. Based on the research that has documented muscle triacylglycerol hydrolysis during exercise as a major source of free fatty acids metabolized during exercise, there must be reactions that occur within skeletal muscle that influence the free fatty acid concentrations in muscle, and the increase or further decrease in the muscle triacylglycerol stores. The mobilized free fatty acids, whether from muscle stores or the blood, must be used during exercise by either reesterifying to triacylglycerols, or catabolized in the β-oxidation pathway of the mitochondria. The role of peripheral mobilization of free fatty acids from adipose tissue during the recovery, and the implications for this to losses in subcutaneous body fat are topics that require further research.

Intense Exercise

During intense exercise to volitional fatigue, blood glucose concentrations are elevated, muscle blood flow is near maximal, several substrates of glycolysis have accumulated in muscle, muscle lactate could have increased from 1 to 30 mmol/kg wet wt (49, 63, 67, 89, 118–120), and blood lactate could have increased from 1 to 25 mmol/L (11, 31, 37, 126). These conditions are very different from blood and muscle conditions following steady-state exercise.

Mitochondrial Respiration   Because of the large oxygen deficit generated during intense exercise, the larger concentrations of circulating catecholamine hormones, and the higher VO_2, EPOC is more elevated during the initial recovery following intense exercise than steady-state exercise.

Glycolysis and Glycogen Synthesis   The perturbed intramuscular environment after intense exercise necessitates the continued flux of intermediates through glycolysis and mitochondrial respiration to normalize muscle concentrations of creatine phosphate and regenerate electrolyte concentration gradients within the muscle fibers and across the sarcolemma. The balance between continued catabolic metabolism and anabolic metabolism is dependent on the type of recovery.

Passive Recovery   Research of glycogen synthesis during the passive recovery after intense exercise has produced varied results on the rate of glycogen synthesis. When confining our interest to the studies with sound methodology, glycogen synthesis has been reported at rates between 12 to 15 mmol/kg

wet wt/h, even without carbohydrate ingestion. This high rate of glycogen synthesis is believed to be evidence for lactate reconversion to pyruvate, with a subsequent reversal of glycolysis producing glucose-6-phosphate, which can then be diverted to glycogen storage (17, 106). Nevertheless, this is a controversial topic because research has not documented adequate activity of the enzymes necessary to avoid the essentially irreversible pyruvate kinase reaction in the conversion of pyruvate to phosphoenolpyruvate. In addition, lactate is known to be removed from skeletal muscle by a transport mechanism (111), and this process is effective as evidenced by the rapid increase in blood lactate during the initial minutes of recovery. However, studies that have used radioactive isotopes have documented that lactate carbons do end as muscle glycogen, as well as carbon dioxide, amino acids, and presumably glycolytic intermediates (121, 122). The high rate of glycogen synthesis after intense exercise is difficult to explain without accounting for endogenous glycogen precursors within skeletal muscle.

Lactate removal and oxidation   When concerned with lactate removal into the circulation, the intensity of exercise, and therefore the muscle lactate concentration, combine to influence the kinetics of the blood lactate response during a passive recovery (37). The greater the increase in muscle lactate, the longer the time to peak blood lactate concentrations, and the more prolonged the decrease in blood lactate concentrations to normal resting values (fig. 6.17). These data support a saturable lactate transporter on the

> **excess postexercise oxygen consumption (EPOC)** the elevated oxygen consumption that is retained immediately after a bout of exercise

FIGURE 6.17

The influence of the intensity of exercise on the kinetics of blood lactate during a passive recovery.

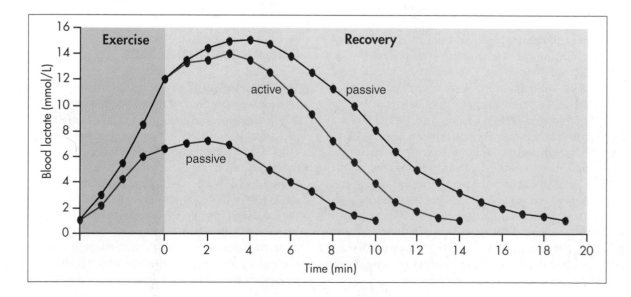

sarcolemma of skeletal muscle, or an inhibition of the transporter with the increasing acidosis that accompanies larger muscle lactate concentrations.

Active Recovery

Glycogen Synthesis   During an active recovery after intense exercise, the accumulated intermediates of glycolysis and muscle lactate are converted to pyruvate and used in mitochondrial respiration. Obviously, an active recovery removes the potential glycogen precursor molecules that have accumulated in skeletal muscle, thus lowering the rate of glycogen synthesis. The glycogen synthesis that occurs during the subsequent passive recovery is therefore similar to that for steady-state exercise.

Lactate Removal   Performing exercise between 35 to 50% VO_{2max} during the recovery from fatiguing exercise increases the removal of lactate from blood (11, 31). Although it is tempting to interpret this as evidence for improved recovery when submaximal exercise is performed, such an interpretation is premature. Recall that lactate is not a molecule that impairs muscle function. The biochemical and physiological detriment of lactate production is the stoichiometric production of hydrogen ions, which, unless buffered, will lower pH. The issues of concern are how muscle and blood acidosis is recovered, and what factors positively and negatively affect these processes.

Acidosis and Creatine Phosphate   The multiple data acquisitions and increased temporal resolution provided by ^{31}P MRS have increased our understanding of the recovery from muscle acidosis and the recovery of creatine phosphate stores. Both muscle acidosis and creatine phosphate recovery need to be discussed together because of the involvement of a free proton (H^+) in the creatine kinase reaction (see chapter 3). The greater and more prolonged the acidosis, the longer the time required for complete recovery of creatine phosphate (5).

Figure 6.18*a* presents the recovery curve of forearm muscle acidosis, and figure 6.18*b* presents the recovery curves of creatine phosphate during minimal and extreme muscle acidosis. Muscle creatine phosphate recovery reveals a biexponential curve, having a fast and a slow component (5, 21, 129). The fast component of CrP recovery is complete within less than 2 min, and represents approximately 80 to 90% of complete CrP recovery. The complete recovery of CrP requires prolonged periods of time that extend beyond the normalization of muscle pH (129), and may be related to the energy requirements of cellular recovery from exercise.

The recovery from muscle acidosis is influenced by the exchange of intracellular protons and other positively and negatively charged molecules and ions between the intracellular and extracellular compartments (78). The recovery from extreme muscle acidosis requires approximately 5 min during a passive recovery; however, little is known of the influence of exercise duration and the severity of muscle acidosis on the kinetics of recovery from acidosis.

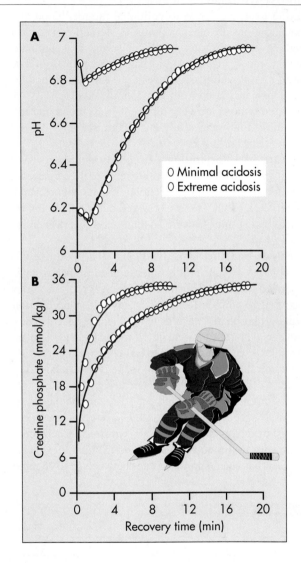

FIGURE 6.18

(a) The recovery of forearm muscle acidosis following forearm wrist flexion exercise to fatigue. *(b)* The recovery of creatine phosphate is known to be influenced by muscle acidosis, as recovery is more rapid during near normal muscle pH conditions.

Chronic Adaptations

The physiological health benefits of exercise, and the improved performance that occurs following training are due in part to **chronic adaptations** of muscle to repeated exercise stress. Chronic muscle adaptations to exercise are specific to the type of exercise performed. Therefore, as with other sections of this chapter, the intensity and duration of exercise will dictate which metabolic pathways adapt, and the extent of their adaptation. However, as training for prolonged exercise often involves intense intervals, and many athletes who compete in high-intensity events also complete endurance training, chronic adaptations will be categorized by metabolic pathways and whether the exercise training is predominantly long term or short term in duration. The chronic training adaptations discussed in this chapter assume that correct training is performed. Discussion of the different training strategies used by athletes is found in chapter 10.

Weight Lifting Exercises

Compared to intense dynamic exercise, such as sprint running and cycling, limited research has been completed on the adaptations of skeletal muscle to weight lifting, or resistance-type exercises. During heavy resistance exercise, muscle fatigue can occur in as little as 30 s. Despite this short time frame, there is adequate stimulation of glycogenolysis and glycolysis to induce a moderate intramuscular lactate accumulation and lactate acidosis. However, the intramuscular accumulation of lactate and the degree of acidosis is significantly less than when performing intense exercise for periods in excess of 1 to 2 min (22, 63, 86, 118, 119).

MacDougall and associates (80) studied the effects of 5 months of heavy resistance training on skeletal muscle metabolic capacities. Resistance training increased resting concentrations of creatine, CrP, ATP, and glycogen. The data were interpreted to indicate an increase in short-term energy stores in skeletal muscle following resistance training. The increased strength resulting from resistance training is known to be a result of improved neuromuscular function (motor unit recruitment and summation) and muscle hypertrophy, as was discussed in chapter 5.

Long-Term Muscular Endurance

Muscular endurance can be defined as the ability of muscle to contract repeatedly over time. Muscular endurance has just as much meaning for short-duration as for long-duration exercise. Consequently, the term endurance exercise has little meaning unless a time frame is clarified. Long-term muscle endurance refers to the ability of skeletal muscle to repeatedly contract for time periods in excess of 5 min. Based on figure 6.1, exercise times in excess of 5 min rely heavily on ATP regeneration from mitochondrial respiration.

The chronic skeletal muscle adaptations to training for long-term muscular endurance are summarized in table 6.1. The subdivisions used in the table are also used to divide the subsequent discussion of research findings.

During muscle contraction, oxygen must be supplied to and utilized by the contracting muscle fibers. When oxygen is released from hemoglobin at the tissue level, it must be transferred from the capillary to within the muscle fiber, where it must then be transferred to within mitochondria. This requirement has raised the question of whether endurance training for long-term endurance increases stores of muscle myoglobin. Despite convincing evidence from animal research, endurance training research with human subjects has not shown

---

chronic adaptations changes in body structure and function resulting from repeated exposure to exercise stress

---

TABLE 6.1

The chronic skeletal muscle metabolic adaptations resulting from long-term muscular endurance

LONG-TERM MUSCULAR ENDURANCE		
METABOLIC PATHWAY	**ADAPTATION**	**CONSEQUENCE**
Mitochondrial respiration	↑Number and size of mitochondria	↑Rate of mitochondrial respiration
		↑Capacity to oxidize carbohydrate
		↑Sensitivity to stimulation
		↓Oxygen deficit
		↓Lactate production
	↑Activity of TCA cycle enzymes	↑Capacity to oxidize acetyl CoA
	↑Activity of β-oxidation enzymes	↑Capacity to oxidize lipid
		↑Sparing of muscle glycogen
Glycogen	↑Concentration	↑Time to exhaustion at steady state
Glycolysis	↑Activity of phosphorylase	↑Capacity of glycogenolysis
	↑Activity of phosphofructokinase	↑Capacity of glycolysis
	↑Lactate threshold	↑Maximal steady-state intensity
	↑Lactate removal	↑Capacity to normalize blood and muscle lactate
	↓Lactate production	↓Acidosis
Creatine phosphate	↑Threshold	↑Maximal steady-state intensity
Buffering capacity	No change	

Sources: Adapted from references 8, 27, 35, 39, 42, 47, 48, 51, 52, 55, 58, 59, 71, 79, 98, 116.

an increase in myoglobin concentrations (69, 92). It is unclear why myoglobin does not increase in human muscle, especially when activities of the enzymes of mitochondrial respiration increase dramatically, and a potential mechanism of the lactate threshold may be decreased in intramuscular oxygen content (75, 76, 126).

Mitochondrial Respiration

Perhaps the most important chronic adaptation increasing long-term muscular endurance is an increase in the number and size of mitochondria (referred to as *mitochondrial mass*). Research that has documented more mitochondria have usually based their findings on an increased density of mitochondria seen by electron microscopy. Because electron microscopy provides a two-dimensional evaluation, it is unclear whether the mitochondria increase in number or increase in size after endurance training, revealing more sections of what might be a continuous mitochondrial matrix. In either case, the adaptation provides a greater mitochondrial surface area exposed to the cytosol, and a greater mitochondrial volume within which are located the enzymes and intermediates of mitochondrial respiration.

The Importance of Mitochondrial Membrane Surface Area

An increase in the surface area of mitochondrial membranes increases the capacity for the exchange of metabolites between the cytosol and mitochondria. As already explained, the metabolites of importance to stimulating mitochondrial respiration are pyruvate, NADH, ADP, Pi, and oxygen. This increased capacity increases the sensitivity for mitochondria to be stimulated by a given metabolic stress (34). Consequently, it is not surprising that the oxygen deficit developed during the transition from rest to steady-state exercise decreases after endurance training (fig. 6.10).

The Importance of Mitochondrial Volume

The increased volume of mitochondria provides a greater concentration of mitochondrial enzymes, which includes enzymes of the TCA cycle, β-oxidation, the electron transport chain coupled to ADP phosphorylation, and also cellular concentrations of the iron-containing electron transfer molecules of the electron transport chain. Because enzyme concentration is proportional to enzyme activity, it is no surprise that research has shown large increases in mitochondrial enzyme activity after chronic training for long-term muscular endurance.

Figure 6.19 illustrates the increases in the activity of important TCA cycle enzymes after several weeks of training for long-term muscular endurance in different modes of exercise. Increases in mitochondrial volume also increase the activity of the enzymes of lipolysis, mitochondrial transport (NADH shuttles), and β-oxidation. The functional importance of these adaptations is to increase the ability to catabolize both fat and carbohydrate during exercise. An increased capacity to catabolize carbohydrate in mitochondrial respiration results in an increased maximal rate of ATP regeneration from oxidative phosphorylation, and an increased

maximal steady-state intensity. During submaximal exercise, an increased capacity to catabolize lipid spares muscle and liver glycogen and conserves the body's carbohydrate stores (26, 39, 42, 65, 109).

Hurley and colleagues (65) trained nine subjects for 12 weeks by training 6 times per week at intensities between 75 and 100% VO_{2max}, with durations of exercise between 5 to 40 min. After training, the subjects could perform a given bout of exercise using less muscle glycogen and more muscle triglyceride compared to pretraining. As will be discussed below, the aforementioned muscle metabolic responses to endurance training can be explained by improvements in one or both of VO_{2max} and the lactate threshold.

VO_{2max}   An increased mitochondrial volume provides skeletal muscle with the ability to increase VO_{2max}. However, cardiovascular adaptations are also involved in increasing VO_{2max} after training, and *muscle adaptations should not be viewed as the sole determinants of VO_{2max}*.

The extent of improvement in VO_{2max} depends on the initial value of VO_{2max} prior to training. Figure 6.20 illustrates

---

FIGURE 6.19

The increase in key enzymes of the mitochondrial oxidation of carbohydrate and lipid after training for long-term muscular endurance.

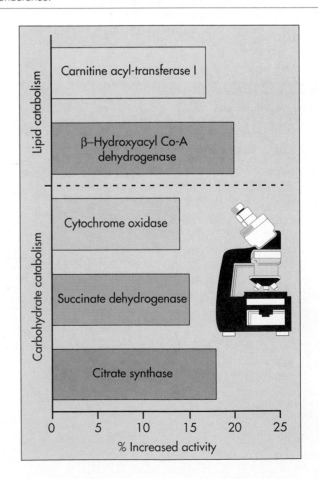

that for individuals with high VO_{2max} values, the extent of improvement possible by training for long-term endurance may be less than 5%. The largest training response reported for VO_{2max} has been 57%, and was accomplished by individuals who had sustained a myocardial infarction, and who then trained for and completed a marathon (77). Although figure 6.20 indicates that training improvement in VO_{2max} decreases as an exponential decay of the initial VO_{2max} value, some evidence exists to disprove this. When training intensity was kept constant relative to VO_{2max}, subjects demonstrated a linear increase in VO_{2max} during 10 weeks of training (52). VO_{2max} values increased on average from 38 to 55 mL/kg/min, a 45% increase. Obviously there would eventually be a plateau in VO_{2max} improvement, but it appears that the type and quality of training is also important (see chapter 10).

The ability to improve VO_{2max} should not be confused with submaximal oxygen consumption. After long-term endurance training, a person's VO_2 for a given exercise intensity remains unchanged, unless there are improvements in economy.

Improvements in Metabolic Thresholds   The combination of an increased mitochondrial volume and mass result in increases in each of the blood and muscle lactate thresholds, and the muscle creatine phosphate threshold. Coggan and associates (24) reported a high negative correlation (−0.63) between muscle mitochondrial enzyme activity (citrate synthase) and the slope of the increase in Pi/CrP, which indicates that an increased mitochondrial capacity must also

increase the rate of ATP demand necessary to tax muscle creatine phosphate stores.

Similar findings to creatine phosphate metabolism during incremental exercise have been obtained for the lactate thresholds. In fact, long-term endurance training has been shown to increase the lactate threshold without increasing VO_{2max}, suggesting that the mechanisms for adaptation of these capacities are different (30). An increased lactate threshold would allow a person to exercise at a higher intensity, while still being at steady state. Consequently, a runner, cyclist, cross-country skier, or swimmer would be able to maintain a faster pace for longer, resulting in a decreased finishing time and improved performance.

Running Economy

As explained in chapter 4, *running economy* refers to the oxygen consumption utilized during a given intensity of steady-state exercise. Good running economy relates to a relatively low VO_2 for a given running pace. Although no study has demonstrated improvements in running economy after training, the duration of training for these studies has been relatively short (< 15 weeks). Comparisons between well-trained long-distance runners compared to well-trained middle-distance runners, and to untrained individuals, indicates large differences in running economy, and suggest that long-term (years) training may be required to induce decreases in submaximal oxygen consumption (improved economy) (29). The determinants of improved running economy are believed to be biomechanical rather than biochemical or physiological (29).

Joyner (70) combined the importance of the lactate threshold, VO_{2max}, and running economy in the development of a model to predict optimal race performance in the marathon. Optimizing VO_{2max} (85 mL/kg/min), lactate threshold (85% VO_{2max}), and using an air resistance and oxygen drift–corrected estimate of running economy resulted in a calculated optimal average marathon running pace of 21.46 km/h. These estimates could lead to a new world record marathon time of 1:57:58 (h:min:s) (current record is 2:06:50) and would emphasize the applied importance of muscle adaptations to training. Time will tell if the genetically gifted human body can adapt to training to attain this "optimal" marathon time.

Glycogen

Experimental evidence exists to support a long-term endurance training–associated increase in muscle glycogen concentrations. For example, Piehl and colleagues (99) measured muscle glycogen concentrations in contralateral trained and untrained legs (cycling) of four subjects. Resting muscle glycogen concentrations were higher in the trained compared to untrained leg (119 vs. 81 mmol/kg wet wt). Similar findings have been reported for runners and swimmers (27, 39).

Hickner and associates (53) recently compared trained and untrained subjects in postexercise (2 h at 75% VO_{2max},

---

FIGURE 6.20

The relationship between the improvement in VO_{2max} and the initial VO_{2max} prior to training. For a given individual, the larger the initial VO_{2max}, the less the improvement for a given training program.

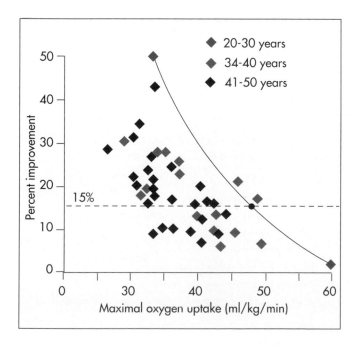

ending with five 1-min sprints) muscle glycogen synthesis after 6 and 72 h of recovery. Trained subjects had more than double the rate of muscle glycogen synthesis in the first 6 h of recovery, and this response was associated with a threefold higher muscle GLUT4 (glucose transport protein) content. After 72 h of recovery, muscle glycogen had increased to 164 vs. 99 mmol/kg wet wt in the trained and untrained subjects, respectively. However, as the trained subjects had higher type I muscle fiber proportions than the untrained subjects, it remains unclear how the muscle glycogen and GLUT4 muscle content results reflect the fiber type versus training differences among the groups.

Glycogenolysis and Glycolysis

Long-term endurance training increases the activities of the two main regulated enzymes of the glycogenolytic and glycolytic pathways: phosphorylase (PHOS) and phosphofructokinase (PFK) (fig. 6.21) (27, 40). The increased activity of these enzymes is not as great as for the enzymes of the mitochondria; nevertheless, when combined with the larger store of muscle glycogen they reflect an increased capacity for glycolysis to produce pyruvate for subsequent mitochondrial respiration.

Creatine Phosphate and Buffering Capacity

Long-term endurance exercise predominantly uses skeletal muscle creatine phosphate for the shuttling of phosphate molecules from the mitochondria to the contractile proteins. Data presented on the acute adaptations of creatine phosphate during incremental exercise indicated that creatine phosphate stores do not decrease at exercise intensities corresponding to less than 60% VO_{2max}. These intensities do not provide a stimulus for increased creatine phosphate stores. As will be discussed in the section on buffering capacity during short-term intense exercise, *muscle buffering capacity* of endurance-trained individuals is no greater than that of untrained individuals.

Short-Term Intense Exercise

For exercise that is terminated because of muscular fatigue, the intensity must have been too high to maintain a steady-state condition, and endurance is more dependent on the nonmitochondrial sources of ATP regeneration as well as the ability to retard and/or tolerate acidosis. Consequently, the chronic adaptations to intense exercise are very different from those that have been documented for long-term less-intense exercise conditions (see table 6.2).

Mitochondrial Respiration

During intense exercise, exercise duration is limited by the development of muscle acidosis and the depletion of creatine phosphate, resulting in exercise durations less than 2 to 3 min. These time frames are inadequate for the development of large metabolic adaptations in mitochondrial respiration. However, research on strength-trained individuals has reported small increases in citrate synthase activity (68), but it is unclear how this change influences the development of muscle fatigue.

Glycogenolysis and Glycolysis

As for long-term endurance training, short-term endurance training stimulates increased resting concentrations of muscle glycogen. In addition, the enzymes phosphorylase and phosphofructokinase also increase in activity to levels comparable to long-term endurance training (fig. 6.21).

Creatine Phosphate and ATP

Studies evaluating chronic adaptations to weight training have reported significant (but small) increases in resting muscle concentrations of creatine phosphate and ATP (81). However, similar results have not been found for sprint training (68, 93). A larger store of creatine phosphate would theoretically provide added potential for a high rate of ATP regeneration during the initial seconds of intense exercise. However, as the increase in creatine phosphate is only minor, it is doubtful that this adaptation is physiologically meaningful.

More recent research has addressed the increase in muscle creatine phosphate and the improved intense exercise performance resulting from the ingestion of creatine monhydrate. As creatine ingestion represents a nutritional ergogenic aid, this information is presented in chapter 11. However, given that muscle creatine phosphate stores do not

TABLE 6.2

The chronic skeletal muscle metabolic adaptations resulting from exercise training for short-term muscular strength and power

METABOLIC PATHWAY	ADAPTATION	CONSEQUENCE
Mitochondrial respiration	Small ↑	No importance during intense exercise. May improve recovery
Glycogen	↑Concentration	↑Store of substrate to fuel glycolysis
Glycolysis	↑Phosphorylase	↑Rate of glycolysis
	↑PFK	↑Rate of glycolysis
ATP	Small ↑	↑Tolerance of intense exercise
Creatine phosphate	Small ↑	↑Capacity to rapidly regenerate ATP
Buffering capacity	↑Capacity	Delays fatigue from acidosis, ↑ ATP capacity of glycolysis

Sources: Adapted from references 67, 70, 80, 93, 115.

FIGURE 6.21

The increase in enzyme activity from glycogenolysis and glycolysis resulting from training for long-term endurance and short-term intense exercise. PHOS = phosphorylase, PFK = phosphofructokinase, CS = citrate synthase.

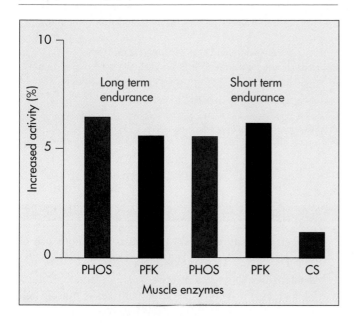

FIGURE 6.22

The influence of training for short-term intense exercise on muscle buffer capacity.

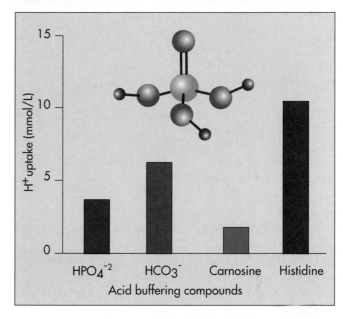

adapt to training like other energy stores, any additional gain in creatine phosphate stores would provide significant exercise performance advantages during intense exercise.

Buffering Capacity

The term **buffering capacity** refers to the ability to bind free protons, and therefore resist increases in the free hydrogen ion concentration ($[H^+]$). As the negative logarithm of the free $[H^+]$ represents pH ($pH = -\log[H^+]$), an increased buffering capacity retards decreases in pH. The physiology of acid-base buffering is presented in chapter 7.

As previously described, during intense exercise muscle contraction increases lactate production with a stoichiometric increase in H^+ production. Hultman and Sahlin (63) have proposed that 94% of the H^+ release during exercise comes from lactic acid. However, comment has already been given to alternative sources of acidosis during exercise (see chapter 3). Given the potentially large increases in lactate production in skeletal muscle, a large exercised muscle mass could result in an H^+ release that would decrease the pH of an unbuffered solution to less than 1.5 (98). This obviously does not happen, and the reason is the buffering capacity of muscle and blood.

The potential buffers in muscle and blood comprise molecules that can receive a proton, and this buffering system is referred to as physicochemical buffering. The main potential

buffers of protons in skeletal muscle are phosphate (HPO_4^{-2}), bicarbonate (HCO_3^-), carnosine, and protein (certain amino acids, especially histidine).

A summary of research based on the biopsy and titration method of muscle pH determination are presented in figure 6.22. It is clear that training for short-term endurance increases the muscle buffer capacity, whereas long-term endurance training results in a muscle buffer capacity no different than that in untrained control subjects (100, 111). In addition, Parkhouse and colleagues (98) demonstrated that the increased buffer capacity of short-term endurance-trained athletes was associated with increased concentrations of carnosine. Carnosine is a histidine-containing dipeptide that, because of the histidine content and relatively unknown function within muscle, was hypothesized to be important as a buffer. Consequently, the improved muscle buffer capacity associated with training may be due to an increased amino acid and protein content of skeletal muscle fibers.

buffering capacity the capacity to remove free hydrogen ions from solution

WEBSITE BOX

Chapter 6: Muscle Metabolic Adaptations to Exercise

The newest information regarding exercise physiology can be viewed at the following sites.*

curtin.edu.au/curtin/dept/phyiol/pt/edres/exphys/ep552_96/Lactate/
   Lecture notes and reports on metabolism during exercise.

arfa.org/index./htm
   Excellent site providing comprehensive information on many topics within exercise physiology.

mediconsult.com/
   Information source for any medical condition, including diabetes.

tees.ac.uk/sportscience/PDA_PDRS/lect6/sld001.htm
   Powerpoint slide presentation on the use of knowledge of muscle metabolism for improved exercise training.

*Unless indicated, all URLs preceded by http://www.

Note: These URLs were valid at the time of publication, but could have changed or been deleted from Internet access since that time.

SUMMARY

- The reactions involved in increasing muscle metabolism during exercise, and altering muscle metabolism in the recovery from exercise, are termed **acute adaptations.**

- **Maximal oxygen consumption (VO_{2max})** is the maximal rate at which the body can consume oxygen during exercise. It is detected as a plateau in VO_2 despite further increases in intensity, and an RER that exceeds 1.1, and is best attained using a protocol duration between 8 to 12 min. VO_{2max} values can be expressed as an absolute volume of oxygen per unit time (L/min) or relative to body mass (mL/kg/min). For comparing VO_{2max} values between genders, the relative expression of VO_{2max} should use lean body mass (LBM,kg) rather than body mass (kg).

- VO_{2max} values are dispersed between extremely low capacities, like those of chronically ill individuals (< 20 mL/kg/min) and well-trained and elite endurance athletes (> 80 mL/kg/min). The factors that combine to influence VO_{2max} are a high proportion of slow-twitch motor units, high central and peripheral cardiovascular capacities, and the quality and duration of training. Added knowledge of how muscle metabolism changes during exercise has been gained from phosphorus magnetic resonance spectroscopy (^{31}P MRS).

- VO_{2max} is known to differ depending on the type of exercise, and the type and extent of training performed by the individual. Generally, VO_{2max} is greatest during running and stepping and lowest during arm ergometry. Adding increased work by the upper-body to lower-body exercise will eventually result in a decrease in VO_{2max} because of cardiovascular limitations.

- As the increase in VO_2 is a linear function of exercise intensity, exercise intensities below VO_{2max} can be expressed as a percent of VO_{2max} (% VO_{2max}), thus *allowing metabolic responses at the same relative intensity to be compared between individuals who may have very different VO_{2max} values.* In addition, the linear relationship between intensity and VO_2 enables synonymous use of the expression %VO_{2max} and % workload at VO_{2max}.

- At intensities in excess of 60% VO_{2max}, lactate production increases and coincides with increases in muscle **acidosis.** During **incremental exercise,** blood and muscle lactate concentrations increase abruptly at a certain exercise intensity, which has been termed the **lactate threshold (LT).** Research indicates that *the intensity at the lactate threshold represents the maximal intensity that steady-state exercise can be maintained.*

- There are several proposed explanations for lactate threshold.

  - The decreased removal of lactate from the circulation
  - An increased recruitment of fast-twitch glycolytic motor units
  - An imbalance between the rate of glycolysis and mitochondrial respiration
  - A decreased redox potential (increased NADH relative to NAD^+)
  - Muscle hypoxia (lowered muscle oxygen content, or anaerobiosis)
  - Ischemia (lowered blood flow to skeletal muscle)

- The NAD^+/NADH, or **redox potential,** is an indirect reflection of the oxygen availability in muscle. Because most of the NAD^+ and NADH are found in the mitochondria, a total muscle measure of NAD^+/NADH reflects the mitochondrial redox potential.

- Because of the time delay in attaining steady-state VO_2, ATP must be regenerated by creatine phosphate hydrolysis and glycolysis to enable continued muscle contraction. The energy provided by creatine phosphate and glycolysis that supplements mitochondrial respiration is called the **oxygen deficit.** As endurance training can decrease the time to steady state, it also decreases the oxygen deficit.

■ The oxygen deficit during exercise can be used as a measure of the capacity of the anaerobic sources of ATP regeneration for a given bout of intense exercise, or **anaerobic capacity**. When calculating the ATP provision from accumulated muscle lactate and decreases in creatine phosphate, and comparing this to the ATP provision calculated from the *accumulated oxygen deficit*, the correlation obtained was 0.94. The ability to generate a large oxygen deficit during intense exercise should correspond to an increased capacity to perform intense exercise.

■ After exercise during a passive recovery, the body's VO_2 decreases in an exponential manner, with an initial fast component followed by a slow component. Researchers have abbreviated the **excess postexercise oxygen consumption** as EPOC. Several factors contribute to EPOC:

1. Replenishment of creatine phosphate and the metabolism of lactate
2. Muscle glycogen and protein metabolism
3. Reoxygenation of venous blood
4. Increased body temperature
5. Increased heart rate
6. Increased ventilation rate
7. Increased circulating concentrations of catecholamine hormones

■ During steady-state exercise muscle glycogen can be decreased to low levels if exercise is performed for long enough. During the recovery, if adequate carbohydrate is ingested (0.7 g CHO/kg body wt/h), the maximal rate of synthesis approximates 7 to 10 mmol/kg wet wt/h, with minimal synthesis occurring without carbohydrate ingestion. Research of glycogen synthesis during the passive recovery after intense exercise has been reported at rates between 12 and 15 mmol/kg wet wt/h, even without carbohydrate ingestion.

■ Muscle creatine phosphate recovery reveals a biexponential curve having a fast and a slow component. The fast component of CrP recovery is complete within less than 2 min, and represents approximately 80 to 90% of complete CrP recovery. The complete recovery of CrP requires prolonged periods of time that extend beyond the normalization of muscle pH (134), and may be related to the energy requirements of cellular recovery from exercise.

■ The physiological health benefits of exercise, and the improved performance that occurs following training are due in part to **chronic adaptations** of muscle to repeated exercise stress. Chronic muscle adaptations to exercise are specific to the type of exercise performed.

■ Resistance training can increase resting concentrations of muscle creatine, CrP, ATP, and glycogen, therefore increasing the short-term energy stores in skeletal muscle. The increased strength resulting from resistance training is known to be a result of improved neuromuscular function (recruitment and summation) and muscle hypertrophy.

■ An increase in the surface area of mitochondrial membranes increases the capacity for the exchange of metabolites between the cytosol and mitochondria. The increased volume of mitochondria provides a greater concentration of mitochondrial enzymes, which includes enzymes of the TCA cycle, β-oxidation, the electron transport chain coupled to ADP phosphorylation, and also cellular concentrations of the iron-containing electron transfer molecules of the electron transport chain.

■ The extent of improvement in VO_{2max} depends on the initial value of VO_{2max} prior to training. For individuals with high VO_{2max} values, the extent of improvement possible by training for long-term endurance may be less than 5%. The largest training response reported for VO_{2max} has been 57%, and was accomplished by individuals who had sustained a myocardial infarction and who then trained for and completed a marathon.

■ The combination of an increased mitochondrial volume and mass result in increases in each of the blood and muscle lactate thresholds, and the muscle creatine phosphate threshold. An increased lactate threshold would allow a person to exercise at a higher intensity, while still being at steady state, resulting a decreased finishing time and improved performance.

■ Long-term endurance training increases the activities of the two main regulated enzymes of the glycogenolytic and glycolytic pathways: phosphorylase (PHOS) and phosphofructokinase (PFK). The increased activity of these enzymes is not as great as for the enzymes of the mitochondria; nevertheless, when combined with the larger store of muscle glycogen they reflect an increased capacity for glycolysis to produce pyruvate for subsequent mitochondrial respiration.

■ Studies evaluating chronic adaptations to weight training have reported significant (but small) increases in resting muscle concentrations of glycogen, creatine, creatine phosphate, and ATP. Similar results have not been found for sprint training.

■ The term **buffering capacity** refers to the ability to bind free protons, and therefore resist increases in the free hydrogen ion concentration ($[H^+]$). Training for short-term endurance increases the muscle buffer capacity, whereas long-term endurance training results in a muscle buffer capacity no different than that in untrained control subjects. The improved muscle buffer capacity associated with training may be due to an increased amino acid and protein content of skeletal muscle fibers.

STUDY QUESTIONS

1. In contracting skeletal muscle, what determines which pathway predominates in ATP regeneration? Why?

2. List all the metabolic events that change during incremental exercise to VO_{2max}.

3. Explain why there is a controversy over the measurement of VO_{2max}.

4. What factors will combine to determine the magnitude of the oxygen deficit during a transition of an increased exercise intensity?

5. What is the lactate threshold and why is it important for long-term endurance exercise performance?

6. Compared to muscle adaptations to long-term muscular endurance, why do you think muscle is so limited in its chronic adaptability to intense exercise training?

7. Explain the factors that contribute to the excess postexercise oxygen consumption (EPOC).

APPLICATIONS

1. Evidence indicates that the LT responds to endurance training differently than VO_{2max}. If this is true, then attempt to explain the different mechanisms that cause improvements in these two capacities.

2. How might an inability to use muscle glycogen influence energy metabolism during (a) long-duration submaximal exercise and (b) short-term intense exercise?

3. Muscle myoglobin stores in ocean mammals that dive to great depths are more than double that of humans. Why do you think exercise training by humans doesn't increase muscle myoglobin if it is so important to oxygen provision to mitochondria?

4. Individuals with diabetes can develop ketosis, caused by the overproduction of ketone bodies by the liver, which in turn lowers blood pH. How would this condition influence exercise performance?

5. The ingestion of creatine has been shown to increase muscle creatine phosphate, and potentially improve intermittent intense exercise performance (see chapter 11). Explain these findings.

REFERENCES

1. Achten, E., et al. ^{31}P-NMR spectroscopy and the metabolic properties of different muscle fibers. *J. Appl. Physiol.* 68(2):644–649, 1990.

2. Adams, G. R., J. M. Foley, and R. A. Meyer. Muscle buffer capacity estimated from pH changes during rest-to-work transitions. *J. Appl. Physiol.* 69(3):968–972, 1990.

3. Bahr, R., I. Ingnes, O. Vaage, O. M. Sejersted, and E. A. Newsholme. Effect of duration of exercise on excess postexercise O_2 consumption. *J. Appl. Physiol.* 62(3):485–490, 1987.

4. Bahr, R., and O. M. Sejersted. Effect of feeding and fasting on excess postexercise oxygen consumption. *J. Appl. Physiol.* 71(6):2088–2093, 1991.

5. Baker, A. J., K. G. Kostov, R. G. Miller, and M. W. Weiner. Slow force recovery after long-duration exercise: Metabolic and activation factors in muscle fatigue. *J. Appl. Physiol.* 74(5):2294–2300, 1993.

6. Bangsbo, J., et al. Anaerobic energy production and O_2 deficit-debt relationship during exhaustive exercise in humans. *J. Physiol. London* 422:539–559, 1990.

7. Bangsbo, J., L. Johansen, B. Quistorff, and B. Saltin. NMR and analytic biochemical evaluation of CrP and nucleotides in the human calf during muscle contraction. *J. Appl. Physiol.* 74(4):2034–2039, 1993.

8. Bassett, D. R., P. W. Merrill, F. J. Nagel, J. A. Agre, and R. Sampedro. Rate of decline in blood lactate after cycling exercise in endurance-trained and untrained subjects. *J. Appl. Physiol.* 70(4):1816–1820, 1991.

9. Bassett, D. R., Jr., and E. T. Howley. Maximal oxygen uptake: "Classical" versus "contemporary" viewpoints. *Med. Sci. Sports Exerc.* 29(5):591–603, 1997.

10. Beaver, W. L., K. Wasserman, and B. J. Whipp. Improved detection of lactate threshold during exercise using a log-log transformation. *J. Appl. Physiol.* 59(6):1936–1940, 1985.

11. Belcastro, A. N., and A. Bonen. Lactic acid removal rates during controlled and uncontrolled recovery exercise. *J. Appl. Physiol.* 39(6):932–936, 1975.

12. Beneke, R., and S. P. von Duvillard. Determination of maximal lactate steady-state response in selected sports events. *Med. Sci. Sports Exerc.* 28(2):241–246, 1996.

13. Bertocci, L. A., J. L. Fleckenstein, and J. Antonio. Human muscle fatigue after glycogen depletion: A ^{31}P magnetic resonance study. *J. Appl. Physiol.* 73(1):75–81, 1992.

14. Bielinski, R., Y. Schutz, and J. Jequier. Energy metabolism during the postexercise recovery in man. *Am. J. Clin. Nutr.* 42:69–82, 1985.

15. Binzoni, T., G. Ferretti, K. Schenker, and P. Cerretelli. Phosphocreatine hydrolysis by ^{31}P–NMR at the onset of constant-load exercise in humans. *J. Appl. Physiol.* 73(4):1644–1649, 1992.

16. Bonen, A., G. W. Ness, A. N. Belcastro, and R. L. Kirby. Mild exercise impedes glycogen repletion in muscle. *J. Appl. Physiol.* 58(5):1622–1629, 1985.

17. Bonen, A., J. C. McDermott, and C. A. Hutber. Carbohydrate metabolism in skeletal muscle: An update of current concepts. *Int. J. Sports Med.* 10:385–401, 1989.

18. Brooks, G. A. Lactate production under fully aerobic conditions: The lactate shuttle during rest and exercise. *Federation Proc.* 45:2924–2929, 1986.

19. Buchfuhrer, M. J., et al. Optimizing the exercise protocol for cardiopulmonary assessment. *J. Appl. Physiol.* 55:558–564, 1983.

20. Carlson, L. A., L. Ekelund, and S. O. Froberg. Concentration of triglycerides, phospholipids and glycogen in skeletal muscle and of free fatty acids and β-hydroxybutyric acid in blood in man in response to exercise. *Europ. J. Clin. Invest.* 1:248–255, 1971.

21. Chance, B., et al. Fatigue in retrospect and prospect: ^{31}P NMR studies of exercise performance. In H. G. Knuttgen, J. A. Vogel, and J. Poortmans (eds.), *Biochemisty of exercise.* International Series on Sport Sciences: Vol. 13, Human Kinetic Publishers, Champaign, IL, 1982, pp. 895–908.

22. Cheetham, M. E., L. H. Boobis, S. Brooks, and C. Williams. Human muscle metabolism during sprint running. *J. Appl. Physiol.* 61(1):54–60, 1986.

23. Chwalbinska-Moneta, J., R. A. Roberge, D. L. Costill, and W. Fink. Threshold for muscle lactate accumulation during progressive exercise. *J. Appl. Physiol.* 66(60):2710–2716, 1989.

24. Coggan, A. R., et al. Muscle metabolism during exercise in young and older untrained and endurance-trained men. *J. Appl. Physiol.* 75(5):2125–2133, 1993.

25. Connett, R. J., T. E. J. Gayeski, and C. R. Honig. Energy sources in fully aerobic rest-work conditions: A new role for glycolysis. *Am. J. Physiol.* 248(17): H922–H929, 1985.

26. Costill, D. L., W. J. Fink, H. Getchell, J. L. Ivy, and F. A. Witzmann. Lipid metabolism in skeletal muscle of endurance-trained males and females. *J. Appl. Physiol.* 47(4):787–791, 1979.

27. Costill, D. L., W. J. Fink, M. Hargreaves, D. S. King, R. Thomas, and R. Fielding. Metabolic characteristics of skeletal muscle detraining from competitive swimming. *Med. Sci. Sports Exerc.* 17(3):339–343, 1985.

28. Costill, D. L., D. D. Pascoe, W. J. Fink, R. A. Roberge, S. I. Barr, and D. Pearson. Impaired muscle glycogen resynthesis after eccentric exercise. *J. Appl. Physiol.* 69(1):46–50, 1990.

29. Daniels, J. T. A physiologist's view of running economy. *Med. Sci. Sports Exerc.* 17(3):332–338, 1985.

30. Davis, J. A., P. Vodak, J. H. Wilmore, J. Vodak, and P. Kurtz. Anaerobic threshold and maximal aerobic power for three modes of exercise. *J. Appl. Physiol.* 41(4):544–550, 1976.

31. Dodd, S., S. K. Powers, T. Callender, and E. Brooks. Blood lactate disappearance at various intensities of recovery exercise. *J. Appl. Physiol.* 57(5):1462–1465, 1984.

32. Dohn, L. G., G. J. Kasperek, E. B. Tapscott, and H.A. Barakat. Protein metabolism during endurance exercise. *Federation. Proc.* 44:348–352, 1985.

33. Doyle, J. A., and W. M. Sherman. Eccentric exercise and glycogen synthesis. *Med. Sci. Sports Exerc.* 24(4):(Abstract 587)S98, 1991.

34. Dudley, G. A., P. C. Tullson, and R. L. Terjung. Influence of mitochondrial content on the sensitivity of respiratory control. *J. Biol. Chem.* 262(19):9109–9114, 1987.

35. Flynn, M. G., D. L. Costill, J. P. Kirwan, W. J. Fink, and D. R. Dengal. Muscle fiber composition and respiratory capacity in triathletes. *Int. J. Sports Med.* 8(6):383–386, 1987.

36. Forster, J., et al. Glucose uptake and flux through phosphofructokinase in wounded rat skeletal muscle. *Am. J. Physiol.* 256(19):E788–E797, 1989.

37. Freund, H., et al. Work rate–dependent lactate kinetics after exercise in humans. *J. Appl. Physiol.* 61(3):932–939, 1986.

38. Gaesser, G., and G. Brooks. Metabolic bases of postexercise oxygen consumption: A review. *Med. Sci. Sports Exerc.* 16:29–43, 1984.

39. Gollnick, P. D., R. B. Armstrong, C. W. Saubert IV, K. Piehl, and B. Saltin. Enzyme activity and fiber composition in skeletal muscle of untrained and trained men. *J. Appl. Physiol.* 33(3):312–319, 1972.

40. Gollnick, P. D., R. B. Armstrong, B. Saltin, C. W. Saubert IV, W. L. Sembrowich, and R. E. Shepherd. Effect of training on enzyme activity and fiber composition of human skeletal muscle. *J. Appl. Physiol.* 34(1):107–111, 1973.

41. Gollnick, P. D., K. Piehl, and B. Saltin. Selective glycogen depletion pattern in human muscle fibers after exercise of varying intensity and at varying pedal rates. *J. Physiol. London* 241:45–57, 1974.

42. Gollnick, P. D. Metabolism of substrates: Energy substrate metabolism during exercise and as modified by training. *Federation Proc.* 44:353–357, 1985.

43. Gore, C. J., and R. T. Withers. Effects of exercise intensity and duration on postexercise metabolism. *J. Appl. Physiol.* 68(6):2362–2368, 1990.

44. Green, H. J., R. L. Hughson, G. W. Orr, and D. A. Ranney. Anaerobic threshold, blood lactate, and muscle metabolites in progressive exercise. *J. Appl. Physiol.* 54(4):1032–1038, 1983.

45. Green, S., B. T. Dawson, C. Goodman, and M. F. Carey. Anaerobic ATP production and accumulated O_2 deficit in cyclists. *Med. Sci. Sports Exerc.* 28(3):315–321, 1996.

46. Hagberg, H. A., J. P. Mullin, and F. J. Nagle. Oxygen consumption during constant-load exercise. *J. Appl. Physiol.* 45(3):381–384, 1978.

47. Hagberg, J. M., R. C. Hickson, A. A. Ehsani, and J. O. Holloszy. Faster adjustment to and recovery from submaximal exercise in the trained state. *J. Appl. Physiol.* 48:218–224, 1980.

48. Harms, E. H., and R. C. Hickson. Skeletal muscle mitochondria and myoglobin, endurance, and intensity of training. *J. Appl. Physiol.* 54(3):798–802, 1983.

49. Harris, R. C., E. Hultman, and K. Sahlin. Glycolytic intermediates in human skeletal muscle after isometric contraction. *Pflugers Arch.* 389:277–282, 1989.

50. Heck, H., A. Mader, G. Hess, S. Mucke, R. Muller, and W. Hoolman. Justification of the 4 mmol/L lactate threshold. *Int. J. Sports Med.* 6:117–130, 1985.

51. Henriksson, J. Training induced adaptation of skeletal muscle and metabolism during submaximal exercise. *J. Physiol.* 270:661–675, 1977.

REFERENCES

52. Henriksson, J., and J. S. Reitman. Time course of changes in human skeletal muscle succinate dehydrogenase and cytochrome oxidase activities and maximal oxygen uptake with physical activity and inactivity. *Acta Physiol. Scand.* 99:91–97, 1977.

53. Hickner, R. C., et al. Muscle glycogen accumulation after endurance exercise in trained and untrained individuals. *J. Appl. Physiol.* 83(3):897–903, 1997.

54. Hickson, R. C., H. A. Bomze, and J. O. Holloszy. Linear increase in aerobic power induced by a strenuous program of endurance exercise. *J. Appl. Physiol.* 42(3):372–376, 1977.

55. Hickson, R. C., H. A. Bomze, and J. Holloszy. Faster adjustment of O_2 uptake to the energy requirement of exercise in the trained state. *J. Appl. Physiol.* 44(6):877–881, 1978.

56. Hill, A. V., and H. Lupton. Muscular exercise, lactic acid, and the supply and utilization of oxygen. *Q J. Med.* 16:135–171, 1923.

57. Hirvonen, J., S. Rehunen, H. Rusko, and M. Harkonen. Breakdown of high-energy phosphate compounds and lactate accumulation during short supramaximal exercise. *Eur. J. Appl. Physiol.* 56:253–259, 1987.

58. Holloszy, J. O., L. B. Oscai, I. J. Don, and P. A. Mole. Mitochondrial citric acid cycle and related enzymes: Adaptive response to exercise. *Biochem. Biophys. Res. Comm.* 40(6):1368–1373, 1970.

59. Holloszy, J. O., and E. F. Coyle. Adaptations of skeletal muscle to endurance training and their metabolic consequences. *J. Appl. Physiol.* 56(4):831–838, 1984.

60. Howley, E. T., D. R. Bassett and H. G. Welch. Criteria for maximal oxygen uptake: Review and commentary. *Med. Sci. Sports Exerc.* 27(10):1292–1301, 1995.

61. Hughson, R. L., K. D. Weisiger, and G. D. Swanson. Blood lactate concentration increases as a continous function in progressive exercise. *J. Appl. Physiol.* 62(5):1975–1981, 1987.

62. Hughson, R. L., J. E. Cochrane,, and G. C. Butler. Faster O_2 uptake kinetics at the onset of supine exercise with and without lower body negative pressure. *J. Appl. Physiol.* 75(5):1962–1967, 1993.

63. Hultman, E. H., and K. Sahlin. Acid-base balance during exercise. *Exerc. Sport Sci. Rev.* 7:41–128, 1980.

64. Hultman, E. H. Carbohydrate metabolism during hard exercise and in the recovery period after exercise. *Acta Physiol. Scand.* 128(Suppl. 556):75–82, 1986.

65. Hurley, B. F., P. M. Nemeth, W. H. Martin III, J. M. Hagberg, G. P. Dalsky, and J. O. Holloszy. Muscle triglyceride utilization during exercise: Effect of training. *J. Appl. Physiol.* 60(2):562–567,1986.

66. Ivy, J. L., R. T. Withers, P. J. Van Handel, D. H. Elder, and D. L. Costill. Muscle respiratory capacity and fiber type as determinants of the lactate threshold. *J. Appl. Physiol.* 48(3):523–527, 1980.

67. Jacobs, I. Lactate in human skeletal muscle after 10 and 30 s of supramaximal exercise. *J. Appl. Physiol.* 55(20:365–367, 1983.

68. Jacobs, I., M. Esbjornsson, C. Sylven, I. Holm, and E. Jansson. Sprint training effects on muscle myoglobin, enzymes, fiber types, and blood lactate. *Med. Sci. Sports Exerc.* 19(4):368–374, 1987.

69. Jansson, E., C. Sylven, and B. Sjodin. Myoglobin concentration and training in humans. In H. G. Knuttgen, J. A. Vogel, and J. Poortmans (eds.), *Biochemisty of exercise.* International Series on Sport Sciences: Vol. 13, Human Kinetic Publishers, Champaign, IL, 1982, p. 821–825.

70. Joyner, M. J. Modeling: Optimal marathon performance on the basis of physiological factors. *J. Appl. Physiol.* 70(2):683–687, 1991.

71. Karlsson, J., L. Nordesjo, L. Jorfeldt, and B. Saltin. Muscle lactate, ATP, and CP levels after physical training in man. *J. Appl. Physiol.* 33(2):199–203, 1972.

72. Karlsson, J., L.-O. Nordesjo, and B. Saltin. Muscle glycogen utilization after physical training. *Acta Physiol. Scand.* 90:210–217, 1974.

73. Katz, A., S. Broberg, K. Sahlin, and J. Wahren. Muscle ammonia and amino acid metabolism during dynamic exercise in man. *Clin. Physiol.* 6:365–379, 1986.

74. Katz, A., and K. Sahlin. Effects of decreased oxygen availability on NADH and lactate contents in human skeletal muscle during exercise. *Acta Physiol. Scand.* 131:119–128, 1987.

75. Katz, A., and K. Sahlin. Regulation of lactic acid production during exercise. *J. Appl. Physiol.* 65(2):509–518, 1988.

76. Katz, A., and K. Sahlin. Role of oxygen in regulation of glycolysis and lactate production in human skeletal muscle. *Exerc. Sport Sci. Rev.* 18:1–28, 1990.

77. Kavanagh, T., R. Shephard, and V. Pandit. Marathon running after myocardial infarction. *J. Am. Med. Assoc.* 229:1602–1605, 1974.

78. Kowalchuk, J. M., G. J. F. Heigenhauser, M. I. Lindinger, G. Obminski, J. R. Sutton, and N.L. Jones. Role of lungs and inactive muscle in acid-base control after maximal exercise. *J. Appl. Physiol.* 65(5):2090–2096, 1988.

79. LaFontaine, T. P., B. R. Londeree, and W. K. Spath. The maximal steady state versus selected running events. *Med. Sci. Sports Exerc.* 13(3):190–192, 1981.

80. MacDougall, J. D., G. R. Ward, D. G. Sale, and J. R. Sutton. Biochemical adaptation of human skeletal muscle to heavy resistance exercise training and immobilization. *J. Appl. Physiol.* 43(4):700–703, 1977.

81. MacDougall, J. D., G. R. Ward, D. G. Sale, and J. R. Sutton. Muscle glycogen repletion after high intensity intermittent exercise. *J. Appl. Physiol.* 42(2):129–132, 1977.

82. MacLean, D. A., L. L. Spriet, E. Hultman, and T. E. Graham. Plasma and muscle amino acid and ammonia responses during prolonged exercise in humans. *J. Appl. Physiol.* 70(5):2095–2103, 1991.

83. Madden, A., M. O. Leach, J. C. Sharp, D. J. Collins, and D. Easton. A quantitative analysis of the accuracy of in vivo pH measurements with ^{31}P NMR spectroscopy: Assessment of pH measurement methodology. *NMR in Biomedicine.* 4(1):1–11, 1991.

84. Mader, A., and H. Heck. A theory of the metabolic origin of the "anaerobic threshold." *Int. J. Sports Med.* (Suppl. 1): 45–65, 1986.

85. Maelum, S., M. Grandmontagne, E. A. Newsholme, and O. M. Sejersted. Magnitude and duration of excess postexercise oxygen consumption in young healthy subjects. *Metabolism* 35:425–429, 1986.

86. McCartney, N., L. L. Spriet, G. J. F. Heigenhauser, J. M. Kowalchuk, J. R. Sutton, and N. L. Jones. Muscle power and metabolism in maximal intermittent cycling. *J. Appl. Physiol.* 60(4):1164–1169, 1986.

87. McKenzie, D. C., et al. Skeletal muscle buffering capacity in elite athletes. In H. G. Knuttgen, J. A. Vogel, and J. Poortmans (eds.), *Biochemisty of exercise*. International Series on Sport Sciences: Vol. 13, Human Kinetic Publishers, Champaign, IL, 1982, pp. 584–589.

88. Medbo, J. I., A. Mohn, I. Tabata, R. Bahr, O. Vaage, and O. M. Sejersted. Anaerobic capacity determined by maximal accumulated O_2 deficit. *J. Appl. Physiol.* 64(1):50–60, 1988.

89. Medbo, J. I., and I. Tabata. Anaerobic energy release in working muscle during 30 s to 3 min of exhausting exercise. *J. Appl. Physiol.* 75(4):1654–1660, 1993.

90. Minotti, J. R., et al. Forearm metabolic asymmetry detected by ^{31}P-NMR during submaximal exercise. *J. Appl. Physiol.* 67(1):324–329, 1989.

91. O'Brien, M. J., C. A. Viguie, R. S. Mazzeo, and G. A. Brooks. Carbohydrate dependence during marathon running. *Med. Sci. Sports Exerc.* 25(9):1009–1017, 1993.

92. Nemeth, P. M., N. M. Chi, C. S. Hintz, and O. H. Lowry. Myoglobin content of normal and trained human muscle fibers. In H. G. Knuttgen, J. A. Vogel, and J. Poortmans (eds.), *Biochemisty of exercise*. International Series on Sport Sciences: Vol. 13, Human Kinetic Publishers, Champaign, IL, 1982, pp. 826–831.

93. Nevill, M. E., L. H. Boobis, S. Brooks, and C. Williams. Effect of training on muscle metabolism during treadmill sprinting. *J. Appl. Physiol.* 67(6):2376–2382, 1989.

94. Noakes, T. D. Implications of exercise testing for prediction of athletic performance: A contemporary perspective. *Med. Sci. Sports Exerc.* 20(4):319–330, 1988.

95. Noakes, T. D. Challenging beliefs: Ex Africa semper aliquid novi. *Med. Sci. Sports Exerc.* 29(5):571–590, 1997.

96. Noakes, T. D. Maximal oxygen uptake: "Classical" versus "contemporary" viewpoints: A rebuttal. *Med. Sci. Sports Exerc.* 30(9):1381–1398, 1998.

97. Pacy, P. J., J. D. Webster, G. Isaacs. S. Hunter, and J. S. Garrow. The effect of aerobic exercise on subsequent 24 h resting metabolic rate in normal male subjects. *Proc. Nutr. Soc.* 46(Abstract):4A, 1987.

98. Parkhouse, W. S., et al. The relationship between carnosine levels, buffering capacity, fiber type and anaerobic capacity in elite athletes. In H. G. Knuttgen, J. A. Vogel, and J. Poortmans (eds.), *Biochemisty of exercise*. International Series on Sport Sciences: Vol. 13, Human Kinetic Publishers, Champaign, IL, 1982, pp. 590–594.

99. Piehl, K., S. Adolfsson, and K. Nazar. Glycogen storage and glycogen synthase activity in trained and untrained muscle of man. *Acta Physiol. Scand.* 90:779–788, 1974.

100. Pollock, M. L., et al. Comparative analysis of physiological responses to three different maximal graded exercise protocols in healthy women. *Am. Heart J.* 103:363–373, 1982.

101. Ravussin, E., C. Bogardus, K. Scheidegger, B. LaGrange, E. D. Horton, and E. S. Horton. Effect of elevated FFA on carbohydrate and lipid oxidation during prolonged exercise in humans. *J. Appl. Physiol.* 60(3):893–900, 1986.

102. Ren, J. M., J. Henriksson, A. Katz, and K. Sahlin. NADH content in type I and type II human muscle fibers after dynamic exercise. *Biochem. J.* 25:183–187, 1988.

103. Rennie, M. J., W. W. Winder, and J. O. Holloszy. A sparing effect of increased plasma free fatty acids on muscle and liver glycogen content in the exercising rat. *Biochem. J.* 156:647–655, 1976.

104. Renaud, J. M., Y. Allard, and G. W. Mainwood. Is the change intracellular pH during fatigue large enough to be the main cause of fatigue? *Can. J. Physiol. Pharmacol.* 64:764–767, 1986.

105. Robergs, R. A., et al. Effects of warm-up on muscle glycogenolysis during intense exercise. *Med. Sci. Sports Exerc.* 23(1):37–43, 1991.

106. Robergs, R. A. Nutritional and exercise determinants of postexercise muscle glycogen synthesis. *Int. J. Sports Nutr.* 1(4):307–337, 1991.

107. Robergs, R. A., et al. Muscle glycogenolysis during differing intensities of weight-resistance exercise. *J. Appl. Physiol.* 70(4):1700–1706, 1991.

108. Robergs, R. A. An exercise physiologist's "contemporary" interpretations of the "ugly and creaking edifices" of exercise physiology. *J. Exerc. Physiol.* online (in review), http://www.css.edu/users/tboone2/asep/toc.htm, 1999.

109. Romjin, J. A., et al. Regulation of endogenous fat and carbohydrate metabolism in relation to exercise intensity and duration. *Am. J. Physiol.* 265(28): E380–E391, 1993.

110. Romjin, J. A., E. F. Coyle, L. S. Sidossis, X.-J. Zhang, and R. R. Wolfe. Relationship between fatty acid delivery and fatty acid oxidation during strenuous exercise. *J. Appl. Physiol.* 79(6):1939–1945, 1995.

111. Roth, D. A., and G. A. Brooks. Facilitated lactate transport across muscle membranes. *Med. Sci. Sports Exerc.* 21(2):(Abstract 206)S35, 1989.

112. Sahlin, K. NADH in human skeletal muscle during short-term intense exercise. *Pfluegers Arch.* 403:193–198, 1985.

113. Sahlin, K., A. Katz, and J. Henriksson. Redox state and lactate accumulation in human skeletal muscle during dynamic exercise. *Biochem. J.* 245:551–556, 1987.

114. Sahlin, K., A. Katz, and S. Broberg. Tricarboxylic acid cycle intermediates in human muscle during prolonged exercise. *Am. J. Physiol.* 259(28): C834–C841, 1990.

115. Sale, D. G., I. Jacobs, J. D. MacDougall, and S. Garner. Comparison of two regimens of concurrent strength and endurance training. *Med. Sci. Sports Exerc.* 22(3):348–356, 1990.

116. Saltin, B., et al. The nature of the training response: Peripheral and central adaptations to one-legged cycling. *Acta Physiol. Scand.* 96:289–305, 1976.

REFERENCES

117. Shearer, J. D, J. F. Amarai, and M. D. Caldwell. Glucose metabolism of injured skeletal muscle: Contribution of inflammatory cells. *Circulatory Shock*. 25:131–138, 1988.

118. Spriet, L. L., K. Sonderland, M. Bergstrom, and E. Hultman. Anaerobic energy release in skeletal muscle during electrical stimulation. *J. Appl. Physiol.* 62(2):611–615, 1987.

119. Spriet, L. L., K. Soderlund, M. Bergstrom, and E. Hultman. Skeletal muscle glycogenolysis, glycolysis, and pH during electrical stimulation in men. *J. Appl. Physiol.* 62(2):616–621, 1987.

120. Spriet, L. L., M. L. Lindinger, R. S. McKelvie, G. J. F. Heigenhauser, and N. L. Jones. Muscle glycogenolysis and H^+ concentration during maximal intermittent cycling. *J. Appl. Physiol.* 66(1):8–13, 1988.

121. Stainsby, W. N., and G. A. Brooks. Control of lactic acid metabolism in contracting muscles and during exercise. *Exerc. Sport Sci. Rev.* 18:29–64, 1990.

122. Stanley, W. C., E. W. Gertz, J. A. Wisneski, D. L. Morris, R. A. Neese, and G. A. Brooks. Systematic lactate kinetics during graded exercise in man. *Am. J. Physiol.* 249(12):E595–E602, 1985.

123. Stromme, S. B., F. Ingjer, and H. D. Meen. Assessment of maximal aerobic power in specifically trained athletes. *J. Appl. Physiol.* 42(6):833–837, 1977.

124. Svedenhag, J. Maximal and submaximal oxygen uptake during running: How should body mass be accounted for? *Scand. J. Med. Sci. Sports* 5(4):175–180, 1995.

125. Tarnopolsky, L. J., J. D. MacDougall, S. A. Atkinson, M. A. Tarnopolsky, and J. R. Sutton. Gender differences in substrate for endurance exercise. *J. Appl. Physiol.* 68(1):302–308, 1990.

126. Terrados, N., E. Jansson, C. Sylven, and L. Kaijser. Is hypoxia a stimulus for synthesis of oxidative enzymes and myoglobin? *J. Appl. Physiol.* 68(6):2369–2372, 1990.

127. Tesch, P. A., B. Collainder, and P. Kaiser. Muscle metabolism during intense, heavy resistance exercise. *Eur. J. Appl. Physiol.* 55:362–366, 1986.

128. Tesch, P. A., A. Thorsson, and N. Fujitsuka. Creatine phosphate in fiber types of skeletal muscle before and after exhaustive exercise. *J. Appl. Physiol.* 66(40):1756–1759, 1989.

129. Tonokura, M., and K. Yamada. Changes in intracellular pH and inorganic phosphate concentration during and after muscle contraction as studied by time-resolved ^{31}P-NMR. *Fed. Eur. Biochem. Soc.* 171(2):165–168, 1984.

130. Vollestad, N. K., O. Vaage, and L. Hermansen. Muscle glycogen depletion pattern in type I and subgroups of type II fibers during prolonged severe exercise. *Acta Physiol. Scand.* 122:433–440, 1984.

131. Vollestad, N. K., and P. C. S. Blom. Effect of varying exercise intensity on glycogen depletion in human muscle fibers. *Acta Physiol. Scand.* 125:395–405, 1985.

132. Vollestad, N. K., P. C. S. Blom, and O. Gronnerod. Resynthesis of glycogen in different muscle fiber types after prolonged exhaustive exercise in man. *Acta Physiol. Scand.* 137:15–21, 1989.

133. Wasserman, K., W. L. Beaver, and B. J. Whipp. Mechanisms and patterns of blood lactate increase during exercise in man. *Med. Sci. Sports Exerc.* 18(3):344–352, 1986.

134. Weicker, H., H. Bert, A. Rettenmeier, U. Oettinger, H. Hagele, and U. Keilholz. Alanine formation during maximal short-term exercise. In H. G. Knuttgen, J. A. Vogel, and J. Poortmans (eds.), *Biochemisty of exercise*. International Series on Sport Sciences: Vol. 13, Human Kinetic Publishers, Champaign, IL, 1982, pp. 385–394.

135. Westerlind, K. C., W. C. Byrnes, and R. S. Mazzeo. A comparison of the oxygen drift in downhill vs. level running. *J. Appl. Physiol.* 72(20):796–800, 1992.

136. Whipp, B. J., and K. Wasserman. Oxygen uptake kinetics for various intensities of constant-load work. *J. Appl. Physiol.* 33(3):351–356, 1972.

137. Wolfe, R. R. Does exercise stimulate protein breakdown in humans? Isotopic approaches to the problem. *Med. Sci. Sports Exerc.* 19(15): S172–S178, 1987.

138. Wolfe, R. R., M. H. Wolfe, E. R. Nadel, and J. H. F. Shaw. Isotopic determination of amino-acid-urea interactions in exercise in humans. *J. Appl. Physiol.* 56(1):221–229, 1984.

139. Zachwieja, J. J., D. L. Costill, D. D. Pascoe, R. A. Robergs, and W. J. Fink. Influence of muscle glycogen depletion on the rate of resynthesis. *Med. Sci. Sports Exerc.* 23(1):44–48, 1990.

140. Zanconato, S., S. Buchthal, T. J. Barstow and D. M. Cooper. ^{31}P-magnetic resonance spectroscopy of leg muscle metabolism during exercise in children and adults. *J. Appl. Physiol.* 74(5):2214–2218, 1993.

RECOMMENDED READINGS

Cheetham, M. E., L. H. Boobis, S. Brooks, and C. Williams. Human muscle metabolism during sprint running. *J. Appl. Physiol.* 61(1):54–60, 1986.

Gaesser, G., and G. Brooks. Metabolic bases of post-exercise oxygen consumption: A review. *Med. Sci. Sports Exerc.* 16:29–43, 1984.

Hirvonen, J., S. Rehunen, H. Rusko, and M. Harkonen. Breakdown of high-energy phosphate compounds and lactate accumulation during short supramaximal exercise. *Eur. J. Appl. Physiol.* 56:253–259, 1987.

Howley, E. T., D. R. Bassett, and H. G. Welch. Criteria for maximal oxygen uptake: Review and commentary. *Med. Sci. Sports Exerc.* 27(10):1292–1301, 1995.

Hurley, B. F., P. M. Nemeth, W. H. Martin III, J. M. Hagberg, G. P. Dalsky, and J. O. Holloszy. Muscle triglyceride utilization during exercise: Effect of training. *J. Appl. Physiol.* 60(2):562–567,1986.

Medbo, J. I., A. Mohn, I. Tabata, R. Bahr, O. Vaage, and O. M. Sejersted. Anaerobic capacity determined by maximal accumulated O_2 deficit. *J. Appl. Physiol.* 64(1):50–60, 1988.

Robergs, R. A. Nutritional and exercise determinants of postexercise muscle glycogen synthesis. *Int. J. Sports Nutr.* 1(4):307–337, 1991.

Robergs, R. A. An exercise physiologist's "contemporary" interpretations of the "ugly and creaking edifices" of exercise physiology. *J. Exerc. Physiol.* online (in review), http://www.css.edu/users/tboone2/asep/toc.htm, 1998.

Romjin, J. A., et al. Regulation of endogenous fat and carbohydrate metabolism in relation to exercise intensity and duration. *Am. J. Physiol.* 265(28):E380–E391, 1993.

Saltin, B., et al. The nature of the training response: Peripheral and central adaptations to one-legged cycling. *Acta Physiol. Scand.* 96:289–305, 1976.

Spriet, L. L., K. Soderlund, M. Bergstrom, and E. Hultman. Skeletal muscle glycogenolysis, glycolysis, and pH during electrical stimulation in men. *J. Appl. Physiol.* 62(2):616–621, 1987.

Tesch, P. A., A. Thorsson, and N. Fujitsuka. Creatine phosphate in fiber types of skeletal muscle before and after exhaustive exercise. *J. Appl. Physiol.* 66(40):1756–1759, 1989.

Wasserman, K., W. L. Beaver, and B. J. Whipp. Mechanisms and patterns of blood lactate increase during exercise in man. *Med. Sci. Sports Exerc.* 18(30):344–352, 1986.

Whipp, B. J. and, K. Wasserman. Oxygen uptake kinetics for various intensities of constant-load work. *J. Appl. Physiol.* 33(3):351–356, 1972.

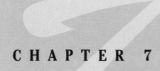

CHAPTER 7

Cardiovascular Function and Adaptation to Exercise

uring exercise, the cellular demand for oxygen requires that the body increase the transfer of oxygen in atmospheric air into the blood, and increase the rate at which blood is circulated around the body. The increasing circulation of blood around the body occurs as a result of the complex and sensitive regulation of the body's heart and blood vessels. As soon as we start to exercise, heart rate increases, the volume of blood pumped at each beat of the heart increases, and there is a decreased resistance to blood flow in arteries, arterioles, and capillaries that supply blood to the contracting muscle. To add complication to how our cardiovascular system functions during and following exercise, the heat stress of exercise involves cardiovascular changes to aid in the dissipation of heat to the surroundings. Heat release from the body is mainly dependent on sweating, which can result in appreciable fluid loss or dehydration, which in turn influences cardiovascular function. Because the cardiovascular system is integral in the regulation of blood oxygen transport, body temperature, fluid balance, and blood pressure, and exercise alters each of these functions, the cardiovascular responses to exercise represent a crucial body of knowledge in exercise physiology. The purpose of this chapter is to briefly outline the components of the cardiovascular system, explain the regulation of cardiovascular function during exercise, and detail the acute and chronic adaptations of cardiovascular structure and function to exercise.

OBJECTIVES

After studying this chapter, you should be able to:

- List the components of the cardiovascular system.
- Describe the diverse functions of blood and its importance to the optimal function of the cardiovascular system.
- Identify approximate volumes of blood and plasma and their relationships to fitness and body mass.
- Identify the changes that occur for cardiac output, stroke volume, and heart rate during different exercise conditions.
- List the several factors that regulate blood flow to skeletal muscle.
- Explain how cardiovascular structure and function changes in response to endurance and strength training.

KEY TERMS

cardiovascular system	anemia	Fick equation
systemic circulation	osmolality	vasoconstriction
blood	cardiac cycle	vasodilation
hematocrit	preload	blood pressure
erythrocytes	afterload	Korotkoff sounds
polycythemia	stroke volume	hemoconcentration
	ejection fraction	hyperemia
	cardiac output	

Components of the Cardiovascular System

*A*natomical and functional aspects of the heart are referred to as *cardiac,* whereas anatomical and functional aspects of the circulation of blood around the body are referred to as *vascular,* hence the term *cardiovascular.* The **cardiovascular system** (or *circulatory system*) is composed of blood, the heart, and the vasculature within which blood is pumped throughout the body. The heart is a biological pump that generates the pressure that drives blood throughout the vasculature, and therefore life is dependent on its continual effective function. Within the cardiovascular system exists the *pulmonary circulation* of the lungs, and the **systemic circulation** of the remainder of the body. Within the systemic circulation are local circulation beds, such as that of the head and brain (*cranial* circulation), liver (*hepatic* circulation), kidney (*renal* circulation), abdominal viscera and intestinal tract (*splanchnic* circulation), skin (*cutaneous* circulation), and *skeletal muscle* circulation. The combined function of the cardiovascular system and lungs (chapter 8) is referred to as *cardiorespiratory* function.

A brief review of the components of the cardiovascular system will be presented so that the full implications of cardiovascular function during exercise can be appreciated.

Blood

Blood is the liquid medium that circulates within the vascular system. Blood can be divided into cellular and noncellular components, as illustrated in figure 7.1. The general functions of the cellular and liquid components of blood are presented in table 7.1.

It is clear that blood serves many functions, and that although the transport of blood gases is crucial to life, other functions of blood can be equally important during rest (e.g., immune functions) and certain exercise conditions (e.g., thermoregulation, water exchange).

Cellular Components

The cell content of blood (hematocrit) constitutes approximately 45% of the total blood volume. Hematocrit is lower in females than males, and will vary with hydration status. For the average individual, total blood volume approximates 5 L, but will be greater for larger, more endurance-trained, and altitude-acclimated individuals. As will be discussed in later sections, the finite store of blood in the body, and the potentially large muscle mass that can be recruited during exercise can severely challenge the capacity of the heart and blood to transport oxygen to contracting muscle during intense exercise.

Blood consists of several types of cells which all emanate from a stem cell located in bone marrow. The original stem cell can differentiate into precursors of white blood cells

FIGURE 7.1

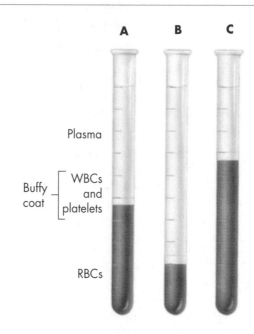

The cellular and liquid components of blood, as they appear after centrifugation.

(*leukocytes*), red blood cells (**erythrocytes**), or cell fragments known as *platelets.* During the synthesis of erythrocytes (*erythropoiesis*), the stem cell is differentiated into nucleated cells that synthesize hemoglobin. These cells are released into the circulation when they have lost their nucleus, and are then termed *reticulocytes.* The reticulocyte has remnants of RNA and continues to synthesize hemoglobin. The differentiation of the stem cell to a reticulocyte requires 2 days, and maturation of the reticulocyte to a mature erythrocyte may take an additional 2 days (6, 20). The stimulation of erythropoiesis is under the control of the hormone *erythropoietin,* as will be discussed in chapter 9.

The shape of the erythrocyte resembles a biconcaved disk, and in humans is approximately 8 μm in diameter, and

cardiovascular system the heart and blood vessels of the body

systemic circulation the vasculature of the body other than the pulmonary circulation

blood the fluid medium that contains cells that function to transport oxygen and carbon dioxide, cells involved in immunity, certain proteins involved in blood clotting and the transport of nutrients, and electrolytes necessary for optimal cell function

hematocrit (hem'a-to-krit) the ratio of the volume of blood cells and formed elements of blood to total blood volume; usually expressed as a percentage

erythrocyte (e-rith'ro-syt) red blood cell

TABLE 7.1

The main functions of the cellular and liquid components of blood

COMPONENT	FUNCTIONS
Cellular	Transport of oxygen and carbon dioxide
	Blood clotting
	Acid-base buffering
	Immune functions
	Tissue repair and destruction
Liquid	Blood clotting
	Circulation of cellular components and their contents
	Heat transfer and thermoregulation
	Water exchange and transport
	Circulation of hormones
	Acid-base buffering
	Circulation of metabolites, nutrients, and waste products

FIGURE 7.2

The size and shape of an erythrocyte resembles that of a bi-concave disc. Hemoglobin molecules are located within the erythrocytes, and can bind oxygen, carbon dioxide and hydrogen ions.

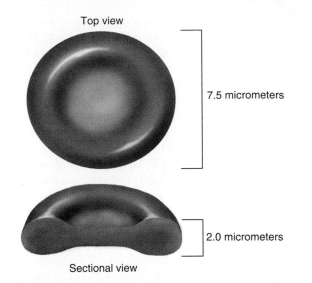

Top view

7.5 micrometers

2.0 micrometers

Sectional view

2 μm thick at the perimeter (6) (fig. 7.2). Molecules of hemoglobin are located on and inside the membrane surface of erythrocytes and function by transporting oxygen and carbon dioxide and buffering protons (see chapter 8). As erythrocytes have an average life span of 120 days, *erythropoiesis* is a continual process that occurs in the bone marrow and spleen. The iron from hemoglobin of the destroyed erythrocytes is recycled by the liver, and along with the nutritional intake of iron, the iron stores are transported in the blood bound to *transferrin* (iron-binding globulin). Iron can be stored in plasma and certain tissues (heart, liver, spleen) as *ferritin,* which is a complex of water-soluble protein and reduced iron (ferrous hydroxide).

An increased production of erythrocytes can result in elevated red blood cell counts, and this condition is termed **polycythemia.** Conversely, an inadequate ion intake, excessive bleeding, or exaggerated erythrocyte destruction can result in a lowered red blood cell count, or **anemia.**

Liquid Component

The liquid component of blood is termed *plasma*. Plasma is the medium within which the blood cells, metabolites, hormones, and nutrients are circulated around the body, body heat and water are redistributed, and certain reactions occur. When blood is drawn from the body, the clotting process forms fibrinogen and the remaining fluid component of blood is termed *serum.*

Because plasma represents 55% of total blood volume (1.00 − 0.45 [hematocrit] = 0.55), it approximates a volume of 3 L in the average adult. Plasma volume can be measured by injecting a substance that is known to remain in the vascular compartment. The total blood volume is then calculated from simple dilution equations, and plasma volume is obtained after adjustment for hematocrit. Plasma volume

varies in proportion with the lean body mass, more so than either of total body mass or even fitness (53). However, plasma volume is highly variable and changes very rapidly with alterations in posture, exercise, dehydration, and acute altitude exposure. For healthy young men (age range 18–35) plasma volume at rest and when seated can be estimated from the following equation. Unfortunately, an equation specific to females has not been produced from research.

7.1 $$PV\ (L) = 0.042\ (LBM, kg) + 0.567$$

where PV = plasma volume,
LBM = lean body mass [from Sawka and associates (53)].

The presence of electrolytes and proteins in plasma generates an osmotic force to attract and retain water within the vasculature. This osmotic force is best reflected by the number of particles in solution, which is termed **osmolality.** Changes in osmolality are detected by several specialized cells in the central nervous system and also in peripheral tissues such as the kidney. Changes in osmolality are important for the processes involved in the control of hydration and kidney function (see chapter 9).

The Heart

The heart is a muscular organ that is required to contract without voluntary control. You can estimate for yourself the number of times the heart must beat in a lifetime, and the volume of blood pumped in a lifetime (assume an average heart rate of 100 b/min, an average volume pumped per beat of 100 mL, and an average life span of 75 years). What is all the more amazing about the heart is that it can be regulated

FOCUS BOX 7.1

Using Heart Rate to Monitor Exercise Intensity and Training Progress

The heart rate monitor works by using a conductive chest strap to detect the small voltage changes from heart contraction that are conducted to the surface of the skin. These small voltage changes are converted to a radio signal and transferred through the air to a watch worn on the wrist by a process termed *telemetry*. The watch has computer software which then converts the received signals to heart rates that are displayed, and can be stored in the watch memory, in previously programmed intervals. This method of using the body's voltage changes during muscle contraction is the basis of the science of electrocardiography, and will be discussed in chapter 16.

The use of a personal heart rate monitor is a relatively simple and inexpensive method for the recording of heart rates during exercise. The heart rate monitor also allows many athletes to bring the laboratory to their training track. However, care must be used in how these heart rates are interpreted. Although heart rate does increase in proportion with increases in exercise intensity, other factors also alter the heart rate response to exercise—such as exercise duration, hydration, body temperature, terrestrial altitude, air pollution, overtraining, illness, and to a lesser extent the phase of the menstrual cycle. All these additional factors must be considered when interpreting the heart rate response to exercise.

to rapidly increase its rate of beating (heart rate) from what could be resting values less than 50 b/min to maximal values that could reach 200 b/min. In increasing the rate of pumping, blood has less time to fill the heart chambers, and there is less time to eject the blood from the heart. Nevertheless, heart function improves with exercise-induced increases in heart rate, as more blood is received and pumped each beat during incremental exercise. The use of heart rate monitors during exercise is described in focus box 7.1.

While pumping blood the healthy heart can generate average circulation pressures that increase from 90 to over 140 mmHg without signs or symptoms of impaired function. The ability to generate pressure is crucial for the function of the heart and the function of the rest of the body for, as will be explained in later sections, the blood circulates throughout the body down a pressure gradient where pressures are largest where blood leaves the heart and lowest where blood returns to the heart.

The heart is illustrated in figure 7.3 to reveal the flow of blood through the four chambers. Blood returns to the right atrium of the heart via the superior and inferior vena cava veins, passes into the right ventricle through the tricuspid valve, and is pumped by the right ventricle through the pulmonary valve into the *pulmonary circulation* where it returns to the left atrium. The blood then passes through the mitral valve into the left ventricle, where it is then pumped though the aorta artery to the circulation of the remainder of body, or *systemic circulation*. As indicated, *the heart functions as a double pump*, and the special one-way valves exist to prevent backflow of blood and the decreased effectiveness of the pump. One pump, the right side of the heart, receives blood from the systemic circulation and pumps it through the pulmonary circulation of the lungs. The other pump, the left side of the heart, receives blood from the pulmonary circulation and pumps it through the systemic circulation. The right and left sides of the heart contract and pump blood together, resulting in a closed-loop circulation. In be-

ing a closed-loop pump, the volume of blood pumped by the right and left sides of the heart must be equal, or else a backlog of blood would occur in either of the pulmonary or systemic circulations and cause serious impairments to pulmonary and cellular respiration.

The Cardiac Cycle

The previous description of blood flow through the heart and vasculature is referred to as the **cardiac cycle.** During the cardiac cycle, the volumes and pressures of blood in the atria and ventricles change in an organized and repeatable fashion, as do the blood pressures within each of the systemic and pulmonary circulations.

The phase of the cardiac cycle when the myocardium is relaxed is termed *diastole,* and blood flows passively into the right and left atrium and then into the respective ventricles. When the atria contract, termed *atrial systole* (or "atrial kick"), an additional 30% of total ventricular filling occurs. The volume of blood in each ventricle at the end of diastole is referred to as *end-diastolic volume* (EDV), and exerts a stretch on the ventricular myocardium. This stretch can be interpreted as a load, and is known as **preload** in clinical cardiology and cardiac rehabilitation. The greater the EDV and the greater the

polycythemia (pol'i-si-the'mi-ah) above-normal increase in the erythrocyte content of the blood

anemia (a-ne'mi-ah) abnormally low erythrocyte content, hemoglobin concentration, or hematocrit of the blood

osmolality (oz'mo-lal'i-ti) the number of particles per kg of solvent

cardiac cycle the events in a functional heart that occur between successive heart beats

preload the load to which a muscle is subjected before shortening; usually explained as the stretch induced on the mycoardium by the filling of the ventricles of the heart

FIGURE 7.3

Blood flow through the valves and chambers of the heart to the pulmonary and systemic circulations.

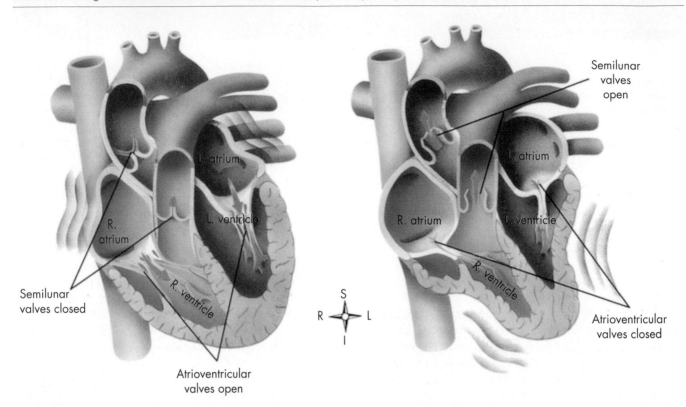

stretch, the faster is the resultant ventricular myocardial contraction, and this relationship is known as the *Frank-Starling law* of the heart (fig. 7.4). Catecholamine stimulation of the myocardium increases contractile force and velocity for a given EDV, and this response is termed *contractility*.

FIGURE 7.4

The relationship between end, diastolic volume (EDV), the velocity of myocardial contraction and contractility. Increasing EDV (increasing venous return) causes an increase in myocardial contraction velocity. In addition, stimulation by catecholamines generates a different curve for EDV and contraction velocity, thereby increasing contractility.

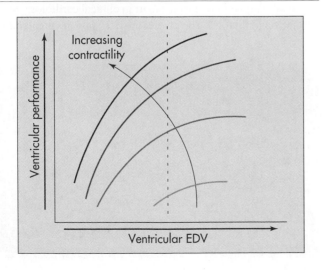

In the average heart, the EDV may approximate 120 mL but, as will be discussed in later sections, genetically gifted individuals may have a large heart and an end-diastolic volume that may exceed 180 mL. Endurance training is also known to increase EDV.

The action potential that is propagated throughout the atrial myocardium begins at the sinoatrial node (SA node) and progresses to the atrioventricular node (AV node). The propagation of the action potential is delayed in the AV node by up to 0.1 s. This delay allows for the time required to complete the atrial kick and resultant increased ventricular filling. The action potential then progresses through the Bundle of His to where the neural tissue branches into a right, left anterior, and left posterior branch, or *bundle branch*. These branches extend inferiorly toward the apex of the heart, where they then diverge to spread the action potential to the apical myocardium. The neural tissue of the diverging bundle branches are referred to as the *Purkinje fibers*, and are important for causing the contraction of the ventricular myocardium to occur in an inferior to superior direction.

The action potentials spread rapidly throughout the ventricular myocardium because of the diffuse presence of specialized low-resistance conducting tissue, termed *intercalated disks*. Blood is ejected from the ventricles during ventricular contraction, or *ventricular systole*. For the right ventricle, the pulmonary arterial pressure prior to ventricular systole (or *end diastole*) approximates 8 mmHg, whereas the end-diastolic pressure of the aorta artery approximates 80 mmHg. These end-diastolic pressures are also termed the **afterload.** Thus the left ventricle must generate more pressure than the right ventricle, causing it to perform more work for a given volume of blood pumped, and accounts for the larger myocardial mass surrounding the left compared to the right ventricle (fig. 7.5).

During ventricular systole, not all blood is ejected from each ventricle. The volume of blood pumped from each ventricle per beat is termed **stroke volume** (SV), and when expressed relative to the EDV is known as the **ejection fraction.** The ejection fraction for a healthy heart at rest approximates 0.6, or 60%. As will be discussed in later sections, the ejection fraction can increase to 80% during exercise. The product of stroke volume and heart rate (HR) quantifies the volume of blood pumped by the heart per unit time, and is referred to as **cardiac output** (Q).

7.2 $Q \text{ (L/min)} = SV \text{ (L)} \times HR \text{ (b/min)}$

At rest, the normal value for cardiac output approximates 5 L/min, but may increase in excess of 35 L/min during the exercise intensities at or close to VO_{2max}.

Once the ventricular pressures return below the respective artery pressures and momentum of ejected blood is overcome, the one-way valves of each ventricle close and the ventricular myocardium relax (*ventricular diastole*), and passive filling from the atrium occurs. The cardiac cycle is then complete and continues over and over again (see focus box 7.2 for another application for understanding cardiovascular function).

The Vasculature

The flow of blood through almost all the circulatory beds within the body proceeds in the order of arteries, arterioles, capillaries, venules, veins. However, there are a few exceptions to this rule in tissues such as the pituitary gland and liver, where one capillary bed is connected to another by an intermediate vein, and each of these special circulation beds is referred to as a *portal circulation.*

The artery has the thickest wall and the greatest ability to stretch and then recoil to its original dimension, a property termed *elasticity*. Conversely, arteries have a limited ability to be distended and increase their vascular volume, a property termed *compliance*. Arterioles possess similar properties to arteries, but in addition can be surrounded circumferentially by layers of smooth muscle fibers. The contraction of this smooth muscle is regulated by nerves, hormones from the circulation, local metabolites, and perhaps even local pressure and electrical changes that result in either the constriction or relaxation of the muscle (3, 6, 21, 28, 33, 49). Contraction of smooth muscle surrounding an arteriole will decrease the diameter of the lumen, increase resistance to blood flow and thereby decrease flow, a process termed **vasoconstriction.** Conversely, smooth muscle relaxation

FIGURE 7.5

A cross-section of the heart, showing the larger muscle mass surrounding the left compared to the right ventricle. Note that the heart is positioned upside down. RA = right atrium, LA = left atrium, IVS = interventricular septum.

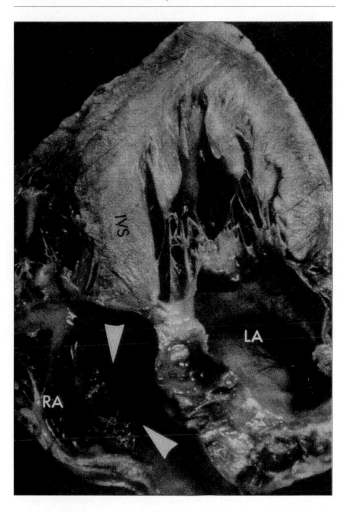

afterload the blood pressure exposed to the aortic valve immediately prior to ventricular contraction

stroke volume the volume of blood ejected from the ventricle each beat

ejection fraction the volume of blood pumped by the heart per beat, expressed relative to the end-diastolic volume of the ventricle

cardiac output the blood volume pumped by the heart each minute

vasoconstriction (vas'o-kon-strik'shun) narrowing of the lumen diameter of blood vessels

FOCUS BOX 7.2

Application of the Fick Equation to Understanding Cancerovascular Function

The function of the central cardiovascular system during rest and exercise can be understood by application of the Fick principle (50). The Fick principle is based on simple physiological principles. The consumption of oxygen by the body is dependent on blood flow and the amount of oxygen extracted from blood, which is expressed as the arterial-venous oxygen difference (a-vO$_2\Delta$). The Fick principle can be applied to the whole body, where VO$_2$ represents total body oxygen consumption, as calculated by indirect gas analysis calorimetry (see chapter 4), cardiac output (Q) represents blood flow, and the difference between arterial and mixed venous blood oxygen content represents the a-vO$_2\Delta$.

$$VO_2 = Q \times \text{a-vO}_2\Delta \text{ (7.3)} \qquad \textbf{7.3}$$

$$Q = VO_2 / \text{a-vO}_2\Delta \text{ (7.4)} \qquad \textbf{7.4}$$

The **Fick equation** can also be applied to regional circulations. Because all blood flow to the contracting thigh and lower leg muscles is provided by the femoral artery, and all blood flow from the leg occurs in the femoral vein, sampling

blood from each vessel would provide an oxygen content difference that reflects oxygen extraction by the leg, For example, when blood flow to the leg is measured in the femoral artery and blood is sampled from the femoral artery and vein for measurement of oxygen content, the a-vO$_2\Delta$ across the leg can be calculated, and using the Fick equation, VO$_2$ can be calculated.

A classic example of the application of the Fick equation to exercise physiology is a recent study published by Knight and associates (34). These researchers wanted to verify that the exercising muscle mass contributed most to the increase in VO$_2$ during exercise. Consequently, the researchers measured total body VO$_2$ during cycle ergometry by indirect calorimetry, while simultaneously sampling blood from the femoral artery and vein of one leg and measuring blood flow in the femoral artery. In the process of accounting for both legs, they noted that the increase in VO$_2$ during exercise to VO$_{2max}$ during cycle ergometry could be more than 90% accounted for by the VO$_2$ measured across the legs, with the remaining VO$_2$ coming from additional muscles used in posture and ventilation.

---

around an arteriole will increase the diameter, decrease resistance, and increase blood flow, a process termed **vasodilation.**

Capillaries are the smallest-diameter blood vessels, and possess a wall comprised of a single cell layer. The cells of the capillary wall are not tightly connected, and pores exist that allow the movement of fluid into and from the vascular compartment, as well as certain white blood cells and small proteins and metabolites. In certain regions of the circulatory bed, smooth muscle may also be present around the junctions between arterioles and capillaries. The walls of venules and veins are not as thick as those of the arteries or arterioles, do not have high elasticity, but have high compliance. Veins are also surrounded by smooth muscle which, because of the compliance of the venous circulation, function to regulate the cross-sectional dimensions of the veins and therefore the volume of blood that is in the venous circulation.

Acute Adaptations to Exercise

During exercise the contracting skeletal muscles contribute more than 90% of the increased demand for oxygen consumption (34). The more rapidly the oxygen is circulated to the contracting muscle, the more rapid will be the increase in VO$_2$, and the lower the oxygen deficit as was discussed in chapter 6. The immediate response of the cardiovascular

system to differing types of exercise will be discussed relative to changes in heart (cardiac) function, changes in blood, and changes in peripheral blood flow.

Cardiac Function

The heart responds to exercise by increasing heart rate, ejection fraction, stroke volume, and cardiac output. The frequency of heart contractions (heart rate) is controlled by neural and hormonal changes to the intrinsic discharge from the SA node. Parasympathetic innervation causes this neural tissue to become hyperpolarized, thus delaying the occurrence of the threshold potential required to propagate an action potential, causing a slower rate of discharge and a slower heart rate. Conversely, sympathetic stimulation from neural secretion of norepinephrine or hormonal stimulation by circulating norepinephrine and epinephrine increases the leakiness of the membranes to sodium, decreasing the time to reach a threshold potential, and increasing the rate of action potential discharge. Sympathetic stimulation also increases the excitability of the nerves within the AV node, resulting in less of a delay in the propagation of the action potential through the AV node and to the ventricular myocardium.

Increases in ejection fraction and stroke volume result from increases in blood flow back to the heart (*venous return*), and improved performance of the myocardium (fig. 7.4).

FIGURE 7.6

The changes in oxygen consumption (VO$_2$), heart rate, stroke volume, and cardiac output during several intermittent steady-state exercise intensities. The sudden increases and decreases in heart rate reflect its intricate regulation. When the steady-state heart rate and VO$_2$ responses are graphed both measures increase linearly with intensity.

Changes in Cardiac Function During Exercise

Not all exercise elicits the same cardiac response. Dynamic exercise induces increases in heart rate, stroke volume, cardiac output, and blood pressures that differ from those of isometric exercise. Similarly, dynamic upper-body exercise, which involves a smaller muscle mass than the dynamic exercise of the larger muscles of the legs, also elicits a slightly unique cardiac response.

Dynamic Lower-Body Exercise *Heart Rate* Figure 7.6 presents the increases in heart rate, oxygen consumption (VO$_2$), cardiac output, and stroke volume during several submaximal steady-state exercise intensities during cycle ergometry. The rapidity of the increases in heart rate and oxygen consumption are obvious. When viewing the steady-state values for VO$_2$ and heart rate, it is clear that both appear to increase linearly with intensity. However, when looking at the heart rate response during incremental exercise to evaluate the relationship between heart rate and exercise intensity, many individuals have only a small portion of the heart rate curve that is linear (11, 25, 47, 59) (fig. 7.7). Furthermore, there is also individual variation in the curvilinear heart rate response to increasing exercise intensities (59), and it is therefore not surprising that considerable error exists in evaluating exercise intensity or predicting VO$_2$ (a more linear response) from heart rate (see chapter 13).

Stroke Volume and Cardiac Output The dramatic increase in muscle metabolic demand during exercise is complemented by near-immediate increases in cardiac output. As previously explained for heart rate, the increased circulation of blood around the body also increases venous return, which in turn increases end-diastolic volume, which for a given ejection fraction will increase stroke volume. In addition, because of the increased contractility of the ventricular myocardium, there is an increased ejection fraction of the heart during exercise, which further increases stroke volume. For example, at rest ejection fraction approximates 60% and stroke volume may equal 80 mL. During exercise at 60% VO$_{2max}$ ejection fraction approximates 85% and stroke volume can equal 150 mL. As

Fick equation the equation based on the Fick principle where, VO$_2$ = Q × a-vO$_2$Δ

vasodilation (vas'o-di-la'shun) widening of the lumen diameter of blood vessels

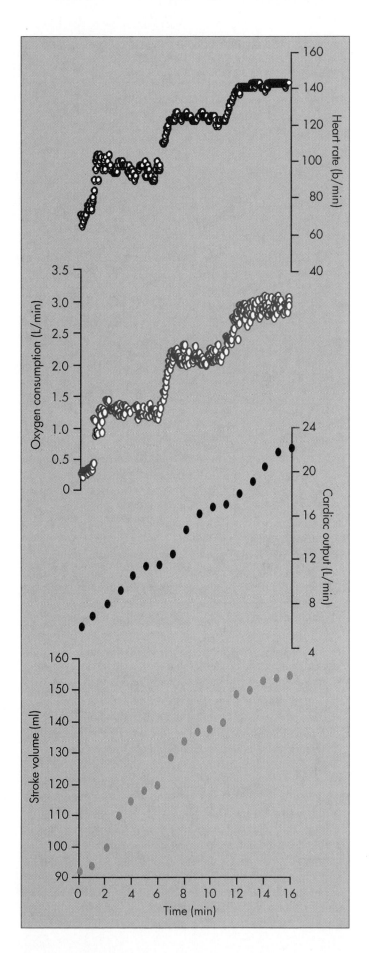

FIGURE 7.7

During increases in exercise intensity to VO_{2max}, the majority of individuals have a non-linear increase in heart rate.

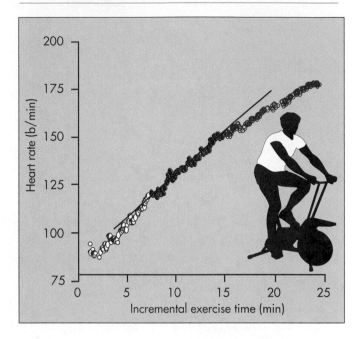

FIGURE 7.8

The increase in stroke volume during incremental exercise to VO_{2max} differs between untrained and endurance-trained individuals. Untrained individuals experience a plateau in stroke volume at relative intensities approximating 50% VO_{2max}. Endurance training enables the heart to increase stroke volume to VO_{2max} and thereby allows for further increases in cardiac output and improved exercise performance.

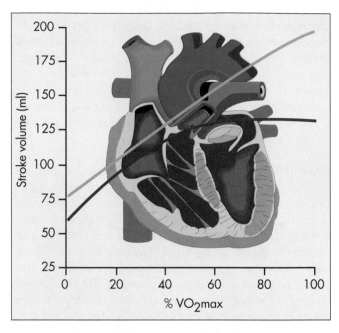

will be explained, endurance training and genetics can alter the maximal values of these capacities.

As indicated in figure 7.8 stroke volume increases as exercise intensity increases from rest to approximately 50% VO_{2max} in relatively untrained individuals and thereafter plateaus. In trained individuals, stroke volume continues to increase to VO_{2max}, which coincides with significant increases in maximal cardiac output and VO_{2max} (19, 35). These responses are only typical for exercise performed in the vertical position. Research conducted on individuals exercising in a recumbent or supine position have shown that maximal stroke volumes are attained at the onset of exercise (9, 40), presumably because of lower hydrostatic pressures which decrease the resistance to venous return to the heart.

The importance of an increased myocardial contractility for increasing or maintaining stroke volumes cannot be overemphasized. For example, figure 7.9 compares the durations of diastolic filling and left ventricular ejection for differing heart rates for untrained and endurance-trained individuals. At increasing heart rates there is less time for diastolic filling and ventricular ejection, with the duration of diastolic filling being less than ventricular ejection. Endurance-trained individuals have an even shorter diastolic filling time, which is accounted for by a longer ventricular ejection period because of their greater stroke volume. This means that the heart must receive blood flow at a higher rate during exercise to ensure faster filling, which in turn means that the ventricular myocardium must generate pressures faster to eject larger volumes of blood from the ventricles.

The increased heart rates and stroke volumes that accompany exercise result in an increase in cardiac output. This increase is linear with increases in exercise intensity and plateaus close to maximal heart rate and VO_{2max}.

Given these demands on the heart during exercise, it is no surprise that individuals with heart disease, or previous damage to the heart from myocardial infarction, have a much lower capacity to exercise than individuals with a healthy cardiovascular system.

Blood Pressure   The increasing cardiac output that occurs during exercise has the potential to increase blood pressure. The potential for such blood pressure increases can be explored with the following equation:

7.5   Q (L/min) = mBP(mmHg) / PVR (arbitrary units)

where mBP = mean blood pressure
PVR = peripheral vascular resistance.

Under resting conditions, Q approximates 6 L/min, and mBP approximates 95 mmHg. Thus, PVR approximates 15.8 units. With exercise to VO_{2max}, Q may increase to 25 L/min, and mBP may increase to 110 mmHg. Even at this increased mBP, to accommodate such an increase in Q, PVR must have decreased to approximately 4.5 units, more than a threefold decrease.

FIGURE 7.9

As heart rate increases there is less time for blood to fill the ventricular chambers (diastolic filling time) and less time for blood to be ejected from the ventricles (ejection time). Due to the larger stroke volumes of endurance-trained individuals, more time is needed for ejection, which reduces the time available for diastolic filling. However, in a healthy heart these constraints do not impair heart function, even when exercising to a maximal heart rate.

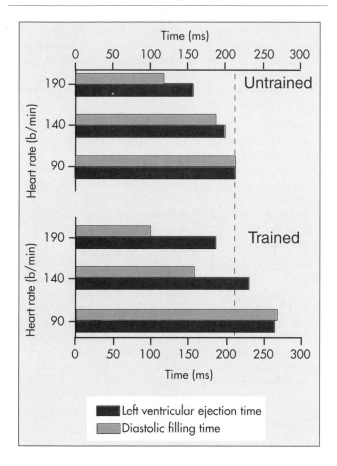

FIGURE 7.10

The change in arterial systolic, diastolic, and mean blood pressures during an incremental cycle ergometer test. Note the steady diastolic blood pressure. The increase in mean arterial blood pressure is therefore due to the increase in systolic blood pressure.

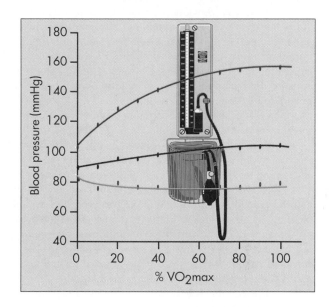

Figure 7.10 presents the change in systolic, diastolic, and mean arterial blood pressures during an incremental exercise test. Mean arterial blood pressure is not the average of systolic (SBP) and diastolic (DBP) blood pressures because the duration of systole and diastole differ. At rest, mean arterial blood pressure (mBP) is estimated from the calculation:

7.6 $mBP \text{ (mmHg)} = DBP + [(SBP - DBP)/3]$

This calculation is based on the duration of diastole being approximately threefold that of systole. However, as indirectly indicated in figure 7.9, this time relationship changes with increases in heart rate. During exercise, arterial systolic and mean pressures increase, whereas diastolic pressure remains close or slightly higher than resting values (< 80 mmHg) (20). This information indicates that during conditions of increasing cardiac output, ejection of blood from the left ventricle exceeds the compliant properties of the arterial vasculature, yet the reduced peripheral vascular resistance maintains a low diastolic pressure, despite the reduced interval between successive ejections from the left ventricle.

Research of pulmonary blood pressures during exercise indicate that there is only a minimal increase in pulmonary mBP of approximately 10 mmHg during even intense exercise. This is understandable, given the proximity of the pulmonary vasculature to the heart, the large divergence and capillary network, and therefore the low resistance to flow that would exist even at high flow rates (see focus box 7.3).

Upper-Body Exercise   The cardiovascular responses to upper-body dynamic exercise invokes a different heart rate, stroke volume, and blood pressure response compared to lower-body dynamic exercise (fig. 7.11).

For a given submaximal steady-state VO_2, heart rate, ventilation, and systemic blood pressures are higher during arm ergometry than during lower-body exercise (40, 46, 60, 61). Cardiac output is the same, and understandably stroke volume is lower. The higher blood pressures are due to the small muscle mass involved in arm exercise, and the large lower-body vasculature that remains undilated and provides resistance to peripheral circulation (42). For a given submaximal exercise intensity expressed relative to heart rate, muscle blood flow is similar between upper- and lower-body exercise (77); however, the VO_2 is lower because of a lower extraction of oxygen as indicated by Δa-vO_2 (46). Conversely, for a given VO_2, heart rate is higher during upper-body exercise.

The pressure within the cardiovascular system is termed **blood pressure.** As previously stated, arterial blood pressure is greater in the systemic compared to pulmonary circulations. Knowledge of how exercise alters blood pressure has important medical applications, as excessive blood pressure causes the heart to work harder by generating greater pressures to drive blood flow throughout the body. Chronic exposure to increased arterial blood pressure can damage the heart, blood vessels of the heart, and even certain organs of the body (e.g., the kidney).

Arterial blood pressure is represented by three pressures: systolic, mean, and diastolic. It has been assumed that when accounting for hydrostatic pressure differences between different arteries, all arterial blood pressure values are the same. However, this is not true. There is no one systolic blood pressure within the arterial systemic circulation at any point in time (20, 42). Systolic blood pressures of the ascending aorta are lower than those of peripheral arteries (e.g., brachial, radial, femoral) (20, 50), whereas diastolic and mean blood pressures are similar in most arteries (20). The more peripheral the artery, the greater the increase in systolic blood pressure (42, 40). These systolic blood pressure differences are due to complex interactions between fluid flow and the elastic properties of arteries. Despite the differences in the systolic and diastolic blood pressures between central and peripheral arteries, mean blood pressures are similar because of differences in the shape of the blood pressure waveform (mean arterial blood pressure is equal to the integrated area under the blood pressure waveform).

Despite the variability in systolic blood pressures within the arteries of the systemic circulation, a common method used to noninvasively measure blood pressure is sphygmomanometry, which can be completed manually (by a technician), or automatically (by computerized mechanical devices). During sphygmomanometry, the brachial artery is occluded by the inflation of a pressure cuff placed around the upper arm. As pressure is slowly released from the cuff, a stethoscope is used to hear *(auscultation)* the change in sounds (**Korotkoff sounds**) generated by the turbulent flow of blood within the artery. The Korotkoff sounds are interpreted as follows:

- Korotkoff sound I occurs when blood first rushes through the previous occlusion. The corresponding pressure = systolic blood pressure
- Korotkoff sound IV occurs when blood has a sudden decrease in resistance to flow through the artery. The corresponding pressure = diastolic blood pressure
- Korotkoff sound V is when sound is no longer audible. It is incorrect to use the corresponding pressure to represent diastolic blood pressure.

Even though manual sphygmomanometry is used routinely during rest and exercise blood pressure measurement, this method is not without error. Because the accuracy of the method is based on the detection of sounds, there is an increased likelihood for erroneous values to be detected as exercise intensity increases. In fact, the detection of diastolic blood pressure by manual sphygmomanometry is known to underestimate true values because of the difficulty in detecting the fourth Korotkoff sound (20).

For maximal exercise, upper-body exercise has a 30% lower cardiac output, a slightly lower maximal heart rate, 30 to 40% lower stroke volumes, and maximal ventilations that are 80% of those during lower-body values. Despite these differences, systemic blood pressures are similar.

Isometric Exercise Muscle blood flow, systemic blood pressures, and central cardiac function also differ between dynamic and static, or isometric, exercise. Sustained isometric contractions are characterized by increased vascular resistance within the exercised muscle mass. The intensity of isometric contractions are expressed relative to the maximal voluntary contraction (MVC) of the muscle(s) concerned. Sustained contractions at 20% MVC induce a rapid increase in both systolic and diastolic blood pressures, whereas blood pressure responses during dynamic exercise with loads of 10% MVC are much lower.

When isometric exercise is performed, additional increases in blood pressure may also occur if the person attempts to exhale against a closed trachea. This maneuver is very similar to a clinical procedure known as *Valsalva maneuver,* where subjects exhale at greatly increased airway pressures. The result is to increase thoracic pressures because of the added muscular contraction of the muscles of expiration against a near-constant lung volume. These pressures raise systemic diastolic arterial blood pressure, lower stroke volumes, and make the heart work harder for a given cardiac output.

Blood

A known acute effect of exercise on blood is to cause a release of fluid from the vascular compartment, which decreases the volume of plasma and blood. This fluid loss from the plasma decreases plasma volume, and causes the hematocrit and plasma metabolite concentrations to increase, which is termed **hemoconcentration.** In fact, a significant hemoconcentration occurs when moving from a supine to vertical posture. Furthermore, the added hemoconcentration of exercise is predominantly confined to the transition from

FIGURE 7.11

Differences between the cardiovascular responses to upper-body and lower-body exercise requiring a similar VO_2.

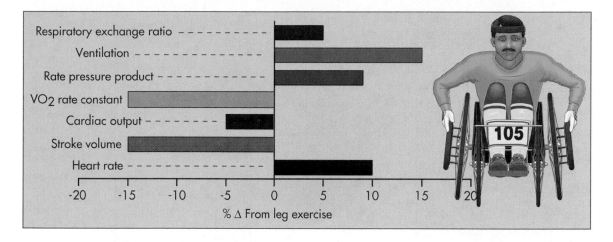

FIGURE 7.12

Exercise and the accompanied increases in blood pressure force fluid from plasma out of the vascular system. This response causes an increase in hematocrit and osmolality, which is termed hemoconcentration.

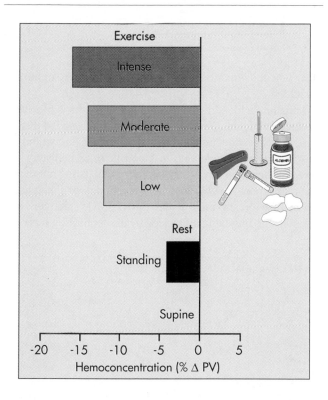

Peripheral Blood Flow

The finite blood volume of the body and limited increase in cardiac output present potential limitations to increased blood flow to peripheral tissues. For example, a cardiac output of 5 L/min and a blood volume of 5 L requires the complete recirculation of the entire blood volume every minute. During exercise, cardiac output may increase to 30 L/min, and the blood volume must be recirculated six times per minute. When compared to the potential 20-fold increase in demand for oxygen during exercise, the sevenfold potential increase in blood flow appears meager.

We can tolerate the increased metabolic demand of intense exercise because the systemic circulation is regulated to *redistribute blood flow* to the more metabolically active skeletal muscle tissue. In addition, the acute metabolic adaptations that occur in skeletal muscle result in an *increased extraction of oxygen* from the capillary blood, causing an increased a-v$O_2\Delta$ (see focus box 7.2).

Blood Flow Redistribution

Figure 7.13 compares the relative contribution of the cardiac output to the main tissue beds of the body during rest and exercise conditions. During exercise, the vasoconstriction of arterioles supplying the brain, gut, and kidney reduces the percent of the cardiac output that perfuses these tissues. However, because of the increased cardiac output, actual blood flow remains the same or increases slightly. The result is to allow an increasing percent of total blood

rest to exercise (9, 17, 26, 37, 38, 41). This response is followed by a more gradual hemoconcentration that occurs with increases in exercise intensity (fig. 7.12), and these changes are greater during the larger blood pressures associated with resistance exercise than during more prolonged dynamic exercise.

blood pressure the pressure within the cardiovascular system generated by the circulation of blood by the heart

Korotkoff sounds the sounds heard by auscultation during the measurement of blood pressure by sphygmomanometry

hemoconcentration increased hematocrit due to the loss of plasma volume

FIGURE 7.13

The distribution of cardiac output to the main tissues of the body during rest and exercise conditions.

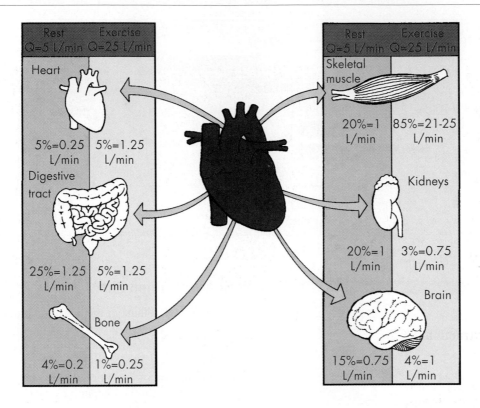

flow to be directed to the working skeletal muscle. Consequently, blood flow to skeletal muscle (assuming 20 kg of muscle) can increase from 50 mL/kg muscle/min, representing 15 to 20% of cardiac output at rest, to over 1000 mL/kg/min, which represents 80% of maximal cardiac output. Furthermore, when exercising a smaller muscle mass, maximal muscle blood flow has been measured at over 2000 mL/kg/min (3).

Peripheral Artery and Skeletal Muscle Blood Flow

As with cardiac output, peripheral artery and muscle blood flow increases linearly with increases in exercise intensity (fig. 7.14). However, this response should not be interpreted to indicate a uniform flow to skeletal muscle, or that the entire skeletal muscle mass is uniformly perfused. Animal research has identified a marked blood flow heterogeneity in contracting skeletal muscle, resulting in regions that are over- and underperfused. This inequality can result in regions of the muscle that do not receive adequate oxygenation, and may compromise muscle metabolism. Because of methodological constraints, it is un-

clear whether this nonuniform perfusion occurs in human muscle.

Variation in blood flow during contractions have been documented in humans. Walloe and Wesche (64) reported that intense muscle contractions compress the vasculature within the muscle, causing a reduction in blood flow, immediately followed by increased flow, termed **hyperemia,** during muscle relaxation. Similar findings have been reported from dynamic exercise of the forearm musculature (48) (fig. 7.15) and show that blood flow to muscle is influenced by the contracting muscle.

FIGURE 7.14

The linear increase in peripheral artery blood flow during increases in exercise intensity. A similar linear increase is also evident for cardiac output.

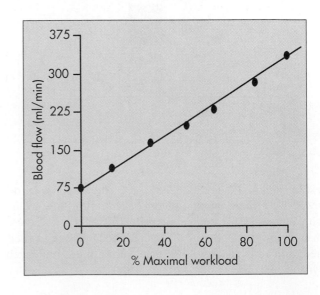

FIGURE 7.15

When blood flow is measured by a Doppler Flowmetry an uneven blood flow to skeletal muscle during dynamic muscle contractions is seen. Beat-to-beat variation in the volume of blood pumped to contracting muscle is dependent on the phase of the contraction cycle: rest, concentric contraction, eccentric contraction. It is clear that as exercise intensity increases, the amount of blood able to flow to the muscle is dramatically reduced during the concentric phase of the contraction because of an increase in intramuscular pressure. Conversely, during the recovery phases there is an exaggerated increase in blood flow, or hyperemia.

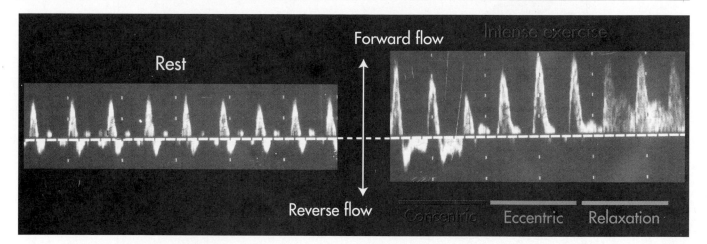

Increased Oxygen Extraction

Under resting conditions blood flow from the central arterial to central venous circulation causes a reduction in the partial pressure of oxygen in the blood from 100 mmHg to 40 mmHg (see chapter 8). Use of the oxy-hemoglobin dissociation curve reveals that such a pressure difference would amount to a 50 mL/L change in oxygen content ($200 - 150$ mL O_2/L blood), which is the arterial-to-mixed venous difference in oxygen content (a-v$O_2\Delta$). During maximal exercise, the a-v$O_2\Delta$ is used to reflect the added uptake of oxygen by the skeletal muscle, and can increase to over 150 mL/L during running and cycling in highly trained endurance athletes.

The use of central blood volume measures of CaO_2 and CvO_2 can be misleading. For example, the previously identified central blood volume values for a-v$O_2\Delta$ indicate that the body is unable to extract all the oxygen from the blood. This is not true for the localized microvasculature, where muscle PO_2 values have been estimated to be as low as 2 mmHg (36, 54, 56). If equilibration between capillary and tissue PO_2 is assumed, these values indicate an almost complete uptake of oxygen from the capillary circulation. Why is there such a high value for CvO_2? The answer is due to the combination of blood returning to the central vasculature from nonactive tissues, and because of the spatial and temporal heterogeneity in blood flow within the exercised muscle mass (27).

The near complete extraction of oxygen from the capillary circulation within muscle during intense exercise provides further evidence of the high capacity of the muscle fibers for oxygen extraction, and that central circulation and oxygen provision to the muscles are the limiting factors to maximal oxygen consumption. In fact, research that has arti-

ficially increased blood flow (4, 5, 7, 8) or artificially increased red blood cell numbers in the circulation (*erythrocythemia*), has shown that the capacity to increase oxygen extraction from the blood increases (55), which is why blood doping and injections of erythropoietin to stimulate polycythemia work and are banned practices in athletic events.

Cutaneous Circulation

The adjustments to skin (cutaneous) blood flow during exercise in a hot environment (see chapter 19) are integral components of the body's ability to dissipate heat to the surroundings. Unlike the splanchnic, renal, and portal circulations, which vasoconstrict during exercise, the start of exercise initially induces an adrenergic vasoconstriction of the skin, which is then followed by a sympathetic cholinergic vasodilation (29, 30, 31). During incremental exercise, skin blood flow decreases as exercise intensity increases above approximately 80% VO_{2max}. This response is interpreted to be due to the increasing circulating catecholamines in the blood at high exercise intensities (32), and increasing systemic blood pressures which further stimulate the baroreceptors causing an inhibition of the cholinergic vasodilator response (29, 30, 31).

A Summary of Acute Cardiovascular Adaptation to Exercise

Figure 7.16 summarizes the acute responses of the cardiovascular system to exercise. Once again the Fick equation is

hyperemia (hi-per-e'mi-ah) increased blood flow above normal; usually expressed relative to a particular tissue

FIGURE 7.16

A summary of the acute cardiovascular adaptations that combine to increase oxygen consumption during exercise.

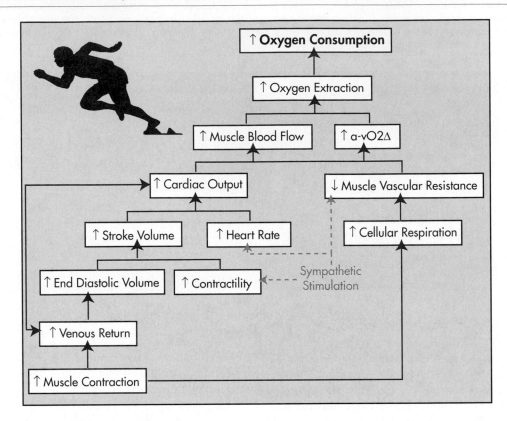

used to differentiate the components responsible for increasing VO_2 at the systemic level, as well as the peripheral level of function.

Systemic function of the cardiovascular system is based on the neural and humoral regulation of heart rate and ventricular contractility. In the periphery, blood flow is determined not only by the increase in cardiac output, but also by redistribution of cardiac output and the local regulators of blood flow (*autoregulation*). The combined effects of local and central regulation of cardiovascular function are crucial for the body to increase tolerance of exercise stress.

Chronic Adaptations to Exercise

Prolonged and repeated exposures to exercise can cause structural and functional changes in the cardiovascular system. The extent of these changes is dependent upon the type and quality of exercise training, and are known to differ between training for long-term endurance and training for short-term muscular endurance, strength, and power. The following description of chronic training adaptations will be organized principally by the type of exercise training and by the component of the cardiovascular system.

Comment must also be made on the influence of genetics to cardiovascular capacities and adaptability. Research that compares two or more groups that differ in training status

(cross-sectional studies) are biased by potential genetic differences that have caused individuals to select certain exercise modes and intensities. Conversely, research that measures changes in cardiovascular parameters in individuals exposed to training (experimental) is more likely to focus on training-induced adaptation. However, these training studies are relatively short term, lasting for several weeks or months, rather than several years, and therefore the full potential of cardiovascular adaptation to exercise alone remains unclear. Where appropriate, clarification will be given as to whether research findings are from cross-sectional or experimental studies.

Adaptations from Training for Long-Term Endurance

Cardiac Structure and Function

Data from cross-sectional studies indicate that heart dimensions and end-diastolic volumes are greater in endurance athletes than athletes involved in activities of a short duration (45) (fig. 7.17). This information has developed the notion of an *athletic heart*, which is larger than that of sedentary individuals. Endurance training has also been shown to elicit increases in cardiac mass and function in previously sedentary individuals (14). The end-diastolic volume of the left ventricle (LVEDV) increases after 9 weeks of endurance training in males, and similar responses have been shown in females (51).

FIGURE 7.17

Data from a cross-sectional evaluation of elite athletes, indicating that the left-ventricular end-diastolic dimension (LVED) and the cardiac mass index (CMI) were larger in athletes involved in more endurance-type activities.

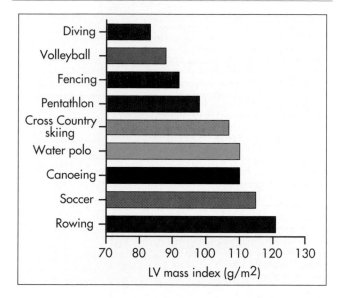

These adaptations occur rapidly: increased measures of ventricular dimensions have been reported after as little as 1 week of endurance training, whereas myocardial mass responds more slowly (16). As will be discussed below, the rapidity of the increase in cardiac dimensions is primarily due to a rapid increase in plasma and blood volume (13, 17, 26).

The larger LVEDV after endurance training is associated with an increased stroke volume and decreased heart rate for a given submaximal exercise intensity. Contradictory information exists as to whether these stroke volume and heart rate responses are cause and effect (10). For example, at rest, the lower heart rate is also accompanied by increased parasympathetic innervation of the heart, and reductions in resting and exercise heart rates have been documented without increases in stroke volume (10). It is logical to interpret the research findings as evidence for combined increases in stroke volume and parasympathetic innervation as the causes of the lower heart rates after training.

Blood Pressure

For individuals who have moderately elevated blood pressure, or *hypertension* (systolic/diastolic blood pressures of 140 to 180/90 to 105 mmHg), an endurance training program that increases VO_{2max} also lowers blood pressure (1). The exercise training must be of low to moderate intensity (40 to 75% VO_{2max}) and be performed for at least 20 to 60 min, 3 to 5 days/week. The maximal reductions in blood pressure associated with this training approximate 10 mmHg for both systolic and diastolic pressures (1, 12, 23, 63). The blood pressure lowering effect of endurance exercise training appears similar for hypertensive men and women of all ages (12, 22, 23).

For individuals with normal blood pressure, continued involvement in endurance training has been shown to provide a protective effect against the development of hypertension later in life (43, 58).

The mechanisms by which the antihypertensive effects of endurance exercise function are unclear, yet are known to be unrelated to reductions in body fat and weight (15, 22, 63). Most evidence indicates that for hypertensive individuals, exercise training lowers resting cardiac output and peripheral vascular resistance (58). The lowered peripheral vascular resistance may result from lowered circulating norepinephrine concentrations (15), or from as yet unexplained exercise-induced alterations in renal function.

Blood

Endurance training increases the volume of plasma in blood. Simultaneous increases in red blood cell counts and hemoglobin

FIGURE 7.18

The changes in plasma volume, hematocrit, and hemoglobin concentration during endurance exercise training. The increased expansion of the plasma volume can decrease hematocrit and hemoglobin, even though total red cell and total hemoglobin masses also increase with training.

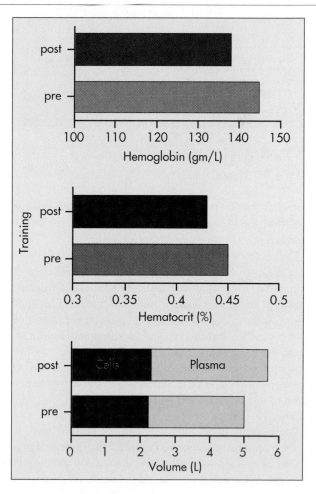

FIGURE 7.19

A summary of the chronic adaptations of the cardiovascular system after exposure to training for long-term endurance. Adaptations are related to their effects during both maximal and submaximal exercise.

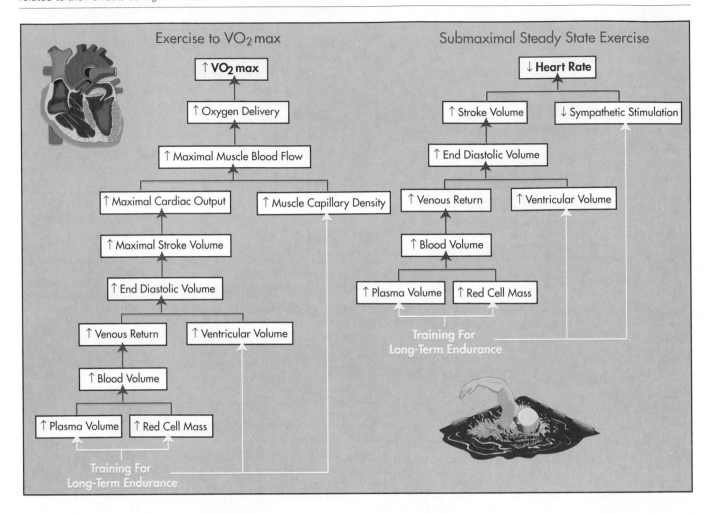

also occur, but their concentration relative to the volume of blood decreases because of the diluting effect of the relatively larger increases in plasma volume (fig. 7.18).

The increase in plasma volume is known to occur without a large training stimulus. For example, Gillen and associates (17) reported that just one session of intense intermittent cycle ergometry exercise performed at 85% VO_{2max} induced a 10% increase in plasma volume after 24 h. This chronic increase was predominantly due to an increase in plasma albumin. The time course of further change in plasma volume during a training program is unknown; however, maximal training-induced increases in plasma volume have been reported between 300 and 800 mL (13, 17, 26).

The benefits of an increased plasma volume have been documented in studies that have artificially increased plasma volume by either saline infusion or increasing the osmolality of blood (e.g., dextran infusion), thereby retaining more fluid in the vascular space. These studies have shown that an increased plasma volume increases venous return to the heart, increases ventricular preload, and thereby increases stroke volume for a given exercise intensity (13, 26). The increased plasma volume also has thermoregulatory benefits, as will be detailed in chapter 18.

During detraining the loss of plasma volume is also rapid, and accounts for the rapid reversal of central cardiac function improvements (increased stroke volume and maximal cardiac output) that accompany the endurance-trained state (13, 16).

Skeletal Muscle Circulation

Anderson and Henriksson (2) performed histology and muscle biopsy tissue sections before and after training and revealed a 20% increase in capillary density which was consistent among the different fiber types, and occurred in combination with a 16% increase in VO_{2max} and a 40% increase in select mitochondrial enzyme activities. Increased capillary density would increase maximal muscle blood flow capacities, improve the distribution of blood flow within a muscle, and prolong the time blood was exposed to the contracting muscle fibers (*capillary transit time*). The latter two responses are probably the more meaningful, as increased oxygen extraction is known to occur after training, even when maximal cardiac output is not increased (10).

A Summary of the Benefit of Cardiovascular Adaptations to Endurance Training

The chronic cardiovascular adaptations to endurance training benefit both maximal and submaximal exercise performance (fig. 7.19). Maximal exercise performance results from an improvement in VO_{2max}, whereas submaximal improvement results from a combined lowering of the relative intensity of given absolute intensities, as well as the raising of the lactate threshold as explained in chapter 6. The most notable chronic training adaptation to cardiovascular function during submaximal exercise is a lowered heart rate. The potential for exercise training to lower systemic blood pressures has important application to the use of exercise as a preventive and rehabilitative prescription against hypertension (see chapter 16).

Adaptations from Training for Short-Term Intense Exercise and Muscular Strength

Generally, far less cardiovascular adaptation occurs from chronic resistance training (or weight lifting). However, the type of resistance training is important in determining the magnitude of potential cardiovascular improvement. Pellicia and colleagues (45) and Urhausen and Kindermann (62) reported that bodybuilders had significantly less total heart volume than endurance-trained athletes. However, with more prolonged resistance training programs involving fewer and shorter rest intervals, such as circuit training, endurance-related cardiovascular adaptation is evident.

The minimal cardiovascular and muscle metabolic adaptations conducive to increased long-term endurance from resistance training prevent significant increases in VO_{2max}. Interestingly, resistance exercise combined with endurance training, especially for relatively untrained individuals, seems to contribute to initial increases in VO_{2max} (24). This may be because of the low muscle mass of untrained individuals. Resistance training may improve muscle recruitment and hypertrophy, thereby allowing improved exercise tolerance during incremental exercise.

WEBSITE BOX

Cardiovascular Function and Adaptation to Exercise

The newest information regarding exercise physiology can be viewed at the following sites.*

lidco.com/cardiac_output.html
  Explanation of cardiac output and how it can be measured.
health.santefe.cc.fl.us/health/vccl/chpt3/HEMODY.html
  Detailed explanation of cardiac metabolism, the hemodynamics of the cardiac cycle, and the Frank-Starling principle.
nbhd.org/services/cardiac/anatomy.htm
  Brief description of the anatomy of the heart, including detailed illustrations of the heart.

mirrors.org.sg/hol/TOC.biosci.html
  Excellent site providing detailed links to written and illustrated explanations of the heart, cardiovascular system, pulmonary system, blood, etc.
arfa.org/iindex.htm
  Excellent site providing comprehensive information on many topics within exercise physiology.
med.jhu.edu/heart/loop.html
  Explanation of the pressure-volume loop of the heart, with emphasis on heart failure.

---

*Unless indicated, all URLs preceded by http://www.

Note: These URLs were valid at the time of publication, but could have changed or been deleted from Internet access since that time.

- The **cardiovascular system** is composed of blood, the heart, and the vasculature within which blood is pumped throughout the body. Within the cardiovascular system are the systemic and pulmonary circulations. Within the **systemic circulation** are local circulation beds, such as those of the head and brain (*cranial* circulation), lungs (*pulmonary* circulation), liver (*hepatic* circulation), kidney (*renal* circulation), abdominal viscera and intestinal tract (*splanchnic* circulation), skin (*cutaneous* circulation), and *skeletal muscle* circulation.

- **Blood** is the liquid medium that circulates within the vascular system. Blood can be divided into cellular and noncellular components, and functions to transport gases, nutrients, and waste products; to clot and decrease injury severity; in acid-base buffering, immune functions, tissue repair and destruction, heat transfer, and thermoregulation.

- The cell content of blood constitutes approximately 45% of the total blood volume, and this measure is termed **hematocrit.** Hematocrit is lower in females than males, and will vary with hydration status. Blood consists of several types of cells which all emanate from a stem cell located in bone marrow. The original stem cell can differentiate into precursors of white blood cells (*leukocytes*), red blood cells (**erythrocytes**), or cell fragments known as *platelets*. During the synthesis of erythrocytes (*erythropoiesis*), the stem cell is differentiated into nucleated cells that synthesize hemoglobin.

- An increased production of erythrocytes can result in elevated red blood cell counts, and this condition is termed **polycythemia.** Conversely, an inadequate ion intake, excessive bleeding, or exaggerated erythrocyte destruction can result in a lowered red blood cell count, or **anemia.**

- The liquid component of blood is termed *plasma*. When blood is drawn from the body, the clotting process forms fibrinogen and the remaining fluid component of blood is termed *serum*. The presence of electrolytes and proteins in plasma generates an osmotic force to attract and retain water within the vasculature. This osmotic force is best reflected by the number of particles in solution, which is termed **osmolality.**

- The cycle of blood flow through the heart and vasculature is referred to as the **cardiac cycle.** The volume of blood in each ventricle at the end of diastole is referred to as *end-diastolic volume* (EDV), and exerts a stretch on the ventricular myocardium. This stretch can be interpreted as a load, and is known as **preload** in clinical cardiology and cardiac rehabilitation. The greater the EDV, and the greater the stretch, the faster is the resultant ventricular myocardial contraction, and this relationship is known as the *Frank-Starling law* of the heart. Catecholamine stimulation of the myocardium increases contractile force and velocity for a given EDV, and this response is termed *contractility*.

- Blood is ejected from the ventricles during ventricular contraction, or *ventricular systole*. For the right ventricle, the pulmonary arterial pressure prior to ventricular systole (or *end diastole*) approximates 8 mmHg, whereas the end-diastolic pressure of the aorta artery approximates 80 mmHg. These end-diastolic pressures are also termed the **afterload.**

- During ventricular systole, not all blood is ejected from each ventricle. The volume of blood pumped from each ventricle per beat is termed **stroke volume,** and when expressed relative to the EDV is known as the **ejection fraction.** The ejection fraction for a healthy heart at rest approximates 0.6, or 60%, but can increase to 80% during exercise. The product of stroke volume and heart rate quantifies the volume of blood pumped by the heart per unit time, and is referred to as **cardiac output** (Q).

$$Q(L) = SV(L) \times HR \text{ (b/min)}$$

- At rest, the normal value for cardiac output approximates 5 L/min, but may increase in excess of 35 L/min during the exercise intensities at or close to VO_{2max}.

- The **Fick equation** is based on simple physiological principles. The extraction of oxygen is dependent on blood flow (Q), and the amount of oxygen extracted from blood which is usually expressed as the arterial-venous oxygen difference (a-v$O_2\Delta$).

$$VO_2 = Q \times \text{a-v}O_2\Delta$$

- Contraction of smooth muscle surrounding an arteriole will decrease the diameter of the lumen, increase resistance to blood flow and thereby decrease flow, a process termed **vasoconstriction.** Conversely, smooth muscle relaxation around an arteriole will increase the diameter, decrease resistance and increase blood flow, a process termed **vasodilation.**

- Heart rate and oxygen consumption increase rapidly during the onset of exercise. The heart rate response during incremental exercise is not completely linear. In many individuals, only a small portion of the heart rate curve is linear, with heart rates above an individually specific value revealing a curvilinear relationship with intensity. Stroke volume increases as exercise intensity increases from rest to approximately 50% VO_{2max} in relatively untrained individuals and thereafter plateaus. In trained individuals, stroke volume continues to increase to VO_{2max}, which coincides with significant increases in maximal cardiac output and VO_{2max}.

■ The increasing cardiac output that occurs during exercise has the potential to increase blood pressure. The potential for such blood pressure increases can be explored with the following equation:

$$Q = mBP / PVR$$

where mBP = mean blood pressure, and
PVR = peripheral vascular resistance.

Under resting conditions, Q approximates 6 L/min, and mBP approximates 95 mmHg. Thus, PVR approximates 15.8 units. With exercise to VO_{2max}, Q may increase to 25 L/min, and mBP may increase to 110 mmHg. Even at this increase mBP, to accommodate such an increase in Q, PVR must have decreased to approximately 4.5 units, more than a threefold decrease.

■ Blood pressure can be measured indirectly using sphygmomanometry. Sphygmomanometry involves the placement of a cuff around a limb, inflation of the cuff to a pressure than causes the complete occlusion of an artery, and the detection of sounds (**Korotkoff sounds**) from an artery (auscultation) caused by the return of blood flow as the cuff pressure is allowed to slowly decrease.

■ We can tolerate the increased metabolic demand of intense exercise because the systemic circulation is regulated to *redistribute blood flow* to the more metabolically active skeletal muscle tissue. In addition, the acute metabolic adaptations that occur in skeletal muscle result in an *increased extraction of oxygen* from the capillary blood, causing an increased $\Delta a\text{-}vO_2$. Increased blood flow to a given tissue bed is termed **hyperemia.**

■ A known acute effect of exercise on blood is to cause a release of fluid from the vascular compartment, which decreases the volume of plasma and blood. This fluid loss from the plasma decreases plasma volume, and causes the hematocrit and plasma metabolite concentrations to increase, which is termed **hemoconcentration.**

■ Endurance training increases the volume of plasma in blood. An increased plasma volume increases venous return to the heart, increases ventricular preload, and thereby increases stroke volume for a given exercise intensity. Less cardiovascular adaptation occurs during resistance training compared to endurance training. Generally, the more continuous and less intense the resistance training, the more likely some cardiovascular adaptation will occur.

STUDY QUESTIONS

1. List the components of the cardiovascular system, and briefly explain why their function is important during exercise.

2. What are normal values for blood volume, plasma volume, hemoglobin concentration, and hematocrit? How do these values change with endurance training?

3. How does heart rate, stroke volume, and cardiac output change during incremental exercise to VO_{2max}? Are responses different after endurance training? If so, how?

4. Explain the different cardiovascular responses between exercise performed with the upper body and lower-body exercise.

5. Why is the body's ability to redistribute blood flow (cardiac output) important for exercise tolerance?

6. Why are there minimal cardiovascular adaptations to chronic resistance training?

APPLICATIONS

1. Explain the cardiovascular benefits of ingesting fluid during prolonged exercise, especially in hot or humid climates.

2. Why is the body's regulation of blood flow redistribution important for increasing oxygen delivery to muscle and maximizing VO_{2max}?

3. Would the chronic adaptations of the central cardiovascular system help individuals recovering from a myocardial infarct? Explain.

4. Individuals who have a heart transplant do not have any neural regulation of the heart, and a diminished potential for increases in heart rate and myocardial contractility. How might these changes alter their ability to exercise?

REFERENCES

1. American College of Sports Medicine. Physical activity, physical fitness and hypertension. *Med. Sci. Sports Exerc.* 25(10):i–x, 1993.

2. Anderson, P., and J. Henriksson. Capillary supply of the quadriceps femoris muscle of man: Adaptive response to exercise. *J. Physiol.* 270:677–690, 1977.

3. Anderson, P., and B. Saltin. Maximal perfusion of skeletal muscle in man. *J. Physiol.* 366:233–249, 1985.

4. Barklay, J. K., and W. N. Stainsby. The role of blood flow in limiting maximal metabolic rate in muscle. *Med. Sci. Sports Exerc.* 7(2):116–119, 1975.

5. Barklay, J. K. A delivery-independent blood flow effect on skeletal muscle fatigue. *J. Appl. Physiol.* 61(3):1084–1090, 1986.

6. Berne, R. M., and M. N. Levy. *Physiology,* 3rd ed. Mosby Year Book, St. Louis, 1993.

7. Brechue, W. F., J. K. Barklay, D. M. O'Drobinak, and W. N. Stainsby. Difference between VO₂ maxima of twitch and tetanic contractions are related to blood flow. *J. Appl. Physiol.* 71(1):131–135, 1991.

8. Brechue, W. F., B. T. Ameredes, G. M. Andrew, and W. N. Stainsby. Blood flow elevation increases VO₂ maximum during repetitive tetanic contraction of dog muscle in situ. *J. Appl. Physiol.* 74(4):1499–1503, 1993.

9. Burge, C. M., M. F. Carey, and W. R. Payne. Rowing performance, fluid balance, and metabolic function following dehydration and rehydration. *Med. Sci. Sports Exerc.* 25(12):1358–1364, 1993.

10. Clausen, J. P. Effect of physical training on cardiovascular adjustments to exercise in man. *Physiol. Rev.* 57(4):779–815, 1977.

11. Conconi, F., M. Ferrari, P. G. Ziglio, P. Droghetti, and L. Codeca. Determination of the anaerobic threshold by a noninvasive field test in runners. *J. Appl. Physiol.* 52(4):869–873, 1982.

12. Cononie, C. C., J. E. Graves, M. L. Pollock, M. I. Phillips, C. Summers, and J. M. Hagberg. Effect of exercise training on blood pressure in 70–79 year old men and women. *Med. Sci. Sports Exerc.* 23:505–511, 1991.

13. Coyle, E. F., M. K. Hemmert, and A. R. Coggan. Effects of detraining on cardiovascular responses to exercise: Role of blood volume. *J. Appl. Physiol.* 60(1):95–99, 1986.

14. Cox, M. L., J. B. Bennett III, and G. A. Dudley. Exercise training–induced alterations of cardiac morphology. *J. Appl. Physiol.* 61(3):926–931, 1986.

15. Duncan, J. J., J. E. Farr, J. Upton, R. D. Hagan, M. E. Oglesbay, and S. N. Blair. The effect of aerobic exercise on plasma catecholamine and blood pressure in patients with mild essential hypertension. *J. Am. Med. Assoc.* 254:2609–2613, 1985.

16. Ehsani, A. A., J. M. Hagberg, and R. C. Hickson. Rapid changes in left ventricular dimensions and mass in response to physical conditioning and deconditioning. *Am. J. Cardiol.* 42:52–56, 1978.

17. Gillen, C. M., R. Lee, G. W. Mack, C. M. Tomaselli, T. Nishiyasu, and E. R. Nadel. Plasma volume expansion in humans after a single intense exercise protocol. *J. Appl. Physiol.* 71(5):1914–1920, 1991.

18. Gledhill, N. Blood doping and related issues: A brief review. *Med. Sci. Sports Exerc.* 14(3):183–189, 1982.

19. Gledhill, N., D. Cox, and R. Jamnik. Endurance athlete's stroke volume does not plateau: Major advantage is diastolic function. *Med. Sci.Sports Exerc.* 26(9):1116–1121, 1994.

20. Griffin, S. E., R. A. Robergs, and V. H. Heyward. Blood pressure measurement during exercise: A review. *Med. Sci. Sports Exerc.*, 29(1):149–159, 1997

21. Guyton, A. C. *Textbook of medical physiology.* 8th ed. Saunders, Philadelphia, 1991.

22. Hagberg, J. M., D. Goldring, and A. A. Ehsani. Effect of exercise training on the blood pressure and hemodynamic features of hypertensive adolescents. *Am. J. Cardiol.* 52:763–768, 1983.

23. Hagberg, J. M., S. J. Montain, W. H. Martin, and A. A. Ehsani. Effect of exercise training on 60–69 year old persons with essential hypertension. *Am. J. Cardiol.* 64:348–352, 1989.

24. Hickson, R. C., B. A. Dvorak, E. M. Gorostiaga, T. T. Kurowski, and C. Foster. Potential for strength and endurance training to amplify endurance performance. *J. Appl. Physiol.* 65:2285–2290, 1988.

25. Hofmann, P., V. Bunc, H. Leitner, R. Pokan, and G. Gaisl. Heart rate threshold related to lactate turn point and steady state exercise on a cycle ergometer. *Eur. J. Appl. Physiol.* 58:303–306, 1988.

26. Hopper, M. K., A. R. Coggan, and E. F. Coyle. Exercise stroke volume relative to plasma-volume expansion. *J. Appl. Physiol.* 64(1): 404–408, 1988.

27. Iversen, P. O., M. Standa, and G. Nicolaysen. Marked regional heterogeneity in blood flow within a single skeletal muscle at rest and during exercise hyperaemia in the rabbit. *Acta Physiol. Scand.* 136:17–28, 1989.

28. Joyner, M. J., R. L. Lennon, D. J. Wedel, S. H. Rose, and J. T. Shepherd. Blood flow to contracting muscles: Influence of increased sympathetic activity. *J. Appl. Physiol.* 68(4):1453–1457, 1990.

29. Kellog, D. L. Jr., J. M. Johnson, and W. A. Kosiba. Selective abolition of adrenergic vasoconstrictor responses in the skin by local iontophoresis of bretylium. *Am. J. Physiol.* 257(26): H1599–H1606, 1989.

30. Kellog, D. L. Jr., L. M. Johnson, and W. A. Kosiba. Baroreflex control of the cutaneous active vasodilator system in humans. *Circ. Res.* 66:1420–1426, 1990.

31. Kellog, D. L. Jr., L. M. Johnson, and W. A. Kosiba. Competition between the cutaneous active vasoconstrictor and vasodilator systems during exercise in man. *Am. J. Physiol.* 261(30): H1184–H1189, 1991.

32. Kenney, W. L., and J. M. Johnson. Control of skin blood flow during exercise. *Med. Sci. Sports Exerc.* 24(3):303–312, 1992.

33. Kiens, B., B. Saltin, L. Walloe, and J. Wesche. Temporal relationship between blood flow changes and release of ions and metabolites from muscles upon single weak contractions. *Acta Physiol. Scand.* 136:551–559, 1989.

34. Knight, D. R., et al. Relationship between body and leg VO$_2$ during maximal cycle ergometry. *J. Appl. Physiol.* 73(3):1114–1121, 1992.

35. Krip, B., N. Gledhill, V. Jamnik, and D. Warburton. Effect of alterations in blood volume on cardiac function during maximal exercise. *Med. Sci. Sports. Exerc.* 29(11):1469–1476, 1997.

36. Lundgren, F., K. Bennegard, A. Elander, K. Lundholm, T. Schersten, and A. Bylund-Fellenius. Substrate exchange in human limb muscle during exercise at reduced flow. *Am. J. Physiol.* 255(24): H1156–H1164, 1988.

37. Martin, D. G., E. W. Ferguson, S. Wigutoff, T. Gawne, and E. B. Schoomaker. Blood viscosity responses to maximal exercise in endurance-trained and sedentary female subjects. *J. Appl. Physiol.* 59(2):348–352, 1985.

38. Martin, W. H. III, R. J. Spina, E. Korte, and T. Ogawa. Effects of chronic and acute exercise on cardiovascular-adrenergic responses. *J. Appl. Physiol.* 71(4):1523–1528, 1991.

39. McCartney, N., R. S. McKelvie, J. Marin, D. G. Sale, and J. D. MacDougall. Weight-training-induced attenuation of the circulatory response of older males to weight lifting. *J. Appl. Physiol.* 74(3):1056–1060, 1993.

40. Miles, D. S., M. H. Cox, and J. P. Bomze. Cardiovascular responses to upper body exercise in normals and cardiac patients. *Med. Sci. Sports Exerc.* 21(5):S126–S131, 1989.

41. Montain, S., and E. F. Coyle. Influence of graded dehydration on hyperthermia and cardiovascular drift during exercise. *J. Appl. Physiol.* 73(4):1340–1350, 1992.

42. O'Rourke, M. F. What is blood pressure? *Am. J. Hyperten.* 3:308–310, 1993.

43. Paffenbarger, R. S., Jr. Energy imbalance and hypertension risk. In P. L. White and T. Mondeika (eds.), *Diet and exercise: Synergism in health maintenance.* American Medical Association, Chicago, 1982., pp.115–125.

44. Paulson, W., D. R. Boughner, P. Ko, D. A. Cunningham, and J. A. Persuad. Left ventricular function in marathon runners: Echocardiographic assesment. *J. Appl. Physiol.* 51(4):881–886, 1981.

45. Pellicia, A., B. J. Maron, A. Spataro, M. A. Proschan, and P. Spirito. The upper limit of physiologic cardiac hypertrophy in highly trained elite athletes. *N. Eng. J. Med.* 324(5):295–301, 1991.

46. Pendergast, D. R. Cardiovascular, respiratory, and metabolic responses to upperbody exercise. *Med. Sci. Sports Exerc.* 21(5):S121–S125, 1989.

47. Pokan, R., et al. Heart rate deflection related to lactate performance curve and plasma catecholamine response during incremental cycle ergometer exercise. *Eur. J. Appl. Physiol.* 70:175–179, 1995.

48. Robergs, R. A., M. V. Icenogle, T. L. Hudson, and E. R. Greene. Temporal disparity in arterial blood flow to contracting muscle. *Med. Sci. Sports Exerc.* 29(8):1021–1027, 1997.

49. Rowell, L. B. What signals govern the cardiovascular response to exercise? *Med. Sci. Sports Exerc.* 12(3):307–315, 1980.

50. Rowell, L. B. *Human cardiovascular control.* Oxford University Press, New York, 1993.

51. Rubal, B. J., A.-R. Al-Muhailani, and J. Rosentsweig. Effects of physical conditioning on the heart size and wall thickness of college women. *Med. Sci. Sports. Exerc.* 19(5):423–429, 1987.

52. Sawka, M. N. Physiology of upper body exercise. *Exerc. Sports Sci. Rev.* 14:175–211, 1986.

53. Sawka, M. N., A. J. Young, K. B. Pandolf, R. C. Dennis, and C. R. Valeri. Erythrocyte, plasma, and blood volume of healthy young men. *Med. Sci. Sports Exerc.* 24(4):447–453, 1992.

54. Schumacker, P. T., and R. W. Samsel. Analysis of oxygen delivery and uptake relationships in the Krogh tissue model. *J. Appl. Physiol.* 67(3):1234–1244, 1989.

55. Spriet, L. L., N. Gledhill, A. B. Froese, and D. L. Wilkes. Effect of graded erythrocythemia on cardiovascular and metabolic responses to exercise. *J. Appl. Physiol.* 61(5):1942–1948, 1986.

56. Stainsby, W. N., W. F. Brechue, D. M. O'Drobinak, and J. K. Barclay. Effects of ischaemic and hypoxic hypoxia on VO$_2$ and lactic acid output during tetanic contractions. *J. Appl. Physiol.* 68:574–579, 1991.

57. Stamler, R., et al. Primary prevention of hypertension by nutritional-hygienic means: Final report of a randomized clinical trial. *JAMA* 262:1801–1807, 1989.

58. Tipton, C. M. Exercise, training, and hypertension: An update. *Exerc. Sport Sci. Rev.* 16:447–505, 1991.

59. Tokmakidis, S. P., and L. A. Leger. Comparison of mathematically determined blood lactate and heart rate "threshold" points and relationship with performance. *Eur. J. Appl. Physiol.* 64:309–317, 1992.

60. Toner, M. M., M. N. Sawka, L. Levine, and K. G. Pandolf. Cardiorespiratory responses to exercise distributed between the upper and lower body. *J. Appl. Physiol.* 54:1403–1407, 1983.

61. Toner, M. M., E. L. Glickman, and W. D. McArdle. Cardiovascular adjustments to exercise distributed between the upper and lower body. *Med. Sci. Sports Exerc.* 22(6):773–778, 1990.

62. Urhausen, A., and W. Kindermann. One- and two-dimensional echocardiography in body builders and endurance-trained subjects. *Int. J. Sports Med.* 10:139–144, 1989.

63. Urata, H., Y. Tanabe, and A. Kiyonaga. Antihypertensive and volume-depleting effects of mild exercise on essential hypertension. *Hypertension* 9:245–252, 1987.

64. Walloe, L., and J. Wesche. Time course and magnitude of blood flow changes in the human quadriceps muscles during and following rhythmic exercise. *J. Physiol.* 405:257–273, 1988.

RECOMMENDED READING

American College of Sports Medicine. Physical activity, physical fitness and hypertension. *Med. Sci. Sports Exerc.* 25(10): i–x, 1993.

Barklay, J. K., and W. N. Stainsby. The role of blood flow in limiting maximal metabolic rate in muscle. *Med. Sci. Sports Exerc.* 7(2):116–119, 1975.

Coyle, E. F., M. K. Hemmert, and A. R. Coggan. Effects of detraining on cardiovascular responses to exercise: Role of blood volume. *J. Appl. Physiol.* 60(1):95–99, 1986.

Ehsani, A. A., J. M. Hagberg, and R. C. Hickson. Rapid changes in left ventricular dimensions and mass in response to physical conditioning and deconditioning. *Am. J. Cardiol.* 42:52–56, 1978.

Gillen, C. M., R. Lee, G. W. Mack, C. M. Tomaselli, T. Nishiyasu, and E. R. Nadel. Plasma volume expansion in humans after a single intense exercise protocol. *J. Appl. Physiol.* 71(5):1914–1920, 1991.

Hickson, R. C., B. A. Dvorak, E. M. Gorostiaga, T. T. Kurowski, and C. Foster. Potential for strength and endurance training to amplify endurance performance. *J. Appl. Physiol.* 65:2285–2290, 1988.

Knight, D. R. et al. Relationship between body and leg VO_2 during maximal cycle ergometry. *J. Appl. Physiol.* 73(3):1114–1121, 1992.

Pellicia, A., B. J. Maron, A. Spataro, M. A. Proschan, and P. Spirito. The upper limit of physiologic cardiac hypertrophy in highly trained elite athletes. *N. Eng. J. Med.* 324(5):295–301, 1991.

Robergs, R. A., M. V. Icenogle, T .L. Hudson, and E. R. Greene. Temporal disparity in arterial blood flow to contracting muscle. *Med. Sci. Sports Exerc.* 29(8):1021–1027, 1996.

Spriet, L. L., N. Gledhill, A. B. Froese, and D. L. Wilkes. Effect of graded erythrocythemia on cardiovascular and metabolic responses to exercise. *J. Appl. Physiol.* 61(5):1942–1948, 1986.

Toner, M. M., E. L. Glickman, and W. D. McArdle. Cardiovascular adjustments to exercise distributed between the upper and lower body. *Med. Sci. Sports Exerc.* 22(6):773–778, 1990.

CHAPTER 8

Pulmonary Adaptations to Exercise

t the start of exercise, two of the first sensations we have concerning changes in physiology are the increases in the frequency and depth of breathing. The rapidity of these responses is not surprising, as once we start to exercise we need to rapidly provide oxygen to the working muscles to minimize the oxygen deficit. Unless ventilation increases in concert with increases in cardiac output, an inadequate volume of air will be available in the lungs to replenish oxygen and remove carbon dioxide from the blood. To understand these changes, and the alteration in blood oxygen and carbon dioxide content as blood circulates around the body, the student must learn the basic physical principles that govern relationships among gas volume, pressure, solubility, and diffusion. Once these principles and accompanied facts are known, the importance of pulmonary physiology to exercise, as well as the changes in pulmonary function when exercising at altitude or when lung function is impaired (e.g., asthma, emphysema), can be fully appreciated. This chapter will present the basic anatomy of the lung, the physiology of gas exchange and the transport of gases in blood, and summarize research that has documented the magnitude of changes in lung function during different exercise conditions (acute) and in response to exercise training (chronic).

OBJECTIVES

After studying this chapter, you should be able to:

- Identify the anatomical structure and components for the conducting zone and respiratory zone of the lungs.
- Describe the differences between ventilation, alveolar ventilation, and respiration.
- Explain how oxygen and carbon dioxide are transported in the blood.
- Explain the differences between the Bohr and Haldane effects and the factors that cause them.
- Identify the contributions that skeletal muscle, blood, carbon dioxide, bicarbonate, ventilation, and buffers make to the regulation of acid-base balance.
- Explain the complexity of neural and humoral controls of ventilation.
- Describe the range of ventilation possible from rest to maximal exercise.
- Explain the relationship between ventilation and exercise intensity and how to detect the ventilation threshold.
- Explain the metabolic theory that connects the ventilation threshold to the lactate threshold.

KEY TERMS

conducting zone
respiratory zone
pores of Kohn
pulmonary circulation
anatomical dead space
tidal volume
ventilation
compliance

alveolar ventilation
surfactant
respiration
hemoglobin
blood-gas interface
Bohr effect
carbonic anhydrase
Haldane effect
myoglobin

ventilatory threshold
hypoxemia
exercise-induced hypoxemia
asthma
pulmonary transit time

The Basic Anatomy of Lung and Pulmonary Circulation

*T*he two lungs of the body are located within the thoracic cavity. Air is directed to and from the lungs by the *trachea*, which is a long tube supported by cartilage that extends from the larynx to the diverging bronchi and bronchioles of the lungs (fig. 8.1). The trachea and each of the left and right *bronchi* have circumferentially layered smooth muscle, and are structurally supported by numerous C-shaped rings of cartilage. Collectively, the mouth and nasal passages, trachea, bronchi, and *bronchioles* comprise the **conducting zone** of the lungs (focus box 8.1), whereas the *respiratory bronchioles, alveoli ducts,* and *alveoli*, which are the sites of gas exchange and responsible for the largest lung gas volumes, are referred to as the **respiratory zone** of the lung (fig. 8.2). The respiratory zone of the lung is the location of lung inflation, and as the category name suggests, is the site of gas exchange, or *respiration*.

The average diameter of an alveolus is approximately 0.25 mm, the average membrane thickness of the respiratory structures is 0.5 μm, and there are approximately 300 million respiratory bronchioles that diverge into numerous alveoli within the two lungs (36). The alveoli and respiratory bronchioles are connected by openings or holes in their membranes, termed **pores of Kohn** (fig. 8.2). Originally it was believed that these holes allowed air to flow from one alveolus to another, however, recent research has shown that the pores are normally filled with fluid, and are responsible for the distribution of water and surfactant throughout the respiratory zone (2). Collectively, the respiratory bronchioles and alveoli comprise a surface area of approximately 70 square meters, which is a phenominally large area for gas exchange when considering that it is contained within the thoracic cavity.

Blood from the heart is pumped through the pulmonary arteries to the lungs, and blood is directed back to the left side of the heart via the pulmonary veins. The circulation of blood to and through the lung is termed the **pulmonary circulation.** The pulmonary circulation has a much lower blood pressure than the systemic circulation (25/8 compared to 120/80 mmHg at rest, see chapter 7). The respiratory zone of the lung is engorged with a rich blood supply (fig. 8.2). A dense capillary bed surrounds the structures of the respiratory zone, providing almost as much surface area of blood as that of the respiratory membranes. Obviously, optimal respiration would require a similarity between lung inflation and blood perfusion, and this concept is expressed by the ventilation perfusion ratio (V_E/Q).

Lung Volumes and Capacities

The conducting zone of the lung is often referred to as the **anatomical dead space,** as it does not have a respiratory function. The anatomical dead space comprises an average volume of 150 mL, although this value will vary in a positive relationship with body size.

The remaining volumes of the lung (fig. 8.3) are subdivisions of the total lung capacity and essentially comprise the *residual volume* and *vital capacity*. The vital capacity is the maximal volume of air that can be exhaled from the lungs, and because it is measured during a maximal inspiratory effort followed by a forced expiration, it can be di-

---

FIGURE 8.1

The respiratory system is located within the thoracic cavity and is connected to the facial openings of the nose and mouth by the trachea and pharynx.

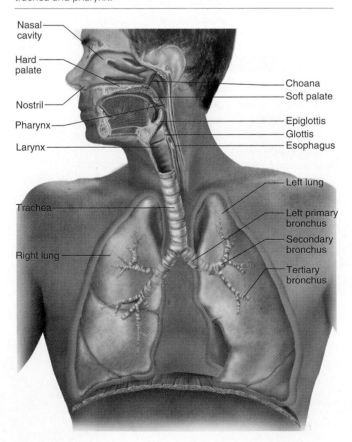

- Nasal cavity
- Hard palate
- Nostril
- Pharynx
- Larynx
- Trachea
- Right lung
- Choana
- Soft palate
- Epiglottis
- Glottis
- Esophagus
- Left lung
- Left primary bronchus
- Secondary bronchus
- Tertiary bronchus

---

conducting zone the zone of the lung where no respiration (gas exchang) occurs

respiratory zone the zone of the lung where respiration (gas exchange) occurs

pores of Kohn the holes within alveoli that allow fluid and surfactant to spread across the alveoli membranes

pulmonary circulation the blood and vessels that connect the heart and the lungs

anatomical dead space the volume of air within the conducting zone of the lung

FIGURE 8.2

Lung structure can be divided into two zones. *(a)* The conducting zone is composed of airways that direct air to and from the regions of the lung involved in gas exchange and the external environment (nose and mouth to alveoli). *(b and c)* The respiratory zone consists of the regions of the lung involved in gas exchange, which are comprised of highly vascularized inflatable structures, termed alveoli. *(c)* The walls of the alveoli are very thin and in close proximity to the blood vessels, which contain the red blood cells and blood gases.

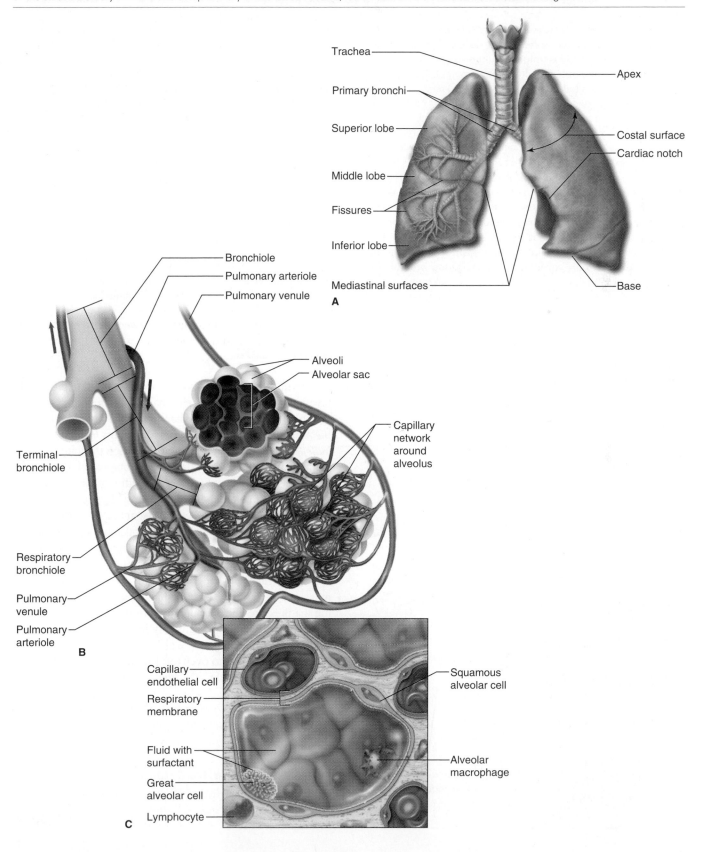

FOCUS BOX 8.1

Do Nasal Strips Improve Ventilation and Exercise Performance?

Because of the narrow passages of the conducting zone of the lung, there is the possibility that resistance to air flowing into the nose and mouth might limit the volume of air we can ventilate into and out of the lungs each minute. Based on this hypothesis, there has been a product sold to competitive athletes that functions to further open the nostrils of the nose so that there is a deceased resistance to airflow during nasal breathing. This product is designed to be adhered to the outer surface of the nostrils, and small springs within the nasal strip function to slightly flare the nostrils.

Since the marketing and sales of the product, several studies have been completed to verify manufacturer claims that the nasal strips will increase ventilation during exercise and improve sports performance (38, 40). Recently, Vermoen and associates (40) measured the resistance to airflow through the nose with and without nasal strips while subjects breathed only through the nose during breathing at rest, and during increased inspiratory and expiratory efforts. Use of the nasal strips did not decrease nasal resistance to

airflow. However, the volume of air ventilated through the nose in 1 s during inspiration was larger when nasal strips were worn.

Despite the increase in the rate of inspired airflow with nasal strips, Thomas and colleagues (38) showed that nasal strips did not result in an increased capacity to generate mechanical power during intense exercise. This latter result is not surprising, because when individuals transition from rest to exercise there is a progressive decreased dependency on nasal breathing and an increased reliance on oral breathing. *The greater the exercise intensity, the greater the contribution of oral ventilation to total ventilation.* This transition occurs because there is less resistance to airflow when breathing through the mouth than the nose (oronasal breathing), and during exercise this breathing transition occurs subconsciously. Consequently, the fact that nasal strips might increase the rate of airflow through the nose is probably redundant given that the contribution of nasal ventilation decreases with increases in ventilation (exercise intensity).

---

vided into inspiratory and expiratory components using the method of *spirometry* (see chapter 14). Normal resting breathing involves the inspiration and expiration of 500 mL of air, termed the **tidal volume,** and it is the sum of the tidal volume and breathing frequency that determines *ventilation.* A detailed description and explanation of the measurement of lung volumes and function, and normal values for these volumes and functional capacities are presented in chapter 14.

FIGURE 8.3

The volumes of the lung can be measured by spirometry. The total lung capacity includes a volume that cannot be exhaled from the lung (residual volume), and a volume that represents the maximal ability for lung inflation (vital capacity). During normal resting breathing, an average of 500 mL of air is inspired and expired, and is termed the tidal volume.

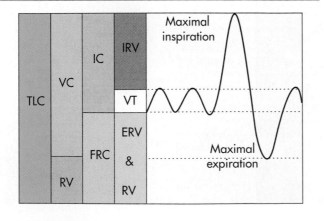

Ventilation

The term **ventilation** is synonymous with the process of breathing, but is very different than the process of respiration which will be described in later sections. *Ventilation involves the movement of air into and from the lungs by the process of bulk flow.* During inspiration and expiration the lung compartments are opened to the external environment and, therefore, to the pressure, temperature, and humidity of atmospheric air. A pressure differential between the air within the lung and the atmospheric air is generated by the muscles of ventilation. During inspiration, the lungs are expanded because of contraction of the muscles of inspiration, forcing the pressure to decrease, and allowing air to move from the atmosphere to within the lungs. During expiration, the contraction of the muscles of expiration force the lung volume to decrease, raising the pressure and forcing air from the lungs to the atmosphere. These events are incredibly important during exercise, when ventilation can increase airflow through the lung from a mere 6 L/min at rest to over 150 L/min during maximal exercise, and in excess of 200 L/min during maximal voluntary breathing (20, 36).

Large changes in lung ventilation occur in as little as a few seconds, and result from increases in each of breathing frequency and tidal volume.

8.1
$$\text{Ventilation } (V_E) \text{ (L/min)} = \text{frequency (br/min)} \times \text{tidal volume (L)}$$

for example, at rest,

$$V_E = 12 \text{ br/min} \times 0.5 \text{ L} = 6 \text{ L/min}$$

and at maximal exercise

$$V_E = 60 \text{ br/min} \times 3.0 \text{ L} = 180 \text{ L/min}$$

The speed at which the lungs can be inflated and deflated is remarkable, and occurs because of the low resistance of the alveoli to inflation and deflation. The property of being able to increase size or volume with only small changes in pressure is termed **compliance.** Thus the lungs must have very high compliance to be able to be inflated and deflated, with changes from 6 L/min to up to 200 L/min in large individuals, with minimal effort.

Alveolar Ventilation

Because of the anatomical dead space, not all of the air inspired actually reaches the respiratory zone and experiences gas exchange. Of the normal 500 mL tidal volume, 350 mL of "fresh" air reaches the respiratory zone, but this value will vary with the size of the individual and therefore the size of the tidal volume. The volume of "fresh" air that reaches the respiratory zone of the lung is termed **alveolar ventilation** (V_A). *The greater the depth of breathing, the less impact the anatomical dead space has on alveolar ventilation.*

For example, for two conditions with identical minute ventilation (V_E):

Normal breathing:

8.2a　$V_A = 12 \text{ br/min} \times (1.0 - 0.15L)$
　　　　$= 12 \times 0.85 = 10.2 \text{ L/min}$

Rapid shallow breathing:

8.2b　$V_A = 60 \text{ br/min} \times (0.2 - 0.15L)$
　　　　$= 60 \times 0.050 = 3.0 \text{ L/min}$

The Importance of Surfactant

*The presence of **surfactant** makes it easier to inflate alveoli.* At normal lung volumes, when the alveoli are not overly inflated and the membrane circumference is small, there is a relatively high surfactant concentration covering the membranes of the alveoli. Surfactant functions to lower the surface tension of the alveoli, thereby decreasing the resistance to inflation and increasing compliance.

During inflation, the size of the alveoli surface area increases, and the concentration of surfactant decreases, so that *at higher lung volumes the resistance to inflation increases.* The latter event is not disastrous because it promotes a more even inflation of neighboring alveoli and respiratory bronchioles, and provides some elastic recoil force during the start of expiration.

Respiration

The three main gases of air are nitrogen, oxygen, and carbon dioxide. All three gases diffuse between the alveolar air and blood, but as gaseous nitrogen is not metabolized within the body (see chapter 3) the latter two gases are of interest for normal physiological conditions. The process of gas exchange, or **respiration,** involves the movement of oxygen and carbon dioxide down pressure gradients that exist between pulmonary capillary blood and the air of the alveoli, and between capillary blood of the systemic circulation and the cells perfused by this blood. Consequently, the locations of respiration can be either in the lung, which is referred to as *external respiration*, or at the level of the systemic tissues, which is referred to as *internal respiration.*

External Respiration

The processes of external respiration result in the movement of gases between alveolar air and the pulmonary capillary blood. This exchange occurs via diffusion through a fluid medium that contains several membranes. The success of this diffusion depends on the characteristics of the gases for diffusion in an aqueous environment, and on the nature of the diffusion medium within the lung.

Gas Partial Pressures in Atmospheric and Alveolar Air

Dry atmospheric air contains 20.93% oxygen, 79.03% nitrogen, 0.03% carbon dioxide, and extremely small percentages of certain rare gases such as argon that comprise the remaining 0.01%. When air contains moisture, or water vapor, the water vapor molecules force the gas molecules to disperse, resulting in an increased volume of air. For constant volumes of gas, the presence of water vapor occupies a pressure within the total gas pressure, and the pressures of the gases decrease. As described in appendix D, the water vapor pressure of air depends on relative humidity and the temperature of the gas.

---

tidal volume the volume of air ventilated into and out of the lung with each breath

ventilation (vent′-l-á-shen) the movement of air into and out of the lungs by bulk flow

compliance (kom′pli-ens) the property of the ease with which an object can increase volume for a given pressure differential

alveolar ventilation the component of ventilation that reaches the respiratory zone of the lungs

surfactant (sir-fak′-tant) the lipoprotein molecule found over alveolar membranes that functions to decrease surface tension and improve compliance

respiration (res′p-ra′shen) gas exchange

FIGURE 8.4

The partial pressures of oxygen and carbon dioxide in air and alveoli when at sea level. Because of the removal of oxygen and the release of carbon dioxide by the body, and the saturation of air with water vapor, alveoli partial presssures of oxygen and carbon dioxide are very different than atmospheric air.

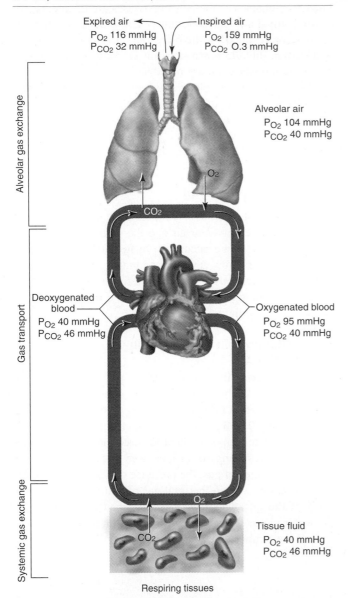

Respiring tissues

TABLE 8.1

Representative concentrations of hemoglobin and oxygen-carrying capacity of the blood in males and females, after blood doping, and when anemic

POPULATION/CONDITION	[HB]	mL O_2/L BLOOD*
Males	14.0	183.8
Females	12.0	157.6
Blood doping	18.0	236.4
Anemia	< 10.0	< 131.3

*Assumes 98% Hb saturation and a blood pH of 7.4

and completely humidified (100% RH), the partial pressure of water vapor increases to 47 mmHg. Consequently, the pressure remaining for the true gases is 700 mmHg.

Diffusion of Gases

Once air is in the alveoli it is subject to gas diffusion between the alveoli and blood, or vice versa. The factors that govern the direction and magnitude of diffusion are:

▪ The diffusion capacity of each of the gases
▪ The gas partial pressure gradient between the alveoli and blood
▪ The characteristics of the medium through which diffusion occurs

These factors are discussed in focus box 8.2.

Transport of Oxygen and Carbon Dioxide in the Blood

To understand how gas partial pressures affect the volume of gases in blood, knowledge of how blood transports oxygen and carbon dioxide must be acquired.

Oxygen Transport

Oxygen is transported in blood bound to a specialized protein, **hemoglobin,** which is located on the surface of red blood cells. The blood hemoglobin concentration is influenced by gender, nutrition, and disease, with reference values provided in table 8.1. A given hemoglobin molecule can bind four oxygen molecules, and *when fully saturated with oxygen, 1 g of hemoglobin can bind 1.34 mL of oxygen.* For example, when the hemoglobin concentration equals 150 g/L, the following calculations result in the maximal volume of oxygen that can be transported in arterial blood:

hemoglobin (he'mo-glo'-bin) the protein within red blood cells that contains four heme (iron)-containing groups that each can bind oxygen

blood-gas interface the anatomical distance that a gas diffuses across

Figure 8.4 presents the partial pressures of gases in air under standard conditions, in atmospheric air at a coastal location, and indicates how these gas pressures change in the alveoli. When accounting for the relative humidity (RH) and temperature of the atmospheric gas sample (at 55% RH and at 22°C, P_{H2O} equals 18 mmHg), the actual pressure occupied by the true gases decreases from 747 to 729 mmHg. Within the alveoli, the pressure remains equal to atmospheric pressure, but as the air is warmed to 37°C

FOCUS BOX 8.2

Factors That Influence the Rate of Gas Diffusion in the Lung

For a gas to diffuse from one region to another, there must be a difference in gas partial pressure. If there is a difference, then the gas will move along this gradient until there is an even distribution of the gas, termed an *equilibrium*. Thus, for the lung, oxygen and carbon dioxide move along each of their partial pressure gradients between the pulmonary arterial blood and alveolar gas until these partial pressures equilibrate.

Not all gases move along a partial pressure gradient in a similar manner. For example, lung gas diffusion is complicated because there is more than just open air between the pulmonary arterial blood and alveolar gas. This anatomical distance, termed the **blood-gas interface,** consists of blood plasma, pulmonary capillary membranes, interstial fluid, and alveolar membranes (fig. 8.5) that can interfere with gas dif-

fusion. For the normal lung, the most important of these components is the liquid of the plasma and interstitial fluid. If a gas has poor water solubility, it will not diffuse rapidly through the blood-gas interface for a given partial pressure gradient.

Compared to carbon dioxide, oxygen is a relatively insoluble gas with a 20.3-fold lower solubility. Despite the small thickness of the alveolar membranes and the large surface area of the respiratory zone (70 m^2), which make the lung suited to gas diffusion, the poor solubility of oxygen causes it to have a relatively low capacity for diffusion. Thus, even though the lung partial pressure gradients of oxygen and carbon dioxide are extremeley different, their different water solubility results in similar times for complete equilibration in the lung.

FIGURE 8.5

The fluid and membranes that determine the distance between the alveolar air and the blood of the pulmonary capillary comprise what is referred to as the "blood-gas interface." The physical principles that influence the diffusion of a gas across this interface depend on the solubility and diffusion coefficients for the respective gas.

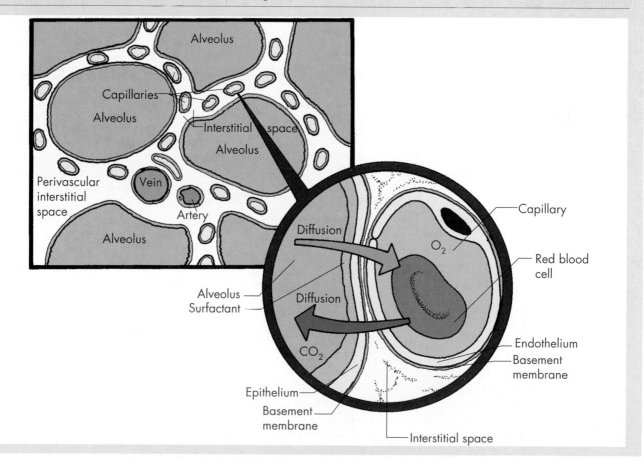

8.3
Blood oxygen carrying capacity
$$= [\text{Hb}] \times O_2/\text{g Hb} \times [\text{Hb}] \text{ - } O_2 \text{ saturation}$$
$$= 150 \text{ g Hb/L} \times 1.34 \text{ mL } O_2/\text{g} \times 0.98$$
$$= 197 \text{ mL } O_2/\text{L}$$

The incomplete $\text{Hb} \cdot O_2$ saturation is due to a combination of (1) diffusion limitation resulting from an average inequality between the lungs' ventilation and perfusion, (2) a *pulmonary arterial-to-venous shunt* because of blood from the bronchioles that drains into the pulmonary veins without passing through the pulmonary capillaries of the respiratory zone, and (3) a *cardiac shunt* involving the drainage of coronary venous blood into the left ventricle. The three deficiencies of pulmonary and cardiac circulation result in minor reductions in average arterial oxy-hemoglobin saturation to 98%.

Another small source of oxygen transport in blood is the volume of dissolved oxygen. Of course, because of the low solubility of oxygen this store is minimal and amounts to 0.003 mL of oxygen for every mmHg of gas partial pressure, or approximately 0.3 mL of oxygen at sea level where PO_2 approximates 104 mmHg.

Oxygen-Hemoglobin Saturation   At sea level, the normal P_AO_2 approximates 104 mmHg. For conditions that lower P_AO_2, such as altitude or air pollution, the partial pressure gradient between the alveoli and blood would decrease. Based on the low-diffusion coefficient of oxygen, this would

be disastrous for the exchange of oxygen between alveolar gas and blood, preventing the ability to equilibrate P_AO_2 and P_aO_2 (39). It is important to understand how a decrease in the partial pressure gradient for oxygen will affect the saturation of hemoglobin, and therefore the oxygen-carrying capacity of the blood.

Figure 8.6 illustrates the oxy-hemoglobin dissociation curve, which essentially describes the change in hemoglobin saturation with a decrease in P_aO_2. For P_aO_2 values that range from 100 to 80 mmHg there are minimal reductions in the saturation of hemoglobin. As P_aO_2 decreases from 80 to 60 mmHg, hemoglobin saturation decreases from 94.9 to 89.3%, and for P_aO_2 values below 60 mmHg, dramatic decreases in hemoglobin saturation occur which can result in large decreases in arterial oxygen transport.

Additional Factors That Alter Oxy-hemoglobin Saturation
Apart from a decreased saturation when the P_aO_2 is reduced, increased dissociation of oxygen and hemoglobin occurs at given PO_2 values by increases in each of blood temperature, PCO_2, and 2,3-bisphosphoglycerate (2,3-BPG, previously abbreviated as 2,3-DPG), and decreases in blood pH.

The molecule 2,3-BPG is a by-product of glycolysis in the red blood cell, and its production increases during conditions of low PO_2 (hypoxia) (24, 26). The 2,3-BPG produced by the red blood cell binds to the deoxygenated form of hemoglobin and therefore assists the unloading of oxygen from

---

FIGURE 8.6

A comparison between oxy-hemoglobin and oxy-myoglobin dissociation curves. For oxygen, the resulting curve is called the oxy-hemoglobin dissociation curve. The curve is moved down and to the right during conditions that increase blood temperature, PCO_2, acidosis, and 2,3-bisphosphoglycerate. As myoglobin retains greater saturation by oxygen at a given partial pressure, it is believed that oxygen moves from hemoglobin to myoglobin within cells. Details of how oxygen moves from myoglobin to within the mitochondria are unclear.

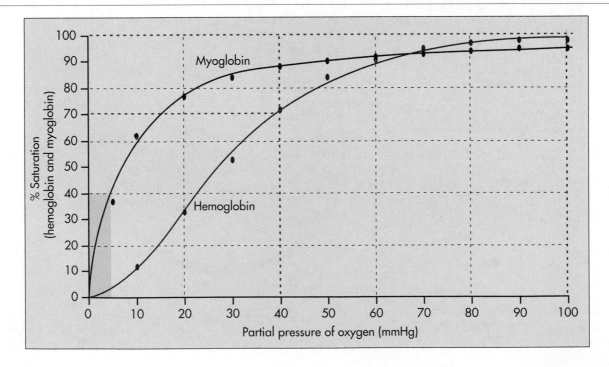

FIGURE 8.7

Carbon dioxide is transported in the blood dissolved in plasma and in the red blood cell, bound to hemoglobin and plasma proteins, and as bicarbonate (HCO_3^-).

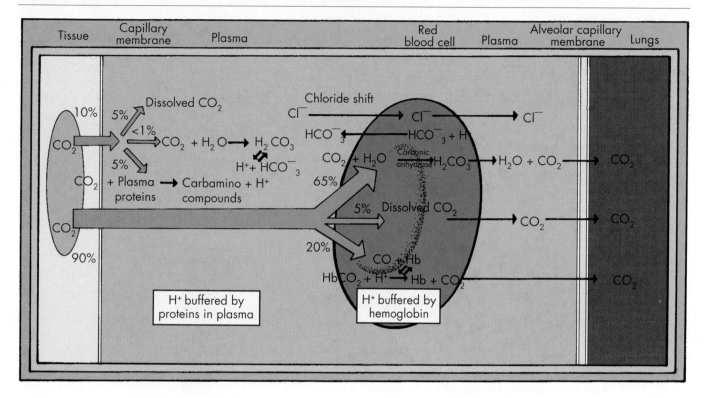

hemoglobin (24, 26). Each of temperature, PCO_2, 2,3-BPG, and pH are conditions that change at the level of the tissues, and the direction of these changes combine to decrease the affinity between oxygen and hemoglobin causing greater unloading of oxygen. The effects of temperature, pH, and PCO_2 on adjusting the oxy-hemoglobin dissociation curve down and to the right is termed the **Bohr effect** in recognition of the scientist who first observed the phenomenon (3, 36).

Carbon Dioxide Transport

The volume of carbon dioxide stored in the body (blood and tissues) is approximately 10-fold greater than oxygen stores (22), and is transported in the blood in several forms (fig. 8.7).

Although carbon dioxide has a greater solubility than oxygen, the majority of CO_2 is not dissolved in plasma or the red blood cell, but reacts with water and is converted to carbonic acid via the **carbonic anhydrase** catalyzed reaction that occurs in red blood cells and the inner walls of the vascular endothelium in the lung. Carbonic acid then dissociates to bicarbonate (HCO_3^-) and a free proton (H^+). The bicarbonate ions are transported in the plasma and under normal acid-base conditions the proton is bound to deoxygenated hemoglobin. The ability of hemoglobin to bind both carbon dioxide and protons is important for acid-base regulation of the blood (see focus box 8.3).

The exchange in hemoglobin binding for carbon dioxide and oxygen is based on the change in partial pressure of oxygen. When the partial pressure of oxygen increases, the affinity between hemoglobin and carbon dioxide decreases and carbon dioxide is forced from hemoglobin. This PO_2 effect on the blood's ability to store carbon dioxide is termed the **Haldane effect** (39).

Internal Respiration

The exchange of gases at the cellular level is influenced by each of the Bohr and Haldane effects. In the tissues the partial pressue of oxygen is low (< 5 mmHg during intense exercise) because of the reduction of oxygen in the electron transport chain, and the partial pressure of carbon dioxide is high because of metabolic production of CO_2. The additional characteristics of an increased temperature and low pH favor the dissociation of oxygen from hemoglobin, and

Bohr effect the decrease in the hemoglobin to oxygen affinity with an increase in temperature, PCO_2, acidosis, and 2,3- BPG

carbonic anhydrase conversion of CO_2 and water to become carbonic acid

Haldane effect the decrease in hemoglobin to carbon dioxide affinity with an increase in the partial pressure of oxygen

FOCUS BOX 8.3

Blood Acid-Base Balance

Acidosis is quantified by the pH scale, where pH equals the negative logarithm of the hydrogen ion concentration (fig. 8.8)

$$pH = -\log [H^+] \quad \text{or} \quad [H^+] = 10^{-pH}$$

Normal arterial blood pH equals 7.4, and normal muscle pH equals 7.0. There are multiple factors that combine to determine each of blood and muscle pH during given nutrition or exercise conditions. The main determinants of pH are:

- The rate of acid production
- The concentration of blood bicarbonate (HCO_3^-) and other weak acids and bases
- The partial pressure of carbon dioxide
- Ventilation of the lung
- The excretion or absorption of acid and base by the kidney

Because reactions of the body occur in an aqueous environment, the characteristics of water are also important in determining pH.

Blood Bicarbonate

The bicarbonate molecule can bind an H^+ to form carbonic acid, as described in the text for carbon dioxide transport in the blood. When acid is produced from metabolism, as it is during conditions accompanied by increased lactate production, protons are removed from the muscle cells and bind with bicarbonate, and eventually form added carbon dioxide and water.

$$Lactate-H^+ + Na^+HCO_3^- \Leftrightarrow Na^+lactate^- + H_2CO_3$$

$$\overset{CA}{H_2CO_3 \Leftrightarrow CO_2 + H_2O}$$

where CA = carbonic anhydrase. Note: there is growing controversy over whether the proton from metabolism comes directly from lactic acid, or is associated with the cellular conditions that lead to increased lactate production.

The production of carbon dioxide from the bicarbonate buffering of acid accounts for the increase in RER above 1.0 during intense or non-steady-state exercise. In addition, the added production of carbon dioxide increases the partial pressure of carbon dioxide in the blood. Consequently, conditions of metabolic acidosis are accompanied by increases in the CO_2 content of venous blood (P_vCO_2) and, as will be discussed in the control of ventilation, severe acidosis may also cause slight increases in the CO_2 content of arterial blood (P_aCO_2).

Because there is a large volume of CO_2 in the body fluids, there is a large source of carbon for the formation of HCO_3^-.

Because of the removal of carbon dioxide from the lungs, large increases in carbon dioxide are prevented, and the metabolic production of CO_2 allows for the reestablishment of normal blood bicarbonate and pH. *The bicarbonate-carbon dioxide system relies on ventilation for proper function as a buffer system.*

FIGURE 8.8

The pH scale, with examples of solutions from everyday life and known changes in blood and muscle pH during exercise.

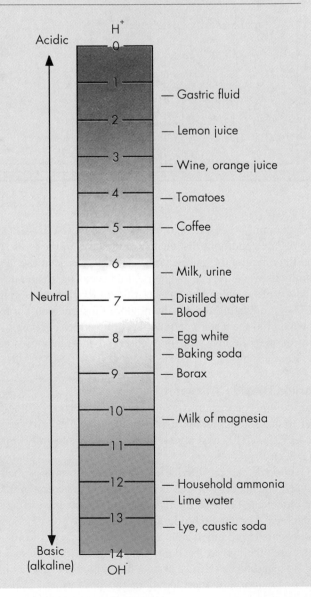

because of the Haldane effect, the affinity between hemoglobin and carbon dioxide increases.

The unloading of oxygen from hemoglobin is also aided by the molecule **myoglobin.** Myoglobin is found within skeletal muscle fibers and is a similar protein to hemoglobin in that it binds oxygen (25). At the cellular level of the circulation where oxygen is consumed and the partial pressure of oxygen in blood decreases, there is a sharp decrease in the affinity between oxygen and hemoglobin. For oxygen partial pressures less than 60 mmHg, myoglobin has a higher affinity for oxygen than does hemoglobin (see fig. 8.6), which allows a unidirectional transfer of oxygen from hemoglobin to myoglobin within the muscle fibers (3, 44). *Myoglobin can therefore be viewed as a "go-between," transferring oxygen molecules between hemoglobin and the mitochondria within the muscle fiber.* The drastic decrease in oxygen and myoglobin affinity below an oxygen partial pressure of 10 mmHg is interesting because the intramuscular PO_2 can get below 10 mmHg during intense exercise. At these low PO_2 values, there is a much higher capacity for oxygen to be released from myoglobin for use in mitochondrial respiration. Having more myoglobin would increase the reservoir of oxygen stored within muscle fibers, and also increase the ability of muscle to continue mitochondrial respiration during intermittent periods of *hypoxia* (low P_aO_2) or *ischemia* (reduced blood flow).

Acute Adaptations of Pulmonary Function During Exercise

The start of exercise is characterized by immediate increases in ventilation. The factors that regulate this increase are numerous and complex, involving neural and blood (humoral) factors. Nerves from the central as well as peripheral nervous systems respond to stimuli to cause increases in the frequency and depth of breathing, thus increasing ventilation. Additional changes in blood, such as increases in partial pressures of carbon dioxide, increased temperature, increased acidosis, and even decreases in partial pressures of oxygen provide the stimuli to nerves or neural tissue involved in increasing ventilation. The rapid and refined nature of ventilatory control result in characteristic responses of ventilation to different types and intensities of exercise.

Ventilation During Transitions from Rest to Steady-State Exercise

As with oxygen consumption, the increase in ventilation during the transition to an increased steady-state exercise intensity is abrupt, exponential, and proportional to the change in intensity (fig. 8.9). Steady-state ventilation is attained earlier than is steady-state VO_2 for a given bout of exercise. As

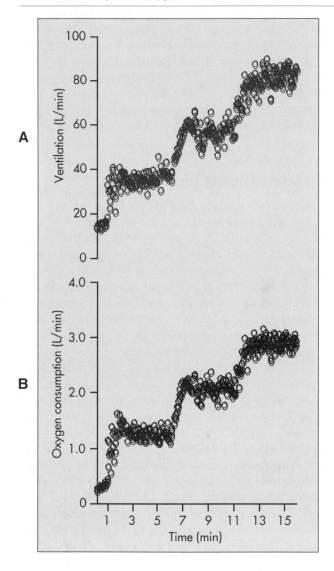

FIGURE 8.9

The increase in *(a)* ventilation during the transition to an increased steady-state exercise intensity is abrupt, exponential, and similar in profile to the change in *(b)* oxygen consumption.

previously explained, the increase in ventilation is because of increases in tidal volume and breathing frequency.

Despite the rapid increase in ventilation at the onset of exercise, there is still a slight increase in P_aCO_2 (45), which indicates that increased ventilation still remains inadequate to remove the sudden increase in CO_2 production by the body. Nevertheless, numerous studies have shown that both ventilation and perfusion of the lungs increase during exercise, become more evenly distributed throughout the lung (6, 7, 13, 22), and improve V_E/Q, and therefore improve the process of external respiration.

myoglobin (mi'o-glo-bin) intramuscular protein that contains one heme (iron)-containing group that enables the binding of oxygen

Ventilation during submaximal exercise at given loads is also known to differ for different types of exercise (17, 29). Arm or upper-body exercise causes a relatively larger ventilation compared to cycling; static exercise also causes ventilation to be larger than dynamic exercise. Data from Paek and McCool (28) indicate that tidal volumes, inspiratory times, and end-expiratory lung volumes may also differ between different types of exercise; however their data were normalized to ventilation and not metabolic load (VO_{2max}). Finally, posture during exercise is also known to affect ventilation, which has been of interest when studying different positions of the upper body during cycling.

Ventilation During Incremental Exercise

The increases in ventilation and oxygen consumption during incremental cycle ergometry exercise are presented in figure 8.10. The variables V_E/VO_2 and V_E/VCO_2 are the *ventilatory equivalents* for oxygen and carbon dioxide, respectively, and are obtained by dividing the VO_2 or VCO_2 by V_E. During the initial intensities, ventilation increases linearly with intensity and VO_2. After an individually specific intensity, the increase in V_E is larger than the increase in VO_2, and by definition there is an abrupt increase in V_E/VO_2. Depending on the protocol used, there is a short time delay (usually 2 min) before V_E/VCO_2 also increases, and this time delay has been explained by the body's large storage capacity for CO_2 and the initial similarity between increased ventilation and VCO_2 at the point of the VT (5).

The Ventilatory Threshold

The exercise intensity at which there is a simultaneous deviation from linearity in ventilation and an increase in V_E/VO_2 is termed the **ventilatory threshold** (VT) (4, 5, 15, 23, 27, 42, 46). Other measures can also be used to detect this point, such as an exponential increase in VCO_2 or RER (respiratory exchange ratio), and an abrupt increase in blood acidosis; however Caizzeo and colleagues (5) have demonstrated that the *joint V_E and V_E/VO_2 criteria are most sensitive in detecting the VT*.

Another method for VT determination is called the V-slope method. Beaver and colleagues (4) introduced this procedure in 1986, which requires a plot of VCO_2 (*y*-axis) versus VO_2 (*x*-axis) (fig. 8.10). The logic behind this approach was based on the assumption that the increased CO_2 produced from acid buffering by bicarbonate would be better detected by graphing the increase in VCO_2 relative to VO_2. Methods that plot changes in ventilation, or are influenced by ventilation, can be influenced by individual differences in the multiple determinants of ventilation during incremental exercise. Nevertheless, the V-slope procedure has not been adequately validated by comparison to blood lactate thresholds (37). Furthermore, evidence indicates that all methods of VT detection are influenced by the exercise protocol, method of detection, and evaluator (37). It appears that no single

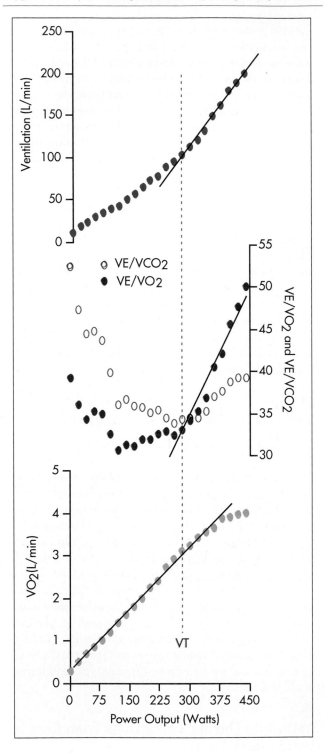

FIGURE 8.10

The increase in ventilation, changes in the ventilatory equivalents for carbon dioxide (V_E/VCO_2) and oxygen (V_E/VO_2), and increase in oxygen consumption during incremental cycle ergometry exercise.

method of VT detection is without error, and therefore the single best method to use.

The traditional explanation of the VT is that as exercise intensity increases, the abrupt increase in lactate acidosis that occurs after the lactate threshold causes an increase in blood acidosis and P_aCO_2. Both the acidosis and the increased P_aCO_2 stimulate the chemoreceptors to induce increased ventilation. This mechanism has been interpreted by many physiologists as evidence that the lactate and ventilatory thresholds occur at the same exercise intensity.

Is the Ventilation Threshold Identical to the Lactate Threshold?

Numerous studies have been conducted to compare the lactate and ventilatory thresholds (15, 17, 27, 42). Researchers have concluded that the two measures are identical (5, 9, 42, 43, 46); however, others have concluded that the two measures can differ under certain conditions, and that the two criteria should not be used interchangeably (1, 16, 17, 20, 27). Factors that can cause the two measures to deviate are:

1. Altered carbohydrate nutrition
2. Different exercise test protocols
3. Enzyme deficiency diseases
4. Methodological errors in detecting each threshold
5. Exercise training
6. Increasing altitude (hypoxia)
7. Altered states of sympathetic stimulation (1, 16, 17, 27)

Gladden and colleagues (17) have estimated that the variation in relative exercise intensity between the LT and VT may be larger than 8% of VO_{2max}, which would be significant when using the measures to prescribe a training exercise intensity.

The Mechanics and Metabolic Costs of Ventilation During Exercise

Both the frequency of ventilation and tidal volume increase during increases in exercise intensity and ventilation. During intense exercise, when ventilation is already high, tidal volume plateaus and further increases in ventilation result from an augmented frequency of breathing. The demands of rapid and deep inflation and deflation of the lungs adds to the work of the muscles of inspiration and expiration.

Do the Muscles of Ventilation Fatigue During Exercise?

The large increase in the work of breathing could cause respiratory muscle fatigue during maximal exercise (see focus boxes 8.1 and 8.4). However, results indicate that for endurance-trained individuals the ability to rapidly ventilate the lungs is not compromised during exercise to VO_{2max} (21). However, whether untrained individuals have near-optimal respiratory muscle and ventilatory function during fatiguing exercise remains to be researched.

Some exercises, such as swimming and deep-water exercise, have the upper body submerged in water, which provides an increased external pressure (compression) to the thoracic cavity. This would theoretically decrease the work of expiration, but potentially increase the work of inspiration. Whether these changes would cause respiratory muscle fatigue and affect the effectiveness of ventilation is unclear. Ventilation and external respiration during swimming is also compromised by forced entrainment of ventilation during specific intervals during a stroke. Although not thoroughly researched, such entrainment causes inspiration and expiration times to be longer but less frequent. It remains unclear how lung function and blood gases and acid-base balance are affected by these constraints in trained or relatively untrained swimmers.

Exercise-Induced Hypoxemia

The partial pressure (P_aO_2) and concentration of oxygen (CaO_2) in arterial blood remain stable in most individuals during all intensities of exercise. However, high altitude can reduce P_aO_2 because of the lowered partial pressure of oxygen, or *hypoxia*, resulting in a reduced C_aO_2, or **hypoxemia.** Interestingly, numerous reports have documented hypoxemia during exhausting exercise at sea level in individuals with healthy lungs.

In 1984 it was observed that highly trained endurance athletes experience significant reductions in C_aO_2 at or near VO_{2max} at sea level, and this condition was termed **exercise-induced hypoxemia** (11). Figure 8.12 reveals the change in arterial oxy-hemoglobin saturation and C_aO_2 in individuals of different cardiorespiratory endurance fitness during an incremental exercise test to volitional fatigue. The more endurance trained the athlete, the larger is the reduction in C_aO_2, which indicates that for these individuals the lungs are not functioning optimally during intense exercise. Powers and colleagues (29, 30, 34) have shown that at sea level, exercise-induced hypoxemia occurs in approximately 50% of well-trained endurance athletes during exercise at intensities above 80% VO_{2max}.

As the healthy lung was always thought to function optimally during exercise, the initial explanation for sea level exercise-induced hypoxemia was an imbalance between cardiac output and maximal effective pulmonary blood flow. It was assumed that endurance athletes were trained to the point where their central blood volume and maximal cardiac output had exceeded the ability of their lungs to maintain pulmonary blood flow at a velocity required to equilibrate P_AO_2 and P_aO_2. The velocity of blood flow in the pulmonary capillaries is important, because a high velocity would decrease the time of a given red blood cell

---

ventilatory threshold the metabolic intensity associated with an increase in the ventilatory equivalent for oxygen (V_E/VO_2)

hypoxemia (hi-pox-see′-mia) lower than normal oxygen availability

exercise-induced hypoxemia a decrease in hemoglobin saturation during exercise

FOCUS BOX 8.4

Asthma, Exercise-Induced Bronchoconstriction, and Exercise

Asthma is an obstructive disorder of the lung that has been difficult to define (35). However, the U.S. Department of Health and Human Services (14) has developed a working definition that recognizes asthma as a lung disease with the following characteristics:

1. Airway obstruction that is reversible (although sometimes not completely) with treatment
2. Airway inflammation
3. Increased airway responsiveness to a variety of stimuli

The airway obstruction is caused by the combination of smooth muscle contraction and inflammation of the tissue surrounding the trachea and bronchioles. This response causes constriction of the large and small airways and a dramatic increase in the resistance to airflow in the conducting zone of the lungs. Some individuals who have mild asthma may be asymptomatic, with their condition detected only with pulmonary function testing (spirometry and peak expiratory flow rate), whereas others with a more severe asthma experience concurrent episodes of cough and wheezing (14). It has been estimated that 10 million individuals in the United States have asthma, that this incidence is increasing, and that up to 25% of the population in the United States have experienced asthma at least once in their lives (14, 25).

Exercise is known to increase the irritability of the bronchial network and increase the likelihood for asthma. However, unlike true asthma, asthma caused by exercise is not accompanied by inflammation, and has therefore been termed *exercise-induced bronchoconstriction*. Exercise-induced bronchoconstriction (EIB) results from irritation of the bronchial lining because of alterations in moisture and tempera-

ture caused by the increased airflow (8). EIB usually does not occur until after exercise, reaching a peak severity after 5 to 10 min of recovery, and becoming completely resolved after 30 min of recovery (fig. 8.11) (14). For individuals with EIB, graded exercise tests are often used to evaluate the onset of the condition or whether certain medications are effective in prevention.

There is some research evidence for the decreased occurrence of EIB when exercise is performed in a warm and humid environment. Consequently, exercise such as swimming is highly recommended, and exercise in cold or dry conditions is to be avoided for individuals susceptible to both EIB and asthma. When medications are used, the inhalation of a bronchodilator immediately prior to exercise, and the use of corticosteroids as a preventive strategy can totally prevent asthma and EIB during and after exercise. Consequently, individuals who are susceptible to asthma and EIB should not refrain from exercise participation. For example, during the 1984 Olympic games, 67 athletes were asthmatics, and many of these individuals received medals (14, 35).

FIGURE 8.11

The changes in FEV_1 (L) (forced expired volume in 1 s) following a bout of exercise by an individual with exercise-induced bronchoconstriction. Note that the most severe restrictions to breathing occur after 5 min of recovery.

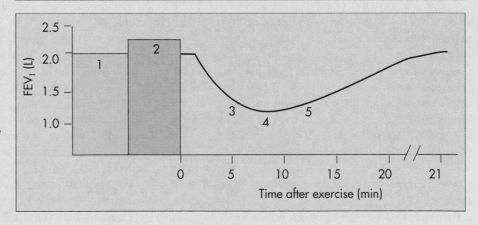

within the blood-gas interface, termed the **pulmonary transit time,** and risk inequilibration. The time required for equilibration between P_AO_2 and P_aO_2 in the healthy lung is believed to be 350 to 400 ms (41). Current research indicates that there is probably sufficient time for equilibration between P_AO_2 and P_aO_2, even in highly trained endurance athletes (41). Consequently, research is currently being pursued to better quantify how other factors could explain the hypoxemia, such as a mild pulmonary edema, or an imbalance in V_E/Q.

Chronic Adaptations

The lungs and pulmonary circulation do not express the degree of long-term adaptation to exercise as was evident for

asthma (az'mah) a condition of the lungs associated with a narrowing of the bronchial airways in response to an irritant

pulmonary transit time the time it takes for a red blood cell to pass through the respiratory zone of the lung

FIGURE 8.12

The decrease in oxy-hemoglobin saturation (hypoxemia) during incremental exercise in individuals with different VO_{2max} capacities. For individuals with larger values for VO_{2max}, there are greater reductions in oxy-hemoglobin saturation, which indicate inadequacies in lung function.

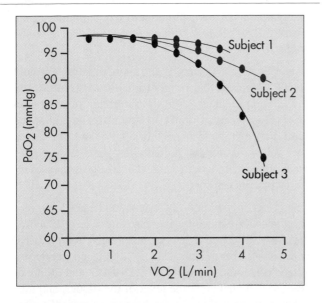

neuromuscular function and skeletal muscle energy metabolism. Efforts have been made to verify whether respiratory muscles can adapt to exercise training and improve lung function during exercise (32). However, although respiratory muscles can adapt to exercise, it appears that their function remains near optimal, and there are no signs to support superior lung function in the trained compared to untrained state.

Numerous studies have shown that the ventilatory threshold improves with endurance training (9, 16, 43). Because the causes for this improvement are more determined by muscular and cardiovascular function, as was explained in chapter 5 for the lactate threshold, no comment will be given for this response in this chapter.

WEBSITE BOX

Chapter 8: Pulmonary Adaptations to Exercise

The newest information regarding exercise physiology can be viewed at the following sites.*

mirrors.org.sg/hol/TOC.biosci.html
    Excellent site providing detailed links to written and illustrated explanations of the heart, cardiovascular system, pulmonary system, blood, etc.
psl.msu.edu/class/501/class8/index.htm
    Lecture material, including PowerPoint slides, on acid-base balance.
lungusa.org/
    Homepage of the American Lung Association, including links to numerous topics such as asthma, tobacco control, lung diseases, smoking cessation, etc.
thoracic.org/
    Homepage of the American Thoracic Society. This is an

extensive site that contains medical, research, educational, and professional information.
nimbus.ocis.temple.edu/~dnowosie/
    Information about asthma and exercise-induced bronchoconstriction.
arfa.org/index.htm
    Excellent site providing comprehensive information on many topics within exercise physiology.
lungnet.org.au/
    Homepage of the Australian Lung Foundation. Provides interesting information on lung health, and support information for the medical practitioner.

---

*Unless indicated, all URLs preceded by http://www.

Note: These URLs were valid at the time of publication, but could have changed or been deleted from Internet access since that time.

SUMMARY

▪ The mouth and nasal passages, trachea, bronchi and bronchioles comprise the **conducting zone** of the lungs, whereas the respiratory bronchioles, alveoli ducts, and alveoli, which are the sites of gas exchange and responsible for the largest lung gas volumes, are referred to as the **respiratory zone** of the lung. The

conducting zone of the lung is often referred to as the **anatomical dead space,** because it does not have a respiratory function. The anatomical dead space comprises an average volume of 150 mL, although this value will vary in a positive relationship with body size.

SUMMARY

- The alveoli and respiratory bronchioles are connected by openings or holes in their membranes, termed **pores of Kohn.** The respiratory bronchioles and alveoli comprise a surface area of approximately 70 square meters.

- The circulation of blood to and through the lung is termed the **pulmonary circulation.** The pulmonary circulation has a much lower blood pressure than the systemic circulation (25/8 compared to 120/80 mmHg at rest). The respiratory zone of the lung is engorged with a rich blood supply, providing almost as much surface area of blood as that of the respiratory membranes.

- The vital capacity is the maximal volume of air that can be exhaled from the lungs. It can be divided into inspiratory and expiratory components using the method of *spirometry*. Normal resting breathing involves the inspiration and expiration of 500 mL of air, termed the **tidal volume**.

- The product of the tidal volume and breathing frequency determines **ventilation**. *Ventilation involves the movement of air into and from the lungs by the process of bulk flow.* Ventilation can increase airflow through the lung from a mere 6 L/min at rest to over 150 L/min during maximal exercise. Of the normal 500 mL tidal volume, 350 mL of "fresh" air reaches the respiratory zone. The volume of "fresh" air that reaches the respiratory zone of the lung is termed **alveolar ventilation** (V_A). *The greater the depth of breathing, the less impact the anatomical dead space has on alveolar ventilation.*

- The property of being able to increase size or volume with only small changes in pressure is termed **compliance.** Thus, the lungs have very high compliance. *The presence of **surfactant** makes it easier to inflate alveoli.* Surfactant functions to lower the surface tension of the alveoli, thereby decreasing the resistance to inflation, and increasing compliance.

- The process of gas exchange, or **respiration**, involves the movement of oxygen and carbon dioxide down pressure gradients that exist between pulmonary capillary blood and the air of the alveoli, and between capillary blood of the systemic circulation and the cells perfused by this blood.

- Once air is in the alveoli it is subject to gas diffusion between the alveoli and blood, or vice versa. The factors that govern the direction and magnitude of diffusion are (1) the diffusion capacity of each of the gases, (2) the gas partial pressure gradient between the alveoli and blood, and (3) the characteristics of the medium through which diffusion occurs.

- The anatomical distance that a gas diffuses across is termed the **blood-gas interface**, and in the lung consists of blood plasma, pulmonary capillary membranes, interstitial fluid, and alveolar membranes that can interfere with gas diffusion. Compared to carbon dioxide, oxygen is a relatively insoluble gas with a 20.3-fold lower solubility.

- Oxygen is transported in blood bound to a specialized protein, **hemoglobin**, which is located on the surface of red blood cells. The blood hemoglobin concentration is influenced by gender, nutrition, and disease. A given hemoglobin molecule can bind four oxygen molecules, and *when fully saturated with oxygen, 1 g of hemoglobin can bind 1.34 mL of oxygen.*

- At sea level, the normal P_AO_2 approximates 104 mmHg. For P_aO_2 values that range from 100 to 80 mmHg there are minimal reductions in the saturation of hemoglobin. As P_aO_2 decreases from 80 to 60 mmHg, hemoglobin saturation decreases from 94.9 to 89.3%, and for P_aO_2 values below 60 mmHg, dramatic decreases in hemoglobin saturation occur, which can result in large decreases in arterial oxygen transport.

- Increased dissociation of oxygen and hemoglobin occurs at given PO_2 values by increases in each of blood temperature, PCO_2, and 2,3-bisphosphoglycerate (2,3-BPG, previously abbreviated as 2,3-DPG), and decreases in blood pH. Temperature, PCO_2, 2,3-BPG, and pH are conditions that change at the level of the tissues, and the direction of these changes combine to decrease the affinity between oxygen and hemoglobin causing greater unloading of oxygen. The adjustment the oxy-hemoglobin dissociation curve down and to the right is termed the **Bohr effect** (3, 54).

- The majority of CO_2 is converted to carbonic acid via the **carbonic anhydrase** catalyzed reaction that occurs on the surface of red blood cells and inner walls of the vascular endothelium. Carbonic acid then dissociates to bicarbonate (HCO_3^-) and a free proton (H^+). The bicarbonate ions are transported in the plasma and under normal acid-base conditions the proton is bound to deoxygenated hemoglobin. When the partial pressure of oxygen increases, the affinity between hemoglobin and carbon dioxide decreases and carbon dioxide is forced from hemoglobin. This PO_2 effect on the blood's ability to store carbon dioxide is termed the **Haldane effect**.

- Acidosis is quantified by the pH scale, where pH equals the negative logarithm of the hydrogen ion concentration (pH $= -\log [H^+]$ or $[H^+] = 10^{-pH}$). Normal arterial blood pH equals 7.4, and normal muscle pH equals 7.0. The main determinants of pH are (1) the rate of acid production, (2) the concentration of blood bicarbonate (HCO_3^-) and other weak acids and bases, (3) the partial pressure of carbon dioxide, (4) ventilation of the lung, and (5) the excretion or absorption of acid and base by the kidney.

- The unloading of oxygen from hemoglobin is also aided by the molecule **myoglobin**. Myoglobin is found within skeletal muscle fibers and is a similar protein to hemoglobin in that it binds oxygen. *Myoglobin can be viewed as a* *"go-between," transferring oxygen molecules between hemoglobin and the mitochondria within the muscle fiber.*

■ Steady-state ventilation is attained earlier than is steady-state VO_2 for a given bout of exercise. The variables V_E/VO_2 and V_E/VCO_2 are the *ventilatory equivalents* for oxygen and carbon dioxide, respectively, and are obtained by dividing the VO_2 or VCO_2 into V_E. The exercise intensity at which there is a simultaneous deviation from linearity in ventilation and an increase in V_E/VO_2 is termed the **ventilatory threshold** (VT). The estimated variation in the relative exercise intensity between the VT and LT may be larger than 8% of VO_{2max}, which would be significant when using the measures to prescribe a training exercise intensity.

■ **Asthma** is an obstructive disorder of the lung that is responsive to pharmacological treatment. The asthma-like condition caused by exercise has been termed exercise-induced bronchoconstriction (EIB). A lowering of blood P_aO_2 is called hypoxemia. During incremental exercise to VO_{2max}, approximately 50% of highly trained endurance athletes experience significant reductions in C_aO_2 at sea level, and this condition is termed **exercise-induced hypoxemia.** As the altitude above sea level increases, exercise-induced hypoxemia increases in occurrence and severity. The velocity of blood flow in the pulmonary capillaries may be influential in causing exercise-induced hypoxemia. A high pulmonary blood flow velocity decreases the time a given red blood cell is within the blood-gas interface, termed the **pulmonary transit time,** and risks inequilibration.

STUDY QUESTIONS

1. What are the two zones of the lung and how do their functions differ?

2. What is surfactant, where is it located within the lung, and what are its functions?

3. How does air move into and from the lung?

4. Why is compliance of the lung important to ventilation at rest and during exercise?

5. Calculate the oxygen transported in the blood every minute for the following conditions:

   a. [Hb] = 135 g/L, P_aO_2 = 98 mmHg, Q = 5 L/min
   b. [Hb] = 135 g/L, P_aO_2 = 95 mmHg, Q = 5 L/min
   c. [Hb] = 135 g/L, P_aO_2 = 98 mmHg, Q = 25 L/min
   d. [Hb] = 135 g/L, P_aO_2 = 95 mmHg, Q = 25 L/min

   When cardiac output is considered, do small changes in hemoglobin concentration or hemoglobin saturation result in large changes in blood oxygen transport? How would small decreases in [Hb] or P_aO_2 influence the ability to exercise at moderate to high intensities?

6. Are the Haldane and Bohr effects simply a reversal of each other? Explain.

7. Why is gas solubility important to diffusion between the alveoli and blood?

8. Explain the importance of CO_2 to blood acid-base balance?

9. How does ventilation change during incremental exercise, and what factors are believed to cause these changes?

10. Is the ventilation threshold identical to the lactate threshold? Explain.

11. What is exercise-induced hypoxemia, what type of individuals mainly experience it, and why does it occur?

APPLICATIONS

1. You are asked by an asthma sufferer why exercise seems to exacerbate the condition. What is your response, and what types of exercise would you recommend?

2. Many clinical exercise tests are conducted that use the ventilation threshold as an index of skeletal muscle metabolism and the lactate threshold. Is this a correct and accurate practice? Explain.

3. If there is 3 mL of O_2 dissolved in plasma for every 1 L of blood at sea level, calculate the amount of O_2 dissolved in blood plasma when breathing pure oxygen at sea level. During this condition, how much extra oxygen circulates around the body when cardiac output is 20 L/min? Do you think this is a meaningful change? Why?

4. During periods between play in American football, many players sit on a bench and breath pure oxygen. This is done with the assumption that it will improve the recovery from intense exercise. However, breathing pure oxygen is known to depress ventilation. How would this practice influence the recovery from acidosis, and could it be doing more harm than good? Explain your answer.

REFERENCES

1. Anderson, G. S., and E. C. Rhodes. The relationship between blood lactate and excess CO_2 in elite cyclists. *J. Sports Sciences* 9:173–181, 1991.

2. Bastacky, J. B., and J. Goerke. Pores of Kohn are filled in normal lungs: Low-temperature scanning electron microscopy. *J. Appl. Physiol.* 73(1):88–95, 1992.

3. Baumann, R., H. Bartels, and C. Bauer. Blood oxygen transport. In L. E. Farhi and S. M. Tenney (eds.), *Handbook of physiology: Sec. 3: The respiratory system. Vol. 1: Gas exchange.* American Physiological Society, Bethesda, MD, 1987, pp. 147–172.

4. Beaver, W., K. Wasserman, and B. Whipp. A new method for detecting anaerobic threshold by gas exchange. *J. Appl. Physiol.* 60(6):2020–2027, 1986.

5. Caiozzeo, V. J., et al. A comparison of gas exchange indices used to detect the anaerobic threshold. *J. Appl. Physiol.* 53(5):1184–1189, 1982.

6. Capen, R., L., W. L. Hanson, L. P. Latham, C. A. Dawson, and W. W. Wagner, Jr. Distribution of pulmonary transmit times in recruited networks. *J. Appl. Physiol.* 69(2):473–478, 1990.

7. Cotton, D. J., F. Taher, J. T. Mink, and B. L. Graham. Effect of volume history on changes in $DL_{CO}{}^{SB}-3EQ$ with lung volume in normal subjects. *J. Appl. Physiol.* 73(2):434–439, 1992.

8. Cox, N. J. M., C. L. A. van Herwaarden, H. Folgering, and R. A. Binkhorst. Exercise and training in patients with chronic obstructive lung disease. *Sports Medicine* 6(3):180–192, 1988.

9. Davis, J. A., P. Vodak, J. Wilmore, J. Vodak, and P. Kurtz. Anaerobic threshold and maximal aerobic power for three modes of exercise. *J. Appl. Physiol.* 41(4):544–550, 1976.

10. Dempsey, J. A., P. G. Hanson, and K. S. Henderson. Exercise-induced arterial hypoxemia in healthy persons at sea level. *J. Physiol.* 355:161–175, 1984.

11. Dempsey, J. A., G. Mitchell, and C. Smith. Exercise and chemoreception. *Am. Rev. Resp. Dis.* 129:31–34, 1984.

12. Dempsey, J. A., E. Virdruk, and G. Mitchell. Pulmonary control systems in exercise: Update. *Federation Proc.* 44:2260–2270, 1985.

13. Dempsey, J. A. Is the lung built for exercise? *Med. Sci. Sports Exerc.* 18(2):143–155, 1986.

14. Department of Health and Human Services. *Guidelines for the diagnoses and management of asthma.* Publication No. 91-3042. National Institutes of Health, 1991.

15. Farrell, S. W., and J. L. Ivy. Lactate acidosis and the increase in V_E/VO_2 during incremental exercise. *J. Appl. Physiol.* 62(4):1551–1555, 1987.

16. Gaesser, G. A., and D. C. Poole. Lactate and ventilatory thresholds: Disparity in time course of adaptations to training. *J. Appl. Physiol.* 61(3):999–1004, 1986.

17. Gladden, L. B, J. W. Yates, R. W. Stremel, and B. A. Stamford. Gas exchange and lactate anaerobic thresholds: Inter- and intraevaluator agreement. *J. Appl. Physiol.* 58(6):2082–2089, 1985.

18. Grucza, R., Y. Miyamoto, and Y. Nakazonto. Kinetics of cardiorespiratory response to rhythmic-static exercise in men. *Eur. J. Appl. Physiol.* 61:230–236, 1990.

19. Guyton, A. C. *Textbook of medical physiology,* 8th ed. Saunders, Philadelphia, 1991.

20. Hagberg, J. M., E. F. Coyle, J. E. Carroll, J. M. Miller, W. M. Martin, and M. H. Brooke. Exercise hyperventilation in patients with McArdle's disease. *J. Appl. Physiol.* 52(4):991–994, 1982.

21. Johnson, B. D., K. W. Saupe, and J. A. Dempsey. Mechanical constraints on exercise hyperpnea in endurance athletes. *J. Appl. Physiol.* 73(3):874–886, 1992.

22. Jones, N. L. *Blood gases and acid-base physiology,* 2nd ed. Thieme Medical Publishers, New York, 1987.

23. Koike, A., D. Weiler-Ravell, D. K. McKenzie, S. Zanconato, and K. Wasserman. Evidence that the metabolic acidosis threshold is the anaerobic threshold. *J. Appl. Physiol.* 68(6):2521–2526, 1990.

24. Loat, C. E. R., and E. C. Rhodes. Relationship between the lactate and ventilatory thresholds during prolonged exercise. *Sports Medicine* 15(2):104–115, 1993.

25. Lehninger, A. L. Principles of biochemistry. Worth Publishers, New York, 1982.

26. Mairbaurl, H., W. Schobersberger, W. Hasibeder, G. Schwaberger, G. Gaesser, and K. R. Tanaka. Regulation of 2,3-DPG and Hb-O_2-affinity during acute exercise. *Eur. J. Appl. Physiol.* 55:174–180, 1986.

27. Neary, P. J., J. D. MacDougall, R. Bachus, and H. A. Wenger. The relationship between lactate and ventilatory thresholds: Coincidental or cause and effect? *Eur. J. Appl. Physiol.* 54:104–108, 1985.

28. Paek, D., and D. McCool. Breathing patterns during varied activities. *J. Appl. Physiol.* 73(3):887–893, 1992

29. Powers, S. K., and J. Williams. Exercise-induced hypoxia in highly trained athletes. *Sports Medicine* 4:46–53, 1987.

30. Powers, S. K., et al. Incidence of exercise induced hypoxemia in the elite endurance athlete at sea level. *Eur. J. Appl. Physiol.* 58:298–302, 1988.

31. Powers, S. K., J. Lawlor, J. A. Dempsey, S. Dodd, and G. Landry. Effects of incomplete pulmonary gas exchange on VO_{2max}. *J. Appl. Physiol.* 66(6):2491–2495, 1989.

32. Powers, S. K., et al. Endurance-training-induced cellular adaptations in respiratory muscles. *J. Appl. Physiol.* 68(5):2114–2118, 1990.

33. Powers, S. K., D. Martin, M. Cicale, N. Collop, D. Huang, and D. Criswell. Exercise induced hypoxemia in athletes: Role of inadequate hyperventilation. *Eur. J. Appl. Physiol.* 65:37–42, 1992.

34. Powers, S. K., D. Martin, and S. Dodd. Exercise-induced hypoxemia in elite endurance athletes: Incidence, causes and impact on VO_{2max}. *Sports Medicine* 16(1):14–22, 1993.

35. Roberts, J. A. Exercise-induced asthma in athletes. *Sports Medicine* 6(4):193–196, 1988.

36. Seeley, R. R., T. D. Stephens, and P. Tate. *Anatomy and physiology.* Times Mirror/Mosby College Publishing, St. Louis, 1989.

37. Shimizu, M., et al. The ventilatory threshold: Method, protocol, and evaluator agreement. *Am. Heart J.* 122:509–516, 1991.

38. Thomas, D. Q., B. A. Bowdoin, D. D. Brown, and S. T. McCaw. Nasal strips, and mouth pieces do not affect power output during anaerobic exercise. *Res. Q. Exerc. Sport.* 69(2):201–204, 1998.

39. Torre-Bueono, J. R., P. D. Wagner, H .A. Saltzman, G. E. Gale, and R. E. Moon. Diffusion limitation in normal humans during exercise at sea level and simulated altitude. *J. Appl. Physiol.* 58(3):989–995, 1985.

40. Vermoen, C. J., A. F. Verbraak, and J. M. Bogaard. Effect of nasal dilator on nasal patency during normal and forced nasal breathing. *Int. J. Sports Med.* 19(2):109–113, 1998.

41. Warren, G., K. J. Cureton, W. F. Middendorf, C. A. Ray, and J. A. Warren. Red blood cell pulmonary transit time during exercise in athletes. *Med. Sci. Sports Exerc.* 23(12):1353–1361, 1991.

42. Wasserman, K., and M. B. McIlroy. Detecting the threshold of anaerobic metabolism in cardiac patients during exercise. *Am. J. Cardiol.* 14:844–852, 1964.

43. Wasserman, K., B. J. Whipp, S. N. Koyal, and W. L. Beaver. Anaerobic threshold and respiratory gas exchange during exercise. *J. Appl. Physiol.* 35(2):236–243, 1973.

44. Wasserman, K., B. J. Whipp, and R. Casaburi. Respiratory control during exercise. In N. S. Cherniak and J. G. Widdicombe (eds.), *Handbook of Physiology: Sec. 3: The respiratory system. Vol. 2: Control of breathing.* American Physiological Society, Bethesda, MD, 1986, pp. 595–620.

45. Weissman, M. L., P. W. Jones, A, Oren, N. Lamarra, B. J. Whipp, and K. Wasserman. Cardiac output increase and gas exchange at the start of exercise. *J. Appl. Physiol.* 52(1):236–244, 1982.

46. Whipp, B. J., and S. Ward. Physiological determinants of pulmonary gas exchange kinetics during exercise. *Med. Sci. Sports Exerc.* 22(1):62–71, 1990.

47. Yeh, M. P., R. M. Gardner, T. D. Adams, F. G. Yanowitz, and R. O. Crappo. "Anaerobic threshold": Problems of determination and validation. *J. Appl. Physiol.* 55(4):1178–1186, 1983.

RECOMMENDED READINGS

Caiozzeo, V. J., et al. A comparison of gas exchange indices used to detect the anaerobic threshold. *J. Appl. Physiol.* 53(5):1184–1189, 1982.

Dempsey, J. A. Is the lung built for exercise? *Med. Sci. Sports Exerc.* 18(2):143–155, 1986.

Dempsey, J. A., P. G. Hanson, and K. S. Henderson. Exercise-induced arterial hypoxemia in healthy persons at sea level. *J Physiol.* 355:161–175, 1984.

Farrell, S. W., and J. L. Ivy. Lactate acidosis and the increase in V_E/VO_2 during incremental exercise. *J. Appl. Physiol.* 62(4):1551–1555, 1987.

Gaesser, G. A. and D. C. Poole. Lactate and ventilatory thresholds: Disparity in time course of adaptations to training. *J. Appl. Physiol.* 61(3):999–1004, 1986.

Johnson, B. D., K. W. Saupe, and J. A. Dempsey. Mechanical constraints on exercise hyperpnea in endurance athletes. *J. Appl. Physiol.* 73(3):874–886, 1992.

Neary, P. J., J. D. MacDougall, R. Bachus, and H. A. Wenger. The relationship between lactate and ventilatory thresholds: Coincidental or cause and effect? *Eur. J. Appl. Physiol.* 54:104–108, 1985.

Powers, S. K., D. Martin, and S. Dodd. Exercise-induced hypoxemia in elite endurance athletes: Incidence, causes and impact on VO_{2max}. *Sports Medicine* 16(1):14–22, 1993.

Shimizu, M., et al. The ventilatory threshold: Method, protocol, and evaluator agreement. *Am. Heart J.* 122:509–516, 1991.

Wasserman, K., B. J. Whipp, S. N. Koyal, and W. L. Beaver. Anaerobic threshold and respiratory gas exchange during exercise. *J. Appl. Physiol.* 35(2):236–243, 1973.

Yeh, M. P., R. M. Gardner, T. D. Adams, F. G. Yanowitz, and R. O. Crappo. "Anaerobic threshold": Problems of determination and validation. *J. Appl. Physiol.* 55(4):1178–1186, 1983.

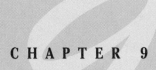

CHAPTER 9

Neuroendocrine Adaptations to Exercise

uring exercise the body must respond rapidly to the increased demands placed upon it. As explained in previous chapters, the increased energy needs of the muscles have to be met, blood flow and ventilation must increase to circulate more oxygen to the muscles and remove wastes, heat must be redistributed to the periphery, and body water must be preserved as best as possible to support the dissipation of heat and maintain cardiovascular function. These and other responses involved in the body's abilities to tolerate exercise are regulated by complex interactions between the autonomic nervous system and the specialized tissues (glands) of the body that release hormones. In addition to neural stimulation, many of the body's glands detect specific chemical or mechanical conditions within the body, and release specific hormones that function to return the condition toward "normal" status. This response can be to increase glucose uptake into muscle cells, reabsorb more water from ducts within the kidneys, or increase the ability of the myocardium to contract powerfully. Clearly, the need to understand how the body responds to exercise requires knowledge of the hormones of the body and how they function. This chapter presents a concise summary of the field of exercise endocrinology. The purpose of the chapter is not to present an overwhelming volume of information, but to organize the known hormonal responses to exercise into discrete biological functions recognized as important to the ability to tolerate exercise stress.

OBJECTIVES

After studying this chapter, you should be able to:

- Describe the complexity of the body's hormonal regulation during rest and exercise.
- Explain the functional differences of how amine, peptide, and steroid hormones alter cellular function.
- List several important hormones essential to the body's ability to respond to exercise, and identify what glands/tissues they are released from.
- Describe the hormonal responses to exercise that influence muscle energy metabolism, energy substrate mobilization, fluid balance, vascular hemodynamics, and protein synthesis.
- Identify the hormones that are released and describe their functions during specific exercise conditions.
- Explain how training for either strength or endurance can alter the hormonal responses to that specific exercise.

KEY TERMS

neuroendocrinology
gland
hormone
second messenger
cyclic AMP (cAMP)
GLUT$_4$

hypoglycemia
diabetes mellitis
hyperglycemia
osmoreceptors
antidiuretic
diuresis

hypertension
hypotension
endogenous opioids
athletic amenorrhea

The Neuroendocrine System

*N*euroendocrinology is the study of the combined function of nerves and *glands* involved in the release of *hormones* that regulate the function of body tissues. Traditionally, the hormones of interest were secreted by glandular tissues grouped and classified as *endocrine* glands. The joint function of nerves and hormones is important, because many of the body's glands are stimulated by nerves. Glands can also be stimulated by chemical conditions (e.g., low blood glucose), resulting in the release, and/or inhibited release, of one or more hormones.

The Glands of the Body

A **gland** is a tissue that secretes a substance within or from the body. The glands of the body can be divided into *exocrine* or *endocrine*. Exocrine glands secrete substances from the body, and are further divided into *apocrine* and *eccrine* glands. Both apocrine and eccrine glands have ducts through which the apocrine gland secretes sebaceous fluid, like the oil that is secreted to the surface of the skin, or the bile ducts of the liver. The eccrine gland secretes sweat. The endocrine gland is ductless and secretes a substance directly into the blood. Traditionally, the substances secreted from endocrine glands were known as **hormones**. Hormones were released in minor amounts resulting in very low concentrations in the blood (< 1 µmole), and they exerted their function on tissues located in other regions of the body. The science of *endocrinology* involves the study of endocrine glands, their hormones, and the effects of specific hormones on various tissues of the body. A list of the traditional endocrine glands and their hormones is provided in table 9.1, and the anatomical locations of these glands are illustrated in figure 9.1.

Are All Hormones Secreted from Glands?

Research during the last decade has revealed that the traditional definition of a hormone may not be appropriate. It is now known that tissues other than true endocrine glands secrete substances that act as hormones. For example, the hypothalamus, heart, kidney, liver, gastrointestinal tract, lymphocytes, and endothelial cells all secrete substances that exert regulatory effects on other tissues (20).

A list of nontraditional hormones and the tissues they are secreted from is also provided in table 9.1. Tissues such as the heart are involved in the regulation of blood pressure and fluid balance via the hormone atrial natriuretic peptide, and substances derived from the endothelial lining of blood vessels can induce vasoconstriction and vasodilation locally as well in distant blood vessels. It is clear that the *traditional approach and definitions of endocrinology are too simplistic and narrow* for application to the now-recognized complex hormonal regulation of many bodily functions.

Hormone Classification

Not all hormones are similar in their methods of stimulation to cells. Hormones can be divided into three main categories: *amine, peptide* and *steroid* hormones.

Amine and Peptide Hormones

Amine hormones are derived from amino acids; peptide hormones are proteins and therefore consist of multiple amino acids connected by peptide bonds (see table 9.1). The more notable amine hormones are epinephrine, norepinephrine, and the thyroid hormones. Notable peptide hormones are antidiuretic hormone, insulin, and erythropoietin.

Because amine and peptide hormones are soluble, most are transported in blood plasma in solution. Steroid hormones are not water soluble and are transported in blood bound to specific transport proteins. The water soluble characteristics of amine and peptide hormones make them easily removed from the circulation by tissues such as the liver, kidneys, and lung, and therefore have only a few minutes to exert their function. The time taken for the removal or destruction of half the hormone is termed a *half-life*. For example, the half-life of epinephrine and norepinephrine is less than 3 min (23), and the half-life of triiodothyronine, although an amine, approximates 7 days because it binds to a special globulin protein in the plasma (23). The half-life of the steroid hormone cortisol approximates 70 to 90 min (20).

Cellular Response Mechanisms   Amine and peptide hormones exert their action on target cells by binding to specific receptors located on the cell membranes of the target tissue(s). Consequently, *the presence of these membrane receptors are essential for the biological response to amine and peptide hormones*. Not only are receptors different and therefore specific for each hormone, but some hormones such as epinephrine and norepinephrine have multiple types of receptors that further differentiate and specialize cellular biological responses. For example, the α- and β-receptors of the neurotransmitter norepinephrine, and the different affinities between norepinephrine and epinephrine for these receptors, explains why some smooth muscle responds by contracting and causing vasoconstriction (α-receptors) because of increased circulating epinephrine and norepinephrine, while other smooth muscle responds by causing

---

neuroendocrinology (nu ro-en do-kri-no'l o-je) the study of the anatomy and function of the endocrine system and the components of the nervous system that regulate endocrine function

gland an organ that secretes one or more substances

hormone a substance secreted from a tissue or cell that exerts a biological effect on that tissue or cell, or on local or distant cells

TABLE 9.1

Traditional and nontraditional glands and hormones.

| | HORMONES | | |
TISSUE/GLAND	AMINE	PEPTIDE	STEROID
Traditional Hormones			
Pituitary			
Anterior		Luteinizing hormone (LH), follicle-stimulating hormone (FSH), prolactin (PRL), growth hormone (GH), adrenocorticotropin (ACTH), β-lipoprotein, β-endorphin, thyroid-stimulating hormone (TSH)	
Intermediate		Melanocyte-stimulating hormone (MSH), β-endorphin	
Posterior		Antidiuretic hormone (ADH, or vasopressin), oxytocin	
Thyroid	Thyroxine (T$_4$), triiodothyronine (T$_3$)	Calcitonin	
Parathyroid		Parathyroid hormone (PTH)	
Adrenal			
Cortex			Cortisol, aldosterone, androstanedione
Medulla	Epinephrine, norepinephrine		
Gonads			
Testes			Testosterone, estradiol, androstanedione
Ovaries			Estradiol, progesterone, testosterone, androstanedione, FSH-releasing peptide
Placenta			Progesterone, estrogen
Pancreas		Insulin, glucagon, somatostatin, vasoactive intestinal peptide (VIP)	
Nontraditional Hormones			
Hypothalamus		[ACTH]-releasing hormone (CRH), thyrotropin-releasing hormone (TRH), LH-releasing hormone (LHRH), GH-releasing hormone (GHRH), somatostatin	
Heart		Atrial natriuretic peptides (ANP)	
Kidney		Erythropoietin, renin, 1,25-dihydroxyvitamin D	
Liver		Insulin-like growth factor I (IGF-I)	
Gastrointestinal tract		Cholecystokinin (CCK), gastrin, secretin, VIP, enteroglucagon	
Lymphocytes		Interleukins	
Vascular endothelium		Endothelin (ET), nitrous oxide (endothelial-derived relaxing factor [EDRF])	

vasodilation (β-receptors). Further response complexity exists because each of α- and β-receptors have subgroups (1, 2).

To elicit a cellular response, the binding of an amine or peptide hormone to a receptor must cause changes in cellular function. The molecules that are produced in a cell in response to hormone binding, and that then stimulate a cellular response are termed **second messengers. Cyclic AMP (cAMP)** is produced in response to the binding of epinephrine to a β$_2$-receptor on the sarcolemma of a skeletal muscle fiber. However, when epinephrine binds to an α$_2$-receptor, the production of cAMP is inhibited. When epinephrine binds to an α$_1$-receptor, an inositol phospholipid is broken

FIGURE 9.1

An overview of the anatomical location of the major glands and gland-like tissues that are involved in the body's acute and chronic responses to exercise.

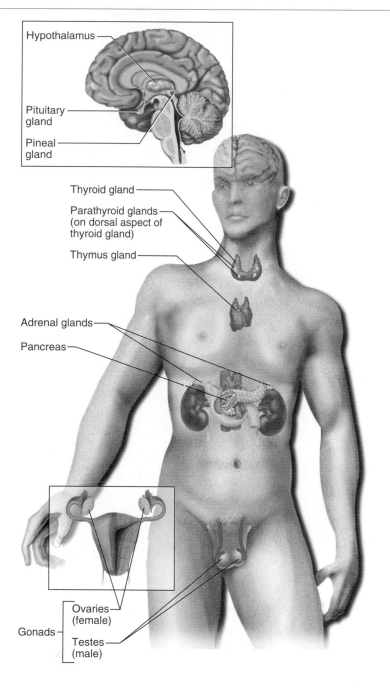

down and two additional second messengers are released (*diacylglycerol* and *inositol triphosphate*), which results in an increase in intracellular calcium and the activation and inhibition of various enzymes. A consistent theme in receptor binding and second messenger production involves the *activation of a membrane-bound enzyme that catalyzes the production of the second messenger*. The second messengers

second messenger an intracellular compound that increases in concentration during the amplification response to the binding of a hormone to its receptor

cyclic AMP (cAMP) the second messenger produced by the activation of adenylate cyclase in response to the binding of certain hormones to their cell receptor(s)

TABLE 9.2

Main functional responses of glandular tissues and hormones involved in acute adaptation to exercise.

GLAND/HORMONES	STIMULANT FOR RELEASE	TARGET TISSUE	RESPONSE
Cellular Energy Metabolism			
Adrenal Medulla			
Epinephrine	Stress, hypotension, moderate to intense exercise	Skeletal muscle	↑ Glycogenolysis
Norepinephrine	Hypoglycemia, moderate to intense exercise	Adipose tissue, liver	↑ Lipolysis, ↑ heart rate, ↑ glycogenolysis, ↑ stroke volume, ↑ vascular resistance
Fuel Mobilization			
Anterior pituitary			
ACTH	Injury, exercise	Adrenal cortex	↑ Cortisol release
GH	Exercise, hypoglycemia	Skeletal muscle, adipose tissue, liver	FFA mobilization, ↑ gluconeogenesis ↓ glucose uptake
Adrenal cortex			
Cortisol	↑ ACTH; intense, prolonged exercise	Skeletal muscle, adipose tissue, liver	↑ Gluconeogenesis, ↓ protein synthesis, ↓ glucose uptake
Pancreas			
Insulin	Hyperglycemia, ↑ circulating amino acids, autonomic nervous system (ANS)	Skeletal muscle, adipose tissue	↑ Glucose, amino acid, FFA uptake
Glucagon	Hypoglycemia, low amino acid concentrations, prolonged exercise	Liver	↑ Gluconeogenesis
Thyroid			
Triiodothyronine (T_3) Thyroxine (T_4)	Low T_3 and T_4 (?)	All	↑ Metabolic rate, GH ↑ serum FFA, amino acids
Testes			
Testosterone	↑ FSH, LH; exercise(?)	Skeletal muscle, testes, bone	↑ Protein synthesis, ↑ sperm production, ↑ sex drive
Ovaries			
Estrogen	↑ FSH, LH; light to moderate exercise	Skeletal muscle, adipose tissue	Inhibition of glucose uptake, fat deposition

then activate and inhibit certain enzymes, which then alter the metabolism of the cell. These processes of enzyme activation and inhibition are extremely fast, and the time between the stimulation for the release of amine and peptide hormones and a resultant cellular response is less than 1 min.

Steroid Hormones

Steroid hormones are named after their chemical structure which is based on four fused carbon rings, termed a *steroid nucleus* (6). Cholesterol is an important substrate in the synthesis of steroid hormones.

Steroid hormones, like other lipid molecules, are *hydrophobic* and therefore insoluble in water. Steroid hormones must therefore be bound to plasma proteins to be transported in the blood to their target tissues. Protein binding compli-

cates the activity and half-life of steroid hormones; as the protein-bound steroid hormone is prevented from being able to enter a cell and stimulate a biological response, the rate of hormone destruction or removal from circulation is decreased, and therefore the half-life is prolonged.

Cellular Response Mechanisms   Steroid hormones do not bind to a cell membrane–bound receptor, but are able to pass through the cell membrane. Steroid hormones then bind to a specific cytoplasmic steroid receptor within the cell. The steroid receptor complex then migrates to the nucleus where it enters and initiates the nuclear and cytosolic events required for the synthesis of specific proteins. The nuclear response to steroid hormones may require more than 45 min for a cellular response to be detected (23).

TABLE 9.2

Main functional responses of glandular tissues and hormones involved in acute adaptation to exercise.

GLAND/HORMONES	STIMULANT FOR RELEASE	TARGET TISSUE	RESPONSE
Fluid Balance			
Posterior pituitary			
Antidiuretic hormone (ADH; arginine vasopressin)	↑ Plasma osmolality	Kidneys	↑ Water reabsorption
Kidneys			
Renin	Urine flow	Blood	Converts angiotensinogen to angiotensin I
Adrenal cortex			
Aldosterone (ADH; arginine vasopressin)	Angiotensin II	Kidneys	↑ Sodium reabsorption, ↑ water reabsorption
Heart			
Atrial natriuretic peptide (ANP)	Hyperhydration ↑ venous return	Pituitary gland	Inhibition of ADH release
Vascular Hemodynamics			
Adrenal medulla			
Norepinephrine	Stress, hypotension, moderate to intense exercise	Peripheral vascular smooth muscle	Vasoconstriction
Epinephrine	Hypoglycemia, moderate to intense exercise	Peripheral vascular smooth muscle	Vasoconstriction
Posterior pituitary			
ADH	↑ Plasma osmolality smooth muscle	Peripheral vascular	Vasoconstriction
Endothelium			
Endothelin	Tissue damage (?)	Local vasculature (??)	Vasoconstriction
Endothelial-derived relaxing factor (EDRF)	(??)	Local vasculature (??)	Vasodilation
Muscle Repair Hypertrophy			
Anterior pituitary			
GH	↑ Stress	Mainly bone	Stimulation of growth
Various cells			
Insulin-like growth factor (IGF-I)	↑ GH	Almost all cells	Stimulation of growth
Testes and adrenal cortex			
Testosterone	↑ Stress	Skeletal muscle tissue	↑ Protein synthesis

Acute Adaptations of the Neuroendocrine System to Exercise

The glandular tissues that are mainly involved in the body's response to different exercise and environmental stresses were presented in figure 9.1. A general summary of the body's responses to exercise that involve hormonal regulation consists of energy metabolism, fuel mobilization, fluid balance, vascular hemodynamics, protein synthesis, and the specific responses to select hormones such as the gonadal hormones and endogenous opioids (table 9.2). These responses differ slightly for exercises of different intensities and between genders and, where appropriate, these differences will be highlighted in the sections to follow. A detailed discussion of gender differences during and in response to exercise are detailed in chapter 20.

Energy Metabolism

Incremental and Intense Exercise

The hormonal regulation of energy metabolism is dependent on exercise intensity and duration. For example, figure 9.2 presents the increase in epinephrine and norepinephrine in the circulation during an incremental cycle ergometer exercise test to VO_{2max}. Each hormone increases in an exponential manner as exercise intensity increases. The increases in the catecholamine hormones stimulate lipolysis inside skeletal muscle and adipose tissue, and increases the activity of phosphorylase which catalyzes the breakdown of glycogen

FIGURE 9.2

The increase in epinephrine and norepinephrine during incremental exercise.

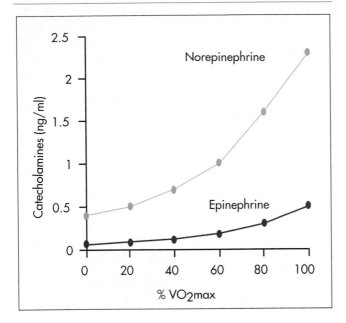

FIGURE 9.3

The change in growth hormone, cortisol, insulin, and glucagon during incremental exercise to fatigue.

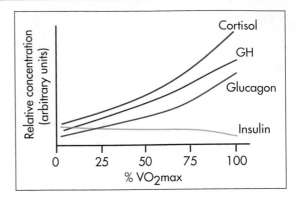

The functions of growth hormone are aided by increases in cortisol. Cortisol also increases the mobilization of free fatty acids from adipose tissue, as well as decreases the uptake of amino acids by peripheral tissues causing an increase in circulating amino acids. The increased amino acids are predominantly used by the liver in gluconeogenesis; however, during incremental or short-term intense exercise, the body's carbohydrate stores are not depleted and there is little need for liver gluconeogenesis. Consequently, the metabolic benefit of cortisol release during intense exercise would also be confined to the immediate recovery period.

Intense exercise actually increases circulating blood glucose concentrations because of the epinephrine-induced increases in liver glycogenolysis. These increases are larger than can be explained by exercise-induced hemoconcentration. Understandably, glucagon does not increase during the normal to increased blood glucose concentrations during incremental exercise. Conversely, the increasing blood glucose concentration would be interpreted as providing a stimulus for increasing insulin release from the β-cells of the pancreas. However, an expected increase in insulin does not happen for two main reasons: (1) exercise increases glucose uptake by skeletal muscle by increasing glucose transporter (**GLUT₄**) protein density on the sarcolemma independent of insulin, thereby increasing insulin sensitivity; and (2) intense exercise is accompanied by increasing blood lactate and acidosis, all of which inhibit the release of insulin (see focus box 9.1).

Prolonged Exercise

Prolonged exercise is accompanied by decreases in the body's skeletal muscle and liver glycogen stores. Low skeletal muscle glycogen increases the reliance of skeletal muscle metabolism on blood glucose concentrations, and can cause decreases in blood glucose below normal (< 3.5 to 4.0 mmol/L), resulting in **hypoglycemia**. Because several tissues of the body are solely reliant on blood as the source of glucose for energy metabolism (e.g., red blood cells, neural tissue), the body must continually regulate blood glucose,

(increased glycogenolysis) in skeletal muscle and the liver. Low-intensity exercise is characterized by low catecholamine concentrations and the predominance of lipid catabolism.

For more intense exercise, like that of sprinting or weight lifting, the increase in catecholamine concentrations in the blood are more extreme. During these exercises the increased catecholamines influence cellular metabolism in skeletal muscle, smooth muscle, the heart, adipose tissue, and the liver.

Growth hormone, cortisol, insulin, and glucagon concentrations in blood change during incremental exercise, as illustrated in figure 9.3. Insulin concentrations initially decrease, with later changes being dependent on carbohydrate ingestion and dehydration (4, 19). In contrast, both growth hormone and cortisol increase; the increase in growth hormone is linear and the increase in cortisol is exponential (4).

The primary function of growth hormone is to increase circulating concentrations of free fatty acids and inhibit glucose uptake by peripheral tissues, thus conserving blood glucose. During intense exercise these effects are made redundant by the increased catecholamines, near total reliance on carbohydrate catabolism in skeletal muscle, and the known increase in glucose uptake in skeletal muscle (8, 13, 22, 24, 31, 37, 49). It would appear that *increasing growth hormone concentrations during exercise would aid in the recovery from exercise* because the half-life for growth hormone is severalfold longer than the catecholamines, which allows for glucose sparing and increased muscle glycogen synthesis and rapid increases in skeletal muscle lipid catabolism.

FOCUS BOX 9.1

The Role of Exercise in the Prevention of and Rehabilitation from Noninsulin-Dependent (Type II) Diabetes Mellitus

Diabetes mellitus, or simply diabetes, is a condition involving the decreased ability of glucose uptake by the tissues of the body. If left untreated, blood glucose concentrations increase dramatically, a condition termed **hyperglycemia**. Sustained hyperglycemia can cause glucose to be bound to membranes of tissues, causing tissue damage and eventually death. For example, hyperglycemia is known to damage peripheral nerves, causing a condition known as peripheral neuropathy, and can damage nerves of the eye causing eventual blindness.

Diabetes is a condition that is expressed in two forms. *Type I diabetes* is characterized by the body's inability to produce and secrete insulin. It requires the administration of insulin, is usually manifested early in life, and is therefore termed *juvenile-onset* or *insulin-dependent* diabetes. *Type II diabetes* is the most common form with a 90% incidence in the total diabetic population (46). Type II diabetes usually occurs later in life and has been termed *adult-onset* diabetes. Type II diabetes can be further divided into two subgroups: (1) individuals with an impaired ability to secrete insulin because of a defect in the βcells of the pancreas, causing decreased insulin responsiveness, and (2) individuals with a decreased ability of cells to respond to insulin, causing decreased insulin sensitivity. Both type II conditions may eventually require insulin administration. The peripheral tissue type II diabetic condition coincides with increases in body fat. Each form of diabetes is associated with elevated blood lipoprotein and triglyceride concentrations resulting from increased glucose conversion to fatty acids in the liver, and increased fatty acid mobilization from adipose tissue that is due to accompanied chronic increases in growth hormone and cortisol (46).

Since the early 1950s, the use of exercise in combination with diet and insulin therapy were recognized treatment alternatives for diabetes (46). Since that time, abundant research has isolated the effects of exercise on blood glucose regulation in individuals with either type I or type II diabetes. As type II diabetes comprises 90% of all diabetic individuals (46), and exercise is a more powerful treatment for the type II diabetic, this condition will be the focus of this section.

Exercise is characterized by an increased glucose uptake by skeletal muscle that is retained for up to 48 h during the recovery from a single bout of exercise in non-diabetics and type II diabetics (18, 34, 36). This response is a combination of increased insulin sensitivity, as well as an endogenous effect in increased GLUT4 transporters on the sarcolemmas of the exercised muscle fibers. The endogenous effect within skeletal muscle is related to the synthesis of muscle glycogen and can last for up to 5 h (34). The exercise-induced increase in insulin sensitivity is greater when there is a larger exercised muscle mass (37). However, for individuals unaccustomed to exercise requiring an eccentric component to muscle contraction (e.g., running, weight lifting) the associated muscle damage causes a transient decrease in insulin sensitivity (29, 30). The known prolonged effect of exercise on improved peripheral glucose disposal and insulin sensitivity is related to the insulin-stimulated mechanism (46). Thus *exercise can acutely alleviate inadequate insulin-mediated glucose disposal*.

Long-term exercise training is also beneficial for the type II diabetic, but not because of a continued improvement in exercise-induced insulin sensitivity. Insulin sensitivity is retained only in individuals who exercise and experience a decrease in body fat content (46). In fact, body fat loss in the overweight type II diabetic can decrease insulin release and increase sensitivity regardless of exercise training. Nevertheless, for individuals who exercise every day, the continued increase in exercise-stimulated insulin sensitivity would be retained from one bout of exercise to the next, and therefore, in reality, be a meaningful improvement in blood glucose control.

---

and if possible decrease the use of glucose by other tissues during low carbohydrate conditions.

Figure 9.4*a* presents the approximate changes in growth hormone, cortisol, insulin, and glucagon during prolonged exercise accompanied by decreases in blood glucose. Similarly, figure 9.4*b* and *c* presents the change in blood β-hydroxybutarate and glycerol during the same exercise condition. As explained in chapter 6, glycerol is used as a marker of increased free fatty acid mobilization, and β-hydroxybutarate is a ketone body that is produced during times of low carbohydrate when the liver is overly reliant on lipid catabolism.

The increased release of growth hormone from the anterior pituitary and cortisol from the adrenal cortex occur simultaneously with an increase in sympathetic activity, as explained previously. The increase in free fatty acid and amino acid concentrations in the blood that accompany increases in

growth hormone and cortisol provide substrates for gluconeogenesis (amino acids) and alternative fuels for skeletal muscle energy metabolism (free fatty acids). However, unless the pathway of gluconeogenesis is stimulated, these responses would have little influence on the liver, and this is one of the main functions of glucagon. Glucagon increases

---

GLUT₄ glucose transporter-4; the predominant glucose transport protein on the sarcolemma of skeletal muscle fiber

hypoglycemia (hi po-gli-se′me-ah) abnormally low blood glucose concentrations (< 3.5 mmol/L)

diabetes mellitus a condition characterized by a reduced ability to regulate blood glucose concentrations by means of insulin.

hyperglycemia (hi per-gli-se′me-ah) abnormally high blood glucose concentrations (> 5 mmol/L)

FIGURE 9.4

The change in *(a)* growth hormone, cortisol, insulin, and glucagon during prolonged exercise, and the accompanied changes in the metabolites *(b)* β-hydroxybutarate and *(c)* glycerol.

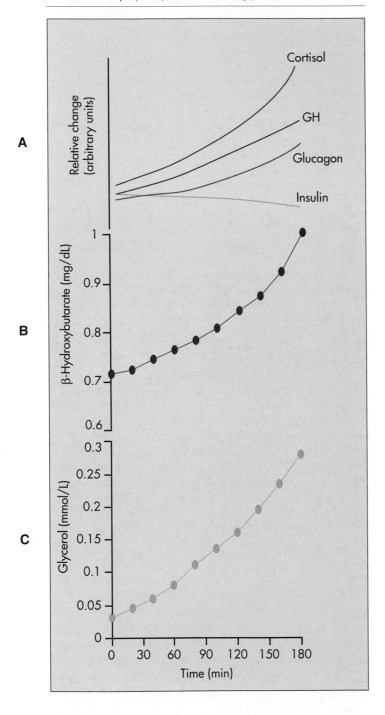

name that applies to a multiple number of hormones released from the ovaries that increase fertility. *The most biologically active estrogen released by the ovary is 17β-estradiol.* The majority of 17β-estradiol in the female is synthesized by the ovaries, however small amounts are also synthesized in the adrenal cortex, and this source accounts for the small amounts of estrogen produced in males. Because males have minimal 17β-estradiol, this hormone and its effect on substrate mobilization and energy metabolism is confined to females and is under the control of the menstrual cycle.

17β-estradiol increases the mobilization of free fatty acids from adipose tissue and inhibits glucose uptake by the peripheral tissues (20, 40). Consequently, 17β-estradiol and growth hormone exert similar metabolic effects during exercise. Exercise is known to increase circulating estrogen in both menstruating (*eumenorrheic*) and nonmenstruating (*amenorrheic*) women (40). Furthermore, the higher circulating concentrations of 17β-estradiol in endurance-trained women compared to equally endurance-trained men has been used to explain the greater dependence on lipid rather than carbohydrate during exercise (40, 45). Chapter 14 will present evidence for differing metabolism between males and females during exercise.

Fluid Balance

Prolonged Exercise and Dehydration

The increase in heat production during exercise initiates several neurally and locally controlled thermoregulatory reflexes that result in increased sweating and blood flow to the skin. Because sweating can occur at rates as high as 2 to 3 L/h during exercise in hot and/or humid environments, the body can experience large losses in body water (*dehydration*). The resulting water loss from the body decreases plasma volume, raises plasma osmolality, and evokes a complex hormonal response to conserve body water and also provide a long-term regulation of blood pressure.

Figure 9.5 illustrates the changing concentrations of antidiuretic hormone (ADH), renin, aldosterone, and atrial natriuretic peptide (ANP) during prolonged exercise. The stimulus for the release of ADH is an increasing plasma osmolality, which is detected by **osmoreceptors** in the hypothalamus. ADH functions by increasing the permeability of the kidney tubule from each of the juxtamedullary nephrons of the kidney. Because this mechanism decreases urine flow and volume, it opposes urine formation (*diuresis*) and is termed an **antidiuretic** function. A reduced urine flow through the kidney is detected by the specialized cells located around the distal tubule (macula densa) in the region of the glomerulus, termed the *juxtaglomerular apparatus.* Low urine flow increases the absorption of sodium and chloride by the cells of the distal tubule, thus reducing the ionic concentrations exposed to the macula densa (23). These conditions cause the neighboring juxtaglomerular cells to secrete *renin.* Renin is actually an enzyme that forms angiotensin I from the prehormone angiotensinogen. Angiotensin I is then

liver glycogenolysis by a cAMP second messenger system that eventually activates glycogen phosphorylase (23). In addition, glucagon increases the rate of gluconeogenesis by allowing an alternative reaction that essentially reverses the PFK (phosphofructokinase) reaction.

Estrogen is another hormone that will influence substrate mobilization during exercise. Actually, *estrogen* is a generic

FIGURE 9.5

The change in renin activity, aldosterone, ADH, and atrial natriuretic peptide during prolonged exercise accompanied by dehydration.

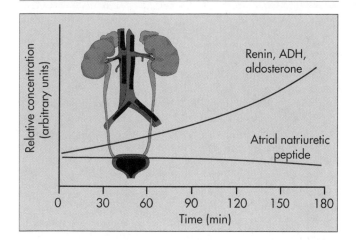

converted to angiotensin II in the circulation by the diffusely located endothelial-bound *angiotensin-converting enzyme* (ACE) (20). Angiotensin II then circulates to the adrenal cortex where it stimulates the release of aldosterone.

Aldosterone is categorized as a *mineralocorticoid* because it is chemically derived from cortisol and regulates not only fluid balance but also the amount of sodium in body fluids. Aldosterone exerts its function by increasing the synthesis of sodium transporter proteins by the epithelial cells of the distal tubule and collecting duct of the kidney, eventually causing an increase in sodium reabsorption and a concomitant osmotic reabsorption of water. Because aldosterone is a steroid hormone, the cellular response to increased aldosterone is relatively slow and approximates 45 min (23). Consequently, unless the exercise duration is at least 2 h long, the biological effects of aldosterone would mainly be in effect in the recovery from exercise.

During conditions of water excess, plasma volume expands, osmolality decreases, and the stimulus for ADH release is decreased. ADH release is further inhibited by the release of atrial natriuretic peptide from the atrial myocardium of the heart in response to the increased filling pressures of the right atrium. Removal of the ADH stimulus for water reabsorption increases urine flow, which in turn decreases renin output from the kidney and the eventual stimulation for aldosterone secretion. These conditions cause the formation of large urine volumes and is termed **diuresis**.

Vascular Hemodynamics

Exercise is accompanied by the regulation of blood vessels, which as explained in chapter 7, is required to regulate peripheral vascular resistance and blood pressures, and to redistribute blood flow to specific tissues. These responses are elicited by neural, hormonal, and local regulators of arterioles and the microvasculature.

The increasing concentrations of the catecholamine hormones during increasing exercise intensities are known to induce a general vasoconstriction of the vasculature because of the overwhelming α-receptor–induced vasoconstriction at high norepinephrine concentrations (39).

Peripheral vascular resistance is also increased by increasing circulating concentrations of angiotensin I, ADH, and to a lesser extent aldosterone (23). Angiotensin I is a potent vasoconstrictor of peripheral smooth muscle, as is ADH, whereas aldosterone exerts a minor role in vascular smooth muscle contraction. The angiotensin, ADH, and aldosterone functions on vascular hemodynamics are more important during resting conditions characterized by dehydration or low blood volume resulting from hemorrhage. The influence of these hormones on vascular hemodynamics during exercise is less clear because of the overriding influence of the catecholamines and locally induced vasodilation in the vasculature of the contracting skeletal muscle (see focus box 9.2).

Protein Synthesis and Reproductive Hormones

During Exercise

Contradictory research has been published concerning whether the gonadotropic stimulatory hormones FSH (follicle-stimulating) and LH (luteinizing) increase during exercise (7, 9, 10, 11). Nevertheless, as the time required for FSH stimulation of the testes and resultant testosterone production may exceed 45 min, acute increases in FSH and LH during short-term exercise cannot account for increases in testosterone (10). Recent findings indicate that testosterone does increase during short-term cycling and weight lifting exercise (10, 41), and has been explained by a direct catecholamine stimulation mechanism (10). Nevertheless, for prolonged exercise there appears to be a cortisol-induced inhibition of testosterone production (24). For the normally menstruating female, exercise-induced increases have also been detected for 17β-estradiol (48). How short-term or prolonged exercise induced changes in estrogen and testosterone influence protein synthesis in males and females is unclear.

The other main androgenic stimulus for protein synthesis is the combined effects of growth hormone and *insulin-like growth factor-1* (IGF-1, or somatomedin C). Although growth hormone does have some independent abilities to induce growth in bone, the majority of the stimulus to protein synthesis and growth by growth hormone results from its

osmoreceptors (oz mo-re-cep'tors) cells that can generate an action potential in response to changes in blood osmolality

antidiuretic (an ti-di u-ret'ik) a substance/condition that causes a decrease in urine volume

diuresis (di u-re'sis) an increase in urine volume

FOCUS BOX 9.2

The Role of Exercise in the Control of Blood Pressure

Exercise is a stress to the body that induces an increased blood pressure, or *hypertensive* response, and during the recovery from exercise the body can experience a dramatic decrease in blood pressure, or *hypotensive* response. As the blood pressure increase during exercise is due to an increased systolic pressure without an increase in diastolic pressure, there is no increase in the afterload of the heart, and therefore, the exercise-induced hypertension is not detrimental to the function of a healthy heart. However, chronic exposure of the heart and vasculature to increases in blood pressures above 140/90 mmHg is termed **hypertension**, and can cause damage to the heart, vasculature, and the organs they perfuse (1). Decreases in blood pressure below normal resting values, or **hypotension**, can occur during the immediate recovery from exercise or be induced by postural adjustment (*orthostatic hypotension*), and can be potentially dangerous to the body. Exposure of the body to hypotension often coincides with a reduced venous return to the heart, which in turn decreases blood flow to the brain. An episode of syncope could, and often will, result. It is clear that the regulation of blood pressure is important for optimal function of body organs and the overall function of the body as a whole.

Blood pressure is regulated by complex interactions among neural, endocrinological, renal, cardiovascular, and behavioral functions (figure 9.6). *The primary determinants of blood pressure are cardiovascular in origin, and consist of cardiac output and peripheral vascular resistance.* Such cardiovascular control of blood pressure by neural regulation is the most immediate, followed by endocrinological regulation, and renal and behavioral factors. The time response is important, as neural regulation must obviously prevail during immediate perturbations that risk immediate alterations in systemic blood pressure. For this reason, the function of the autonomic nervous system in blood pressure regulation is an important area of research.

Endurance-Exercise Training Can Prevent or Reverse Hypertension

For individuals with hypertension, use of diet and exercise are typically used in the first round of treatment. Individuals are required to lower their total calorie and salt intake, and engage in regular daily bouts of increased physical activity. For example, the American College of Sports Medicine has indicated that regular exercise can reduce both systolic and diastolic blood pressures by as much as 10 mmHg in individuals with mild hypertension (BP = 140 to 180/90 to 105 mm Hg) (1). Increased exercise and physical activity should be characterized by the use of large muscle groups, performed for 20 to 60-min duration for 3 to 5 days/week, and at an intensity between 50 to 85% of VO_{2max}.

---

stimulation of the production of IGF-1 in the tissues of interest. Increased concentrations of IGF-1 then induce the cellular growth response. The majority of human research on growth hormone responses during exercise have not included the measurement of IGF-1 in their design. However, IGF-1 does increase during exercise, and this acute role is more for the insulin-like effects of the hormone rather than the anabolic effects. This interpretation is supported by the overwhelming evidence for protein catabolism and amino acid release from muscle during exercise (7, 44, 47).

During Recovery

The protein synthesis response of IGF-1 has been documented in resting individuals (7). Data from Carraro and associates (7) also indicate that *protein synthesis is impaired during exercise, but stimulated during the recovery from exercise*, resulting in a net protein synthesis. More research is needed to elucidate the hormonal regulation of postexercise muscle protein synthesis, document the magnitude of this response, and evaluate its role of net protein synthesis in response to training.

Endogenous Opioids

An opioid substance is one that provides an analgesic effect, similar to that of morphine which is also referred to as opium. The body produces opioid-like substances that can be categorized into three main types; β-endorphins, enkephalins, and α-endorphins (dynorphins) (21). The three molecules are produced in various regions of the brain, but secretion into the systemic circulation mainly occurs from the anterior pituitary. Research of the **endogenous opioids** has been based on blocking their receptors by the molecule *naloxone*, and this strategy mainly focuses on the effects of β-endorphin.

The secretion of β-endorphin from the anterior pituitary is linked to the secretion of ACTH. In fact, β-endorphin and ACTH share the same prehormone. β-endorphin increases during times of hypoglycemia, and is therefore involved in the body's multihormone blood glucose regulation. During exercise, β-endorphin and the enkephalins increase and have been associated with cardiovascular, ventilatory, metabolic, and thermoregulatory effects (16, 17, 21, 42). β-endorphin

hypertension abnormally high blood pressure (< 140/90 mm Hg)

hypotension (hi po-ten' shun) abnormally low blood pressure

endogenous opioids hormones released by the anterior pituitary gland that provide a biological response similar to that of morphine

FIGURE 9.6

A summary of the hormonal regulation of blood pressure and fluid balance.

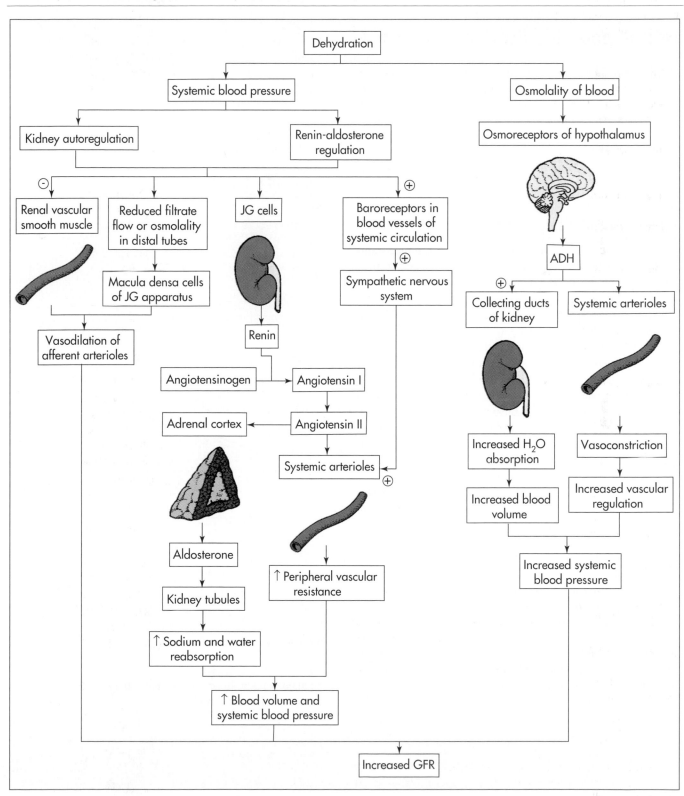

provides a slight inhibition of ventilation, can suppress baroreceptor firing, and is associated with inhibition of the release of ACTH and growth hormone (21). However, the metabolic effects of β-endorphin have not been documented experimentally.

Chronic Adaptations of the Neuroendocrine System to Exercise

Participation in exercise training, no matter what type, has the potential to alter the secretion of hormones by (1) *altering the stimuli that release them*, (2) *altering the ability of cells to respond to hormones*, or (3) *altering the maximal capacity of endocrine tissues to release the hormone*. The chronic adaptations of the neuroendocrine system to exercise will be categorized once again by their general biological responses.

Energy Metabolism and Fuel Mobilization

For a given submaximal exercise intensity, endurance training lowers the catecholamine, growth hormone, and cortisol concentrations in the blood, as illustrated in figure 9.7. As explained in chapter 6, endurance training is also accompanied by an increased reliance on lipid catabolism for a given submaximal exercise intensity (27). At first glance, these hormonal findings appear inconsistent with an increase in lipid catabolism. However, because the main source of free fatty acids during submaximal exercise is the active skeletal muscle rather than adipose tissue, lower cortisol and growth hormone concentrations do not detract from lipid catabolism.

When performing submaximal exercise for longer periods of time, the reduced reliance on carbohydrate spares muscle and liver glycogen, and therefore is not associated with the decreases in blood glucose that would otherwise occur. Consequently, serum glucagon concentrations are also lower after endurance training (4,12). An additional factor that contributes to improved glucose kinetics during exercise is the chronic increase in $GLUT_4$ glucose transport proteins on the sarcolemma of muscle fibers (25, 26).

During resting conditions the hormonal balance between trained and untrained individuals is also different. Dela and colleagues (12) demonstrated that trained individuals have higher catecholamine concentrations during the active day than untrained individuals, and the functional implications of these differences are unclear. In addition, insulin responses to a meal are lower in the trained state, and one would expect consistently lower ACTH, cortisol, ADH, and aldosterone

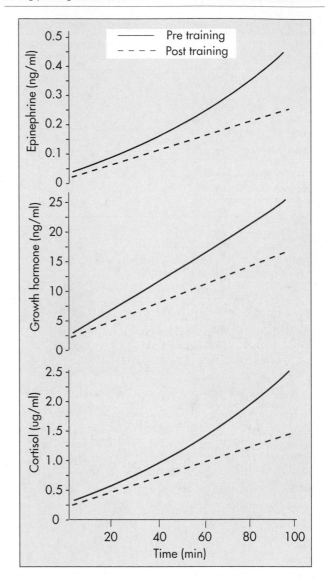

FIGURE 9.7

The influence of endurance training on the circulating concentrations of catecholamines, growth hormone, and cortisol during prolonged exercise.

concentrations during the average day because of the plasma volume expansion and overall improved body hydration that accompanies endurance training (see chapter 7).

Reproductive Hormones

The secretion of LH and FSH from the anterior pituitary regulate gonadal hormone production and secretion. For the female, the gonadal hormones of interest are 17β-estradiol and progesterone, whereas for the male the hormone of interest is testosterone. For each gender, more than 90% of these hormones are secreted from the gonads, whereas the remainder comes from the adrenal cortex.

Athletic Amenorrhea

Women who are biologically capable of menstruating, yet do not, have a condition known as *amenorrhea*. When the cause of the amenorrhea is related directly to exercise participation, the condition is termed **athletic amenorrhea**. Historically, the mechanism that causes athletic amenhorrhea was believed to be a reduced body fat percentage, attributable to the added caloric demands of exercise (3, 14, 28, 32, 35). However, it is now known that *body fat content does not directly cause this condition* (14, 25).

Females who repeatedly train expose themselves to increased concentrations of catecholamines, β-endorphin, and cortisol, which are known to exert some inhibition to anterior pituitary function, and more specifically, to inhibition of the release of gonadotropin-releasing hormone (GnRH). However, the exact mechanism that explains athletic amenorrhea remains obscure (32). Nevertheless, it is known that athletic amenorrhea is due to an altered release of LH and FSH, indicating that the irregularity resides in hypothalamic-pituitary axis regulation of LH and FSH secretion. Decreased levels of FSH and LH prevent the stimulation of the follicle of the ovary, and therefore prevent the synthesis and secretion of estradiol by the ovary. Consequently, women with athletic amenorrhea have lower than normal circulating 17β-estradiol concentrations, and therefore do not have the estradiol-stimulated increases in lipid catabolism during exercise, or the protective qualities of estradiol relative to bone density and HDL concentrations in the blood.

It has been proposed that the development of athletic amenorrhea starts with a decreasing length of the luteal phase (43); however, minimal changes in luteal phase length and menstrual function have been reported for women who engage in exercise training involving moderate distances and intensities (32). Therefore, women who participate in extremes of long-distance or high-intensity exercise may be more likely to develop athletic amenorrhea, and this statement is supported by research that has shown that athletic amenorrhea may be reversed with a reduction in training intensity or volume (3, 5, 14, 28, 32), and that the incidence of athletic amenorrhea (between 1 and 44%) is higher in females who participate in more prolonged or metabolically stressful activities such as long-distance running and ballet dancing (14).

The dramatically reduced ability to secrete 17β-estradiol in the amenorrheic woman decreases the mobilization of free fatty acids and the ability to catabolize lipid during low to moderate exercise intensities. This condition is further supported by reduced growth hormone secretion during exercise, and a disrupted daily growth hormone release profile in the amenorrheic woman (48). The condition of *athletic amenorrhea essentially makes the female "more male-like" in relation to the endocrinological and metabolic responses to exercise.*

Testicular Function

The male version of athletic amenorrhea is characterized by a chronic decrease in resting serum testosterone, and chronically elevated resting cortisol concentrations (9, 15). For the male, lowered testosterone may reduce sperm counts, and could also decrease bone mineral density, although no evidence has documented this fact (2, 33).

An Overview of the Endocrinological Responses to Exercise

The diverse control exerted by the body's hormonal responses to exercise is illustrated in figure 9.8. It is clear that the pituitary gland is pivotal in the regulation of substrate mobilization, fluid balance and kidney function, protein synthesis, and gonadal function during exercise. The previous sections of this chapter clearly revealed the research evidence that proves this to be true. Primary regulation of energy metabolism occurs via the catecholamines, and primary control over blood glucose regulation is exerted by the pancreas. However, prolonged exercise and the secretion of cortisol, growth hormone, and estrogen in the female also alters cellular metabolism and blood glucose regulation. The multiple functions of many of the body's hormones makes the study of neuroendocrinology a difficult task. However, as this chapter has shown, knowledge of hormonal function during exercise is necessary to appreciate how the body can tolerate, and sometimes not tolerate, the various types, intensities, and durations of exercise.

athletic amenorrhea (a-men′ or-e′ah) loss of the menstrual cycle caused by excessive exercise training or psychological stress

FIGURE 9.8

An overview of the hormones released during exercise, and their effects of the body's acute adaptations to exercise.

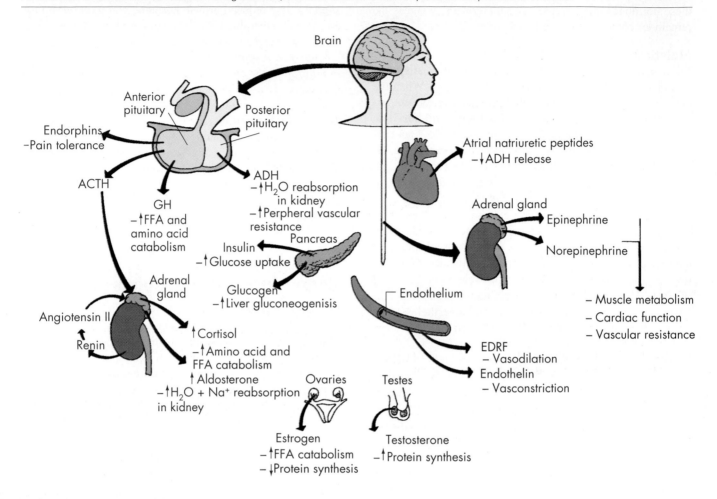

WEBSITE BOX

Chapter 9: Neuroendocrine Adaptations to Exercise

The newest information regarding exercise physiology can be viewed at the following sites.*

endocrineweb.com/
   Detailed site providing education information on endocrine disorders of the thyroid, parathyroid, adrenal, and pancreas glands. Provides excellent illustrations.
jkittredge.com/~jkimball/BiologyPages/H/Hypothalamus.html
   Detailed information and links for the hormones of the hypothalamic-pituitary axis.
mediconsult.com/
   Information source for any medical condition, including diabetes.
uams.edu/physiology/FacultyFolders/Kurten/renal.7H/index.htm
   Provides links to a series of slides concerning the ADH regulation of fluid balance.
shamrockbay.com/~jkimball/BiologyPages/H/HormoneTable.html
   Links to the biochemical structure and physiology of all the hormones.
ir-web.com/english/gp/index.html
   Elaborate site for finding all you need on insulin resistance.
http://diabetesnet.com/irtips.html
   Provides information on risks for diabetes, and links to

other sites for diabetes-related research and other information.
http://webidirect.com/~discover/
   Detailed historical information on the discovery of insulin.
idi.org.au/
   Comprehensive site from the International Diabetes Institute of Australia that provides all you need to know about diabetes.
musculardevelopment.com/oct/andro1.html
   Excellent overview of testosterone and androstanedione, including the biochemical pathway of steroid synthesis.
cdc.gov/diabetes/
   A diabetes and public health resource from the Centers for Disease Control and Prevention (CDC).
ndei.org/
   Homepage for the National Diabetes Education Initiative. Provides detailed information of type II diabetes and insulin resistance.
mediconsult.com/menopause/
   Detailed information on the role of estrogen in menopause, osteoporosis, exercise, and the rationale for estrogen replacement therapy.

----

* Unless indicated, all URLs preceded by http://www.
Note: These URLs were valid at the time of publication, but could have changed or been deleted from Internet access since that time.

SUMMARY

▪ **Neuroendocrinology** is the study of the combined function of nerves and *glands* involved in the release of *hormones* that regulate the function of body tissues. A **gland** is a tissue that secretes a substance within or from the body. The glands of the body can be divided into *exocrine* or *endocrine*. Substances secreted from endocrine glands are known as **hormones,** are released in minor amounts resulting in very low concentrations in the blood (< 1 μm), and typically exert their functions on tissues located in other regions of the body.

▪ Hormones can be divided into three main categories: *amine*, *peptide*, and *steroid* hormones. Amine and peptide hormones exert their action on target cells by binding to specific receptors located on the cell membranes of the target tissue(s). The binding of an amine or peptide hormone to a receptor stimulates a cellular response by causing increases in **second messengers**. For example, **cyclic AMP (cAMP)** is produced in response to the binding of epinephrine to a β_2-receptor on the sarcolemma of a skeletal muscle fiber.

▪ Steroid hormones, like other lipid molecules, are *hydrophobic* and therefore insoluble in water. Steroid hormones bind to plasma proteins to be transported in the blood to their target tissues. Steroid hormones do not bind to a cell membrane–bound receptor, but are able to pass through the cell membrane where they bind to a specific cytoplasmic steroid receptor.

▪ The hormonal regulation of energy metabolism is dependent on exercise intensity and duration. Epinephrine and norepinephrine increase in an exponential manner as exercise intensity increases. The increases in the catecholamine hormones stimulate lipolysis inside skeletal muscle and adipose tissue and increase the activity of phosphorylase which catalyzes the breakdown of glycogen (increased glycogenolysis) in skeletal muscle and the liver.

▪ During incremental exercise, insulin and glucagon concentrations initially decrease, and then return to near-resting values at moderate to maximal exercise intensities. In contrast, both growth hormone and cortisol increase; the increase in growth hormone is linear and the increase in cortisol is exponential. The primary function of growth hormone is to increase circulating concentrations of free fatty acids and inhibit glucose uptake by peripheral tissues, thus conserving blood glucose.

- Intense exercise actually increases circulating blood glucose concentrations because of the epinephrine-induced increases in liver glycogenolysis. An expected increase in insulin does not happen for two main reasons: (1) exercise increases glucose uptake by skeletal muscle by increasing glucose transporter (**GLUT$_4$**) protein density on the sarcolemma independent of insulin, thereby increasing insulin sensitivity, and (2) intense exercise is accompanied by increasing blood lactate and acidosis, all of which inhibit the release of insulin.

- Prolonged exercise is accompanied by decreases in the body's skeletal muscle and liver glycogen stores. Low skeletal muscle glycogen increases the reliance of skeletal muscle metabolism on blood glucose concentrations, and can cause decreases in blood glucose below normal (< 3.5 to 4.0 mmol/L), or **hypoglycemia**. Because several tissues of the body are solely reliant on blood as the source of glucose for energy metabolism (e.g., red blood cells, neural tissue), the body must continually regulate blood glucose, and if possible decrease the use of glucose by other tissues during low carbohydrate conditions.

- Estrogen is another hormone that will influence substrate mobilization during exercise. *The most biologically active estrogen released by the ovary is 17β-estradiol.* 17β-estradiol increases the mobilization of free fatty acids from adipose tissue and inhibits glucose uptake by the peripheral tissues. Consequently, 17β-estradiol and growth hormone exert similar metabolic effects during exercise.

- **Diabetes mellitis,** or simply diabetes, is a condition involving the decreased ability of glucose uptake by the tissues of the body. If left untreated, blood glucose concentrations increase dramatically, a condition termed **hyperglycemia**. Sustained hyperglycemia can cause glucose to be bound to membranes of tissues, causing tissue damage and eventually death. For example, hyperglycemia is known to damage peripheral nerves, causing a condition known as peripheral neuropathy, and can damage nerves of the eye causing eventual blindness.

- Exercise is characterized by an increased glucose uptake by skeletal muscle that is retained for up to 48 h during the recovery from a single bout of exercise in normal and type II diabetics. This response is a combination of increased insulin sensitivity, as well as an endogenous effect in increased GLUT$_4$ transporters on the sarcolemmas of the exercised muscle fibers. Thus, *exercise can acutely alleviate inadequate insulin-mediated glucose disposal.*

- The stimulus for the release of ADH is an increasing plasma osmolality, which is detected by **osmoreceptors** in the hypothalamus. ADH functions by increasing the permeability of the kidney tubule from each of the juxtamedullary nephrons of the kidney. As this mechanism decreases urine flow and volume, it opposes urine formation (*diuresis*), and is termed an **antidiuretic** function. The juxtaglomerular cells of the kidney secrete *renin* during low flow conditions. Renin is actually an enzyme that forms angiotensin I from the prehormone angiotensinogen. Angiotensin I is then converted to angiotensin II in the circulation by the diffusely located endothelial-bound an*giotensin-converting enzyme* (ACE). Angiotensin II then circulates to the adrenal cortex where it stimulates the release of aldosterone.

- Aldosterone is categorized as a *mineralocorticoid*, as is cortisol and the other hormones released by the adrenal cortex. Each of these hormones has a minor role in the regulation of blood potassium and sodium concentrations, hence their category name. Aldosterone exerts its function by increasing the synthesis of sodium transporter proteins by the epithelial cells of the distal tubule and collecting duct, eventually causing an increase in sodium reabsorption and a concomitant osmotic reabsorption of water.

- During conditions of water excess, plasma volume expands, osmolality decreases, and the stimulus for ADH release is decreased. ADH release is further inhibited by the release of atrial natriuretic peptide from the atrial myocardium of the heart in response to the increased filling pressures of the right atrium. Removal of the ADH stimulus for water reabsorption increases urine flow, which in turn decreases renin output from the kidney and the eventual stimulation for aldosterone secretion. These conditions cause the formation of large urine volumes, which is termed **diuresis.**

- The increasing concentrations of the catecholamine hormones during increasing exercise intensities are known to induce a general vasoconstriction of the vasculature because of the overwhelming α-receptor–induced vasoconstriction at high norepinephrine concentrations. Peripheral vascular resistance is also increased by increasing circulating concentrations of angiotensin I, ADH, and to a lesser extent aldosterone.

- Chronic exposure of the heart and vasculature to increases in blood pressures above 140/90 mmHg is termed **hypertension**, and can cause damage to the heart, vasculature, and the organs they perfuse. Decreases in blood pressure below normal resting values, or **hypotension**, can occur during the immediate recovery from exercise or be induced by postural adjustment (*orthostatic hypotension*), and can be potentially dangerous to the body.

■ The body produces opioid-like substances, **endogenous opioids**, that can be categorized into three main types; β-endorphins, enkephalins, and α-endorphins (dynorphins). β-endorphin increases during times of hypoglycemia, and is therefore involved in the body's multihormone blood glucose regulation.

■ For a given submaximal exercise intensity, endurance training lowers the catecholamine, growth hormone, and cortisol concentrations in the blood. When performing submaximal exercise for longer periods of time, the re-

duced reliance on carbohydrate spares muscle and liver glycogen, and therefore is not associated with the decreases in blood glucose that would otherwise occur.

■ Women who are biologically capable of menstruating, yet do not, have a condition known as *amenorrhea*. When the cause of the amenorrhea is related directly to exercise participation, the condition is termed **athletic amenorrhea.** The exact mechanism that explains athletic amenorrhea remains obscure. Nevertheless, it is known that athletic amenorrhea is due to an altered release of LH and FSH, indicating that the irregularity resides in hypothalamic-pituitary axis regulation of LH and FSH secretion. It has been proposed that the development of athletic amenorrhea starts with a decreasing length of the luteal phase.

STUDY QUESTIONS

1. Explain the differences between traditional and nontraditional endocrine functions.

2. What are the structural and functional (cell response) differences between peptide and steroid hormones?

3. Which hormones predominantly provide control over substrate mobilization and energy metabolism during exercise?

4. List the hormones that either directly or indirectly influence the blood glucose concentration during exercise. In addition, list the gland/tissue each hormone is released from, the stimulus for the release, and the mechanism for how it influences blood glucose.

5. Explain the terms *insulin sensitivity* and *insulin responsiveness* with respect to the metabolic and endocrine differences between a type II diabetic and a nondiabetic individual.

6. Explain the multihormonal regulation of fluid balance during exercise.

7. What is exercise amenorrhea, and what are the probable causes of the condition?

8. Explain how endurance training can influence the hormonal response to prolonged submaximal exercise.

APPLICATIONS

1. Why is exercise an important component in the prevention of and rehabilitation from type II diabetes?

2. Some female athletes think that athletic amenorrhea is beneficial as a cheap form of oral contraception. Explain why this is not true for their ability to excel in long-term endurance exercise. Are you aware of any health benefits of estrogen? If so, what are they?

3. How might exercise increase the stimulus for protein synthesis?

4. Why are there so many hormones that function, either directly or indirectly, to regulate the blood glucose concentration during exercise?

REFERENCES

1. American College of Sports Medicine. Physical activity, physical fitness and hypertension. *Med. Sci. Sports Exerc.* 25(10):i–x, 1993.

2. Bagatell, C. J., and W. J. Bremner. Sperm counts and reproductive hormones in male marathoners and lean controls. *Fertility and Sterility* 53:688–692, 1990.

3. Bale, P. Body composition and menstrual cycle irregularities of female athletes: Are they precursors of anorexia? *Sports Medicine* 17(6):347–352, 1994.

4. Bloom, S. R., R. H. Johnson, D. M. Park, M. J. Rennie, and W. R. Sulaiman. Differences in the metabolic and hormonal response to exercise between racing cyclists and untrained individuals. *J. Physiol.* 258:1–18, 1976.

5. Brown, W. H. *Introduction to organic chemistry*. Willard Grant Press, Boston, 1982.

6. Capaldo, B., R. Nappoli, P. Di Bonito, G. Albano, and L. Sacca. Dual mechanism of insulin action on human skeletal muscle: Identification of an indirect component not mediated by FFA. *Am. J. Physiol.* 260(23):E389–E394, 1991.

7. Carraro, F., C. A. Stuart, W. H. Hartl, J. Rosenblatt, and R. R. Wolfe. Effect of exercise and recovery on muscle protein synthesis in human subjects. *Am. J. Physiol.* 259(22):E470–E476, 1990.

8. Cooper, D. M., T. J. Barstow. A. Bergner, and W. N. Paul Lee. Blood glucose turnover during high- and low-intensity exercise. *Am. J. Physiol.* 257(3P+1):E405–E412, 1989.

9. Cumming, D. C., M. E. Guigley, and S. S. C. Yen. Acute suppression of circulating testosterone levels by cortisol in men. *J. Clin. Endocrin. Metab.* 57:671–677, 1983.

10. Cumming, D. C., L. A. Brunsting III, G. Strich, A. L. Ries, and R. W. Rebar. Reproductive hormone increases in response to acute exercise in men. *Med. Sci. Sports Exerc.* 18(4):369–373, 1986.

11. Cumming, D. C., G. D. Wheeler, and E. M. McCall. The effects of exercise on reproductive function in men. *Sports Med.* 7:1–17, 1989.

12. Dela, F., K. J. Mikines, M. V. Linstow, and H. Galbo. Effect of training on response to a glucose load adjusted for daily carbohydrate intake. *Am. J. Physiol.* 260(23):E14–E20, 1991.

13. Dela, F., K. J. Milkines, M. Von Linstow, N. H. Secher, and H. Galbo. Effect of training on insulin-mediated glucose uptake in human muscle. *Am. J. Physiol.* 263(26):E1134–E1143, 1992.

14. De Souza, M. J., and D. A. Metzger. Reproductive dysfunction in amenorrheic athletes and anorexic patients: A review. *Med. Sci. Sports Exerc.* 23(9):995–1007, 1991.

15. Eichner, E. R. Exercise and testicular function. *Sports Science Exchange* 5(38):1–5, 1992.

16. Farrell, P. A., A. B. Gustafson, W. P. Morgan, and C. B. Pert. Enkephalins, catecholamines, and psychological mood alterations: Effects of prolonged exercise. *Med. Sci. Sports Exerc.* 19(4):347–352, 1987.

17. Farrell, P. A., M. Kjaer, F. W. Bach, and H. Galbo. Beta-endorphin and adrenocorticotropin response to supramaximal treadmill exercise in trained and untrained males. *Acta Physiol. Scand.* 130:619–625, 1987.

18. Fell, R. D., S. E. Terblanche, J. L. Ivy, and J. O. Holloszy. Effect of muscle glycogen on glucose uptake following exercise. *J. Appl. Physiol.* 52:434–437, 1982.

19. Galbo, H., J. J. Holst, and N. J. Christensen. Glucagon and plasma catecholamine responses to graded and prolonged exercise in man. *J. Appl. Physiol.* 38(1):70–76, 1975.

20. Griffin, J. E., and S. R. Ojeda. Organization of the endocrine system. In J. E. Griffin and S. R. Ojeda (eds.), *Textbook of endocrine physiology*. Oxford University Press, New York, 1988, pp. 3–16.

21. Grossman, A., and J. R. Sutton. Endorphins: What are they? How are they measured? What is their role in exercise? *Med. Sci. Sports Exerc.* 17(1):74–81, 1985.

22. Gulve, E. A., G. D. Cartee, J. R. Zierath, V. M. Corpus, and J. O. Holloszy. Reversal of enhanced muscle glucose transport after exercise: Roles of insulin and glucose. *Am. J. Physiol.* 259(22):E685–E691, 1990.

23. Guyton, A. C. *Textbook of medical physiology*. 8th ed. Saunders, Philadelphia, 1991.

24. Heath, G. W., J. R. Gavin III, J. M. Hinderliter, J. M. Hagberg, S. A. Bloomfield, and J. O. Holloszy. Effects of exercise and lack of exercise on glucose tolerance and insulin sensitivity. *J. Appl. Physiol.* 55(2):512–517, 1983.

25. Houmard, J. A., et al. Elevated skeletal muscle glucose transporter levels in exercise-trained middle-aged men. *Am. J. Physiol.* 261(24): E437–E443, 1991.

26. Houmard, J. A., et al. Exercise training increases $GLUT_4$ protein concentration in previously sedentary middle-aged men. *Am. J. Physiol.* 264(27): E896–E901, 1993.

27. Hurley, B. F., P. M. Nemeth, W. H. Martin III, J. M. Hagberg, G. P. Dalsky, and J.O. Holloszy. Muscle triglyceride utilization during exercise: Effect of training. *J. Appl. Physiol.* 60(2):562–567, 1986.

28. Keizer, H. A., and A. D. Rogol. Physical exercise and menstrual cycle alterations: What are the mechanisms? *Sports Med.* 10(4):218–235, 1990.

29. Kirwan, J. P., R. E. Bourey, W. M. Kohrt, M. A. Staten, and J. O. Holloszy. Effects of treadmill exercise to exhaustion on the insulin response to hyperglycemia in untrained men. *J. Appl. Physiol.* 70(1):246–250, 1991.

30. Kirwan, J. P., R. C. Hickner, K. E. Yarasheski, W. M. Kohrt, B. V. Wiethop, and J. O. Holloszy. Eccentric exercise induces transient insulin resistance in healthy individuals. *J. Appl. Physiol.* 72(6):2197–2202, 1992.

31. Kjaer, M., B. Kiens, M. Hargreaves, and E. A. Richter. Influence of active muscle mass on glucose homeostasis during exercise in man. *J. Appl. Physiol.* 71(2):552–557, 1991.

32. Loucks, A. B., and S. B. Horvath. Athletic amenorrhea: A review. *Med. Sci. Sports Exerc.* 17(1):56–72, 1985.

33. MacDougall, J. D., et al. Relationship among running mileage, bone density, and serum testosterone in male runners. *J. Appl. Physiol.* 73(3):1165–1170, 1992.

34. Mikines, K. J., B. Sonne, P. A. Farrell, B. Tronier, and H.. Galbo. Effect of physical exercise on sensitivity and responsiveness to insulin in humans. *Am. J. Physiol.* 254(17):E248–E259, 1988.

35. Myerson, M., et al. Resting metabolic rate and energy balance in amenorrheic and eumenorrheic runners. *Med. Sci. Sports Exerc.* 23(1):15–22, 1991.

36. Ploug, T., H. Galbo, and E. A. Richter. Increased muscle glucose uptake during contraction: No need for insulin. *Am. J. Physiol.* 247(10):E712–E731, 1984.

37. Richter, E. A., B. Kiens, B. Saltin, N. J. Christensen, and G. Savard. Skeletal muscle glucose uptake during dynamic exercise in humans: Role of muscle mass. *Am. J. Physiol.* 254(17):E555–E561, 1988.

38. Rogol, A. D. Growth hormone: Physiology, therapeutic use, and potential for abuse. *Exerc. Sport Sci. Rev.* 17:352–378, 1989.

39. Rowell, L. B., and D. S. O'Leary. Reflex control of the circulation during exercise: Chemoreflexes and mechanoreflexes. *J. Appl. Physiol.* 69(20):407–418, 1990.

40. Ruby, B. C., R. A. Roberghs, and D. L. Waters. Effects of estrodiol on substrate turnover during exercise in amenorrheic females. *Med. Sci. Sports Exerc.* 29(9):1160–1169, 1997.

41. Schwab, R., G. O. Johnson, T. J. Housh, J. E. Kinder, and J. P. Weir. Acute effects of different intensities of weight lifting on serum testosterone. *Med. Sci. Sports Exerc.* 25(12):1381–1385, 1993.

42. Schwellnus, M. P., and N. F. Gordon. The role of endogenous opioids in thermoregulation during sub-maximal exercise. *Med. Sci. Sports Exerc.* 19(6):575–578, 1987.

43. Shangold, M., R. Freeman, B. Thysen, and M. Gatz. The relationship between long distance running, plasma progesterone, and luteal phase length. *Fertility and Sterility* 31(20):130–133, 1979.

44. Spencer, M. K., A. Katz, and I. Raz. Epinephrine increases tricarboxylic acid cycle intermediates in human skeletal muscle. *Am. J. Physiol.* 260(23):E436–E439, 1991.

45. Tarnopolsky, L. J., J. D. MacDougall, S. A. Atkinson, M. A. Tarnopolsky, and J. R. Sutton. Gender differences in substrate for endurance exercise. *J. Appl. Physiol.* 68(1):302–308, 1990.

46. Wallberg-Henriksson, H. Exercise and diabetes mellitus. *Exerc. Sport Sci. Rev.* 20:339–368, 1992.

47. Wasserman, D. H., and A. D. Cherrington. Hepatic fuel metabolism during muscular work: Role and regulation. *Am. J. Physiol.* 260(23):E811–E824, 1991.

48. Weltman, A., J. Y. Weltman, R. Schurrer, W. S. Evans, J. D. Veldhus, and A. D. Rogol. Endurance training amplifies the pulsatile release of growth hormone: Effects of training intensity. *J. Appl. Physiol.* 72(6):2188–2196, 1992.

49. Young, A. A., C. Bogardus, K. Stone, and D. M. Mott. Insulin response of components of whole-body and muscle carbohydrate metabolism in humans. *Am. J. Physiol.* 254(17):E231–E236, 1988.

RECOMMENDED READINGS

American College of Sports Medicine. Physical activity, physical fitness and hypertension. *Med. Sci. Sports Exerc.* 25(10): i–x, 1993.

Carraro, F., C. A. Stuart, W. H. Hartl, J. Rosenblatt, and R. R. Wolfe. Effect of exercise and recovery on muscle protein synthesis in human subjects. *Am. J. Physiol.* 259(22): E470–E476, 1990.

Dela, F., K. J. Mikines, M. V. Linstow, and H. Galbo. Effect of training on response to a glucose load adjusted for daily carbohydrate intake. *Am. J. Physiol.* 260(23): E14–E20, 1991.

Dela, F., K. J. Milkines, M. Von Linstow, N. H. Secher, and H. Galbo. Effect of training on insulin-mediated glucose uptake in human muscle. *Am. J. Physiol.* 263(26): E1134–E1143, 1992.

Houmard, J. A., et al. Exercise training increases GLUT$_4$ protein concentration in previously sedentary middle-aged men. *Am. J. Physiol.* 264(27):E896–E901, 1993.

Loucks, A. B., and S. B. Horvath. Athletic amenorrhea: A review. *Med. Sci. Sports Exerc.* 17(1):56–72, 1985.

Mikines, K. J., B. Sonne, P. A. Farrell, B. Tronier, and H.. Galbo. Effect of physical exercise on sensitivity and responsiveness to insulin in humans. *Am. J. Physiol.* 254(17):E248–E259, 1988.

Shangold, M., R. Freeman, B. Thysen, and M. Gatz. The relationship between long distance running, plasma progesterone, and luteal phase length. *Fertility and Sterility* 31(20):130–133, 1979.

Weltman, A., J. Y. Weltman, R. Schurrer, W. S. Evans, J. D. Veldhus, and A. D. Rogol. Endurance training amplifies the pulsatile release of growth hormone: Effects of training intensity. *J. Appl. Physiol.* 72(6):2188–2196, 1992.

Young A. A., C. Bogardus, K. Stone, and D. M. Mott. Insulin response of components of whole-body and muscle carbohydrate metabolism in humans. *Am. J. Physiol.* 254(17): E231–E236, 1988.

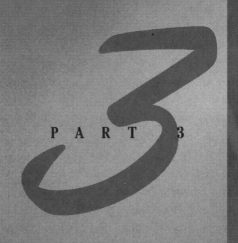

oxygen

$$Q = SV \times HR$$

$$HRmax = 220 - age$$

RQ

fatigue   RER

stress

mmHg

VO_2max

Methods to Improve Exercise Performance

CHAPTER 10

Training for Sport and Performance

hroughout the history of mankind it has been known that the body must be challenged on a regular basis if it is to improve in the ability to tolerate exercise or sustain a given level of conditioning. Consequently, the concept of training is not new and, as you may appreciate, has a history that began prior to any scientific evaluation of the benefit of one method of training over another. Initially, athletes and coaches simply used procedures that seemed to give results, that is, improved performance. However, with the improved scientific investigation of sport and athletics that exists today, we know more of how to optimally train for specific objectives, how to recognize whether there is a need for more or less training, and the physiological and cellular adaptations that contribute to the trained state. Furthermore, we also know that training is a very specific concept that applies not only to given conditions, but also to given individuals. An individual who exercises to improve recovery from a heart attack, and to reduce the likelihood of a second heart attack, trains differently than an Olympic-level marathon runner. Similarly, a triathlete trains differently than a weight lifter, no matter what the level of competition. The purpose of this chapter is to explain the fundamental concepts behind different methods of training, and to present evidence from research of the main adaptations to training for long-term endurance, muscular power, and strength.

OBJECTIVES

After studying this chapter, you should be able to:

- Explain the multiple theories and training concepts.
- Identify the principles behind the methods of training for specific sports and athletic activities.
- Explain the concept of overtraining and provide indirect methods for detecting symptoms of overtraining.
- Explain the importance of a taper to a training program and optimal prerace preparation.
- Describe the process of detraining for each type of fitness component.

KEY TERMS

training	cross-training	reversibility
fitness	overload	detraining
adaptation	overtraining	retraining
specificity	taper	

Defining Fitness and Training

*T*he process of **training** improves **fitness** and athletic performance. Training involves the organized sequence of exercise that stimulates improvements, or **adaptations,** in anatomy and physiology. Depending on the quality of training and the duration between each exercise session, these training-induced improvements are developed and retained, thereby providing improved tolerance of the exercise. In most circumstances, improved exercise tolerance results in improved exercise performance. Throughout this text, these retained training adaptations have been termed *chronic adaptations.*

The term *fitness* is more difficult to define. Fitness involves many components, including cardiorespiratory endurance, muscular endurance, muscular strength, muscular power, flexibility, body composition, and emotional/psychological qualities. Typically, the term fitness is used to express components of cardiorespiratory and muscle function, whether the components be endurance, strength, or power. Thus an athlete may be concerned with training any one or more of these components for the purpose of improving exercise performance. As will be explained, the term fitness will mean different things to different people and athletes. For example, an elite rower may train to improve fitness for rowing distances greater than 2000 m, but would not be classified as fit for the marathon running race.

An understanding of the important connections among training, chronic adaptation, and improved exercise performance is crucial if a high-quality training program is to be developed. In addition, this knowledge has to be applied to the specific demands of an exercise stress for the development of a successful training program. Therefore, knowledge of what types, intensities, durations, and frequencies of exercise are required to optimize training adaptations is essential. This knowledge is acquired from the study of skeletal muscle energy metabolism, systems physiology, and the principles and terminology of training. Furthermore, a successful athlete or coach not only has these attributes, but also has experience or a familiarity with the sport/event that optimizes the application of this knowledge. It is for this reason that many past athletes make excellent coaches.

Important Principles of Training and Training Terminology

Optimizing training requires knowledge of such principles as specificity, overload, progression, recovery, diminishing returns, the taper, reversibility, detraining, and overtraining. In addition, knowledge of specific types of training programs is also required.

Specificity

Specificity implies that the training should be devised to "train" the specific muscles and systems of the body, in a manner that is similar to how these systems are used during competition. Thus, the specificity principle has implications to anatomy, neuromuscular recruitment, motor skill patterns, cardiorespiratory function, and muscle energy metabolism. The different components of the specificity principle are illustrated in figure 10.1.

Traditionally, the component of specificity most emphasized has been skeletal muscle metabolism. In chapter 3, figure 3.1 illustrated the time dependence of the reliance on specific energy pathways for ATP regeneration. Such an approach is useful for categorizing the metabolic demands of specific events. The shorter the time duration, the greater the dependence on glycolytic and creatine phosphate (CrP) ATP (adenosine triphosphate) regeneration. The longer the duration, the greater the reliance on ATP regeneration from mitochondrial respiration.

Figure 10.2 is a modification of figure 10.1, revealing the types of events that predominantly use each metabolic pathway, along with the main limitations to exercise performance associated with these time frames. The metabolic objectives of training for an activity of a given duration would therefore be to optimize the capacity of ATP regeneration from the pathways most relied on for ATP regeneration and/or stimulate adaptations that decrease the limitations (causes of fatigue) (table 10.1). Of course, the difficulty is that very few events have a near-total reliance on just one metabolic pathway. Furthermore, one could also argue that for the activities that do rely heavily on one metabolic pathway, such as throwing or jumping events, metabolic capacities are not the determining factor for success. In throwing events, muscle power, strength, and technique could be argued to be most important. However, for the 100-m sprint, which is of a duration that can completely tax muscle creatine phosphate stores, metabolic factors may limit performance. In addition, for prolonged endurance events, where VO_{2max} and the lactate threshold combine to determine exercise performance, metabolic limitations are obvious.

Research on Training Specificity

When concerned with cardiorespiratory endurance and prolonged exercise performance, researchers have asked the question of whether the mode of exercise training is important (27, 29, 34). For example, is training by cycling as effective as running training for running exercise performance? Obviously, the measures of VO_{2max} and the lactate threshold

training an organized program of exercise designed to stimulate chronic adaptations

fitness a state of well-being that provides optimal performance

adaptation a modification in structure or function that benefits life in a new or altered environment

specificity (spes'i-fis'i-ti) having a fixed relation to a single cause or definite result

FIGURE 10.1

The different components of the specificity principle applied to exercise training.

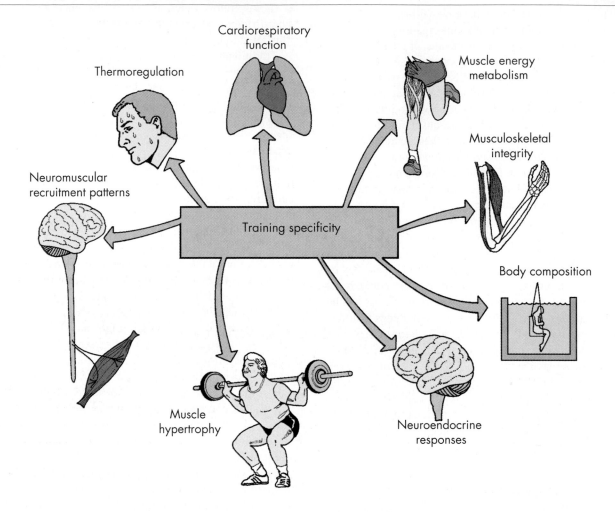

have been evaluated to answer this question. This question is also important for athletes involved in multimode events, such as biathlons, triathlons, and quadrathlons, because it is important to know how to distribute training among the multiple exercise modes for optimal performance.

VO_{2max}   When concerned with either run or cycle training, VO_{2max} improvements are largest in the exercise mode that is trained (31, 33). Consequently, *there is a transfer of fitness from one mode to another if the training stimulus and muscles used are similar.* Furthermore, despite the fact that VO_{2max} is greater for running than cycling in recreationally trained individuals, well-trained cyclists have a larger VO_{2max} during cycling than running, which further emphasizes the importance of training specificity.

For individuals who train in both cycling and running, VO_{2max} results in well-trained triathletes have shown that running VO_{2max} is larger than that in cycling (38). Conversely, for moderately trained triathletes VO_{2max} is similar between running and cycling (1). It is unclear whether the level of fitness and training of an individual will influence

the specificity of training adaptations in a given exercise mode.

Lactate Threshold   In well-trained individuals, the lactate and ventilation thresholds (LT and VT) are more sensitive indices of training improvement than VO_{2max}. Moreira and colleagues (30) and Withers and associates (43) reported that trained runners had a significantly higher VT during treadmill running compared to cycle ergometry, whereas the VT in trained cyclists did not differ between running and cycling. One would hypothesize fewer differences between the LT during running and cycling for triathletes or biathletes because these individuals are trained in both modes. Although minimal research has been done on this topic (1), results indicate that no differences exist in the VT or LT between running and cycling in triathletes, thereby supporting the hypothesis.

Intense Exercise and Weight Lifting   Research of the specificity of exercise training has mainly been focused on cardiorespiratory endurance and prolonged exercise perform-

FIGURE 10.2

The activities that predominantly rely on given energy systems and their main causes of fatigue.

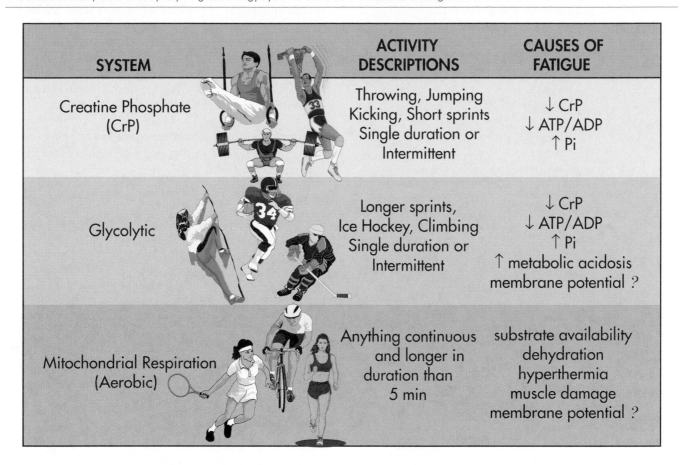

SYSTEM	ACTIVITY DESCRIPTIONS	CAUSES OF FATIGUE
Creatine Phosphate (CrP)	Throwing, Jumping Kicking, Short sprints Single duration or Intermittent	↓ CrP ↓ ATP/ADP ↑ Pi
Glycolytic	Longer sprints, Ice Hockey, Climbing Single duration or Intermittent	↓ CrP ↓ ATP/ADP ↑ Pi ↑ metabolic acidosis membrane potential ?
Mitochondrial Respiration (Aerobic)	Anything continuous and longer in duration than 5 min	substrate availability dehydration hyperthermia muscle damage membrane potential ?

ance. Whether intense exercise training should be performed in a specific mode, and how much carryover occurs between different modes is unknown. Furthermore, the influence of resistance exercise on muscular endurance, or endurance exercise on muscle strength, are topics that have not received considerable research attention.

It is known that long-distance running training decreases muscle power, so much so that endurance-trained individuals have lower muscle power than sedentary individuals. This information indicates that although training for muscular strength and power as well as endurance may at first seem in opposition, and therefore have low specificity, both training strategies may combine to improve running performance by maintaining a more optimal muscle power. Thus, *the concept of specificity must always be used in reference to the demands of the exercise* rather than the main metabolic pathway used during exercise.

For exercise and sports involving short bouts of intense exercise, the need to train to optimize muscle power is important. As discussed in chapter 5, research has shown that the velocity of muscle contraction during training can optimize gains in muscle power at specific contraction velocities (6). Consequently, resistance training should be done with rapid contractions for sports/events that involve high muscle power. Thus there seems to be a specificity of training in

muscle contraction velocity that obviously involves the neuromuscular system (42).

Cross-Training   An interesting topic that pertains to the principle of specificity is that of **cross-training.** This term can be defined in several ways because of different exercise mode, intensity, and duration options. Training in different modes of exercise can be performed to stimulate similar metabolic adaptations in the same or different muscles (e.g., cardiorespiratory and muscular endurance for long-term running and cycling, or weight lifting and swimming for the development of muscle power) or can involve the practice of completing resistance exercise by muscles that are being trained for long-term endurance.

On the basis of the previous description of research, the concept of cross-training is really a means to improve the quality of training (4, 35). It may do this by increasing the stimulus/overload for adaptation, preventing overuse and maintaining muscle power (especially for runners), and preventing overuse injuries. For example, Ruby and associates (35) compared the training improvements of previously

cross-training the practice of exercise training with more than one exercise mode

TABLE 10.1

Objectives for improving the metabolic functions of skeletal muscle for the three different energy systems

ENERGY SYSTEM	OBJECTIVES	MECHANISMS
Creatine phosphate (CrP)	↑ Potential ATP regeneration from CrP ↑ Rate of CrP regeneration during recovery	↑ Muscle CrP concentration ↑ Muscle fiber sizes
Glycolytic	↑ Potential ATP regeneration from glycolysis	↑ Muscle glycogen concentration ↑ Glucose uptake ↑ Muscle fiber sizes ↑ Blood and muscle buffer capacity
Mitochondrial respiration	↑ Maximal oxygen delivery ↑ The exercise intensity that can be sustained from mitochondrial respiration ↑ Prolong the exercise duration that can be sustained from mitochondrial respiration	↑ Maximal cardio-respiratory function ↑ Blood volume ↑ Muscle capillary density ↑ Muscle mitochondrial density ↑ Muscle glycogen store ↑ Muscle damage

sedentary women who trained by either running or cycling, or both (cross-training). All groups increased VO_{2max} and the LT similarly, indicating that there was adequate crossover in cardiorespiratory and muscular endurance between cycling and running in this low to moderate fitness population.

Overload and Overtraining   Training implies improved exercise tolerance and performance. Obviously, even if specificity principles are applied and therefore appropriate intensities are used, unless sufficient durations and frequencies of training are performed there may be no improvement in fitness components and performance. There must be a level of training above which there is a sufficient training stimulus for chronic improvement. The principle of **overload** is based on the need to train above this stimulus threshold for the development of chronic training adaptations. In short, *the body does not improve unless it experiences more stress than it is accustomed to.* The talent required by a coach or an athlete is to determine the training program that provides an overload stimulus to optimize training adaptation rather than overstress the athlete and develop a condition known as **overtraining.**

The overload principle is based in part on the research of Dr. Hans Selye (37, 39). Dr. Selye identified a pattern of physical stress referred to as the *general adaptation syndrome* (GAS). The GAS reveals how the human body responds and adapts to physical stress over time. Initially, a stress to the body causes the body to respond and adapt to that stress. With exercise, chronic adaptation results in improvements in muscle and cardiorespiratory function. When the stress is too great, for too long a period, the body is not able to respond adequately, and the stress leads to exhaustion and losses in muscle and cardiorespiratory function.

Minimal Training Intensities and Frequencies

The nature of the overload stimulus depends on a variety of factors which include:

- Exercise intensity
- Exercise duration
- Frequency of exercise sessions and duration of recovery
- Type of exercise
- Initial level of fitness

Exercise intensity can be expressed relative to VO_{2max} or maximal heart rate for endurance exercise, or relative to maximal muscle strength (maximal voluntary contraction), peak torque, or peak power for strength- and power-related activities. For endurance exercise, a minimal training overload stimulus is attained at exercise intensities that elicit greater than 50% VO_{2max}, 70% of maximum heart rate, or 60% of the heart rate reserve, and is maintained for greater than 15 min (2). Although evidence exists to indicate training improvements from less exercise, or the accumulation of exercise throughout the day (2), this minimal training stimulus has limited application to recreational or elite athletes.

Exercise performed at or slightly above the lactate threshold (LT) is most beneficial in increasing both VO_{2max} and the LT. However, the transition in the gains in cardiorespiratory endurance with further increases in exercise intensity are unclear.

For muscular strength and power, the specific nature of overload that favors strength, power, or muscular endurance is manipulated by altering the number of repetitions, the resistance lifted, and the recovery duration (see focus box 10.1). A similar approach can be used to train for muscular power in cycling, running, swimming, rowing, and other activities. However, rather than resistance being modified, speed and exercise duration are altered.

Planning the Overload Stimulus

The principle of overload requires developing a training program to provide a training stimulus that increases in conjunction with improvements in training adaptation, yet still provides adequate recovery time. This requires knowledge of the rate of training adaptation for long-term cardiorespiratory and muscular endurance, muscular strength, or muscular power (figs. 10.3 and 10.4).

As discussed in chapters 5 to 8, chronic adaptations to exercise involve alterations in neuromuscular, skeletal muscle,

FOCUS BOX 10.1

Application of the Interval Concept to Training Programs

Interval training requires the completion of exercise bouts, separated by a recovery period. The relationship between the intensity and duration of exercise to the duration of recovery will determine the specific training stimulus. For dynamic exercises, interval training can be used to develop varying degrees of endurance or power, whereas for resistance exercise, interval training can be used to develop strength, power, or general physical conditioning.

Training for Endurance and Power

Typically, interval training is suited to dynamic activities such as running, cycling, rowing, and wrestling. A training session would involve standard features of training, such as a warm-up, stretching, the training session, and a cool down and further stretching. The training session involves a given number of *work intervals*, each followed by a *rest interval*.

An example of a weekly training schedule for a marathon runner that includes interval training on day 4 is provided in table 10.2.

Training for Muscular Strength and Hypertrophy

The practice of weight lifting involves the organization of exercises into the resistance (weight) used, the number of times the weight is lifted (repetitions), the number of times a given repetition number is completed (sets), and the recovery between sets.

Manipulating any component will alter the specific training stimulus. Typically, repetition numbers less than 10 are used with heavy weights for the development of muscular strength and hypertrophy. Increasing the number of repetitions decreases the amount of weight that can be lifted and

decreases the stimulus for hypertrophy, but further increases metabolism and the development of improved muscular endurance and tone. Weight lifting can also be organized by the body parts (muscles) trained, especially in reference to agonists and antagonists, or upper vs. lower body. For example, a person may train the upper body on one day and the lower body the next day. Conversely, body builders often try to maximize the training stimulus on the muscles acting on a joint by first training one side of the joint (agonists) and completing the other side (antagonists) on the next day, or in the second session of a given day.

The following terms are used frequently in weight training:

- **Load**—the amount of resistance or weight used
- **Repetition**—the number of times an exercise is performed without recovery
- **Sets**—the number of times a series of repetitions is completed
- **Volume**—the total number of repetitions performed in a given time period
- **Recovery**—the duration between sets, which can be either active or passive
- **Frequency**—the number of training sessions per week

An example of a weekly schedule for weight training is provided in table 10.3.

TABLE 10.3

An example of a training schedule using weight lifting to increase general muscle conditioning

DAY	TRAINING
1	20 repetitions × 2 intervals of main actions for lower legs, upper legs, chest, shoulders, arms, etc. (5-min rest between sets and stations)
2	Rest day
3	20 repetitions × 2 intervals of main actions for lower legs, upper legs, hips (5-min rest between sets)
4	20 repetitions × 2 intervals of main actions for abdominals, back, chest, shoulders, arms (5-min rest between sets and stations)
5	Rest day
6	1 h of sport/activity of choice (e.g., hiking, swimming, cycling, squash, sailing)
7	20 repetitions × 1 interval of main actions for lower legs, upper legs, hips, back, abdominals, chest, shoulders, arms (30-s rest between stations)

TABLE 10.2

An example of a training schedule for a marathon runner

DAY	TRAINING
1	0.5 h easy run in morning; leg weight workout in afternoon
2	1.0 h easy run
3	1.5 h road run, approximating 12–15 mi
4	6-mi run in morning (easy); track interval workout in afternoon— 3 × 1000 m, 1 × 5000 m, 2 × 1,000 m (110% race pace); 5-min rest intervals
5	1.0 h run at desired pace
6	Rest
7	5 mi in morning; 50 min of hard running in afternoon

overload exposure of the body to stress that it is unaccustomed to

overtraining training that causes excess overload that the body is unable to adapt to, resulting in decreased exercise performance

FIGURE 10.3

Training programs provide a gradual increase in training volume that includes periods of constant or decreased training. As a person adapts to training, further improvements either require larger increases in training volume or more time at a given training volume.

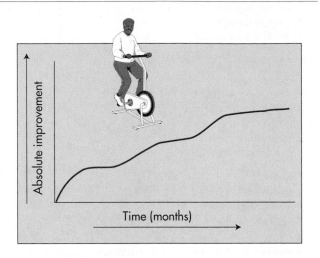

FIGURE 10.4

The improved function and exercise performance resulting from endurance and strength training. Cardiovascular adaptations to endurance training occur rapidly and explain the initial improved exercise performance. Later improvements are related to adaptations in skeletal muscle. For strength training, initial improvement has neuromuscular determinants, and subsequent increases in strength are slow and due to muscle hypertrophy.

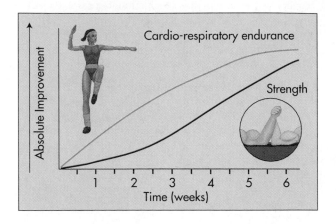

pulmonary, and cardiovascular structure and function. Figure 10.4 presents the relative changes that occur in specific aspects of body function during endurance and strength training. Cardiovascular adaptations to endurance training are very immediate, with evidence of an increased plasma volume as early as after the first bout of exercise (8, 19), a polycythemia that may take approximately 2 weeks, and skeletal muscle metabolic adaptations that are detected as early as 6 weeks into a training program and that persist after a plateau in cardiorespiratory endurance (10, 13, 16, 28). As discussed in chapter 6, research indicates that the initial improvements in VO_{2max} and endurance exercise performance are more attributable to the initial cardiovascular adaptations than to muscle metabolic adaptations (8, 14). These training improvements are of a larger magnitude for individuals who begin the training at lower relative levels of specific fitness.

The rapidity of exercise-induced training adaptations is astounding, and stresses not just the need for a rapid progression in training quality, but also the needed recovery time to allow these adaptations to occur. It is important to remember that *training provides the stimulus to adapt, and adaptation occurs during the recovery.*

For strength training, the initial increase in strength occurs from improved neuromuscular function (see chapter 5), followed by muscular hypertrophy. The dose-response curve for strength training is considerably slower in time development than that of cardiorespiratory endurance, especially after the initial neuromuscular improvement. The rate of strength improvement is variable depending on gender, hormonal status, genetics, and diet. In any case, the overload used in training must be applied progressively by manipulating the exercise intensity, duration, and frequency of training.

Research on Overload and Overtraining

Unfortunately, limited research exists that evaluates the volume of training performed by athletes. Costill and colleagues (12) studied swimmers to determine whether decreasing the volume of training lowered conditioning and worsened race performance. Interestingly, swimmers who trained once a day at 15,000 m/week rather than twice per day peaking at 30,000 m/week did not decrease in markers of conditioning (VO_{2max}, submaximal blood lactates, race performance). Conversely, the swimmers who trained at the greater distances did experience increased symptoms of overtraining. These findings raised questions concerning the efficacy of swim training using large distances. However, concerns exist regarding whether these results would have been found in more elite athletes, and whether these results can be applied to other forms of exercise such as running, cycling, weight lifting, and so forth.

When there has been too much of an overload training stimulus relative to the recovery, overtraining occurs. During overtraining, exercise performance decreases and there is actually a loss in training adaptations, causing a partial *detraining* effect. Overtraining can be detected by the presence of symptoms which include:

- Increased resting heart rate
- Loss of body weight
- Decrease in appetite
- Muscle soreness that is retained for more than 24 h
- Increased serum enzyme activity for creatine kinase and lactate dehydrogenase
- Worse running economy and thus an increased submaximal heart rate
- Increase in illness, such as colds, flu, and so on
- Constipation or diarrhea

- Decrease in performance
- Lack of desire to train or compete

Most of these aforementioned symptoms indicate overtraining, and therefore when present indicate the need to immediately decrease training volume. Of these symptoms, the resting heart and submaximal exercise heart rate are most sensitive to the development of overtraining, whereas the remainder occur when overtraining is evident. Unfortunately, science has yet to provide a sensitive gauge of overtraining that is noninvasive, inexpensive, and applicable to all athletes.

The Taper

The **taper** involves a period of reduced training, usually timed in the weeks prior to athletic competition. For swimmers, cyclists, and runners, the taper does not decrease conditioning, but actually can increase muscle power, improve psychological states, and improve performance (9).

Research has shown that periods of reduced training do not decrease VO_{2max} (21). For example, after 10 weeks of endurance training, subjects that either decreased training from 6 to 2 days per week or reduced training duration from 40 to 13 min per day, retained cardiovascular conditioning as measured by VO_{2max} for an additional 4 to 8 weeks. Clearly, the maintenance of a given level of conditioning can be done on less training than what is needed to improve fitness. Given these facts, the practice of a taper is supported by research, even for athletes who are currently within a training cycle and need to reduce training to prevent overtraining. An athlete should not fear intermittent periods of reduced training in a long-term training program.

Reversibility and Detraining

When muscles are overloaded, they adapt by getting stronger and larger. When the exercise stimulus is removed, the training adaptations reverse. If athletes do not remain active, changes in strength or aerobic endurance levels occur at a rapid pace.

An extreme example of **reversibility** and **detraining** occurs during bed rest (35). Under this condition of forced inactivity, VO_{2max} has been shown to decrease by 27% (35) in as little as 20 days. Decreases in VO_{2max} have also been shown for prolonged periods where no training has occurred. Based on research on swimmers, runners, and cyclists, decrements in VO_{2max} resulting from training cessation initially result from reductions in plasma volume (14) and then from marked reductions in muscle mitochondrial enzyme activity (7, 10, 13) (fig. 10.5).

As reductions in glycolytic enzyme activities have not been shown during detraining, the metabolic causes of decreased performance during strength or power-related exercises are minimal. Furthermore, because of this fact, it is no surprise that strength and muscle power exhibit slower detraining curves compared to endurance fitness. For example, it has been shown that no loss of strength occurred after 6 weeks of detraining from a strength training program (40, 41).

Retraining

The concept of **retraining** concerns whether previously trained individuals who then detrain have a more rapid rate of gains after a return to training. Research clearly indicates that in both low-moderate (32) and highly trained individuals (22), being previously trained does not alter the rate of

FIGURE 10.5

The physiological events associated with detraining from cardiorespiratory and muscular endurance.

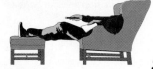

Other
Loss of heat acclimation

Body composition
↑ Body fat
↓ Lean body mass
↑ Body weight

DETRAINING

Pulmonary Function
↓ Respiratory muscle strength & endurance

Cardiovascular function
↓ Red blood cell mass
↓ End diastolic volume
↓ Plasma volume

Skeletal muscle
↓ Mitochondrial density
↓ Capillary density
↓ Muscular strength

taper a period of reduced training prior to athletic competition

reversibility the loss of training adaptations when exercise training ceases

detraining the absence of training, usually occurring after the attainment of training adaptations

retraining the process of regaining training adaptations previously lost from a period of detraining

training improvements from aerobic exercise after a period (2 to 7 weeks) of detraining. Thus, once training adaptations are lost it is as though they were never acquired by the body. This is strong evidence for the need to maintain a consistent training regimen throughout life so that there are fewer difficulties in having to return to previous levels of conditioning.

Training for Specific Performance Improvement

Given the previously explained requirements of a training program, how should an athlete train to optimally develop specific performance capacities, such as long-term endurance, muscular strength, or muscular power?

Cardiorespiratory and Muscular Endurance

Athletes can increase cardiorespiratory and muscular endurance, or muscle power, by performing one or a combination of *interval, continuous,* or *fartlek* training protocols.

Interval training, as was explained in focus box 10.1, pertains to the completion of exercise at an intensity that is above steady state, or race pace, and therefore requires a recovery period between successive exercise bouts. The faster or more intense the exercise, the longer is the recovery interval. Consequently, athletes involved in long-duration exercise typically have short recovery intervals, whereas events of a shorter duration (e.g., the mile) have longer recovery intervals because of the greater need to recover muscle metabolites and restore more normal muscle and blood acid-base balance.

Controversy exists regarding the best way to increase aerobic power. Training programs that stress intensity over duration have been shown to be very effective at increasing aerobic power (5, 15, 18). Lower-intensity, long-duration training was made popular in the 1960s and 1970s. This type of training was referred to as LSD training, or *long slow-distance* training. Today most endurance athletes use a combination of periods of high-intensity training, LSD training, and interval workouts on a track (focus box 10.2).

Muscular Strength and Hypertrophy

Apart from increasing the resistance and lowering the number of repetitions, research has shown that strength gains can be increased when dynamic rather than isometric contrac-

tions are used (17), and when eccentric contractions are incorporated into the training program (26). Similar increases in strength occur from variable resistance and constant resistance exercise (17, 25).

There are numerous ways to design a strength training program, and the definition of terms involved in this training methodology are summarized in focus box 10.3. Essentially, training programs differ depending on the purpose of the weight lifting (strength vs. general conditioning) and the number of body parts used. Different types of weight lifting exercises are presented in table 10.4.

TABLE 10.4
Weight training exercises

Exercises to Develop the Chest Muscles
1. Bench press (barbell)
2. Incline bench press (barbell)
3. Incline bench press (dumbbell)
4. Decline bench press
5. Dumbbell flys

Exercises to Develop the Shoulder Muscles
1. Dumbbell shoulder press
2. Dumbbell lateral raise
3. Dumbbell front raise
4. Medial rotation
5. Lateral rotation

Exercises to Develop the Arm Muscles
1. Tricep extension
2. Arm french curls
3. Dumbbell kickback
4. Seated dumbbell curl
5. Preacher curl with dumbbells
6. Standing dumbbell curl
7. Concentration curl
8. Wrist curls

Exercises to Develop the Upper and Lower Back Muscles
1. Upright rowing (barbell)
3. Upright rowing (dumbbells)
4. Shoulder shrugs
5. Lateral pulls (machine)
6. Extensions

Exercises to Develop the Lower Body Muscles
1. Squats
2. Lunges
3. Calf raises
4. Knee extensions (machine)
5. Hamstring curls (machine)

FOCUS BOX 10.2

Example of a Fartlek Training Schedule

1. Warm-up (dynamic exercise and stretching)
2. Run, with sprint bouts of 50 to 100 m, repeated continuously until fatigue is evident
3. Run at full speed for 100 to 200 m
4. Recover with slow jogging
5. Run, with bouts of increased speed and a duration specific to the race pace and duration, repeated continuously until fatigue is evident

FOCUS BOX 10.3

Different Strength Training Terminology and Protocols

Terminology

Power Lifting

Power lifting, or lifting in a competitive setting to determine the maximum amount of weight an individual can lift is not recommended for young or elderly people, or individuals just starting a strength training program. Power lifting generally involves core weight lifting exercises, such as the bench press, squat, clean and jerk, and the snatch. These types of exercises are commonly used by athletes to develop overall strength and explosive power. Power lifting is effective, but can also be dangerous if not performed correctly. Athletes should be gradually introduced to power lifting over time.

One Repetition Maximum (1RM)

The 1RM is used to establish starting weights for different exercises. It involves an individual lifting the maximum amount of weight he or she can lift for a particular exercise. Once an individual's 1RM is established, different percentages of the 1RM weight are used when performing selected exercises.

Circuit Training

Circuit training is a form of strength training that consists of a series of strength training exercises that collectively involve multiple body parts. Circuit training is an effective way of developing strength and flexibility of a variety of muscle groups, and can cause small increases in cardiorespiratory endurance (VO_{2max}).

Periodization

Periodization is a technique used by virtually all athletes. Periodization is a way to systematically plan training sessions to avoid overtraining and maximize workout sessions. With periodization, athletes vary the type, amount, and intensity of training for several weeks, a month, or a whole year.

Pyramid System

The pyramid system has become a popular technique among athletes and body builders. In this system, the athlete performs multiple sets of exercises, progressing from light to heavy resistance, while decreasing the number of repetitions during the session.

Split Routine System

A split routine system trains different body parts on alternate days in an effort to stimulate hypertrophy of all muscles in a particular area of the body. A typical training routine might be chest, shoulders, and back on Monday, Wednesday, and Friday; and arms, legs, and abdominal muscles on Tuesday, Thursday, and Saturday.

Eccentric Loading

Eccentric loading or performing *negatives* increases the stimulus for the development of strength. However, negatives cause more fatigue and muscle soreness than other methods of resistance training.

Plyometric Training

Plyometric training is a technique used to develop explosive strength and power. A plyometric exercise consists of a quick eccentric stretch followed by a powerful concentric contraction.

Super Set System

With the super set system, opposing muscle groups are worked through exercises performed with one following immediately after the other. An example of a super set workout would be to perform bicep curls immediately followed by tricep extensions, or leg extensions immediately followed by leg curls. Supersetting is a popular way to increase muscle hypertrophy.

(Adapted from references 3, 20, 23.)

WEBSITE BOX

Chapter 10: Training for Sport and Performance

The newest information regarding exercise physiology can be viewed at the following sites.*

tees.ac.uk/sportscience/PDA_PDRS/lect6/sld001.htm
    PowerPoint slide presentation on the use of knowledge of muscle metabolism for improved exercise training.

arfa.org/index.htm
    Excellent site providing comprehensive information on many topics within exercise physiology.

curtin.edu.au/curtin/dept/physio/pt/edres/exphys/e552_96/
    Index of brief reviews of exercise physiology by students from Curtin University, Australia. Topics include nutrition, ergogenic aids, environmental physiology, training, and clinical applications.

brainmac.demon.co.uk/whatsnew.htm
    Excellent site intended for coaches to have access to exercise-related information, including field tests of phys-

ical fitness, training strategies, nutrition, and coaching strategies.

http://fitnesslink.com/nutri.htm
    Information-packed site on exercise and the mind and body, nutrition, fitness programs, how to train, and more.

sportsci.org/
    Large site for sports scientists. In particular check out the "TrainGain," "Training and Technology," and the "Training" links within the "Net Links" sections.

_____

*Unless indicated, all URLs preceded by http://www.

Note: These URLs were valid at the time of publication, but could have changed or been deleted from Internet access since that time.

SUMMARY

▪ The process of **training** is performed to improve **fitness.** Training involves the organized sequence of exercises that stimulate improvements, or **adaptations,** in anatomy and physiology. Fitness involves many components, including cardiorespiratory endurance, muscular endurance, muscular strength, muscular power, flexibility, body composition, and emotional/psychological qualities.

▪ **Specificity** implies that training should be devised to "train" the appropriate muscles and systems of the body, in a manner that is similar to how these systems are used during competition. The specificity principle has implications to anatomy, neuromuscular recruitment, motor skill patterns, cardiorespiratory function, and muscle energy metabolism.

▪ When concerned with either run or cycle training, VO_{2max} improvements are largest in the exercise mode that is trained. Consequently, *there is a transfer of fitness from one mode to another if the training stimulus and muscles used are similar.* In well-trained individuals, the LT and VT are more sensitive indices of training improvement than VO_{2max}.

▪ **Cross-training** can be defined in several ways because of different exercise mode and exercise intensity/duration options. Training in different modes of exercise can be performed to stimulate similar metabolic adaptations in the same muscles (e.g., cardiorespiratory and muscular endurance for long-term running and cycling, or weight lifting and swimming for the development of muscle power) or can involve the practice of completing resistance exercise by muscles that are being trained for long-term endurance.

▪ The principle of **overload** is based on the need to train above a stimulus threshold for the development of chronic training adaptations. In short, *the body does not improve unless it experiences more stress than it is accustomed to.* The talent required by a coach or an athlete is to determine the training program that provides an overload stimulus to optimize training adaptation rather than overstress the athlete and develop a condition known as **overtraining.**

▪ The nature of the overload stimulus depends on a variety of factors that include exercise intensity, exercise duration, frequency of exercise sessions and duration of recovery, the type of exercise, and the initial level of fitness. Overtraining can be detected by the presence of symptoms, which include but are not limited to, increased resting heart rate, a loss of body weight, a decrease in appetite, muscle soreness that is retained for more than 24 h, worse running economy, and increased submaximal heart rate.

▪ Research has shown that exercise performed at or slightly above the lactate threshold (LT) is most beneficial in increasing both VO_{2max} and the LT. However, the transition in the gains in cardiorespiratory endurance and further increases in exercise intensity are unclear.

▪ The **taper** involves a period of reduced training, usually timed in the weeks prior to athletic competition. An extreme example of **reversibility** and **detraining** occurs during bed rest. Under this condition of forced inactivity, VO_{2max} has been shown to decrease by 27% in as little as 20 days. Decrements in VO_{2max} resulting from training cessation initially result from reductions in plasma volume, and then from marked reductions in muscle mitochondrial enzyme activity.

▪ There is no difference between athletes and more sedentary individuals in the rate of training gains after a period of detraining. Thus the process of **retraining** occurs at the same pace for all healthy individuals.

▪ Athletes can increase cardiorespiratory and muscular endurance, or muscle power, by perfoming one or a combination of *interval, continuous,* or *fartlek* training protocols. Strength gains can be increased when dynamic rather than isometric contractions are used, and when eccentric contractions are incorporated into the training program. Similar increases in strength occur from variable resistance (e.g., isokinetic) and constant resistance (e.g., external load) exercise.

STUDY QUESTIONS

1. Why is overload required to induce chronic training adaptations?

2. Why are the risks and repercussions of overtraining so severe in elite athletes?

3. What differentiates the taper from detraining?

4. Why is the taper an important component of a training program for competitive athletes?

5. What is cross-training?

6. Explain how changing repetition number, resistance, and the number of sets can alter the specificity of resistance training.

7. Why is interval training so widely used by athletes involved in training that ranges from resistance training to sprint cycling to marathon running?

APPLICATIONS

1. How would you plan a training schedule for a runner preparing to compete in a 15-km road race (hilly course) in 4 months? How would this training program change if the event was for a weight lifter preparing for a power lifting competition?

2. Do you think the extra training completed by competitive athletes compared to recreationally active individuals adds to increased health and disease prevention?

3. How would you change a cardiorespiratory endurance training program to suit a more elderly individual with risk factors for coronary artery disease? Why?

RECOMMENDED READINGS

American College of Sports Medicine. *ACSM's guidelines for exercise testing and prescription.* Williams & Wilkins, Baltimore, 1995.

Convertino, V. A., P. J. Brock, L. C. Keil, and E. M. Bernauer. Exercise training-induced hypervolemia: Role of plasma albumin, renin, and vasopressin. *J. Appl. Physiol.* 48(4):665–669, 1980.

Costill, D. L., W. J. Fink, M. Hargreaves, D. S. King, R. Thomas, and R. Fielding. Metabolic characteristics of skeletal muscle during detraining from competitive swimming. *Med. Sci. Sports Exerc.* 17(3):339–343, 1985.

Costill, D. L., et al. Adaptations to swimming training: Influence of training volume. *Med. Sci. Sports Exerc.* 23(3):371–377, 1991.

Coyle, E. F., M. K. Hemmert, and A. R. Coggan. Effects of detraining on cardiovascular responses to exercise: Role of blood volume. *J. Appl. Physiol.* 60(1):95–99, 1986.

Coyle, E. F., W. H. Martin III, D. R. Sinacore, M. J. Joyner, J. M. Hagberg, and J. O. Holloszy. Time course of loss of adaptations after stopping prolonged intense endurance training. *J. Appl. Physiol.* 57(6):1857–1864, 1984.

Hickson, R. C., and M. A. Rosenkoetter. Reduced training frequencies and maintenance of aerobic power. *Med. Sci. Sports Exerc.* 13:13–19, 1981.

Kirwan, J. P., D. L. Costill, and M. G. Flynn. Physiological responses to successive days of intense training in competitive swimmers. *Med. Sci. Sports Exerc.* 20(3):255–259, 1988.

Pierce, E. F., R. L. Seip, D. Snead, and A. Weltman. Specificity of training on the lactate threshold (LT) and VO_{2max}. *Med. Sci. Sports Exerc.* 20(2):S38, 1988.

Withers, R. T., W. M. Sherman, J. M. Miller, and D. L. Costill. Specificity of the anaerobic threshold in endurance trained athletes. *Eur. J. Appl. Physiol.* 47:93–104, 1981.

REFERENCES

1. Albrecht, T. J., V. L. Foster, A. L. Dickinson, and J. M. De-Bever. Triathletes: Exercise parameters measured during bicycle, swim bench, and treadmill testing. *Med. Sci. Sports Exerc.* 18(2):S86, 1986.

2. American College of Sports Medicine. *ACSM's guidelines for exercise testing and prescription.* Williams & Wilkins, Baltimore, 1995.

3. Barnett, A. Periodization training with exercise machines. *NSCA Journal* 15(5):14–16, 1993.

4. Boutcher, S. S., R. L. Seip, R. K. Hetzler, E. F. Pierce, D. Snead, and A. Weltman. The effects of specificity of training on rating of perceived exertion at the lactate threshold. *J. Appl. Physiol.* 59:365–369, 1989.

5. Burke, E., and B. D. Franks. Changes in VO_{2max} resulting from bicycle training at different intensities holding total mechanical work constant. *Res. Quart.* 46:31–37, 1975.

6. Caiozzeo, V. J., J. J. Pernie, and V. R. Edgerton. Training-induced alterations of the in vivo force-velocity relationship of human muscle. *J. Appl. Physiol.* 51(3):750–754, 1981.

7. Chi, M. Y., et al. Effects of detraining on enzymes of energy metabolism in individual human muscle fibers. *Am. J. Physiol.* 244(13):C276–C287, 1983.

8. Convertino, V. A., P. J. Brock, L. C. Keil, and E. M. Bernauer. Exercise training-induced hypervolemia: Role of plasma albumin, renin, and vasopressin. *J. Appl. Physiol.* 48(4):665–669, 1980.

9. Costill, D. L., D. S. King, R. Thomas, and M. Hargreaves. Effects of reduced training on muscular power of swimmers. *Phys. Sports Med.* 13:94–101, 1985.

10. Costill, D. L., W. J. Fink, M. Hargreaves, D. S. King, R. Thomas, and R. Fielding. Metabolic characteristics of skeletal muscle during detraining from competitive swimming. *Med. Sci. Sports Exerc.* 17(3):339–343, 1985.

11. Costill, D. L., M. G. Flynn, and J. P. Kirwan. Effects of repeated days of intensified training on muscle glycogen and swimming performance. *Med. Sci. Sports Exerc.* 20(3):249–254, 1988.

12. Costill, D. L., et al. Adaptations to swimming training: Influence of training volume. *Med. Sci. Sports Exerc.* 23(3):371–377, 1991.

13. Coyle, E. F., W. H. Martin III, D. R. Sinacore, M. J. Joyner, J. M. Hagberg, and J. O. Holloszy. Time course of loss of adaptations after stopping prolonged intense endurance training. *J. Appl. Physiol.* 57(6):1857–1864, 1984.

14. Coyle, E. F., M. K. Hemmert, and A.R. Coggan. Effects of detraining on cardiovascular responses to exercise: Role of blood volume. *J. Appl. Physiol.* 60(1):95–99, 1986.

15. Davies, C., and A. Knibbs. The training stimulus: The effects of intensity, duration and frequency of effort on maximum aerobic power output. *Int. Z. Angew. Physiol.* 29:299–305, 1971.

16. Dudley, G., W. Abraham, and R. Terjung. Influence of exercise intensity and duration on biomechanical adaptations in skeletal muscle. *J. Appl. Physiol.* 53(4):844–850, 1982.

17. Fleck, S. J., and W. J. Kraemer. Designing resistance training programs. Human Kinetics Books, Champaign, IL, 1987.

18. Fox, E. L., R. L. Bartels, C. Billings, D. Mathews, R. Bason, and W. Webb. Intensity and distance of interval training programs and changes in aerobic power. *J. Appl. Physiol.* 38(3):481–484, 1975.

19. Gillen, C. M., R. Lee, G. W. Mack, C.M. Tomasellia, T. Nishiyasu, and E.R. Nadel. Plasma volume expansion in humans after a single intense exercise protocol. *J. Appl. Physiol.* 71(5):1914–1920, 1991.

20. Gonyea, W. J., and D. Sale. Physiology of weightlifting. *Arch. Phys. Med. Rehab.* 63:235–237, 1982.

21. Hickson, R. C., and M. A. Rosenkoetter. Reduced training frequencies and maintenance of aerobic power. *Med. Sci. Sports Exerc.* 13:13–19, 1981.

22. Houston, M., E. H. Bentzen, and H. Larsen. Interrelationships between skeletal muscle adaptations and performance as studied by detraining and retraining. *Acta Physiol. Scand.* 105:163–170, 1979.

23. Jensen, C. R., and A. G. Fisher. *Scientific basis of athletic conditioning.* Lea & Febiger, Philadelphia, 1979.

24. Kirwan, J. P., D. L. Costill, and M. G. Flynn. Physiological responses to successive days of intense training in competitive swimmers. *Med. Sci. Sports Exerc.* 20(3):255–259, 1988.

25. Kojima, T. Force-velocity relationship of human elbow flexors in voluntary isotonic contraction under heavy loads. *Int. J. Sports Med.* 12:208–213, 1991.

26. Komi, P. V., and E. R. Buskirk. Effect of eccentric and concentric muscle conditioning on tension and electrical activity of human muscle. *Ergonomics* 15:417–434, 1972.

27. Kravitz, L., R. A. Roberg, V. H. Heyward, D. R. Wagner, and K. Powers. Exercise mode and gender comparisons of energy expenditure at self-selected intensities. *Med. Sci. Sports Exerc.* 28(8):1028–1035, 1997.

28. MacDougall, J. D., G. R. Ward, D. G. Sale, and J. R. Sutton. Biochemical adaptation of human skeletal muscle to heavy resistance training and immobilization. *J. Appl. Physiol.* 43(3):700–703, 1985.

29. McKenzie, D. C., E. L. Fox, and D. Cohen. Specificity of metabolic and circulatory responses to arm and leg training. *Eur. J. Appl. Physiol.* 39:241–248, 1978.

30. Moreira, C. M., A. K. Russo, I. C. Picarro, T. L. Barros Neto, A. C. Silva, and J. Tarasantchi. Oxygen consumption and ventilation during constant-load exercise in runners and cyclists. *J. Sports Med. Phy. Fit.* 29(1):36–44, 1980.

31. Pechar, G. S., W. D. McArdle, F. I. Katch, J. R. Magel, and J. Deluca. Specificity of cardiorespiratory adaptation to bicycle and treadmill running. *J. Appl. Physiol.* 36(6):753–756, 1974.

32. Pedersen, P., and J. Jorgensen. Maximal oxygen uptake in young women with training, inactivity and retraining. *Med. Sci. Sports Exerc.* 10(4):233–237, 1979.

33. Pierce, E. F., R. L. Seip, D. Snead, and A. Weltman. Specificity of training on the lactate threshold (LT) and VO_{2max}. *Med. Sci. Sports Exerc.* 20(2):S38, 1988.

34. Roberts, J. A., and J. W. Alspaugh. Specificity of training effects resulting from programs of treadmill running and bicycle ergometer riding. *Med. Sci. Sports Exerc.* 4(1):6–10, 1972.

35. Ruby, B., R. A. Robergs, G. Leadbetter, C. Mermier, T. Chick, and D. Stark. Cross-training between cycling and running in untrained females. *J. Sports Med. Phys. Fit.* 36:246–254, 1996.

36. Saltin, B., G. Blomqvist, J. H. Mitchell, R. L. Johnson, K. Wildenthal, and C. B. Chapman. Response to submaximal and maximal exercise after bed rest and training. *Circulation* 38(S Suppl.):VII 1–78, 1968.

37. Schafer, W. *Wellness through stress management.* International Dialogue Press, Davis, CA, 1983.

38. Schnieder, D. A., K. A. Lacroix, G. R. Atkinison, P. J. Troped, and J. Pollacl. Ventilatory threshold and maximal oxygen uptake during cycling and running in triathletes. *Med. Sci. Sports Exerc.* 22(2):257–264, 1990.

39. Selye, H. *The stress of life.* McGraw-Hill, New York, 1956.

40. Thorstensson, A., L. Larsson, P. Tesch, and J. Karlsson. Muscle strength and fiber composition in athletes and sedentary men. *Med. Sci. Sports Exerc.* 9:26–30, 1977.

41. Thorstensson, A. L. Observations on strength training and detraining. *Acta Physiol. Scand.* 100:491–493, 1977.

42. Tesch, P. A., and L. Karlsson. Muscle fiber type and size in trained and untrained muscles of elite athletes. *J. Appl. Physiol.* 59(9):1716–1723, 1985.

43. Withers, R. T., W. M. Sherman, J. M. Miller, and D. L. Costill. Specificity of the anaerobic threshold in endurance-trained athletes. *Eur. J. Appl. Physiol.* 47: 93–104, 1981.

CHAPTER 11

Nutrition and Exercise

hen we contract skeletal muscle, molecules are broken down to release energy that is needed during the process of contraction. These reactions were detailed in chapter 2. The molecules used by cells to release energy have been termed *energy substrates.* The body must have a continual supply of these energy substrates for optimal exercise performance. In addition, molecules exist that are needed by cells in order to more effectively break down energy substrates. The molecules needed by cells can be made by the body from other molecules ingested in food or can be ingested in their needed form. Exercise increases the demand for these molecules and, therefore, the type and quantities of food eaten must be suited to the particular exercise stresses placed on the body. The purpose of this chapter is to present the recommended dietary needs of the body before, during, and after different types of exercise.

OBJECTIVES

After studying this chapter, you should be able to:

- List the main macronutrients and micronutrients of the body.
- Explain why and for which exercise conditions the macronutrients of the body serve as fuel for energy metabolism in contracting skeletal muscle.
- Identify the dietary strategies required for optimizing muscle and liver glycogen during the days preceding prolonged endurance exercise.
- Explain the importance of ingesting fluid and carbohydrate during prolonged exercise.
- Explain the relative amount of carbohydrate intake required to prevent hypoglycemia during prolonged exercise.
- Provide nutritional and exercise recommendations that will increase the rate of muscle glycogen synthesis after exercise.
- List the additional nutritional ergogenics other than carbohydrate that athletes can use to improve performance (endurance, strength, or power), and explain why each is or is not beneficial.

KEY TERMS

nutrients
nutrition
micronutrients
macronutrients
vitamins
minerals
complete proteins
glycogen supercompensation
rebound hypoglycemia
glycemic index
hyperhydration
glucose polymers
gastric emptying
intestinal absorption
dehydration
water intoxication
hyponatremia
rehydration
free radicals
antioxidants
3-methylhistidine
nitrogen balance
ferritin

Nutrition

*T*he molecules needed by cells to function optimally are termed **nutrients.** The study of nutrients and their roles in the body is the science of **nutrition.** Nutrients can be divided into the small compounds that are not catabolized to release free energy during energy metabolism: the **micronutrients,** and those used during energy metabolism: the **macronutrients.** As will be discussed in the sections to follow, *many of the micronutrients are necessary for optimal catabolism of macronutrients.*

Micronutrients

The important micro- and macronutrients of the body, and their major functions are presented in table 11.1. The micronutrients can be divided into *vitamins* and *minerals.*

Vitamins are organic compounds that the body requires in small amounts for health. Vitamins are not used as substrates for energy metabolism, but as indicated in table 11.1, they are required for the catabolism of carbohydrates, fats, and protein. In fact, vitamins are the principle component of most coenzymes.

The vitamins are grouped based on their solubility characteristics. The *water soluble* vitamins consist of the B-group vitamins and vitamin C. The *fat soluble* vitamins consist of vitamins A, D, E, and K. Water soluble vitamins can be stored in the body in small amounts bound to protein structures; however, as this capacity is small the majority of excess intake is excreted in the urine. Except for vitamin K, fat soluble vitamins are stored in adipose tissue fat, and excess intake can lead to symptoms of toxicity. Of the fat soluble vitamins, vitamins D and K are produced in the body.

Minerals are elements that the body needs for a diverse number of functions. There are minerals that the body requires relatively large amounts of (calcium, phosphorus, potassium, sulfur, sodium, chloride, and magnesium), and there are minerals that the body needs in only small, or trace amounts (iron, iodine, manganese, copper, zinc, cobalt, fluorine, selenium, and chromium) and these are termed *trace elements.* The functions of the vitamins and minerals of the body and their main nutrient sources are listed in table 11.1.

The recommended daily allowance (RDA) of vitamins and minerals are determined by the Food and Nutrition Board of the National Academy of Sciences (app. F). The RDAs are small, vary for individuals of different gender and age, and can range from between 0.002 mg for vitamin B_{12} to more than 1 g each of sodium, calcium, and phosphorus.

Macronutrients

The macronutrients of the body comprise carbohydrates, lipids, and proteins. The functions of the macronutrients in the body are presented in table 11.1.

It is recommended that a normal balanced diet should have 60% of total kcal from carbohydrate, 30% from fat, and 10% from protein (133) (focus box 11.1). Of the carbohydrate component, 48% should be from complex carbohydrates and 12% from simple carbohydrates (sucrose, fructose, glucose). Of the fat component, 10% should be from saturated fat, 10% from monounsaturated fat, and the remaining 10% from polyunsaturated fat. As will be discussed in chapter 20, saturated fats have a greater risk for the development of increased blood cholesterol and atherosclerotic cardiovascular disease. In reality, the average citizen in the United States ingests a diet of 46% carbohydrate (24% from simple carbohydrate), 42% fat, and 12% protein (133). *The absolute amount of calories provided from each food source depends on the total caloric intake,* which may vary between 1200 kcal/day for a dieting small individual, to over 5000 kcal/day for a competitive athlete involved in 3 to 4 hours of vigorous exercise each day.

Of the three macronutrients—carbohydrate, fat, and protein—there is an RDA only for protein, which equals 0.8 g/kg body wt/day (133). As the protein RDA is expressed relative to body weight, it accounts for the increased protein needs of larger individuals. Ironically, the average citizen of the United States ingests protein equivalent to twice the RDA for protein. Not all protein is identical in nutrient content, as the adult body cannot synthesize eight amino acids: leucine, isoleucine, threonine, lysine, methionine, phenylalanine, tryptophan, and valine. These amino acids are termed *essential amino acids.* For individuals who do not consume animal or dairy products, which are the main sources of **complete protein** (contain all essential amino acids), careful selection of grains, nuts, and legumes is required to receive all essential amino acids (see table 11.1).

Fat is categorized into saturated, monounsaturated, and polyunsaturated forms. These divisions relate to the presence of carbon-carbon double bonds. The absence of double bonds enables greater hydrogen atoms to bind to the carbon chain, thus causing it to be saturated. When there is one double bond in the fatty acid chain, the fat is termed monounsaturated, and when there are more than two double bonds it is a polyunsaturated fat. The greater the number of double bonds, and the more polyunsaturated the fat, the more likely it is to be a liquid (oil) at room temperature. The division of fats based on saturation also has practical application because of the association of saturated fat intake to the development of high blood cholesterol concentrations, and an increased risk for atherosclerotic cardiovascular diseases (see chapters 16 and 21).

An intake of fat is required for the acquisition of the one essential fatty acid, linoleic acid. However, minimal fat ingestion is required to meet this need. For the majority of individuals, lowering the fat contribution of the diet is of focal interest.

Water

Water is an important nutrient of the body because it comprises approximately 70% of the lean body mass (53). Water provides the aqueous medium within which the reactions of the body occur, and the interactions between charged and un-charged regions of proteins in an aqueous environment are responsible for the structure of many of the body's proteins and many lipid-containing structures such as the cell membrane.

The body continually replenishes its water content. Water is lost through the excretion of urine, the evaporation of sweat, and the humidification of inhaled air. Water is used as a substrate in many chemical reactions, and also is a product of other chemical reactions. It is recommended that for normally active people in a temperate climate, approximately 2.5 L of water should be ingested each day (133). This value increases for individuals who live in a hot, humid, or high-altitude environment, or who exercise on a daily basis. The specific details of the types of fluid, and the amounts required to be ingested during and after exercise will be presented in the sections to follow.

Meeting the Body's Nutrient Needs

The need to ingest calories, vitamins, minerals, and water, yet restrict the intake of fat and protein requires that individuals be selective in their choices of food and liquid. This is true even for athletes because a sound diet provides the foundation from which the tolerance of exercise training and optimal performance can develop.

Categorizing foods into food groups has proven to be a time-tested successful approach to selecting food and establishing a balanced diet. Foods have been divided into six main classes: whole grain cereals, vegetables, fruits, dairy, meat and poultry, and fats and simple carbohydrates (mainly glucose, sucrose, and fructose). The macro- and micronutrients provided from each food category are used to determine the amount of food from each group needed to attain the RDA for micronutrients. For a healthy low-fat diet that provides at least 60% of kcal from carbohydrate, the whole grain cereals should provide the majority of calories, followed by fruits and vegetables, dairy, meat and poultry, and finally, fats and simple carbohydrates should provide minimal calories (fig. 11.1).

For individuals who exercise regularly, the need for a sound diet based on the previously mentioned food groups is also paramount. However, as will be discussed in the following sections, *participation in regular exercise for extended periods of time places additional nutritional demands on the body*, and depending on the type of exercise performed, *minor nutritional modifications can improve exercise performance*, as well as the *recovery from exercise*.

Optimizing Nutrition for Exercise

Exercise can be performed at different intensities, durations, and frequencies during the day or week. In addition, exercise can be organized in such a way as to stimulate specific changes or adaptations in the body, such as those that occur from training. The specific demands that each type of exercise condition places on nutritional needs must be understood in order to prescribe appropriate alterations in dietary intake. For these reasons, the information to follow will be broadly categorized into the type of nutrient (macro- and micronutrients), time frames of reference (before, during, and after exercise, and long-term exercise), as well as the type of exercise (short-term intense vs. long-term steady-state).

Macronutrient Concerns Before, During, and After Exercise

From an exercise perspective, the intake of macronutrients serves to replenish muscle and liver glycogen, maintain normal blood glucose concentrations, replenish muscle and adipose tissue triglycerides, maintain cell membrane integrity, and maintain or increase muscle protein. The importance of each of these components changes for exercise of different intensities and the time of ingestion relative to when the exercise is performed (111).

Prolonged Submaximal Exercise

During prolonged exercise muscle and liver glycogen, blood glucose, blood free fatty acids, muscle free fatty acids, and blood and muscle amino acids are the substrates used to fuel muscle energy metabolism. The relative priority of these substrates changes for different intensities and durations of exercise. During low-intensity exercise lipid predominates as the primary substrate. As much as 60% of this lipid comes from within skeletal muscle lipid droplets (endogenous stores) (114, 115, 129). However, the reliance on carbohydrate increases as exercise intensity increases. When the body's stores of carbohydrate become low, there is an increased use of lipid and amino acids as substrates for energy metabolism (131).

Because of the general need to conserve the body's stores of amino acids, low-carbohydrate conditions are not recommended for the body during exercise. Low-carbohydrate conditions for the body also decrease exercise performance and

nutrients a food component that can be utilized by the body

nutrition the science involving the study of food and liquid requirements of the body for optimal function

micronutrient essential food component required only in small quantities

macronutrient essential food component required in large quantities

vitamins organic micronutrient of food, essential for normal body functions

minerals inorganic micronutrients, essential for normal bodily functions

complete proteins proteins that contain all of the essential amino acids

TABLE 11.1

Major micronutrients and macronutrients and their functions that support exercise

NUTRIENT	FUNCTIONS SUPPORTING EXERCISE	MAIN NUTRIENT SOURCES
MICRONUTRIENTS		
Vitamins		
Water soluble		
Thiamine (B_1)	Coenzyme in cellular metabolism	Pork, organ meats, whole grains, legumes
Riboflavin (B_2)	Component of FAD^+ and FMN of the electron transport chain	Most foods
Niacin	Component of NAD^+ and $NADP^+$	Liver, lean meats, grains, legumes
Pyridoxine (B_6)	Coenzyme in metabolism	Meat, vegetables, whole grains
Pantothenic acid	Component of coenzyme A (e.g., acetyl CoA, fatty acyl-CoA	Most foods
Folacin	Coenzyme of cellular metabolism	Legumes, green vegetables, whole wheat
Cobalamin (B_{12})	Coenzyme of metabolism in nucleus	Muscle meat, eggs, dairy products
Biotin	Coenzyme of cellular metabolism	Meats, vegetables, legumes
Ascorbic acid (C)	Maintains connective tissue; immune protection (?)	Citrus fruits, tomatoes, green peppers
Fat Soluble		
β–carotene (provitamin A)		Green vegetables
Retinol (A)	Sight; component of rhodopsin (visual pigment); maintains tissues	Milk, butter, cheese
Cholecalciferol (D)	Bone growth and maintenance; calcium absorption	Cod liver oil, eggs, dairy products
Tocopherol (E)	Antioxidant; protects cellular integrity	Seeds; green, leafy vegetables; margarine
Phylloquinone (K)	Role in blood clotting	Green, leafy vegetables; cereals; fruits; meat
Major Minerals		
Calcium (Ca^{2+})	Bone and tooth formation; muscle contraction; action potentials	Milk, cheese, dark green vegetables
Phosphorus (PO^{3-})	Bone and tooth formation; acid-base; chemical energy	Milk, cheese, yogurt, meat, poultry, grains, fish
Potassium (K^+)	Action potential; acid-base; body water balance	Leafy vegetables, cantaloupe, lima beans, potatoes, milk, meat
Sulfur (S)	Acid-base; liver function	Proteins, dried food
Sodium (Na^+)	Action potential; acid-base; osmolality; body water balance	Fruits, vegetables, table salt
Chlorine (Cl^-)	Membrane potential; fluid balance	Fruits, vegetables, table salt
Magnesium (Mg^{2+})	Cofactor for enzyme function	Whole grains; green, leafy vegetables
Minor Minerals		
Iron (Fe)	Component of hemoglobin, myoglobin, and cytochromes	Eggs; lean meats; legumes; whole grains; green, leafy vegetables
Fluorine (F)	Bone structure (?)	Water, sea food
Zinc (Zn)	Component of enzymes of digestion	Most foods

increase perceptions of fatigue (1, 2, 32, 89). Understandably, importance is placed on receiving adequate carbohydrate prior to exercise to ensure optimal muscle and liver glycogen reserves and decrease the catabolism of amino acids.

Preexercise Nutrition   The importance of muscle glycogen to exercise performance was first documented by Scandinavian researchers in 1967 (7–9, 61, 70). The Scandinavian researchers provided evidence that a modified diet strategy in the days preceeding an athletic event could increase skeletal muscle glycogen stores (9), and this regimen was termed

glycogen supercompensation. As indicated in figure 11.2, this regimen involved the depletion of the body's carbohydrate stores by a combination of exhaustive exercise and a low-carbohydrate diet. After this, the athlete was required to decrease training, ingest a high-carbohydrate diet, and have a rest day prior to competition. This regimen required approximately 1 week. The problem was that the process of carbohydrate depletion is physically and mentally uncomfortable, especially in the week prior to competition. For this reason, other researchers studied the ability of athletes to increase muscle glycogen stores by simply altering training

TABLE 11.1

Major micronutrients and macronutrients and their functions that support exercise

NUTRIENT	FUNCTIONS SUPPORTING EXERCISE	MAIN NUTRIENT SOURCES
MACRONUTRIENTS		
Copper (Cu)	Component of enzymes of iron metabolism	Meat, water
Selenium (Se)	Functions with vitamin E	Seafood, meat, grains
Iodine (I)	Component of thyroid hormones	Marine fish and shellfish, dairy products, vegetables, iodized salt
Chromium (Cr)	Required for glycolysis	Legumes, cereals, organ meats
Molybdenum (Mo)	Cofactor for several enzymes	Fats, vegetable oils, meats, whole grains
Carbohydrates		
Monosaccharides		
Glucose	Essential for neural tissue and blood cell metabolism; required for optimal cellular metabolism	Candies, fruit, processed food, soda
Fructose	Metabolic substrate for the liver	Honey, corn, fruit
Galactose	Metabolic substrate for the liver	Breast milk
Disaccharides		
Sucrose	Provides glucose and fructose for energy metabolism	Table sugar, maple syrup, sugar cane
Lactose	No essential role in nutrition	Dairy products
Maltose	No essential role in nutrition	Formed during digestion
Polysaccharides		
Starch	Source of glucose, for storage as glycogen or conversion to fat	Corn, cereal, pasta, bread, beans, peas, potatoes
Fiber	Increases intestinal motility	Fruits, vegetables
Lipids		
Cholesterol	Component of cell membrane; precursor for steroid hormone synthesis	Beef liver, eggs, butter, shrimp
Triglycerides and fatty acids	Energy source; insulation; organ protection	Meats, oils, nuts, cheese, whole milk and other dairy products
Omega-3 fatty acids	May improve blood cholesterol and decrease atherosclerosis	Cold-water fish oils
Saturated fat	?	Coconut oil, butter, cream, animal fat
Monounsaturated fat	?	Olives, almonds, avocados, peanuts
Polyunsaturated fat	?	Safflower and sunflower oil, sesame seeds
Protein		
Complete proteins	Cell maintenance, structure, and repair; immune function	Meats, poultry, eggs, cheese, fish, milk
Incomplete proteins	Cell maintenance, structure, and repair; immune function	Legumes, cereal, seeds, leafy vegetables
Water	Medium for cell reactions, blood, circulation, thermoregulation	Drinking water, juices, sodas, fruits, vegetables

volumes and intensities and increasing the carbohydrate content of the diet during the final week prior to competition (121) (fig. 11.2). For trained athletes, this modified regimen was as beneficial in increasing muscle glycogen stores as the original Scandinavian approach. Recommendations for optimizing muscle glycogen stores prior to exercise are presented in focus box 11.2.

The guidelines for maximizing preevent muscle glycogen stores raise questions concerning the amount of carbohydrate that should be in a diet for endurance athletes, the extent to which this proportion should be increased during the

days prior to competition, and what types of carbohydrate should be ingested.

Recommended Quantities and Types of Carbohydrate For the athlete, the macronutrient recommendations based on a % of total kcal are inappropriate because a 5000-kcal diet

glycogen supercompensation a regimen of increased carbohydrate ingestion and modified exercise training that results in maximal storage of glycogen in skeletal muscle

Recommendations for the Percent Caloric Intake of Macronutrients: Which Recommendation Is Correct?

Traditionally, recommendations for macronutrient quantities and proportions in the diet have been to ingest a diet with an energy content balanced to energy need with a proportion of carbohydrate (CHO), fat, and protein equivalent to 60, 30, and 10% of total calories. Additional recommendations within each macronutrient category are presented in the text.

This basic recommendation may not be suitable for athletes, as there is a need to raise the CHO and protein proportions (see text). However, other strategies for balancing macronutrient intake also exist, and most have involved raising fat and lowering carbohydrate intake.

The 40, 30, 30 "Zone Diet"

In 1995 Barry Sears (118) published a book, referenced with scientific research, that advocated that CHO intake at 60% of total calories is far too excessive, can be potentially harmful to long-term health, and even for athletes may detrimentally influence exercise performance. Sears recommends that a diet characterized by severe caloric restriction with a macronutrient percentage closer to a CHO, fat, and protein equivalent of 40, 30, and 30% of total calories be ingested. Obviously, this macronutrient approach differs from that recommended by the American Dietetics Association and, because it provides less CHO and more fat, initially appears to be unsuitable for athletes. Similarly, even for sedentary individuals, initial concern must also be placed on the relatively high-protein component and the fact that most meat protein sources are associated with more saturated than unsaturated fat. Could this diet also increase the likelihood for the development of cardiovascular diseases?

It is important to realize that Sears didn't just "make up" these macronutrient proportions or base these values solely on his own research. There is considerable research in clinical nutrition on the application of such macronutrient proportions and caloric restrictions to individuals with diabetes mellitus. Basically, when an individual has an impaired ability of tissues (especially skeletal muscle) to use CHO (e.g., diabetics), dietary CHO intake can cause excessive increases in blood glucose, forcing the liver to process more of the glucose. Based on the content of chapter 3, the student should realize that liver handling of glucose results in increased fatty acid production. These fats are converted to triacylglycerols, packaged into lipoprotein molecules, and increase blood lipids (triacylglycerols and cholesterol) and fat storage in adipocytes. Thus, for diabetics, a diet high in CHO may be worse than a diet higher in fat and protein because of elevations in blood lipids and increased risk for cardiovascular diseases.

Sears applied the proven facts of dietary intake for diabetics to individuals without metabolic diseases. The rationale for this, as described by Sears, is that a high-CHO intake, especially when of simple CHO, can excessively raise blood glucose causing increased insulin release. The increased blood glucose and insulin increases liver glucose disposal, increases liver fatty acid production, and thereby also contributes to increased blood lipoproteins. For athletes and nonathletes alike, the negative of a high–simple CHO diet is that the increased blood glucose and insulin conditions increase the uptake of glucose into adipocytes, where glucose is also converted to fatty acids. When combined with the increased blood fatty acids and triacylglycerols, there is greater likelihood of fat deposition and greater difficulty in fat loss. Sears also proposes that for athletes, another problem of a high-CHO diet is that it increases the CHO dependence of metabolism. This fact is well supported by research because high-CHO diets are associated with increases in RER (respiratory exchange ratio) and total CHO oxidation for given intensities of exercise, thereby suppressing fat oxidation (60). Sears's logic is that if CHO is so important to athletes for endurance exercise, then why stimulate a metabolic condition that increases CHO catabolism? Why not stimulate

---

would require that these athletes consume 167 g of fat, 125 g of protein, and restrict carbohydrate intake to 750 g. For a 75-kg person, this protein intake would be more than twice the RDA of 0.8 g/kg, would waste caloric intake in excess fat, and would relate to a *daily carbohydrate intake* of 10 g/kg. Because the primary nutrient used during prolonged exercise at moderate to high intensities is carbohydrate, and for most people there is adequate triglyceride stored in adipose tissue, athletes should try to increase caloric intake by ingesting added carbohydrate to 70% of total kcal, with fat intake approximating 20% and protein intake remaining at 10% of total kcal. The increase in calories from carbohydrate may be in the form of complex or simple carbohydrates, in either a liquid or solid form (54, 56, 71, 84).

One could argue that for individuals expending more than 5000 kcal per day less fat intake could be recommended, however, a diet lower than 20% fat in today's society would require considerable effort in planning and preparation, and therefore be time-consuming. One has to admire the individuals who succeed in devising a diet where fat contributes less than 20% of total kcal. However, as discussed in focus box 11.1, recent research indicates that relatively high-fat diets that do not provide excess energy may not have the negative health consequences that were previously thought, and research evidence exists to show the added performance benefits of a relatively high-fat and low-carbohydrate diet (15, 65, 66, 79, 131). Clearly more research needs to be done comparing the influence different diet strategies have on exercise performance.

a metabolic condition that is more conducive to sparing muscle and liver glycogen stores, and thus preserving blood glucose?

Exercise-Related Research of Diets Low in Carbohydrate and Higher in Fat and Protein

The exercise-related logic of Sears's approach has been well researched, and has provided inconsistent results. For example, fat feeding immediately prior to exercise, causing blood free fatty acids to raise to above 1.0 mmol/L, has been consistently shown to increase fatty oxidation and even spare muscle glycogen during prolonged steady-state exercise (15, 106, 130). Consequently, the potential for increased fat intake to lower CHO oxidation during exercise is not at question. Conversely, the question of whether the same is true for exercise intensities during competition is a totally different issue. Okano, Sato, and Murata (102) had subjects complete two trials of cycle ergometry exercise (2 h at 67% VO_{2max} followed by exercise to fatigue at 78% VO_{2max}) 4 h after either a high-fat [30% CHO, 61% fat, and 9% protein (kcal = 4711 kJ] or a high-CHO meal (58% CHO, 31% fat, 11% protein). Although the high-fat meal increased fat oxidation early in exercise, there was no difference between the trials for total endurance time and work production. The researcher's conclusions were that increasing fat intake could alter macronutrient catabolism during lower-intensity exercise, but that more intense exercise, closer to those attained during performance, does not seem to be improved by increased fat ingestion.

The other issue is the longer-term effects of an increased fat component of the diet on exercise metabolism and exercise performance. Is there a chronic adaptation to higher fat intakes (fat adaptation) that can be beneficial for endurance exercise performance? This is the question that still requires further research before a clear answer can be provided. For example, Lambert and associates (79) have shown that increasing the fat intake for a period of 7 days can significantly increase exercise endurance at intensities < 70% VO_{2max}. Such benefits also transfer to improvements in 20-km cycling time trials when there is a period of CHO loading prior to the event (79). Similarly, ingesting medium-chained triacylglycerols with CHO during exercise can result in similar endurance and performance improvements (79).

Despite these research findings, Hawley, Brouns, and Jeukendrup (59) state that prolonged high-fat diets have yet to be shown to spare muscle glycogen, and consistently improve exercise performance. Similarly, Jeukendrup and colleagues (65) also researched the influence of the ingestion of medium-chain triaclyglycerols (MCT) with CHO on exercise metabolism and showed that it did not decrease CHO oxidation or spare muscle glycogen. Furthermore, because of the gastrointestinal distress that can accompany MCT ingestion, such a nutritional practice may even be detrimental to exercise performance (66, 99).

Finally, nutritional surveys of elite-level cyclists show that the typical nutrient intake pattern remains one of a moderate CHO intake, reduced fat intake, and elevated protein intake (60, 14.5, and 25.5%, respectively) (42). Currently, recommendations for macronutrient intake should remain focused on providing adequate CHO, especially during the immediate days prior to an event and in the immediate hours after exercise. Except for the immediate postexercise period, the majority of the CHO ingested should be complex rather than simple sugars. The need for increased protein should also be recognized (< 1.2 g/kg/day). Although the research on longer-term ingestion of higher-fat diets suggests that the body does respond by lowering CHO catabolism, there is contradictory evidence on how these diets may improve endurance exercise performance. Until long-term studies on how these diets alter risk factors for cardiovascular diseases are completed, it is prudent to avoid the recommendation to ingest high-fat diets to stimulate "fat adaptation" for purposes of sparing muscle glycogen and improving competitive exercise performance.

The ingestion of fat or protein in the hours prior to exercise is not beneficial for optimizing muscle and liver glycogen stores. In addition, high fat and protein contents in a meal delay gastric emptying, and can detrimentally affect blood acid-base balance in the resting state, and impair subsequent exercise performance (50–52, 86). Nevertheless, research done on the basis of increasing blood free fatty concentrations during exercise by either ingesting lipid or infusing heparin to increase blood free fatty acid mobilization from circulating triglycerides, or both, have shown that high–free fatty acid concentrations in the blood increase lipid catabolism for a given submaximal exercise intensity, and even spare muscle glycogen (27, 57, 130). These findings are tempting as recommendations because not even glucose ingestion during exercise spares muscle glycogen.

However, there is no evidence that such a dietary strategy can support exercise performance in a manner similar to carbohydrates, and on the basis of muscle biochemistry and the higher rates of ATP regeneration from carbohydrate than from fat, a reduction in exercise performance would be expected from a decreased capacity of contracting skeletal muscle to catabolize carbohydrate.

Timing of Carbohydrate Ingestion Prior to Exercise Evidence exists to question the use of carbohydrates at certain times prior to the start of exercise. In 1977 Costill and colleagues (27) reported that the ingestion of carbohydrate and increased blood glucose 30 to 60 min prior to exercise can increase blood insulin concentrations. When exercise commences, the increased uptake of glucose by skeletal muscle

FIGURE 11.1

The USDA's Food Guide Pyramid, which lists and illustrates the recommended number of servings of each major food group for adults.

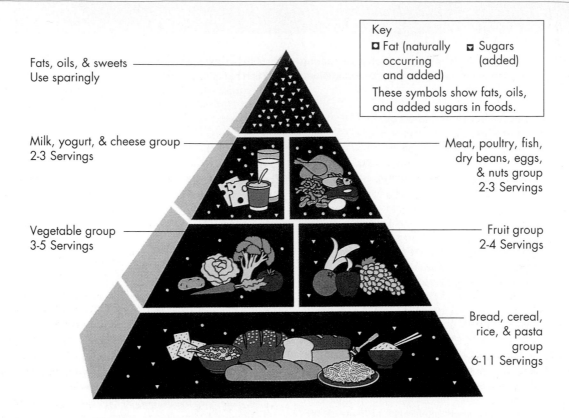

Key

▫ Fat (naturally occurring and added)   ◩ Sugars (added)

These symbols show fats, oils, and added sugars in foods.

Fats, oils, & sweets
Use sparingly

Milk, yogurt, & cheese group
2-3 Servings

Meat, poultry, fish, dry beans, eggs, & nuts group
2-3 Servings

Vegetable group
3-5 Servings

Fruit group
2-4 Servings

Bread, cereal, rice, & pasta group
6-11 Servings

FIGURE 11.2

The original and modified regimens for increasing skeletal muscle glycogen concentrations prior to exercise.

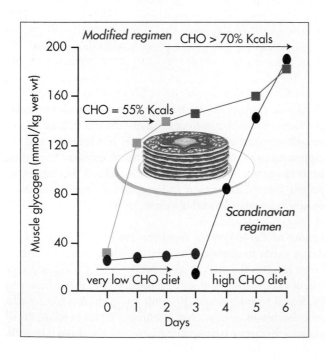

from contraction and the increased insulin can rapidly lower blood glucose concentrations, causing what was termed **rebound hypoglycemia** (fig. 11.3). Evidence has also been presented that muscle glycogenolysis increases under these conditions, resulting in the risk of prematurely lowered muscle glycogen concentrations and accompanied decreases in prolonged exercise performance (27).

Despite the risk of rebound hypoglycemia, ingesting carbohydrates prior to exercise should not be totally avoided. A large meal can be eaten up to 6 h prior to competition, and smaller meal volumes providing less than 100 g of carbohydrate can be ingested up to 45 min before exercise without detriment to performance (33, 40, 48, 49, 55, 76, 90, 123, 124). Such added carbohydrate ingestion can further ensure maximal muscle and liver glycogen stores. Added carbohydrate can also be ingested in a liquid or carbohydrate form within 15 min prior to exercise. This short time interval, especially if it includes a warm-up, does not provide enough time for insulin to increase in the blood. In addition, exercise performed during or shortly after carbohydrate ingestion depresses the body's insulin response to a given increase in blood glucose, and the rebound hypoglycemic response is avoided. The ingestion of fructose prior to exercise does not have the same time constraints as glucose because of the low-glycemic response (101) (focus box 11.3).

FOCUS BOX 11.2

Recommendations for Increasing Muscle Glycogen Stores in the Days Prior to Prolonged Exercise

1. Plan to taper at least 1 week prior to the event.
2. In the final week, train as planned and eat your typical diet during the first 3 days.
3. For the 3 days prior to the day of the event, increase the carbohydrate content of the diet to approximately 10 g/kg body weight/day.

4. Refrain from training the day prior to the event.
5. Eat your final meal at least 3 h prior to the event.

Adapted from references (9 and 121).

Hydration and Fluid Ingestion Before Exercise During exercise the body continually loses water because of sweating. This fluid must be replaced to decrease the development of dehydration and its accompanied detriments to endurance performance. Athletes who intend to exercise for prolonged periods of time can prepare themselves by ensuring adequate hydration prior to starting exercise (table 11.3).

One strategy for ensuring optimal nutrition is to ingest excess fluid the day and evening prior to the prolonged event. This will ensure adequate hydration, and excess fluid will then be removed from the body by the kidney. However, research has also identified procedures to increase the body's fluid stores, which has been termed **hyperhydration.**

For hyperhydration to occur, the intravascular and/or extravascular compartments must be able to attract and retain added water and in doing so, prevent it from being filtered by the kidney (41, 113). Experimental procedures have succeeded in doing this by infusing an osmotic agent into the blood to retain water in the vascular space; this method has been shown to increase blood volume by 400 mL (91). The expansion of the blood volume by this method results in increased venous return and associated improvements in cardiovascular function (increased stroke volume, lowered heart rate), and enhances endurance performance. However, the artificial osmotic retention of water in the vascular space does not increase the body's ability to dissipate heat and dampen the increase in core temperature during prolonged exercise (91). In addition, the infusion of a foreign substance into the vasculature space of the body to enhance exercise performance can be questioned on medical and ethical grounds, and should not be condoned.

A hyperhydration procedure based on nutritional supplementation involves the ingestion of glycerol, a metabolite of the body, prior to exercise. Robergs and Griffin (113) have completed a thorough review of glycerol ingestion and how it influences body functions. The ingestion of glycerol (> 1.0 g/kg) with added water (26 mL/kg) can increase total body water compared to the ingestion of an equal volume of water, and like artificial plasma volume expansion, may icrease venous return during exercise and enhance exercise performance (82, 92, 109) (fig. 11.5). Unlike artificial plasma volume expansion, glycerol hydration does dampen the increase in core temperature during prolonged exercise, and therefore has thermoregulatory as well as cardiovascular benefits (82). When combined with carbohydrate ingestion during exercise (see sections to follow), hyperhydration may provide the athlete with a distinct advantage during prolonged exercise or exercise in a hot or humid environment, compared to athletes who rely on fluid ingestion during exercise to offset dehydration (91, 109, 112, 113). Nevertheless, symptoms associated with glycerol ingestion can include headache, blurred vision, light-headedness, and mild feelings of nausea (113).

FIGURE 11.3

When exercise is performed within 30 to 45 min after the ingestion of simple carbohydrates, the muscle contraction combined with increased circulating insulin can lower blood glucose concentrations. This hypoglycemia can be accompanied by increased perceptions of fatigue, or ratings of perceived exertion and impaired exercise performance.

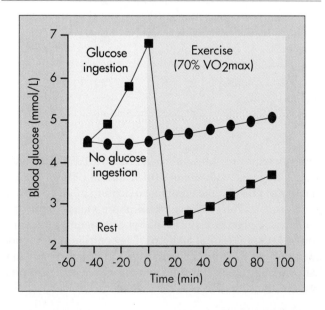

rebound hypoglycemia the decrease in blood glucose when exercising at least 30 min after the ingestion of carbohydrate

hyperhydration the increase in body water content above normal values

FOCUS BOX 11.3

Glycemic Index: Clinical and Applied Use

Nutritionists have developed a rating that compares different foods on their ability to raise blood glucose concentrations. This method is termed the **glycemic index**, and the blood glucose response to the ingestion of different foods is illustrated in figure 11.4. The reference standard for the glycemic index is the blood glucose response to the ingestion of white bread (133). This reference value is the area under the blood glucose concentration curve, and is denoted a value of 100. Other foods that have the same quantity of carbohydrate are compared as a percentage of this reference. For example, table 11.2 lists the glycemic index for several carbohydrate-containing foods.

In general, more complex carbohydrates will cause a lower glycemic index compared to simple forms. However, the glycemic index is not just a reflection of the type of carbohydrate in the food. For foods that have greater fat or fiber content than white bread, the digestion of carbohydrate will be slowed and there will be less of an increase in blood glucose. The same is true when mixing foods of a different glycemic index.

The use of the glycemic index has been applied to maximizing muscle glycogen synthesis during the immediate hours after exercise (18, 64, 72). As explained in the text, high-glycemic index foods are better for optimizing muscle glycogen synthesis in the first 2h or recovery (18, 62).

TABLE 11.2

The glycemic index of several sources of carbohydrate

FOOD ITEM	GLYCEMIC INDEX
Cornflakes	121
Instant mashed potatoes	120
Whole wheat bread	100
Baked beans	70
Skim milk	46
White pasta (boiled)	45
Lentils (boiled)	36

Source: Adapted from Burke, Collier, and Hargreaves (18)

FIGURE 11.4

The different blood glucose responses to the ingestion of equal carbohydrate amounts from different food sources. The expression of the blood glucose response as a percentage of the glucose response to white bread ingestion is referred to as the glycemic index.

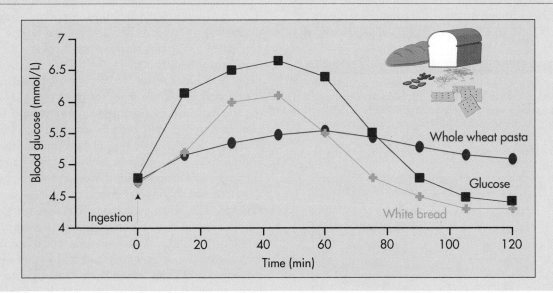

Nutrition During Exercise   The store of glycogen is limited in skeletal muscle and the liver, and approximates 150 to 250 mmol/kg and 300 to 350 mmol/kg wet wt, respectively. Because of the much larger mass of muscle tissue relative to the liver, far greater total glycogen stores are found in skeletal muscle. The duration that optimal muscle glycogen stores can supply substrate for energy metabolism can be estimated. For running, we can assume a prime moving muscle mass of 20 kg, and if running at an exercise intensity requiring 2.0 L/min at an RER of 1.0, there would be an energy expenditure of 10.1 kcal/min (90). For an efficiency of 40% for the complete oxidation of glucose from glycogen (–277.4/–686 kcal/mol), these values would enable muscle glycogen stores to support running for a duration of 110 min (see calculation). The contribution of blood glucose derived from the liver to skeletal muscle metabolism would prolong this time, but only by a small duration (< 20 min).

FIGURE 11.5

Prior to exercise, increased total body water stores can be attained from the ingestion of fluid containing less than 50 g/L of glycerol. This process of hyperhydration can decrease urine output and increase total body weight (body fluid content), and result in improved exercise performance as measured by decreased heart rates, lower rectal temperatures, and prolonged exercise durations until volitional fatigue.

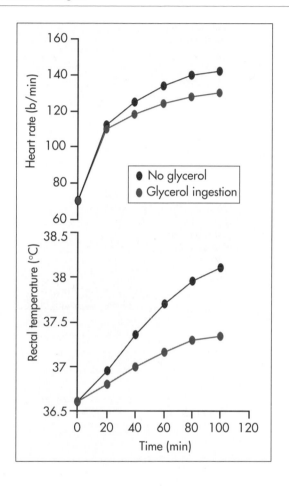

kcal from glycogen:

277.4 kcal/mol × 0.2 mol glycogen/kg muscle × 20 kg
= 1109.6 kcal

kcal expended during exercise when VO_2 = 2.0 L/min and RER = 1.0:

2.0 LO_2/min × 5.05 kcal/min = 10.1 kcal/min

Exercise duration:

1109.6 kcal / 10.1 kcal/min = 110 min

The main interpretation of the previous calculation is that *exercise performed when predominantly reliant on carbohydrate as a substrate cannot be maintained for much longer than 2 h.* After this time muscle and liver glycogen stores are at risk of being depleted, and continued exercise will require the ingestion of carbohydrate to prevent hypoglycemia and delay fatigue and the accompanied detriments to exercise performance.

Figure 11.6 illustrates the ergogenic benefit provided by the ingestion of carbohydrate during prolonged exercise. Research has shown that this benefit can be obtained when carbohydrate is ingested at repeated intervals during exercise (25, 32, 36, 82), during the initial 60 min (127, 128), or simply 30 min prior to the expected time of fatigue (24). A previously accepted interpretation of the latter finding is that *carbohydrate ingestion during prolonged continuous exercise at between 65 and 75% VO_{2max} does not spare muscle glycogen*, but simply provides an added supplement to blood glucose that only becomes important when muscle glycogen stores are near depletion and blood glucose becomes the main source of glucose for the contracting muscle (24, 25, 31). However, this interpretation has been questioned by Tsintzas and associates (127), who demonstrated that CHO ingestion during the intial hour of prolonged exercise resulted in a sparing of glycogen in type I muscle fibers. The implication of fiber type specific muscle glycogen changes to exercise performance and impending fatigue requires further investigation.

Research of continuous exercise performed at low intensities (< 60% VO_{2max}) indicates that muscle glycogen is spared because of a larger insulin reponse from ingesting carbohydrate compared to exercise performed at or above 70% VO_{2max} (55, 135). When continuous exercise during competition is performed at or above 70% VO_{2max}, the latter findings of glycogen sparing during carbohydrate ingestion have limited practical significance. In addition, carbohydrate ingestion during intermittent exercise may have the ability to increase muscle glycogen synthesis during the recovery intervals, and thereby act to prolong the time until muscle and liver glycogen stores are depleted (135).

Optimal Fluid and Carbohydrate Ingestion During Exercise

Liquid carbohydrate There are various types of carbohydrate, and these can be ingested in either liquid or solid forms. Research of liquid carbohydrate ingestion during exercise reveals the preference of glucose as the main form of carbohydrate. Drinks too high in fructose content may irritate the stomach and small intestine, thereby decreasing gastric emptying (16, 26, 87). In addition, fructose is poorly taken up by skeletal muscle and incorporated into glycolysis, and is not effective in raising blood glucose concentrations. Conversely, *fructose is a good gluconeogenic substrate for the liver.* Sports beverages (focus box 11.4) can also contain chains of glucose molecules that are connected, called **glucose polymers.** *Multidextran* is one such glucose polymer.

glycemic index a rating of the increase in blood glucose after the ingestion of a standard amount of carbohydrate, based on a comparison to the blood glucose response following the ingestion of an equivalent amount of carbohydrate in the form of white bread

glucose polymers glucose residues connected to form a chain structure

TABLE 11.3

Recommendations and guidelines for fluid ingestion before, during, and after exercise

CONDITION	EXERCISE TYPE AND DURATION	CONTENTS	DOSAGE	VOLUME
Preexercise*	Continuous or intermittent, < 60 min	Carbohydrate		7 mL/kg
		Glucose	6g/100 mL	
		Fructose	0	
		Electrolytes		
		Na^+	10–20 mEq/L	
		Cl^-	10–20 mEq/L	
		K^+	5–10 mEq/L	
		Glycerol	0	
	Continuous or intermittent, > 60 min	Carbohydrate		26 mL/kg
		Glucose	6–8 g/100 mL	
		Fructose	0.5–1.0g /100 mL	
		Electrolytes		
		Na^+	20–30 mEq/L	
		Cl^-	20–30 mEq/L	
		K^+	5–10 mEq/L	
		Glycerol	1.2 g/kg	
	Continuous or intermittent, short-term intense	Carbohydrate		7 mL/kg
		Glucose	6–8 g/100 mL	
		Fructose	0	
		Electrolytes		
		Na^+	10–20 mEq/L	
		Cl^-	10–20 mEq/L	
		K^+	0	
		Glycerol	0	
During exercise	Continuous or intermittent, < 60 min	Carbohydrate		7 mL/kg
		Glucose	0	water only
		Fructose	0	
		Electrolytes		
		Na^+	0	
		Cl^-	0	
		K^+	0	
		Glycerol	0	
	Continuous or intermittent, > 60 min	Carbohydrate		7–15 mL/kg/h‡
		Glucose	6–8 g/100 mL	
		Fructose	0.5–1.0g /100 mL	
		Electrolytes		
		Na^+	10–20 mEq/L	
		Cl^-	10–20 mEq/L	
		K^+	5–10 mEq/L	
		Glycerol	2 g/100 mL§	

Originally, these forms of carbohydrate were theorized to aid gastric emptying by providing carbohydrate calories with fewer particles in solution, or a lower *osmolality*. However, research has shown that drinks with this form of carbohydrate do not empty faster than pure glucose or glucose/fructose mix solutions of a similar carbohydrate content (87, 89).

The amount of carbohydrate needed to be ingested to provide an ergogenic effect approximates 45 to 60 g CHO/h (25, 35). Presumably, sufficient carbohydrate is needed to raise blood glucose concentrations and in turn increase glucose uptake by skeletal muscle.

The optimal carbohydrate concentration for a drink that is to be ingested during exercise is specific to the individual and environmental conditions that predominate during the exercise session. Research has presented contradictory findings of the carbohydrate concentrations that result in decreased rates of **gastric emptying** compared to water/electrolyte solution. When different sampling methods are considered, it is generally accepted that drink concentrations in excess of 80 g/L empty slower from the stomach than water, may cause gastric distress, and obviously may be detrimental to exercise performance (31, 87, 94, 95). Research of **intestinal absorption** also supports these findings (36, 44–47, 87). However, there is marked individual variability in the gastric emptying of carbohydrate solutions, and in the incidence of gastrointestinal distress (4, 87). *A carbohydrate concentration approximating 60 g/L or less is more appropriate for fluid delivery than more concentrated solutions.*

Table 11.6 presents a range of drink carbohydrate concentrations and drink volumes that can be ingested to hy-

TABLE 11.3

Recommendations and guidelines for fluid ingestion before, during, and after exercise

CONDITION	EXERCISE TYPE AND DURATION	CONTENTS	DOSAGE	VOLUME
	Continuous or intermittent, short-term intense	Carbohydrate		7–10 mL/kg/h[‡]
		Glucose	6–8 g/100 mL	
		Fructose	0	
		Electrolytes		
		Na$^+$	10–20 mEq/L	
		Cl$^-$	10–20 mEq/L	
		K$^+$	0.5–1.0 mEq/L	
		Glycerol	0	
Immediate[†] recovery from exercise	Continuous or intermittent, < 60 min	Carbohydrate		7 mL/kg
		Glucose	0	
		Fructose	0	
		Electrolytes		
		Na$^+$	0	
		Cl$^-$	0	
		K$^+$	0	
		Glycerol	0	
	Continuous or intermittent, > 60 min	Carbohydrate		7–15 mL/kg/h[‖]
		Glucose	6–8 g/100 mL	
		Fructose	0.5–1.0g /100 mL	
		Electrolytes		
		Na$^+$	30–40 mEq/L	
		Cl$^-$	30–40 mEq/L	
		K$^+$	5–10 mEq/L	
		Glycerol	5 g/100 mL[§]	
	Continuous or intermittent, short-term intense	Carbohydrate		7–10mL/kg/h[‖]
		Glucose	6–8 g/100 mL	
		Fructose	0	
		Electrolytes		
		Na$^+$	10–20 mEq/L	
		Cl$^-$	10–20 mEq/L	
		K$^+$	5–10 mEq/L	
		Glycerol	0.5–1.0g /100 mL	

*Within 2 h prior to exercise.
[†]Within 2 h after exercise.
[‡]Depends on rate of fluid loss.
[§]Not yet verified by research.
[‖]Depends on total amount of fluid loss.

Source: Based on data from Freund et al. (41), Gisolfi (47), Maughan et al. (88), Montner et al. (92), Nose et al. (98, 99), and Robergs and Griffin (113).

drate the body and support energy metabolism during exercise. The higher the carbohydrate concentration of the drink, the greater is the carbohydrate delivery to the body, but the lower is the fluid delivery to the body because of impaired gastric emptying, especially for drinks providing more than 120 g/L of carbohydrate (fig. 11.7). Nevertheless, because of the overriding influence of the volume of a drink on gastric emptying, it is unclear whether frequent ingestion that maintains a larger gastric volume, or infrequent larger fluid intakes is most desirable for fluid delivery.

As research has shown that carbohydrate provision may not be important until late in exercise for prolonged continuous exercise events (24, 25), a low-concentration drink may be recommended for the first 60 to 90 min for fluid replenishment purposes. During the last 30 to 60 min of a long-term activity, a drink with an increased carbohydrate concentration would be needed. Similarly, if environmental conditions are hot and/or humid, a drink composition low in carbohydrate would favor fluid delivery to the body, and therefore assist in the prevention of dehydration and hyperthermia. As the maximal rate of gastric emptying approximates 1200 mL/h (35), a carbohydrate concentration and drink volume association that provides close to 1 L/h would be recommended for hydration purposes. As indicated in table 11.6, drinks at a concentration

gastric emptying the emptying of stomach contents into the small intestine

intestinal absorption the absorption of water and organic and inorganic nutrients from the small intestine

FOCUS BOX 11.4

Commercial Sports Beverages and Energy Bars: Are They All They Claim to Be?

The increased popularity and need for daily physical activity and exercise has spawned a diverse exercise nutrition market. On the shelves of supermarkets are numerous drinks and solid food items that are proposed to not just provide fluid, but also essential nutrients that will improve muscle metabolism and exercise performance (tables 11.4 and 11.5).

The contents of a sports drink have been discussed in the text. However, it should be stated that there is nothing "magical" about any sports beverage. Research has clearly shown that the ingestion of carbohydrate (CHO) solutions during exercise can be beneficial, but there is no evidence that any drink is superior for any reason other than the carbohydrate content (table 11.6). Thus, drinks that provide the sufficient amount of carbohydrate, with the majority of the CHO source as glucose, flavored and lightly salted to improve taste, is all that is required. Obviously, these drinks can be made by any enthusiastic recreational or elite athlete, at a fraction of the cost of the commercial beverage!

The solid food items that are commercially available have been spawned by the need to provide a calorically dense, yet light-weight source of fuel for athletes/individuals involved in extremely prolonged exercise (> 2 h) who cannot afford to haul a water-based caloric supplement. As research has shown that solid carbohydrate is as effective in providing CHO as a liquid source (54, 62, 84), a solid food alternative to liquid CHO is valid.

The solid food alternative to a liquid carbohydrate is also advantageous in providing calories from fat and protein. In addition, some nutrition companies are including antioxidant ingredients to improve protection from oxidant stress (vitamins C and E and selenium), choline to support neural function, and further supplementing vitamin intake. As such, many of the solid food items are not just food bars to ingest during exercise, but can also be used as a meal replacement.

TABLE 11.4

Nutrient and electrolyte content of commercial sports beverages and other solutions

DRINK	TOTAL CHO (g/100 mL)	SODIUM (mEq/L)	POTASSIUM (mEq/L)	CAFFEINE (mg/L)	OSMOLALITY (mOsmol/kg)
10K	6.3	52	26		350
Coca-Cola	10.7	2	0	136.8	554
Cranberry juice	10–15	2	7		890
Dioralyte	1.6	60	20		?
Exceed	6.0	21	3		250
Gatorade	6.0	21	3		280
Isostar	7.6	24	4		305
Orange juice	11.8	0.5	58		690
Sprite	10.2	5	0		695
Water	0	Trace	Trace		0–20

Adapted from Gisolfi and Duchman (47), and Brouns, Kovacs, and Senden (17).

between 40 to 80 g/L carbohydrate would satisfy these requirements.

It must be understood that research has only shown that carbohydrate ingestion during exercise is beneficial during prolonged exercise when muscle glycogen concentrations are near depletion and blood glucose concentrations decline to below 3 mmol/L (25, 32). *When preexercise nutrition has been adequate, there is no metabolic or ergogenic need to ingest carbohydrate during continuous exercise lasting less than 90 min* (table 11.4, focus box 11.4). This is important, because carbohydrate ingestion during short-term exercise involves excess caloric intake, which for the majority of individuals who exercise is counterproductive to using exer-

cise as a means to generate a caloric deficit. However, because carbohydrate and fluid intake during exercise have independent benefits to exercise performance (6), fluid intake should always be of concern during exercise.

Solid carbohydrate   Although the research of carbohydrate ingestion before, during, and after exercise has predominantly used liquid beverages, blood glucose is also maintained during exercise when solid carbohydrate supplementation is provided (54, 62, 84). Of course, water should be ingested to aid in the digestion of the food and emptying the stomach, and to prevent exercise-induced dehydration (see focus box 11.4).

TABLE 11.5

Caloric content and additional nutrients provided in "energy bars"

ITEM	TOTAL WEIGHT (g)	TOTAL KCAL*	TOTAL CHO (g)	TOTAL FAT (g)	TOTAL PROTEIN (g)	FIBER (g)	Na⁺ (mg)	K⁺ (mg)	OTHER NUTRIENTS
Cliff Bar™	68	245	42	4	9	5	50	230	Ca, Fe, B_6, B_{12}, A, $C^\dagger$, $E^\dagger$, selenium†
High Protein Steel Bar	85	330	52	6	16	1	210	?	Ca, P, Mg, Zn, Fe, Cu, A, $C^\dagger$, D, $E^\dagger$, B_1, B_2, B_3, B_6, B_{12}, D, folate, biotin, pantothenic acid, iodine
Power Bar™	65	230	45	2.5	10	?			Ca, P, Mg, Zn, Fe, Cu, A, $C^\dagger$, D, $E^\dagger$, B_1, B_2, B_3, B_6, B_{12}, folate, biotin, pantothenic acid
PR Ironman Triathlon	56.8	230	25	7	16	0	220	130	Ca, P, Mg, Zn, Fe, Cu, A, $C^\dagger$, D, $E^\dagger$, B_1, B_2, B_3, B_6, B_{12}, folate, biotin, pantothenic acid
Tiger Bar	35	145	18	5	7	1	70	?	Ca, P, Mg, Zn, Fe, Cu, A, $C^\dagger$, D, B_1, B_2, B_3, B_6, B_{12}, biotin, pantothenic acid
Tiger Sport	65	230	43	2.5	10	3	110	?	Ca, P, Mg, Zn, Fe, Cu, A, $C^\dagger$, $E^\dagger$, B_1, B_2, B_3, B_6, B_{12}, folate, biotin, chromium, pantothenic acid

*Per serving (1 bar).
† Antioxidants.
Note: A = vitamin A, C = vitamin C, D = vitamin D, E = vitamin E, B_1 = vitamin B_1 (thiamin), B_2 = vitamin B_2 (riboflavin), B_3 = vitamin B_3 (niacin), B_6 = vitamin B_6 (pyridoxine), B_{12} = vitamin B_{12} (cobalamin), Ca = calcium, Cu = copper, P = phosphorus, Fe = iron, Zn = zinc.

Source: From manufacturer's food labels.

Hydration and fluid ingestion during exercise   Previous comment has been given to the importance of fluid ingestion before exercise. When exercising in a hot or humid environment, the body can lose water at a maximal rate of between 2 and 3 L/h through sweat (fig. 11.8), and the majority of this fluid comes from the cells and interstitial spaces of the body (97), resulting in **dehydration**. However, the largest relative decrease in fluid volume occurs from the vascular compartment (decreased plasma volume). Obviously, without fluid replacement, these rates of water loss cannot be maintained for long and the rate of sweating decreases, which, as will be explained in chapter 19, further adds to the risks of heat illness.

Despite the difficulty in ingesting large fluid volumes during prolonged exercise, some individuals have accomplished this. If the fluid ingested at such large volumes has a low osmolality, individuals can become at risk for the development of **water intoxication** (97). This condition can be dangerous as large volumes of fluid with a low osmolality

dehydration a decreased water content of the body below normal

water intoxication water ingestion that causes decreased blood concentrations of electrolytes, especially sodium

FIGURE 11.6

The ingestion of carbohydrate high in glucose content during exercise can increase blood glucose concentrations, and prolong the exercise duration to volitional fatigue. Carbohydrate ingestion late in exercise can produce similar results.

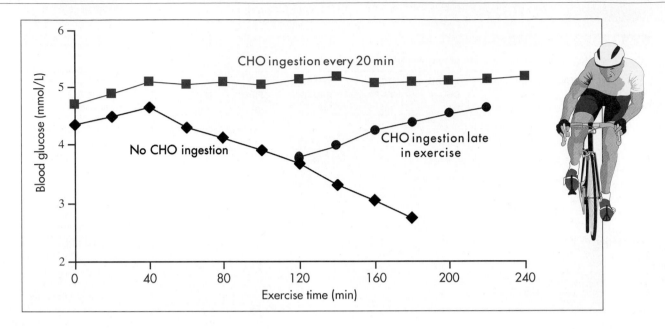

leach electrolytes from the blood bathing the stomach and small intestine, resulting in a lowering of the serum sodium concentration to below 130 mmol/L, a condition termed **hyponatremia** (94, 96). During ultraendurance events, the incidence of hyponatremia has been reported to be 0.03% of the total number of competitors, with at least a 10% incidence in those runners who collapse and require medical assistance (96).

Postexercise Nutrition   Many athletes need to train several times a day, or compete with the need to perform prolonged exercise bouts on consecutive days (e.g., Tour DeFrance Cycle Race). These demands require that the individual attempt to optimize the recovery process regarding hydration and muscle glycogen synthesis.

Rehydration Following Exercise   Of course, the best strategy to treat dehydration is prevention. However, as previously explained, it is difficult for most individuals to replace fluid equal to its loss during prolonged exercise, and especially in a competitive environment. Therefore, exercise-induced dehydration is always a concern and, for this reason, research has been conducted to determine procedures for optimal fluid replacement or **rehydration** during the recovery.

Ingestion of pure water causes less fluid retention in the body when dehydrated compared to carbohydrate-electrolyte drinks and relatively high-concentration (80–100 mmol/L) electrolyte drinks (41, 45, 47, 113). The reason for this difference is that the ingestion of carbohydrate and electrolyte drinks maintains a higher osmolality of the blood than does water. A higher osmolality retains more of the antidiuretic hormone stimuli for water conservation by the kidney and, therefore, less fluid is lost in the urine. Data also ex-

ist that show carbonated beverages are as beneficial for rehydration as noncarbonated beverages (78). Based on the evidence that glycerol ingestion can increase the osmalality of body fluids and decrease urine volume, even when compared to electrolyte solutions (109), added ingestion of glycerol with carbohydrate-electrolyte solutions may further benefit rehydration (113).

Factors That Determine Postexercise Muscle Glycogen Synthesis   Unfortunately, research has provided only estimations of the maximal rate of postexercise muscle glycogen synthesis after 2 h of recovery (107, 111). Nevertheless, on the basis of in vitro research on the regulation of glycogen synthetase and the fact that glucose uptake and synthetase activity are inversely affected by the amount of glycogen present (39, 75, 136), it is likely that muscle glycogen synthesis is maximal immediately after exercise and then decreases exponentially (111). Optimal nutrition conditions for muscle glycogen synthesis need to be fostered as soon after exercise as possible.

Exercise determinants   The rate of postexercise muscle glycogen synthesis will depend on whether the previous bout of exercise damaged skeletal muscle. Exercise that has an eccentric component such as running, or involves body contact such as football (American or Australian) or ice hockey, can result in microscopic damage to skeletal muscle fibers. This damage is known to stimulate the infiltration of white blood cells, which rely on blood glucose as their sole energy substrate. Consequently, the local increase in white blood cells within skeletal muscle will compete for blood glucose, resulting in a decreased rate of muscle glycogen synthesis.

TABLE 11.6

Volume of drink at given carbohydrate concentrations that must be ingested every 20 min to provide certain amounts of carbohydrate per hour

| | HOURLY AMOUNT OF CHO INGESTION (g) | | | | | | |
| | DRINK VOLUME (mL) | | | | | | |
CHO (g/L)	30	35	40	45	50	55	60
20	500	583	667	750	833	917	1000
30	333	389	444	500	555	611	667
40	250	291	333	375	416	458	500
50	200	233	267	300	333	367	400
60	167	194	222	250	278	306	333
70	142	167	190	214	238	262	286
80	125	145	166	187	208	227	250
90	111	130	148	167	185	204	222
100	100	116	133	150	166	183	200
110	91	106	121	135	151	167	182
120	83	97	111	125	139	153	166
150	67	78	89	100	111	122	133
200	50	65	74	75	83	91	100

Source: Adapted from Coyle and Montain (35).

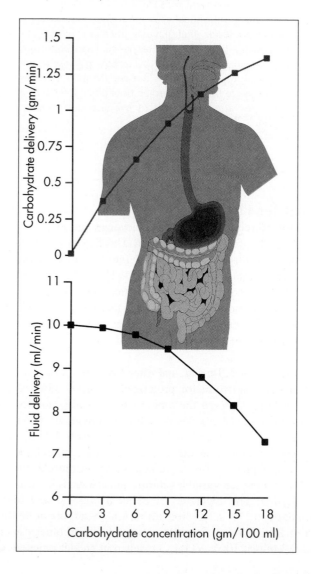

FIGURE 11.7

The relationship between the carbohydrate content of a drink and each of carbohydrate and fluid delivery to the body.

However, because the infiltration of white blood cells requires at least 12 h (30, 37, 120), it is known that carbohydrate intake during the immediate hours after exercise can sustain rates of glycogen synthesis comparable to conditions of no muscle damage. In addition, increasing the carbohydrate ingested during recovery can further increase blood glucose, which in turn provides added glucose availability for the muscle despite increasing white blood cell proliferation (30, 37).

Muscle glycogen synthesis is decreased during an active recovery (11, 14); however, if the active recovery is at a low intensity (< 35% VO$_{2max}$), some glycogen can be stored in fast-twitch muscle, which is not being recruited at these low intensities (99, 105, 132).

Nutritional determinant The optimal rate of carbohydrate ingestion after exercise approximates 0.7 g/kg body wt/h (10–12, 63, 64, 103, 107, 116, 122, 136) and is associated with a rate of glycogen synthesis approximating between 7

hyponatremia (hi'po-na-tre'mi-ah) a decrease in the serum concentration of sodium below 135 mmol/L

rehydration the return of water to the body during recovery from dehydration

FOCUS BOX 11.5

Nutritional Concerns for Athletes Involved In Weight Maintenance, Body Weight Reduction, or Increased Body Weight

For athletes who participate in wrestling, boxing, ballet dancing, horse racing, rowing, or other sports requiring performance categories based on body weight or aesthetics, practices to rapidly lose weight are promoted and condoned. In certain circumstances, the routine completion of these practices may be detrimental to long-term nutrition and health. Conversely, some individuals are required to increase body mass, preferably by a selective increase in lean body weight. Unfortunately, for some sports the health and body composition implications of weight gain are not always the most performance-enhancing end objective (e.g., sumo wrestling). The specific nutritional demands of either dietary and exercise intervention require clarification.

Body Weight Maintenance and Reduction

The mass of water (1g/mL), its contribution to total body mass (65 to 75% by weight), and relative ease of removal from the body (exercise-induced sweating can lose between 1 to 3 L/h), result in dehydration as a preferred means of weight loss. Dehydration is problematic to individuals who must exercise. Dehydration to levels where more than 2% of the body weight has been lost is known to be detrimental to prolonged as well as short-term intense exercise (125).

The more serious nutritional concern for individuals who must constantly lose or retain a low weight is the development of malnutrition (125). Numerous studies have reported that athletes who routinely lose weight rapidly have poor diets, resulting in the ingestion of micronutrients at amounts less than the RDA, and have clinically diagnosed eating disorders (21, 125). The main micronutrients of concern are iron and calcium, which for females is bothersome because of the already relatively low iron stores and the connection between low dietary calcium and an increased risk of osteoporosis. For these individuals, it is not the exercise that demands increased macro- and micronutrient intake, but the presence of an unbalanced diet that is mainly caused by an insufficient caloric intake (125).

Gaining Weight

Unfortunately, the specific dietary and exercise strategies best used for weight gain while still promoting cardiovascular health has not been researched with the fervor of weight loss. For the athlete and nonathletic individual, weight gain by increasing lean body mass is the most desirable for health reasons. Commonsense recommendations would include selecting foods that have high-caloric density but will not induce a high-glycemic response. Lean body mass increases would be maximized by including a resistance-exercise training program into the weight gain program. Research needs to be conducted on the interaction between different types and intensities of exercise and diets on weight gain.

---

and 9 mmol/kg/h (10, 12, 63, 64, 103, 108, 111, 122, 136). Increase of carbohydrate does not increase glycogen synthesis (10, 63, 107, 111); however, addition of protein to the liquid carbohydrate solution may further increase the rate of glycogen synthesis because of an increased release of insulin (137). The carbohydrate should be in the form of glucose, sucrose, or glucose polymers in liquid form, or if in solid form, should be of a high-glycemic index (16, 29, 84) (focus box 11.3).

If there is a delay in ingesting the carbohydrate, the rate of glycogen synthesis is reduced considerably. For example, delaying the carbohydrate ingestion until 2 h postexercise can decrease the rate of synthesis from 7 mmol/kg/h to less than 3 mmol/kg/h (62).

Demands of Exercise Performed on Consecutive Days   When exercise is performed on consecutive days there is a need to replenish muscle glycogen within a 24-h period (90). Research has clearly shown that muscle glycogen can be returned to normal resting values within 24 h (9, 78, 100, 107); however, when there is muscle damage muscle glycogen replenishment may take several days (28, 38, 122).

Short-Term Intense Exercise

Intense exercise requires the rapid degradation of muscle glycogen as explained in chapter 6. This fact is true, even for exercise performed to volitional fatigue for durations as short as several minutes (110, 111). These facts stress that carbohydrate nutrition may also be important for intense exercise (13). In addition, the muscle damage experienced during intense exercise and the subsequent hypertrophy may also increase the need for protein in the diet.

Nutrition Before, During, and After Exercise   Compared to preexercise nutrition for prolonged exercise, minimal research has addressed the topic of nutritional needs for intense exercise (13, 50–52), or for those individuals who need to lose weight or gain lean body mass (focus box 11.5). In a series of studies conducted by scientists in Scotland, the influence of preexercise diet composition on muscle, blood, and performance variables during intense exercise was investigated. The ingestion of either a high-fat and high-protein diet (3% CHO in kcal) or a high-carbohydrate diet (87% kcal) for 4 days prior to intense cycle ergometer exercise (3 min at 100% VO_{2max}) resulted in greater preexercise muscle glycogen concentrations in the high-carbohydrate diet trial, and greater use of glycogen during the exercise (50–52). During the high-fat and high-protein diet, muscle acidosis was more severe after exercise than on the carbohydrate diet, which indicated that the muscle and/or blood buffer capacity is lowered by a high-fat and high-protein diet. When comparing a normal carbohydrate diet to a high-carbohydrate diet, greater acidosis occurred during the high-carbohydrate diet (50). These results indicate that intense exercise may be deterimentally affected by either a low- or very high-carbohydate diet. It is therefore recommended that *individuals involved in intense exercise should eat moderate amounts of carbohydrate, and should not complete a regimen of carbohydrate supercompensation in preparation for intense exercise.*

Finally, as explained in chapter 6, muscle glycogen stores as low as 50 mmol/kg wet wt have not been shown to detrimentally affect intense exercise performance. This provides further evidence that supports the decreased importance of preexercise carbohydrate nutrition for intense compared to prolonged steady-state exercise.

Factors That Determine Postexercise Muscle Glycogen Synthesis   The large degradation of muscle glycogen during intense exercise demands that glycogen stores be replenished as rapidly as possible during the recovery from exercise. However, research has shown that carbohydrate ingestion during the recovery from high-intensity exercise is not necessary because glycogen synthesis rates as high as 15 mmol/kg wet wt/h have been reported without carbohydrate ingestion (61, 110).

Micronutrient Concerns Before, During, and After Exercise

From the previous discussions it should be clear that a well-balanced diet that provides sufficient calories also provides all the micronutrients, in adequate amounts, that are required to sustain exercise of different types, intensities, and durations. Nevertheless, questions remain as to whether vitamin and mineral supplementation can improve exercise performance.

On the basis of the research on fluid ingestion during or after exercise and body hydration, an argument can be made for the need for sodium. However, this need applies only to prolonged exercise performed in an environment that causes high sweat rates resulting in losses of body water between 1 and 3 L/h. In these circumstances sodium ingestion in liquid beverages improves drink palatability (84), assists in the absorption of fluid from the small intestine (41–43, 78), and prevents excess fluid loss in urine (67, 98, 99, 117). Although it has been theorized that sodium should increase glucose absorption by the small intestine, there is no experimental evidence for this effect (58).

Another issue that is raised concerning electrolytes is whether sufficient electrolytes are lost in sweat to require

FIGURE 11.8

During prolonged exercise inducing profuse sweating, the body can become dehydrated, resulting in increases in heart rate, core temperature, and perceptions of fatigue. When liquid is ingested during exercise, the increase in heart rate, core temperature, and perceptions of fatigue are depressed and exercise can be performed for longer durations until volitional fatigue.

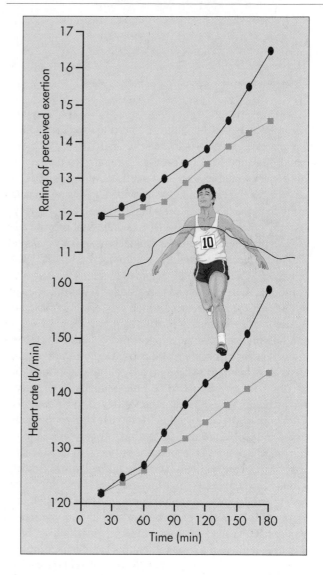

supplementation for replacement during or after exercise. Table 11.7 presents the concentration of the electrolytes in sweat and plasma, and the amounts of these electrolytes lost during exercise-induced dehydration. Because the duct of the sweat gland absorbs most of the electrolyes before excretion to the surface of the skin, electrolyte loss through sweat is minimal. The main electrolyte of concern is sodium and, as has been previously discussed, sodium decreases in blood are caused by a combination of loss through sweat and redistribution within the body. Sodium redistribution into the small intestine increases when ingesting hypotonic (drink osmolality less than blood osmolality) drinks (86).

TABLE 11.7

The concentrations of electrolytes in plasma, sweat, and the loss of electrolytes during exercise[*]

ELECTROLYTE	PLASMA [] (mEq/L)	SWEAT [] (mEq/L)	LOSSES[*] (mEq)
Na^+	140	40-60	155
K^+	4	4-5	16
Cl^-	101	30-50	137
Mg^{++}	1.5	1.5-5	13
Osmolality	302	80-185	

[*]From exercise-induced dehydration of –5.8%, from Costill (28).

FIGURE 11.9

Intense exercise, such as weight lifting, can increase markers of the catabolism of muscle contractile proteins (3-methylhistidine). Similar evidence of increased protein catabolism exists during endurance training.

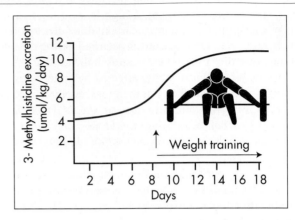

This evidence does not indicate a need to ingest salt tablets during exercise, which would cause a large loss of water into the small intestine to decrease the osmolality of the chyme, which in turn would exacerbate the effects of dehydration on exercise performance. Similarly, the evidence does not indicate a need to increase the intake of sodium after exercise. Ingesting a rehydration beverage that contains sodium will provide adequate sodium replenishment in the initial hours of recovery and, because the typical diet provides sodium in excess of the RDA, body sodium stores are rapidly returned to normal.

Although there are claims that added vitamins can increase exercise performance, which are probably based on their major roles in energy metabolism (see table 11.1), no research evidence exists to support these claims (5). However, current research interest has focused on the potential need to destroy tissue-damaging by-products of metabolism called **free radicals** (68). Free radicals have only a very short half-life (< 1 s), but are believed to be responsible for some of the microscopic tissue damage accompanying exercise (3). Vitamin E, vitamin C, β-carotene, and selenium are known to protect the body against tissue damage from free radicals and are termed **antioxidants.** The body increases its own antioxidant function in response to exercise training; however, it is thought that during strenuous bouts of exercise antioxidant supplementation may reduce tissue damage (119). Nevertheless, other researchers believe the research on this topic is incomplete, and a clear statement on the benefit of antioxidant supplementation by individuals who perform strenuous exercise cannot be made as yet (69).

Long-Term Macronutrient Concerns for Those Who Exercise

Comment has already been given to the need for raising the carbohydrate content and lowering the fat content of the diet for individuals who participate in prolonged exercise. Of more interest to long-term dietary macronutrient needs of athletes is the amount of ingested protein.

Traditionally, the RDA for protein has been refuted to be adequate, even for individuals involved in intense exercise to induce increases in muscle mass. However, recent research has indicated that the RDA may not be appropriate for highly trained endurance athletes, as well as athletes involved in intense exercise training (80, 81). For highly trained individuals, there is an increase in protein catabolism that must be compensated for by an increased protein intake. For example, during training involving weight resistance exercise, the urinary excretion of **3-methylhistidine,** a marker of skeletal muscle actin and myosin catabolism, increased after only 3 days of training (104) (fig. 11.9). Research using **nitrogen balance** techniques (81), which are required to determine if subjects are either gaining or losing protein, has shown that weight training exercise may require a protein intake approximating 1.6 to 1.7 g/kg/day to be in nitrogen balance, which is more than double the RDA. Current evidence indicates that additional strength or hypertrophy does not occur when the RDA is exceeded for periods of less than 6 weeks. However, it remains to be proved that added hypertrophy does not occur when athletes are in positive nitrogen balance for extended periods of time, as is the claim by those individuals who train for body building.

Because a well-balanced diet that is sufficient in calories generally provides almost double the RDA for protein, these results indicate that although an increased RDA is necessary, the typical diet does not need supplementation to attain this (19). Consequently, although some research has indicated that increases in protein intake to 2 g/kg body wt/day may be inadequate for some individuals (23), the combined effects of caloric intake, energy expenditure, and training adaptation on influencing nitrogen balance make a definitive recommendation of protein needs for athletes impossible at this time (126).

Long-Term Micronutrient Concerns for Those Who Exercise

Long-term micronutrient concerns mainly apply to individuals who exercise and have poor dietary habits. For example, the need for vitamins C and B_6 may increase during exercise, but usually there are adequate stores within the body. For individuals with low vitamin C or B$_6$ intake, supplemental ingestion of these vitamins is known to be beneficial (77). Also, added vitamin C intake for individuals who train and compete in marathon and ultraendurance events has been shown to decrease the incidence of upper–respiratory tract infection and reduce the duration of the infection (20, 43). Similar long-term benefits may also exist for antioxidant intake, although this remains to be proved.

Of greatest concern to individuals is the intake of iron. Iron is an important component of hemoglobin and myoglobin, and is therefore essential for the transport of oxygen in blood, and the delivery of oxygen from the blood to the muscle tissues, and then to the mitochondria of the muscle fibers. Depleted iron stores have been reported in both male and female runners (22, 83, 84), although the incidence is greater in females and, ironically, the incidence in athletes is generally no greater than that of sedentary controls (22). Early stages of iron deficiency are measured as a decrease in serum **ferritin** levels (the main storage form of iron). Serum ferritin levels are known to decrease during periods of intense training (83), but these decreases are not associated with decrements in exercise performance (85). Supplementation of iron improves body iron

stores, but only increases exercise performance in individuals who are diagnosed as being iron deficient (anemic) with low serum ferritin and blood hemoglobin concentrations (22, 74).

Despite the reported incidence of vitamin and mineral supplementation by athletes of 72% (51), studies that have been conducted on the effects of vitamin and mineral supplementation on exercise performance have shown no benefit (134). For athletes who consume a balanced diet, there is no need for micronutrient supplementation (3, 5, 77).

---

free radicals small molecules within the body that have an extremely high affinity for electrons

antioxidants substance that provides electrons to reduce free radicals, thus preserving other, more important molecules

3-methylhistidine (3-meth'il-his'ti-deen) methylated amino acid that is used as a urine marker for muscle protein catabolism

nitrogen balance equal nitrogen intake versus excretion from the body

ferritin (ferr'i-tin) the form of iron that is stored in the body

---

WEBSITE BOX

Chapter 11: Nutrition and Exercise

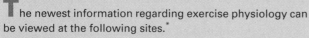

The newest information regarding exercise physiology can be viewed at the following sites.*

sportsci.org/
    Large site for sports scientists. In particular check out the "CompEat," "Training and Technology," and the "Nutrition" links within the "Net Links" sections.
http://arborcom.com/
    Huge site providing basic nutrition information—food, food science, and clinical and applied nutrition information.
nutribase.com/
    Interactive online food nutrient information database.
arfa.org/index.htm
    Excellent site providing comprehensive information on many topics within exercise physiology.
brainmac.demon.co.uk/whatsnew.htm
    Excellent site intended for coaches to have access to exercise-related information, including field tests of physical fitness, training strategies, nutrition, and coaching strategies.
gssi.web.com/membership/toc-sse.html
    Gatorade Sports Science Index—lists all publications of the Gatorade Sports Science Exchange.
curtin.edu.au/curtin/dept/physio/pt/edres/exphys/e552_96/
    Index of brief reviews of exercise physiology by students from Curtin University, Australia. Topics include nutrition,

ergogenic aids, environmental physiology, training, and clinical applications.
http://nimbus.ocis.temple.edu/~sklein/
    Summary on the use and abuse of creatine supplementation.
http://137.142.42.95/Students/Bio380/Flinton/Seminar/seminar2.html
    Slide format lecture material about caffeine as an ergogenic aid.
mediconsult.com
    Information source for any medical condition, including vitamins and nutrition.
vhttp://fitnesslink.com/nutri.htm
    Information-packed site on exercise and the mind and body, nutrition, fitness programs, how to train, and more.
playtextampons.com/doctor.htm
    Site that provides information on the menstrual cycle, and general questions and anwsers

---

*Unless indicated, all URLs preceded by http://www.

Note: These URLs were valid at the time of publication, but could have changed or been deleted from Internet access since that time.

SUMMARY

- **Nutrients** can be divided into the small compounds that are not catabolized to release free energy during energy metabolism: **micronutrients,** which consist of **vitamins** and **minerals,** and those nutrients that can be used during energy metabolism; **macronutrients,** which consist of carbohydrate, fat, protein, and water. The study of the nutrients needed by the body is termed **nutrition.**

- Of the three macronutrients, carbohydrate, fat, and protein, there is only an RDA for protein, which equals 0.8 g/kg body wt/day. Proteins that contain all the essential amino acids are termed **complete proteins.**

- For trained athletes, simply reducing the duration and frequency of training and increasing the carbohydrate content of the diet to above 10 g/kg/day during 3 days prior to competition increases muscle glycogen stores to their maximal values. This process has been termed **glycogen supercompensation.**

- Carbohydrate ingestion between 20 and 60 min prior to the start of exercise can increase both blood glucose and insulin concentrations, and result in a rapid fall in blood glucose after the start of exercise, or **rebound hypoglycemia.**

- Procedures to optimize fluid status have been termed **hyperhydration** and the ingestion of fluid-retaining substances, such as solutions of glycerol (< 50 g/L) have been shown to increase body water, improve thermoregulation during exercise, and prolong the time until fatigue during cycling at less than 70% VO_{2max}.

- When exercising for periods longer than 1.5 h, the ingestion of carbohydrate prevents hypoglycemia, delays fatigue, and therefore can improve exercise performance. This benefit can be obtained when carbohydrate is ingested at repeated intervals during exercise, before exercise, or simply 30 min prior to the expected time of fatigue. The amount of carbohydrate required is estimated at between 30 to 60 g/h and can be in liquid or solid form. Foods that cause a large increase in blood glucose, termed high **glycemic index** foods, are preferred sources of carbohydrate during, and immediately after exercise.

- The ingestion of drinks too high in fructose content may irritate the stomach, thereby decreasing **gastric emptying.** Drinks can also contain connected chains of glucose molecules, called **glucose polymers.** However, research has shown that drinks with this form of carbohydrate do not empty from the stomach faster than pure glucose or glucose/fructose–mix solutions of a similar carbohydrate content and drink volume.

- Drinks with carbohydrate concentrations in excess of 80 g/L empty slower from the stomach than water, may cause gastric distress, and obviously may be detrimental to exercise performance. Research of **intestinal absorption** also supports these findings. As the maximal rate of gastric emptying approximates 1200 mL/h, a carbohydrate concentration and drink volume association that provides close to 1 L/h would be recommended to decrease **dehydration.**

- Despite the difficulty in ingesting large fluid volumes during prolonged exercise, some individuals have accomplished this. If the fluid ingested at such large volumes has a low osmolality, individuals can become at risk for the development of **water intoxication,** which can lead to a life-threatening reduction in serum sodium concentrations, or **hyponatremia.**

- For purposes of **rehydration,** the ingestion of pure water causes less fluid retention in the body when dehydrated compared to a carbohydrate-electrolyte drink. The optimal rate of carbohydrate ingestion after exercise for muscle glycogen synthesis approximates 0.7 g/kg/h.

- A well-balanced diet that provides sufficient calories also provides all the micronutrients, and in adequate amounts, that are required to sustain exercise of different types, intensities, and durations. Although vitamins E and C, and selenium are known as **antioxidants** and can protect the body against tissue damage from **free radicals,** it is unknown how this protection functions, and what levels of these micronutrients offer greatest protection.

- For highly trained individuals there is an increase in protein catabolism, as measured by increased urinary **3-methylhistidine** and amino acid release from skeletal muscle, that must be compensated for by an increased protein intake that exceeds the RDA for protein. For example, weight training exercise may require a protein intake of 2 g/kg/day to be in **nitrogen balance,** which is more than double the RDA. Although an increased protein RDA is necessary for many athletes, the typical diet already provides protein ingestion in excess of the RDA, and therefore protein supplementation is not necessary.

- For athletes who consume a well-balanced diet, vitamin and mineral supplementation is not necessary. However, for athletes known to be low in iron stores (**ferritin**), or who have been diagnosed as anemic, iron supplementation is recommended.

STUDY QUESTIONS

1. Is there controversy over the recommended percentages of total caloric intake for each of the macronutrients in a healthy diet? Explain the reasons why the 60, 30, and 10% (CHO, fat, protein) recommendation may not be correct for athletes and nonathletes alike.

2. For healthy individuals who are concerned with exercise performance, why is carbohydrate the main macronutrient of interest?

3. What is the recommended procedure for maximizing muscle glycogen stores prior to exercise?

4. What is rebound hypoglycemia?

5. What is the glycemic index? Why and when are high-glycemic foods recommended for athletes?

6. What is the optimal carbohydrate concentration of a drink to increase fluid intake by the body, thereby delaying dehydration? Why?

7. What would be your dietary recommendations to an individual who must replenish muscle glycogen as rapidly as possible after exercise because of the need to compete/train again the same day?

8. Is the RDA for protein adequate for all individuals? Explain.

9. Why are free radicals and antioxidants of interest to exercise physiologists?

10. Is there any research evidence on the need to supplement micronutrient intake of certain populations in order to improve exercise performance? If so, explain.

APPLICATIONS

1. If you could prepare your own sports drink, what would it contain and in what concentrations?

2. Most individuals who exercise ingest sports beverages. Should all individuals ingest these beverages when they exercise? Explain.

3. If fat feeding during exercise can spare muscle glycogen, why isn't this a recommended strategy to improve athletic performance?

REFERENCES

1. Ahlborg, B., J. Bergstrom, L. G. Ekelund, and E. Hultman. Muscle glycogen, and muscle electrolytes during prolonged physical exercise. *Acta Physiol. Scand.* 70:129–142, 1967.

2. Ahlborg, G., and P. Felig. Substrate utilization during prolonged exercise preceded by ingestion of glucose. *Am. J. Physiol.* 233(3):E188–E194, 1977.

3. Anderson, R. A. New insights on the trace elements, chromium, copper and zinc, and exercise. In F. Brouns (ed.), *Advances in nutrition and top sport. Int. J. Sports Med.* 32:38–58, Karger, Basel, 1991.

4. Beckers, E. T., J. B. Leiper, and J. Davidson. Comparison of aspiration and scintigraphic techniques for the measurement of gastric emptying. *Gut.* 33:115–117, 1992.

5. Belko, A. Z. Vitamins and exercise—An update. *Med. Sci. Sports Exerc.* 19(5):S191–S196, 1987.

6. Below, P. R., R. Mora-Rodriquez, J. Gonzalez-Alonso, and E. F. Coyle. Fluid and carbohydrate ingestion independently improve performance during 1 h of intense exercise. *Med. Sci. Sports Exerc.* 27(20):200–210, 1995.

7. Bendich, A. Exercise and free radicals: Effects of antioxidant vitamins. In F. Brouns (ed.), *Advances in nutrition and top sport. Int. J. Sports Med.* 32:59–78, Karger, Basel, 1991.

8. Bergstrom, J., and E. Hultman. Muscle glycogen synthesis after exercise: An enhancing factor localized to the muscle cells in man. *Nature* 210:309–310, 1967.

9. Bergstrom, J., L. Hermansen, and B. Saltin. Diet, muscle glycogen and physical performance. *Acta Physiol. Scand.* 71:140–150, 1967.

10. Blom, P., O. Vaage, K. Kardel, and L. Hermansen. Effect of increasing glucose loads on the rate of muscle glycogen resynthesis after prolonged exercise. *Acta Physiol. Scand.* 108(2):C12, 1980.

11. Blom, P. C. S., N. K. Vollestad, and D. L. Costill. Factors affecting changes in muscle glycogen concentration during and after prolonged exercise. *Acta Physiol. Scand.* 128(Suppl. 556):67–74, 1986.

12. Blom, P. C. S., A. T. Hostmark, O. Vaage, K. R. Kadel, and S. Maehlum. Effect of different postexercise sugar diets on the rate of muscle glycogen resynthesis. *Med. Sci. Sports Exerc.* 19(5):491–496, 1987.

13. Bonen, A., S. A. Malcom, R. D. Kilgour, K. P. MacIntyre, and A. N. Belcastro. Glucose ingestion before and during intense exercise. *J. Appl. Physiol.* 50(4):766–771, 1981.

14. Bonen, A., G. W. Ness, A. N. Belcastro, and R. L. Kirby. Mild exercise impedes glycogen repletion in muscle. *J. Appl. Physiol.* 58(5):1622–1629, 1985.

REFERENCES

15. Bracy, D. A., B. A. Zinker, J. C. Jacobs, D. Brooks Lacy, and D. H. Wasserman. Carbohydrate metabolism during exercise: Influence of circulating fat availability. *J. Appl. Physiol.* 79(2):506–513, 1995.

16. Brouns, F. Gastrointestinal symptoms in athletes: Physiological and nutritional aspects. In F. Brouns (ed.), *Advances in nutrition and top sport. Int. J. Sport Med.* 32:166–199, Karger, Basel, 1991.

17. Brouns, R., E. M. R. Kovacs, and J. M. G. Senden. The effect of different rehydration drinks on postexercise electrolyte excretion in trained athletes. *Int. J. Sports Med.* 19:56–60, 1998.

18. Burke, L., G. R. Collier, and M. Hargreaves. Muscle glycogen storage after prolonged exercise: Effect of the glycemic index of carbohydrate feedings. *J. Appl. Physiol.* 75(2):1019–1023, 1993.

19. Butterfield, G. E. Whole-body protein utilization in humans. *Med. Sci. Sports Exerc.* 19(5):S157–S165, 1987.

20. Buzina, R., and K. Suboticanec. Vitamin C and physical working capacity. *Int. J. Vitamin Nutr. Res.* (Suppl. 27):157–166, 1985.

21. Calabrese, L. H., et al. Menstrual abnormalities, nutritional patterns, and body composition in female classical ballet dancers. *Phys. Sportsmed.* 11(2):86–98, 1983.

22. Clarkson, P. M. Tired blood: Iron deficiency in athletes and effects of iron supplementation. *Sports Sci. Exchange.* 1(28):1–5, 1990.

23. Clarkson, P. M. Trace mineral requirements for athletes: To supplement or not to supplement. *Sports Sci. Exchange* 4(33):1–6, 1991.

24. Coggan, A. R., and E. F. Coyle. Metabolism and performance following carbohydrate late in exercise. *Med. Sci. Sports Exerc.* 21(1):59–65, 1989.

25. Coggan, A. R., and E. F. Coyle. Carbohydrate ingestion during prolonged exercise: Effects on metabolism and performance. *Exerc. Sport Sci. Rev.* 19:1–40, 1991.

26. Costill, D. L., and B. Saltin. Factors limiting gastric emptying during rest and exercise. *J. Appl. Physiol.* 37:679–683, 1974.

27. Costill, D. L., E. F. Coyle, G. Dalsky, W. Evans, W. J. Fink, and D. Hoopes. Effects of elevated plasma FFA and insulin on muscle glycogen usage during exercise. *J. Appl. Physiol.* 43:695–699, 1977.

28. Costill, D. L. Sweating: Its composition and effect on body fluids. *Annal. New York Acad. Sci.* 301:160–174, 1977.

29. Costill, D. L., W. M. Sherman, W. J. Fink, C. Maresh, W. Witten, and J. M. Miller. The role of dietary carbohydrates in muscle glycogen resynthesis after strenuous running. *Am. J. Clin. Nut.* 34:1831–1836,1981.

30. Costill, D. L., D. D. Pascoe, W. J. Fink, R. A. Robergs, S. I. Barr, and D. Pearson. Impaired muscle glycogen resynthesis after eccentric exercise. *J. Appl. Physiol.* 69(1):46–50, 1990.

31. Coyle, E. F., D. L. Costill, W. J. Fink, and D. G. Hoopes. Gastric emptying rates of selected athletic drinks. *Res. Quart.* 49:119–124, 1978.

32. Coyle, E. F., J. M. Hagberg, B. F. Hurley, W. H. Martin, A. A. Ehsani, and J. O. Holloszy. Carbohydrate feedings during prolonged exercise can delay fatigue. *J. Appl. Physiol.* 55(1):230–235, 1983.

33. Coyle, E. F., A. R. Coggan, M. K. Hemmert, R. C. Lowe, and T. J. Walters. Substrate usage during prolonged exercise following a preexercise meal. *J. Appl. Physiol.* 59(2):429–433, 1985.

34. Coyle, E. F., A. R. Coggan, M. K. Hemmert, and J. L. Ivy. Muscle glycogen utilization during prolonged strenuous exercise when fed carbohydrate. *J. Appl. Physiol.* 61(1):165–172, 1986.

35. Coyle, E. F., and S. J. Montain. Carbohydrate and fluid ingestion during exercise: Are there trade-offs? *Med. Sci. Sports Exerc.* 24(6):671–678, 1992.

36. Davis, J. M., W. A. Burgess, C. A. Slentz, W. P. Bartoli, and R. R. Pate. Effects of ingesting 6% and 12% glucose-electrolyte beverages during prolonged intermittent cycling exercise in the heat. *Eur. J. Appl. Physiol.* 57:563–569, 1988.

37. Doyle, J. A., and W. M. Sherman. Eccentric exercise and glycogen synthesis. *Med Sci. Sports Exerc.* 23(4) (Abstract 587):S98, 1991.

38. Doyle, J. A., W. M. Sherman, and R. L. Strauss. Effects of eccentric and concentric exercise on muscle glycogen replenishment. *J. Appl. Physiol.* 74(4):1848–1855, 1993.

39. Fell, R. D., S. E. Terblanche, J. L. Ivy, J. C. Young, and J. O. Holloszy. Effect of muscle glycogen content on glucose uptake following exercise. *J. Appl. Physiol.* 52:434–437, 1982.

40. Fielding, R. A., D. L. Costill, W. J. Fink, D. S. King, J. E. Kovaleski, and J. P. Kirwan. Effects of preexercise carbohydrate feedings on muscle glycogen use during exercise in well-trained runners. *Eur. J. Appl. Physiol.* 56:225–229, 1987.

41. Freund, B. J., et al. Glycerol hyperhydration: Hormonal, renal, and vascular fluid responses. *J. Appl Physiol.* 79(6):2069–2077, 1995.

42. Garcia-Roves, P. M., N. Terrados, S. F. Fernandez, and A. M. Patterson. Macronutrient intake of top level cyclists during continuous competition: Change in the feeding pattern. *Int. J. Sports Med.* 19(1):61–67, 1998.

43. Gerster, H. The role of vitamin C in athletic performance. *J. Am. Coll. Nutr.* 8(6):636–643, 1989.

44. Gisolfi, C. V., K. J. Spranger, R.W. Summers, H. P. Schedle, and T. L. Bleiler. Effects of cycle exercise on intestinal absorption in humans. *J. Appl. Physiol.* 71(6):2518–2527, 1991.

45. Gisolfi, C. V. Exercise, intestinal absorption, and rehydration. *Sports Sci. Exchange.* 4(32):1–5, 1991.

46. Gisolfi, C. V., R. W. Summers, H. P. Schedl, and T. L. Bleiler. Intestinal water absorption from select carbohydrate solutions in humans. *J. Appl. Physiol.* 73(5):2142–2150, 1992.

47. Gisolfi, C. V., and S. M. Duchman. Guidelines for optimal replacement beverages for different athletic events. *Med. Sci. Sports Exerc.* 24(6):679–687, 1992.

48. Gleeson, M., R. J. Maughan, and P. L. Greenhaff. Comparison of the effects of preexercise feedings of glucose, glycerol, and placebo on endurance and fuel homeostasis in man. *Eur. J. Appl. Physiol.* 55:645–653, 1986.

49. Gollnick, P. D., K. Piehl, C. W. Saubert IV, R. B. Armstrong, and B. Saltin. Diet, exercise and glycogen changes in human muscle fibers. *J. Appl. Physiol.* 33(4):421–425, 1972.

50. Greenhaff, P. L., M. Gleeson, and R. J. Maughan. The effects of a glycogen loading regimen on acid-base status and blood lactate concentration before and after a fixed period of high intensity exercise in man. Eur. *J. Appl. Physiol.* 57:254–259, 1988.

51. Greenhaff, P. L., M. Gleeson, and R. J. Maughan. The effects of diet on muscle pH and metabolism during high intensity exercise. *Eur. J. Appl. Physiol.* 57:531–539, 1988.

52. Greenhaff, P. L., M. Gleeson, and R. J. Maughan. Diet-induced metabolic acidosis and the performance of high intensity exercise in man. *Eur. J. Appl. Physiol.* 57:583–590, 1988.

53. Guyton, A. C. *Textbook of Medical Physiology,* 8th ed. W.B. Saunders, Philadelphia, 1991.

54. Hargreaves, M., D. L. Costill, A. R. Coggan, W. J. Fink, and I. Nishibata. Effects of carbohydrate feedings on muscle glycogen utilization and exercise performance. *Med. Sci. Sports Exerc.* 16:219–222, 1984.

55. Hargeaves, M., D. L. Costill, W. J. Fink, D. S. King, and R. A. Fielding. Effect of preexercise carbohydrate feedings on endurance cycling performance. *Med. Sci. Sports Exerc.* 19:33–36, 1987.

56. Hargreaves, M., and C. A. Briggs. Effects of carbohydrate ingestion on exercise metabolism. *J. Appl. Physiol.* 65:1553–1555, 1988.

57. Hargreaves, M., B. Kiens, and E.A. Richter. Effect of increased plasma free fatty acid concetrations on muscle metabolism in exercising man. *J. Appl. Physiol.* 70(1):194–201, 1991.

58. Hargreaves, M., D. L. Costill, L. Burke, G. McConell, and M. Febbraio. Influence of sodium on glucose bioavailability during exercise. *Med. Sci. Sports Exerc.* 26(3):365–368, 1994.

59. Hawley, J. A., F. Brouns, and A. Jeukendrup. Strategies to enhance fat utilization during exercise. *Sports Med.* 25(4):241–257, 1998.

60. Horowitz, J. F., R. Mora-Rodriguez, L. O. Byerley, and E. F. Coyle. Lipolytic suppression following carbohydrate ingestion limits fat oxidation during exercise. *Am. J. Physiol.* 273(4, Part 1):E768–E775, 1997.

61. Hultman, E. H. Carbohydrate metabolism during hard exercise and in the recovery period after exercise. *Acta Physiol. Scand.* 128(Suppl. 556):75–82, 1986.

62. Ivy, J. L., A. L. Katz, C. L. Cutler, W. M. Sherman, and E. F. Coyle. Muscle glycogen synthesis after exercse: Effect of time of carbohydrate ingestion. *J. Appl. Physiol.* 64(4):1480–1485, 1988.

63. Ivy, J. L., M. C. Lee, J. T. Bronzinick, Jr., and M. C. Reed. Muscle glycogen storage following different amounts of carbohydrate ingestion. *J. Appl. Physiol.* 65(5):2018–2023, 1988.

64. Jarvis J. K., D. Pearsall, C. M. Oliner, and D. A. Schoeller. The effect of food matrix on carbohydrate utilization during moderate exercise. *Med. Sci. Sports Exerc.* 24(3):320–326, 1992.

65. Jeukendrup, A. E., W. H. Saris, F. Brouns, D. Halliday, and J. M. Wagenmakers. Effects of carbohydrate (CHO) and fat supplementation on CHO metabolism during prolonged exercise. *Metabolism* 45(7):915–921, 1996.

66. Jeukendrup, A. E., W. H. Saris, and J. M. Wagenmakers. Fat metabolism during exercise: A review. Part 3: Effects of nutritional interventions. *Int. J. Sports Med.* 19(6):371–379, 1998.

67. Johnson, H. L., R. A. Nelson, and C. F. Consolazio. Effects of electrolyte and nutrient solutions on performance and metabolic balance. *Med. Sci. Sports Exerc.* 20(1):26–33, 1988.

68. Kanter, M. Free radicals and exercise: Effects of nutritional antioxidant supplementation. *Exerc. Sport Sci. Rev.* 23:375–397, 1995.

69. Kanter, M. M., and M. H. Williams. Antioxidants, carnitine, and choline as putative ergogenic aids. *Int. J. Sports. Nutr.* 5:S120–S131, 1995.

70. Karlsson, J., and B. Saltin. Diet, muscle glycogen and endurance performance. *J. Appl. Physiol.* 31:203–206, 1971.

71. Keizer, H. A., H. Kuipers, G. Van Kranenburg, and P. Guerten. Influence of liquid and solid meals on muscle glycogen resynthesis, plasma fuel hormone response, and maximal physical work capacity. *Int. J. Sports Med.* 8:99–104, 1986.

72. Kiens, B., A. B. Raben, A. K. Valeur, and E. A. Richter. Benefit of dietary simple carbohydrates on the early postexercise muscle glycogen repletion in male athletes. *Med. Sci. Sports Exerc.* 22(2)(Abstract 524):S88, 1990.

73. Kirwan, J. P., et al. Carbohydrate balance in competitive runners during successive days of intense training. *J. Appl. Physiol.* 65(6):2601–2606, 1988.

74. Klingshirn, L. A., R. R. Pate, S. P. Bourque, J. Mark Davis, and R. G. Sargent. Effect of iron supplementation on endurance capacity in iron-depleted female runners. *Med. Sci. Sports Exerc.* 24(7):819–824, 1992.

75. Kochan, R. G., D. R. Lamb, S. A. Lutz, C. V. Perrill, E. R. Reimann, and K. K. Schlender. Glycogen synthetase activation in human skeletal muscle: Effects of diet and exercise. *Am. J. Physiol.* 236(6):E660–E666, 1979.

76. Koivisto, V., S. L. Karonen, and E. O. Nikkila. Carbohydrate ingestion before exercise: Comparison of glucose, fructose, and sweet placebo. *J. Appl. Physiol.* 51:783–787, 1981.

77. Kris Etherton, P. M. The facts and fallacies of nutritional supplements for athletes. *Sports Sci. Exchange* 2(18):1–5, 1989.

78. Lambert, C. P., et al. Fluid replacement after dehydration: Influence of beverage carbonation and carbohydrate content. *Int. J. Sports Med.* 13(4):285–292, 1992.

REFERENCES

79. Lambert, E. V., J. A. Hawley, J. Goedecke, T. D. Noakes, and S. C. Dennis. Nutritional strategies for promoting fat utilization aand delaying the onset of fatigue during prolonged exercise. *J. Sports Sci.* 15(3):315–324, 1997.

80. Lemon, P. W. R. Does exercise alter dietary protein requirements? In F. Brouns (ed.), *Advances in nutrition and top sport. Int. J. Sports Med.* 32:15–37, Karger, Basel, 1991.

81. Lemon, P. W. R., M. A. Tarnopolsky, J. D. MacDougall, and S. A. Atkinson. Protein requirements and muscle mass/strength changes during intensive training in novice body builders. *J. Appl. Physiol.* 73(2):767–775, 1992.

82. Lyons, T. P., M. L. Riedesel, L. E. Meuli, and T. W. Chick. Effects of glycerol-induced hyperhydration prior to exercise in the heat on sweating and core temperature. *Med. Sci. Sports Exerc.* 22(4):477–483, 1990.

83. Magazanik, A., Y. Weinstein, R. A. Dlin, M. Derin, and S. Schwartzman. Iron deficiency caused by 7 weeks of intensive physical exercise. *Eur. J. Appl. Physiol.* 57:198–202, 1988.

84. Mason, W. L., G. McConell, and M. Hargreaves. Carbohydrate ingestion during exercise: Liquid vs. solid feedings. *Med. Sci. Sports Exerc.* 25(8):966–969, 1993.

85. Matter, M., et al. The effect of iron and folate therapy on maximal exercise performance in female marathon runners with iron and folate deficiency. *Clin. Sci.* 72:415–422, 1987.

86. Maughan, R. J., and P. L. Greenhaff. High intensity exercise performance and acid-base balance: The influence of diet and induced metabolic acidosis. In F. Brouns (ed.), *Advances in nutrition and top sport. Int. J. Sports Med.* 32:147–165, Karger, Basel, 1991.

87. Maughan, R. J. Gastric emptying during exercise. *Sports Sci. Exchange.* 6(5):1–6, 1993.

88. Maughan, R. J., J. H. Owen, S. M. Sherriffs, and J. B. Leiper. Postexercise rehydration in man: Effects of electrolyte addition to ingested fluids. *Eur. J. Appl. Physiol.* 69:209–215, 1994.

89. Mitchell, J. B., D. L. Costill, J. A. Houmard, R. A. Roberg, and J. A. Davis. Gastric emptying: Influence of prolonged exercise and carbohydrate concentration. *Med. Sci. Sports Exerc.* 21:269–274, 1989.

90. Montain, S. J., M. K. Hooper, A. R. Coggan, and E. F. Coyle. Exercise metabolism at different time intervals following a meal. *J. Appl. Physiol.* 70(2):882–888, 1991.

91. Montain, S. J., and E. F. Coyle. Fluid ingestion during exercise increases skin blood flow independent of increases in blood volume. *J. Appl. Physiol.* 73(3):903–910, 1992.

92. Montner, P., T. Chick, M. Rieddesel, M. Tims, D. Stark, and G. Murata. Glycerol hyperhydration and endurance exercise. *Med. Sci. Sports Exerc.* 24(4):S157, 1992.

93. Natali, A., et al. Effects of acute hypercarnitinemia during increased fatty substrate oxidation in man. *Metabolism* 42(5):594–600, 1993.

94. Noakes, T. D., R. J. Norman, R. H. Buck, J. Godlonton, K. Stevenson, and D. Pittaway. The incidence of hyponatremia during prolonged ultraendurance exercise. *Med. Sci. Sports Exerc.* 22(2):165–170, 1990.

95. Noakes, T. D., N. J. Rehrer, and R. J. Maughan. The importance of volume in regulating gastric emptying. *Med. Sci. Sports Exerc.* 23(3):307–313. 1991.

96. Noakes, T. D. Hyponatremia during endurance running: A physiological and clinical interpretation. *Med. Sci. Sports Exerc.* 24(4):403–405, 1992.

97. Noakes, T. D. Fluid replacement during exercise. *Exerc. Sport Sci. Rev.* 21:297–330, 1993.

98. Nose, H., G. W. Mack, X. Shi, and E. R. Nadel. Role of osmolality and plasma volume during rehydration in humans. *J. Appl. Physiol.* 65:325–331, 1988.

99. Nose, H., G. W. Mack, X. Shi, and E. R. Nadel. Involvement of sodium retention hormones during rehydration in humans. *J. Appl. Physiol.* 65:332–336, 1988.

100. O'Brien, M. J., C. A. Vivuie, R. S. Mazzeo, and G. A. Brooks. Carbohydrate dependence during marathon running. *Med. Sci. Sports Exerc.* 25(9):1009–1017, 1993.

101. Okano, G., H. Takeda, I. Morita, M. Katoh, Z. Mu, and S. Miyake. Effect of preexercise fructose ingestion on endurance performance in fed men. *Med. Sci. Sports Exerc.* 20(2):105–109, 1988.

102. Okano, G., Y. Sato, and Y. Murata. Effect of elevated blood FFA levels on endurance performance after a single fat meal ingestion. *Med. Sci. Sports Exerc.* 30(5):763–768, 1998.

103. Pascoe, D. D., D. L. Costill, W. J. Fink, R. A. Roberg, and D. R. Pearson. Effects of exercise mode on muscle glycogen restorage during repeated bouts of exercise. *Med. Sci. Sports Exerc.* 22(5):593–598, 1990.

104. Pivarnik, J. M., J. F. Hickson, Jr., and I. Wolinsky. Urinary 3-methylhistidine excretion increases with repeated weight training exercise. *Med. Sci. Sports Exerc.* 21(3):283–287, 1989.

105. Peters Futre, E. M., T. D. Noakes, R. I. Raine, and S. E. Terblanche. Muscle glycogen repletion during active postexercise recovery. *Am. J. Physiol.* 253(16):E305–E311, 1987.

106. Ravussin, E., C. Bogardus, K. Scheidegger, B. LaRange, E. D. Horton, and E. S. Horton. Effect of elevated FFA on carbohydrate and lipid oxidation during prolonged exercise in humans. *J. Appl. Physiol.* 60(3):893–900, 1986.

107. Reed, M. J., J. T. Bronzinick, Jr., M. C. Lee, and J. L. Ivy. Muscle glycogen storage postexercise: Effect of mode of carbohydrate administration. *J. Appl. Physiol.* 66(2):720–726, 1989.

108. Rehrer, N. J., E. Beckers, F. Brouns, F. Ten Hoor, and W. H. M. Saris. Exercise and training effects on gastric emptying of carbohydrate beverages. *Med. Sci. Sports Exerc.* 21:540–549, 1989.

109. Riedesel, M. L., D. Y. Allen, G. T. Peake, and K. Al-Qattan. Hyperhydration with glycerol solutions. *J. Appl. Physiol.* 63(6):2262–2268, 1987.

110. Roberg, R. A., et al. Muscle glycogenolysis during differing intensities of weight resistance exercise. *J. Appl. Physiol.* 70(4):1700–1706, 1991.

111. Robergs, R. A. Nutrition and exercise determinants of postexercise glycogen synthesis. *Int. J. Sport Nutr.* 1(4):307–337, 1991.

112. Robergs, R. A. Glycerol hyperhydration to beat the heat. *Training and Technology* online: http://www.sportsci.org

113. Robergs, R. A., and S. E. Griffin. Glycerol: Biochemistry, pharmacokinetics and clinical and practical applications. *Sports Med.* 26(3):145–167, 1998.

114. Romijn, J. A., et al. Regulation of endogenous fat and carbohydrate metabolism in relation to exercise intensity and duration. *Am. J. Physiol.* 265:E380–E391, 1993.

115. Romijn, J. A., E. F. Coyle, L. S. Sidossis, X. J. Zhang, and R. R. Wolfe. Relationship between fatty acid delivery and fatty acid oxidation during strenuous exercise. *J. Appl. Physiol.* 79(6):1939–1945, 1995.

116. Ryan, A. J., T. L. Bleiler, J. E. Carter, and C. V. Gisolfi. Gastric emptying during prolonged cycling exercise in the heat. *Med. Sci. Sports Exerc.* 21(1):51–58, 1989.

117. Sawka, M. N., and J. E. Greenleaf. Current concepts concerning thirst, dehydration, and fluid replacement: Overview. *Med. Sci. Sports Exerc.* 24(6):643–644, 1992.

118. Sears, B. *The zone: A dietary road map*. Regan Books, New York, 1995.

119. Sen, C. K. Oxidants and antioxidants in exercise. *J. Appl. Physiol.* 79(3):675–686, 1995.

120. Shearer, J. D., J. F. Amarai, and M. D. Caldwell. Glucose metabolism of injured skeletal muscle: Contribution of inflammatory cells. *Circulatory Shock* 25:131–138, 1988.

121. Sherman, W. M., D. L. Costill, W. J. Fink, and J. M. Miller. Effect of exercisediet manipulation on muscle glycogen and its subsequent utilization during performance. *Int. J. Sports Med.* 2(2):114–118, 1981.

122. Sherman, W. M., D. L. Costill, W. J. Fink, F. C. Hagerman, L. E. Armstrong, and T. F. Murray. Effect of a 42.2–km foot race and subsequent rest or exercise on muscle glycogen and enzymes. *J. Appl. Physiol.* 55:1219–1224, 1983.

123. Sherman, W. M. Preevent nutrition. *Sports Sci. Exchange* 1(12):1–5, 1989.

124. Sherman, W. M. Muscle glycogen supercompensation during the week before athletic competition. *Sports Sci. Exchange* 2(16):1–6, 1989.

125. Steen, S. N. Nutritional concerns for athletes who must reduce body weight. *Sports Sci. Exchange* 2(20):1–6, 1989.

126. Tarnopolsky, M. A., S. A. Atkinson, J. D. MacDougall, A. Chesley, S. Phillips, and H. P. Schwarcz. Evaluation of protein requirements for trained strength athletes. *J. Appl. Physiol.* 73(5):1986–1995, 1992.

127. Tsintzas, O. K., C. Williams, L. Boobis, and P. Greenhaff. Carbohydrate ingestion and glycogen utilization in different muscle fiber types in man. *J. Physiol. London* 489:243–250, 1995.

128. Tsintzas, O. K., C. Williams, W. Wilson, and J. Burrin. Influence of carbohydrate supplementation early in exercise on endurance capacity. *Med. Sci. Sports Exerc.* 28(11):1373–1379, 1996.

129. Turcotte, L. P., P. Hespel, and E. A. Richter. Circulating palmitate uptake and oxidation are not altered by glycogen depletion in contracting skeletal muscle. *J. Appl. Physiol.* 78(4):1266–1272, 1995.

130. Vukovich, M. D., D. L. Costill, M. S. Hickey, S. W. Trappe, K. J. Cole, and W. J. Fink. Effect of fat emulsion infusion and fat feeding on muscle glycogen utilization during cycle exercise. *J. Appl. Physiol.* 75(4):1513–1518, 1993.

131. Wagenmakers, A. J. M., et al. Carbohydrate supplementation, glycogen depletion, and amino acid metabolism during exercise. *Am. J. Physiol.* 260(23):E883–E890. 1991.

132. Walberg, J. L., V. K. Ruiz, S. L. Tarlton, D. E. Hinkle, and F. W. Thye. Exercise capacity and nitrogen loss during a high or low carbohydrate diet. *Med. Sci. Sports Exerc.* 20(1):34–43, 1988.

133. Wardlaw, G. M., and P. M. Insel. *Perspectives in nutrition*. Mosby-Year Book, St. Louis, 1993.

134. Weight, L. M., et al. Vitamin and mineral status of trained athletes, including the effects of supplementation. *Am. J. Clin. Nutr.* 47:186–191, 1988.

135. Yaspelkis, B. B., III, J. G. Paterson, P. A. Anderla, Z. Ding, and J. L. Ivy. Carbohydrate supplementation spares muscle glycogen during variable-intensity exercise. *J. Appl. Physiol.* 75(4):1477–1485, 1993.

136. Zachweija, J. D. L. Costill, D. D. Pascoe, R. A. Robergs, and W. J. Fink. Influence of muscle glycogen depletion on the rate of resynthesis. *Med. Sci. Sports Exerc.* 23(1):44–48, 1990.

137. Zawadzki, K. M., B. B. Yaspelkis, and J. L. Ivy. Carbohydrate-protein complex increases the rate of muscle glycogen storage after exercise. *J. Appl. Physiol.* 72(5):1854–1859, 1992.

RECOMMENDED READINGS

Coggan, A. R., and E. F. Coyle. Carbohydrate ingestion during prolonged exercise: Effects on metabolism and performance. *Exerc. Sport Sci. Rev.* 19:1–40, 1991.

Coyle, E. F., and S. J. Montain. Carbohydrate and fluid ingestion during exercise: Are there trade-offs? *Med. Sci. Sports Exerc.* 24(6):671–678, 1992.

Doyle, J. A., W. M. Sherman, and R. L. Strauss. Effects of eccentric and concentric exercise on muscle glycogen replenishment. *J. Appl. Physiol.* 74(4):1848–1855, 1993.

Ivy, J. L., A. L. Katz, C. L. Cutler, W. M. Sherman, and E. F. Coyle. Muscle glycogen synthesis after exercse: Effect of time of carbohydrate ingestion. *J. Appl. Physiol.* 64(4):1480–1485, 1988.

RECOMMENDED READING

Ivy, J. L., M. C. Lee, J. T. Bronzinick, Jr., and M. C. Reed. Muscle glycogen storage following different amounts of carbohydrate ingestion. *J. Appl. Physiol.* 65(5):2018–2023, 1988.

Lyons, T. P., M. L. Riedesel, L. E. Meuli, and T. W. Chick. Effects of glycerol-induced hyperhydration prior to exercise in the heat on sweating and core temperature. *Med. Sci. Sports Exerc.* 22(4):477–483, 1990.

Robergs, R. A. Nutrition and exercise determinants of postexercise glycogen synthesis. *Int. J. Sport Nutr.* 1(4):307–337, 1991.

Romijn, J. A., et al. Regulation of endogenous fat and carbohydrate metabolism in relation to exercise intensity and duration. *Am. J. Physiol.* 265:E380–E391, 1993.

Sherman, W. M., D. L. Costill, W. J. Fink, and J. M. Miller. Effect of exercise diet manipulation on muscle glycogen and its subsequent utilization during performance. *Int. J. Sports Med.* 2(2):114–118, 1981.

Tsintzas, O. K., C. Williams, L. Boobis, and P. Greenhaff. Carbohydrate ingestion and glycogen utilization in different muscle fiber types in man. *J. Physiol. London* 489:243–250, 1995.

CHAPTER 12

Ergogenic Aids

he quest to improve exercise performance has characterized athletic competition throughout history. Improved training techniques, improved clothing and equipment, new tactics, improved nutritional practices, medical interventions, and the use of illegal drugs have all characterized the need to win at what seems to be ever-increasing costs to tradition, health, moral beliefs, and a clear conscience. However, not all of these changes should be viewed as unethical. The changes in equipment, such as those seen in cycling, rowing, and skiing, are the results of scientific invention applied to the athletic endeavor to push the limits of human performance. Conversely, the use of certain nutritional practices (ingestion of caffeine, sodium bicarbonate), medical interventions (blood doping), prescription drugs (β-blockers, antihistamines), and nonprescribed medications (anabolic steroids, growth hormone, erythropoietin) by athletes are less accepted, can result in serious injury, and can significantly increase risk of death. The purpose of this chapter is to identify the substances that have been used by athletes for the purpose of improving performance, and present the scientific evidence that has either confirmed or negated a benefit.

OBJECTIVES

After studying this chapter, you should be able to:

- Define the term ergogenic aid.
- Explain the benefits of warm-up to different exercise conditions.
- List the mechanisms of how caffeine ingestion provides ergogenic benefit to exericse.
- Identify the ergogenic aids that have been shown to alter muscle metabolism during exercise and improve exercise performance.
- Identify the substances that have been proposed to improve exercise performance, yet been shown by research not to be ergogenic.
- Explain the concept of central fatigue and why certain substances might decrease this response to prolonged exercise.
- Identify the ergogenic aids that are not deleterious to body function, as well as those that can harm certain body functions.

KEY TERMS

ergogenic aid
warm-up
caffeine
glycerol
carnitine
phosphate loading
sodium bicarbonate
dichloroacetate (DCA)

creatine
branched-chain amino acids
central fatigue
erythropoietin (EPO)
blood doping
autologous transfusion

homologous transfusion
polycythemia
erythrocythemia
growth hormone
anabolic-androgenic steroids
amphetamines

Ergogenic Aids Used in Sports and Athletics

*T*he term *ergogenic* is defined as "tending to increase work." This definition has been modified to suit application to exercise performance, and the term **ergogenic aid** has been created and defined as "...a physical, mechanical, nutritional, psychological, or pharmacological substance or treatment that either directly improves physiological variables associated with exercise performance or removes subjective restraints which may limit physiological capacity" (1, 2, 71). Consequently, *any substance, practice, or piece of equipment that can increase the work performed during exercise, or enhance exercise performance, is an ergogenic aid.* Table 12.1 lists the substances that can be ingested, and practices that can be performed by athletes that adhere to the definition of an ergogenic aid. Focus box 12.1 presents the recommendations of the American College of Sports Medicine concerning the use of ergogenic aids for improved exercise performance.

As indicated in table 12.1, all the main ergogenic aids except for the ingestion of carnitine are known to be effective in improving attributes of function that can influence exercise performance. However, the exercise conditions that are associated with improved function are often limited, and several ergogenic aids are known to impose health risks when used excessively or improperly. The content of this chapter will be structured by each ergogenic aid, with comment given to different exercise intensities and durations.

Warm-up

Exercise is a stress to the body as it forces body functions to differ from those during rest conditions. As detailed in chapter 2, the human body is regulated to be able to respond rapidly to stress, and the metabolism and systems physiology that allows this adaptation have been detailed in chapters 3 through 9.

The process of adaptation to a stress occurs so that the body can alter its level of functioning and tolerate the stressor. When exercise is the stress, body functions change so that the demands of the exercise are met as best (as soon) as possible, thereby decreasing the impact of the stress on the body. Given this, it makes sense that if the body can adapt more readily to a stress, it will minimize the stress on the body. This basic concept is the logic behind a warm-up. *A warm-up has the potential to improve exercise because it enables a person to more rapidly adapt to the exercise stress,* thereby allowing more time at steady state and/or a better ability to focus on additional skills that might accompany the exercise.

The ergogenic benefits of **warm-up** are supported by a vast array of research (7, 18, 24, 38, 41, 56) that even

dates back to the 1950s (53). The benefits of warm-up (table 12.2) are related to increases in muscle temperature and energy metabolism, increased tissue elasticity, increases in cardiac output and peripheral blood flow, and improved function of the central nervous system and neuromuscular recruitment of motor units. Many athletes may also obtain psychological benefits from a warm-up. Consequently, research has attempted to provide evidence for the best types of warm-up for specific types of exercise, including prolonged submaximal exercise, intense short-term exercise, and activities requiring fine-tuned motor control.

What Is the Best Way to Warm-Up?

There are several ways to warm-up the body prior to competition. An important question that was originally answered by research was whether exercise was better than passive methods for increasing body temperature (hot shower or bath). Passive body heating proved better than no means of warm-up, but it was not as effective at increasing the rapidity of the body's responses to exercise as an active warm-up (41).

If exercise was required during a warm-up, how intense and long should the exercise be? The answers are quite simple. Warm-up should be active, not too intense (43), and should use the muscles that will be the prime movers in the exercise bout. General warm-ups, such as muscle stretching and total body exercise can provide some of the benefits of table 12.2, but are not as effective in stimulating increased blood flow and muscle mitochondrial respiration as a specific warm-up.

Warm-up strategies also exist for activities that demand more neuromuscular precision than physiological function, such as gymnastics, dancing, diving, ice skating, and other high-skill activities. These athletes often perform psychological imagery that is believed to stimulate the correct sequence of motor pattern stimulation in the central nervous system. Based on the extent of its use by these athletes, this form of general warm-up seems to be important, but there is no scientific evidence for its effectiveness.

Based on the ability of a specific and active warm-up to increase local blood flow, muscle temperature, and reduce the oxygen deficit, it has been proposed that warm-up may also be beneficial for intense exercise performance (56, 57).

---

ergogenic aid a physical, mechanical, nutritional, psychological, or pharmacological substance or treatment that either directly improves physiological variables associated with exercise performance or removes subjective restraints that may limit physiological capacity

warm-up a general term used for practices performed prior to exercise for the purpose of preparing the body for the exercise

TABLE 12.1

The potential and known ergogenic aids to exercise performance

ERGOGENIC AID	PROPOSED BENEFIT	PROVEN BENEFIT	BEST USE
Warm-up	Stimulates muscle metabolism and cardiorespiratory function	Yes	Perform low-moderate intensity exercise 5–30 min prior to moderate-intense exercise
	↓ Oxygen deficit	Yes	
Caffeine ingestion	↑ Lipid mobilization	Yes	Ingest prior to prolonged exercise
	↑ Muscle glycogen sparing	Yes	
	↑ CNS stimulation	Yes	
Carbohydrate ingestion	Prevents hypoglycemia	Yes	Ingest prior to, during, and after exercise
	↑ CHO dependence	Yes	
	Prolongs time to fatigue	Yes	
Liquid ingestion	Maintains hydration	Yes	Ingest prior to, during, and after exercise, especially in a hot or humid environment
	Improves thermoregulation and cardiovascular function	Yes	
Saline infusion	Maintains hydration	Yes	Ingest prior to, during, and after exercise, especially in a hot or humid environment
	Improves thermoregulation and cardiovascular function	Yes	
Glycerol ingestion	↑ Interstitial and intracellular water	Yes	Ingest with additional water prior to exercise, followed by continued ingestion with water during exercise and recovery
	Improves thermoregulation and cardiovascular function	Yes	
	Prolongs time to fatigue	Yes	
Carnitine ingestion	↑ Lipid catabolism	No	
	Spares muscle glycogen	No	
Phosphate ingestion	Delays muscle fatigue	?	Ingest for 3-6 days prior to event
	↑ VO_{2max} and VT	Yes	
Sodium bicarbonate ingestion	↑ Blood buffering capacity	Yes	Ingest immediately prior to intermittent intense exercise
Dichloroacetate ingestion[†]	↑ Oxidation of pyruvate	Yes	Ingest 2 h prior to exercise
	↓ Lactate production	Yes	
	↓ Peripheral vascular resistance	Yes	
Creatine ingestion	↑ Muscle creatine phosphate stores	Yes	Ingest for at least 5 days for metabolic and hydration benefits; ingest for several weeks for muscle mass and strength benefits
	↑ Rate of CrP resynthesis	Yes	
	↑ Body water	Yes	
	↑ Lean body mass	Yes	
	↑ Muscular strength	Yes	
	↑ Intense exercise performance	Yes	
Blood doping*	↑ Blood oxygen transport	Yes	
	↑ VO_{2max}	Yes	
	↑ Endurance performance	Yes	
Erythropoietin*	↑ Red blood cell mass	Yes	
	↑ Blood oxygen transport	Yes	
	↑ VO_{2max}	Yes	
	↑ Endurance performance	Yes	
Growth hormone*	↑ Muscle mass	Yes	
	↑ Muscle strength	Yes	
Testosterone*	↑ Muscle mass	Yes	
	↑ Muscle strength	Yes	
Amphetamines*	↓ Perception of pain	Yes	

*Detrimental side effects when used in excess or administered incorrectly.
†Not yet approved by the FDA.

Position of the American College of Sports Medicine Concerning the Use of Ergogenic Aids and Alcohol for Improved Exercise Performance

The American College of Sports Medicine (1, 2) has published several statements concerning the use of blood doping, anabolic-androgenic steroids, and alcohol for the purpose of improving exercise performance. Each statement is supported by research, and is written to justify the current opinion of the world's leading experts on the use of the specific substance. The recommendations of the statements follow.

The Use of Alcohol in Sports

Alcohol has been used by athletic and nonathletic individuals for centuries. The reported ability of alcohol to cause increased relaxation and less perception of stress has raised the belief that alcohol may improve exercise performance. However, as explained in the text, alcohol is not classed as an ergogenic aid, but an ergolytic aid. In 1982, the ACSM published this statement concerning the use of alcohol as a potential ergogenic aid:

1. The acute ingestion of alcohol can exert a deleterious effect upon a wide variety of psychomotor skills such as reaction time, hand-eye coordination, accuracy, balance, and complex coordination.
2. Acute ingestion of alcohol will not substantially influence metabolic or physiological functions essential to physical performance such as energy metabolism, maximal oxygen consumption (VO_{2max}), heart rate, stroke volume, cardiac output, muscle blood flow, arteriovenous oxygen difference, or respiratory dynamics.
3. Alcohol consumption may impair body temperature regulation during prolonged exercise in a cold environment. Acute alcohol ingestion will not improve and may decrease strength, power, local muscular endurance, speed, and cardiovascular endurance.
4. Alcohol is the most abused drug in the United States and is a major factor contributing to accidents and their consequences. Also, it has been documented widely that prolonged excessive alcohol consumption can elicit pathological changes in the liver, heart, brain, and muscle, which lead to disability and death.
5. Serious and continuing efforts should be made to educate athletes, coaches, health and physical educators, physicians, trainers, the sports media, and the general public regarding the effects of acute alcohol ingestion upon human physical performance and on the potential acute and chronic problems of excessive alcohol consumption.

The Use of Anabolic-Androgenic Steroids in Sports

Evidence of athletes using steroids to enhance performance was first detected in the early 1950's (53), and despite re-search evidence and medical recommendations of the dangers of the use of exogenous steroid compounds, increased use has occurred in the years to date. Such increased use has also been fueled by the development of steroids that have maximized the anabolic effects, while minimizing (though not completely) the androgenic effects. The following statements have been published by the ACSM, and are based on research that has been completed to 1986.

1. Anabolic-androgenic steroids in the presence of an adequate diet can contribute to increases in body weight, often in the lean mass compartment.
2. The gains in upper body strength achieved through high-intensity exercise and proper diet can be increased by the use of anabolic-androgenic steroids in some individuals.
3. Anabolic-androgenic steroids do not increase aerobic power or capacity for muscular exercise.
4. Anabolic-androgenic steroids have been associated with adverse effects on the liver, cardiovascular system, reproductive system, and psychological status in therapeutic trials and in limited research on athletes. Until further research is completed, the potential hazards of the use of the anabolic-androgenic steroids in athletes must include those found in therapeutic trials.
5. The use of anabolic-androgenic steroids by athletes is contrary to the rules and ethical principles of athletic competition as set forth by many of the sports governing bodies. The American College of Sports Medicine supports these ethical principles and deplores the use of anabolic-androgenic steroids by athletes.

Blood Doping as an Ergogenic Aid

The scientific inquiry into homologous and autologous blood reinfusion has provided extensive evidence of normal physiological function, the body's response to high and low erythrocyte content of blood, and the importance of blood oxygen transport in determining both maximal and submaximal exercise performance. However, the fact that research has proved the benefits of blood reinfusion to endurance exercise performance has resulted in the adoption of this procedure by athletes for the purpose of enhancing training and competitive performance. In 1984 the ACSM published the following statement concerning the use of blood doping by athletes with the intent of improving exercise performance:

"It is the position of the American College of Sports Medicine that the use of blood doping as an ergogenic aid for athletic competition is unethical and unjustifiable, but that autologous RBC infusion is an acceptable procedure to induce erythrocythemia in clinically controlled conditions for the purpose of legitimate scientific inquiry."

TABLE 12.2

The proven and as yet unsubstantiated benefits of an active warm-up prior to submaximal and intense exercise

BENEFIT	VERIFIED BY RESEARCH
Submaximal exercise	
↑ Muscle temperature	Yes
↑ Muscle blood flow	Yes
↓ Oxygen deficit	Yes
Improved neuromuscular function	No
↑ Lipid catabolism	Yes
↓ Carbohydrate metabolism	Yes
Muscle glycogen sparing	No
↓ Risk of musculoskeletal injury	No
Intense exercise	
Improved neuromuscular function	Yes
↑ Lipid catabolism	No
↓ Carbohydrate metabolism	No
Improved acid-base balance	Yes
↓ Oxygen deficit	Yes
Muscle glycogen sparing	No
↓ Risk of musculoskeletal injury	No

FIGURE 12.1

The actions of caffeine on the liver, skeletal muscle, adipose tissue, and central nervous system.

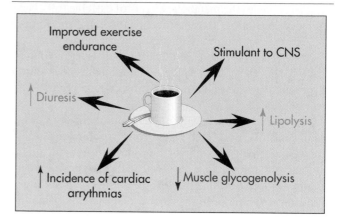

An active warm-up prior to intense swimming or cycling has been shown to increase oxygen consumption and improve muscle metabolism (57), as well as decrease the acid-base disturbance caused by intense exercise (56). Despite these improvements, there is no evidence for improved exercise performance.

Clinical Considerations

Not all people who exercise are young, healthy, or highly trained. Research has revealed that an active warm-up has certain benefits to cardiovascular function that may prevent abnormal heart responses, and in fact save lives (6, 7). When men who had no symptoms of heart disease performed intense treadmill running exercises with or without a warm-up, significantly more arrhythmias occurred without a warm-up, which was interpreted to indicate impaired coronary blood flow. These findings indicate that warm-up may be especially important for individuals with known cardiovascular disease or risk factors for cardiovascular disease.

Nutritional Ergogenic Aids

Caffeine

Caffeine is found in many foods, especially coffee, tea, and cocoa, and because of this it is arguably the most highly consumed drug in North America and Europe (66). Caffeine

functions as a central nervous system (CNS) stimulant, a stimulator of adipocyte lipolysis, a mild diuretic, and a potentiator of muscle contraction (fig. 12.1).

Caffeine functions in the CNS and in adipocytes by binding to adenosine receptors and *increasing intracellular cAMP concentrations*. In the CNS, this function improves alertness, concentration, vigor, and may increase maximal motor unit recruitment. The increase in cAMP concentrations within adipose tissue augments lipolysis, increasing the mobilization of free fatty acids and the availability of FFA for muscle catabolism. In skeletal muscle, caffeine facilitates the release of calcium from the sarcoplasmic reticulum, thereby increasing the ability to promote force generation during contraction (13, 20, 66, 70).

Research of the ergogenic effects of caffeine during exercise were based on the metabolic implications of an increased reliance on lipid for energy catabolism during exercise (14). The hypothesis was that if caffeine increased free fatty acid mobilization and reliance on lipid catabolism, muscle glycogen would be spared and exercise could be performed at higher intensities, or for longer durations. Research has provided contradictory evidence of the ergogenic benefits of caffeine (13, 14, 20, 22, 27, 63, 66, 69, 70). The main reasons for the discrepant findings have been interpreted as the difference in caffeine tolerance of the subjects (65), different doses of caffeine, and the often uncontrolled dietary state of the subjects prior to exercise. For example,

caffeine a naturally occurring substance that acts as a central nervous system (CNS) stimulant and a competitive antagonist for adenosine receptors in the CNS and periphery

subjects who routinely ingest caffeine have a blunted response to caffeine, and recently it has been shown that carbohydrate intake immediately prior to exercise, or during exercise, negates the metabolic effects of caffeine (69). Nevertheless, in studies that measured the effects of preexercise caffeine ingestion on muscle glycogen use during exercise (27, 28, 63), caffeine consistently caused the sparing of muscle glycogen. In addition, caffeine ingestion has been shown to prolong exercise endurance and lower perceptions of effort (14, 27, 32).

The main drawback for the ingestion of caffeine lies in its diuretic function. This response is problematic for exercise performed in a hot or humid environment, or for prolonged exercise, as it will exacerbate the development of dehydration. Caffeine can also be addictive, resulting in withdrawal symptoms of headache, nausea, and irritability (66).

On the basis of the research findings on and subjective feelings about caffeine as an ergogenic aid for long-term endurance events, the International Olympic Committee (IOC) classified caffeine as a banned substance as early as 1962, yet removed caffeine from this list in 1972. Currently, caffeine ingestion resulting in urinary caffeine concentrations of 12 mg/L or greater would be recognized as unethical by the IOC and Olympic medals would be confiscated. Ironically, such urinary concentrations of caffeine would require extreme dosages because a caffeine intake greater than 13.5 mg/kg is generally required to exceed a urinary caffeine concentration of 12 mg/L (a 250-mL cup of instant coffee contains approximately 80 mg of caffeine) (66). In addition, the lowest caffeine dosage used in research that demonstrated an ergogenic effect has been 4.4 mg/kg (9).

For example, for a 75-kg person,

IOC ban dosage
13.5 mg/kg = 13.5 × 75 = 1012.5 mg of caffeine

Ergogenic benefit dosage
4.4 mg/kg = 4.4 × 75 = 330 mg of caffeine

One cup of coffee provides 80 mg, therefore,

1012/80 = 12.7 cups of coffee   330/80 = 4.1 cups of coffee

Research has indicated that caffeine is not a positive ergogenic aid for short-term intense exercise conditions (66).

Glycerol Ingestion
The importance of muscle glycogen, the maintenance of blood glucose, and the prevention of dehydration during prolonged exercise already received extensive comment in chapter 11. Furthermore, the practice of consuming carbohydrates and liquid during exercise is accepted in most athletic competitions, and is therefore not at question regarding ethics. Students should refer to chapter 11 for research results on exercise performance following carbohydrate and fluid ingestion.

Recently, researchers have shown that compared to carbohydrate ingestion, the time to fatigue during prolonged exercise is increased by as much as 22% when a **glycerol** solution is ingested (54). These increases do not directly relate to increased performance, but have been estimated to coincide with 3 to 5% increases in competitive performance times during events such as cycling or running in hot or humid environments (58, 59).

The mechanism of glycerol's ergogenic benefits is that it causes increased water reabsorption in the kidney (30, 47, 59). Because of the widespread distribution of glycerol in the body, this increased water is distributed within cellular, interstitial, and vascular spaces, and can amount to between 600 to 700 mL 2 h after the ingestion of 26 mL/kg of fluid (fig. 12.2). Glycerol hyperhydration has been shown to improve cardiovascular function and thermoregulation during exercise, especially in a hot or humid environment (51, 55).

Despite the minimal research on improved hydration following glycerol ingestion (glycerol hyperhydration), current recommendations are for the ingestion of a concentrated solution of glycerol 200 to 300 g/L providing 1.2 g glycerol/kg body wt (see table 12.3) up to 2 h prior to exercise (54). This glycerol solution should be followed immediately by water ingestion, with a total fluid intake approximating 26 mL/kg body wt. The duration of the hyperhydration could be prolonged with added ingestion of glycerol and water (50 to 100 g/L) during exercise in volumes and frequencies similar to standard liquid carbohydrate ingestion (47).

Carnitine Ingestion
Carnitine is a molecule that is essential for the transportation of acylated free fatty acids into mitochondria (see chapter 3). During exercise of increasing intensity, there is a metabolic transition from a reliance on fat catabolism to carbohydrate catabolism. It has been proposed that the limiting step for continued fatty acid entry into mitochondria and its subsequent degradation in β-oxidation is the availability of carnitine. However, research that has evaluated this hypothesis has shown no ergogenic benefit to the ingestion of carnitine (36, 67).

Phosphate Ingestion
During intense exercise, muscle fatigue develops because of the inability of the muscles to regenerate ATP from oxidative phosphorylation at a rate that matches demand. ATP regeneration therefore is more reliant on glycolysis and creatine phosphate. It has been hypothesized that if added phosphate

FIGURE 12.2

The greater body water retention when glycerol is ingested with water compared to water ingestion. Adapted from Robergs and Griffin (59).

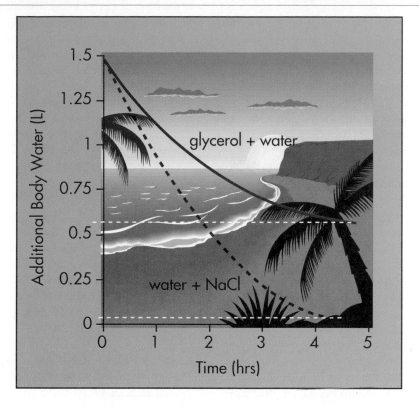

can be provided to the muscles during intense exercise, it would take longer to exhaust creatine phosphate stores, and intense exercise could be performed for longer periods prior to fatigue. In addition, added phosphate levels in blood have been hypothesized to increase 2,3-bisphosphoglycerate production and facilitate oxygen dissociation from hemoglobin, thereby improving oxygen delivery to skeletal muscle.

Despite evidence of no benefit of **phosphate loading** during intense isokinetic resistance exercise and treadmill running to exhaustion (214.4 m/min at 6%) (21), Kreider and colleagues (44) reported that phosphate ingestion significantly improved VO_{2max} and the ventilation threshold, and may improve 5-mi run performance. It appears that further research is needed, especially at the level of the muscle, to clarify the influence of phosphate loading on exercise performance.

Sodium Bicarbonate Ingestion

During intense exercise performed for between 1 to 4 min, the development of metabolic acidosis can contribute to the eventual deterioration in muscle force and power, and the resultant decrease in exercise performance (40). Because bicarbonate (HCO_3^-) is the main molecule in blood that

TABLE 12.3

Glycerol hyperhydration procedure

TIME (MIN)	INGESTION	COMMENT
0	5 mL/kg of 20% glycerol	Glycerol dose = 1.0 g/kg
30	5 mL/kg of water	
45	5 mL/kg of water	
60	1 mL/kg of 20% glycerol	Glycerol dose = 0.2 g/kg
90	5 mL/kg of water	
150		COMMENCE EXERCISE†

*Procedure used by Montner and colleagues (54).
†Exercise was commenced 1 h after the end of the hydration regimen. However, it remains unclear whether this delay is optimal, or whether added hydration benefits would occur with continued glycerol and water ingestion during exercise.

glycerol (glis'er-ol) a by-product of glycolysis that is used in triacylglycerol synthesis; released during the mobilization of fatty acids in lipolysis, and often used as an indirect reflection of the mobilization of fatty acids in blood and adipose tissue

carnitine (kar'ni-teen) a molecule required for the transport of medium- to long-chain fatty acids in the mitochondria

phosphate loading the practice of ingesting phosphate for the purpose if improving exercise performance

buffers acid, research has evaluated the potential for increases in blood HCO_3^- to improve intense exercise performance.

A common method of increasing blood HCO_3^- is to ingest **sodium bicarbonate** (baking soda). However, the ingestion of baking soda can be accompanied by an increased likelihood for gastrointestinal distress. Initial research on the use of bicarbonate for intense exercise was not supportive of an ergogenic benefit (39, 48, 49). However, when intense exercise is performed for between 1 and 7 min, and when the exercise is intermittent, definite improvements in performance have been documented (15, 50, 52, 62, 68, 71). The reason for the importance of intermittent exercise is that without a recovery there is minimal blood flow in intensely contracting skeletal muscle. It is during recovery from intense exercise that muscle receives a large hyperemia, allowing the HCO_3^- to become available to buffer the acid that accumulates in muscle and the interstitial space.

Dichloroacetate Ingestion

Dichloroacetate (DCA) is an artificial derivative of a substrate that occurs in the body (acetate) during lipid catabolism in the liver. DCA does not have approval from the Food and Drug Administration (FDA); however, approval has been granted to many researchers for its use in combating metabolic acidosis in humans for several clinical disorders such as heart failure, and certain kidney and liver conditions that contribute to metabolic acidosis. DCA has also been used in research that has used exercise to stress muscle metabolic and cardiovascular function. Evidence exists that DCA decreases peripheral vascular resistance, thereby increasing muscle blood flow, and stimulates pyruvate dehydrogenase which increases pyruvate oxidation, decreases lactate production, and theoretically should increase the rate of ATP regeneration from oxidative phosphorylation (10, 19, 50). Unfortunately, minimal human subject research has been completed using DCA during exercise, and it is unclear whether DCA improves exercise performance (10, 64).

Creatine Ingestion

Skeletal muscle has a finite store of creatine phosphate (CrP), approximately 26 mmol/kg wet wt. Because the muscle CrP store, via the creatine kinase reaction (chapter 3), is a rapid means to rephosphorylate ADP during muscle contraction, exercise involving very intense short-term exercise (< 30 s) is influenced by the muscle CrP store. Theoretically, the larger the CrP store the greater the ability of skeletal muscle to maintain ATP concentrations and sustain muscle contractions during intense exercise.

Creatine is an amino acid that forms the main component of CrP. Dietary creatine intake is typically large in the non-vegetarian, with the largest sources of dietary creatine being meat and fish (46). Creatine can also be synthesized in the body from other amino acids.

Supplementing the diet with with at least 15 g/day of creatine (creatine monohydrate) for between 2 to 7 days ele-vates skeletal muscle total creatine by between 10 and 20% (5, 33, 34), with up to 40% of the increased creatine present in the form of CrP (33–35). These gains occur in individuals with an adequate nutritional intake of creatine and are not the result of correcting a dietary insufficiency (46). Thus, *the supplemental intake of creatine can increase both free creatine and CrP in skeletal muscle in as little as 2 days in individuals with a well-balanced diet* (fig. 12.3).

Given the biochemical benefits arising from creatine ingestion, it is not surprising that research has shown that creatine ingestion can improve high-intensity exercise performance during a variety of activities including rowing, running, cycling, swimming, and weight lifting (3, 4, 8, 17, 33, 46, 60). In addition, creatine ingestion has been associated with rapid increases in body mass, which have been shown to be due to fluid retention (74). Longer durations of creatine ingestion (up to 28 days) have caused increases in lean body mass in athletes involved in intense resistance and power training (23, 44), presumably because of an increase in protein synthesis. It is unclear whether the increased protein synthesis occurs via a direct cellular mechanism or because of an improved quality of training seconday to the increase in muscle creatine and CrP (45).

Branched-Chain Amino Acid Ingestion (BCAAs)

Branched-chain amino acids (BCAAs, leucine, isoleucine, valine) are a subgroup of the large neutral amino acids (16). It has been proposed that BCAAs provide a means to combat the signals in the brain that result in perceptions of fatigue (known as **central fatigue**). Central fatigue is associated with increased concentrations of the neurotransmitter seratonin, which in turn increases when the molecule tryptophan accumulates in the blood (16). During prolonged exercise, the lowered blood glucose and greater reliance on fatty acids displace tryptophan from blood proteins (albumin), causing

FIGURE 12.3

The biochemical and physiological results of creatine ingestion.

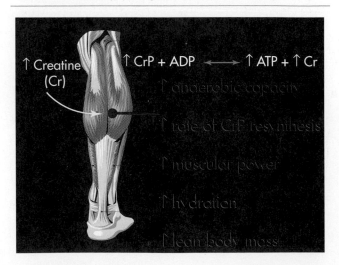

"free" tryptophan to increase. The ingestion of BCAAs causes their concentrations to increase in blood and compete with tryptophan for crossing the blood-brain barrier, thus decreasing the formation of seratonin in the brain and reducing central fatigue (12, 16).

Interestingly, the mere ingestion of carbohydrate during exercise has been shown to decrease free tryptophan in blood, and may also be important in decreasing the onset of central fatigue. Given the fact that the ingestion of large quantities of BCAAs during exercise is likely to cause gastrointestinal distress, and also increase ammonia production, there is little experimental support for a benefit from the ingestion of BCAAs prior to or during prolonged exercise.

Pure Oxygen Inhalation

The inhalation of pure oxygen has been used by athletes to better prepare themselves immediately prior to an athletic event, improve performance during exercise, and improve recovery from intense exercise. The justification for using pure oxygen is based on its increased partial pressure relative to oxygen in normal atmospheric air. Inhalation of pure oxygen will raise the partial pressure of arterial oxygen from approximately 98 mmHg to over 600 mmHg, depending on the barometric pressure and extent of mixing that occurs with atmospheric air during inhalation.

For example, increasing the P_aO_2 from 104 to 600 mmHg increases the oxygen dissolved in plasma to:

$$104 \text{ mmHg} \times 0.03 \text{ mL/L/mmHg} = 3.12 \text{ mL/L}$$
$$600 \text{ mmHg} \times 0.03 \text{ mL/L/mmHg} = 18 \text{ mL/L}$$
$$18 - 3.12 = 14.88 \text{ mL/L}$$

The increase in oxygen transport of approximately14.9 mL/L with the use of pure oxygen may not seem like much, but when multiplied by the cardiac output, which increases from 5 L/min at rest to over 25 L/min at maximal exercise in large trained individuals, this additional oxygen store can amount to an increase in oxygen transport of 0.37 L/min at maximal exertion. Given these numbers it is no surprise that research conducted on the use of pure oxygen during exercise has shown significant increases in VO_{2max}, VO_2 during the initial minutes of intense exercise, and time to exhaustion (72) (fig. 12.4).

The use of supplemental oxygen for improving recovery from intense exercise has no experimental support. In fact, the inhalation of pure oxygen is known to depress ventilation, which could confound the postexercise hyperventilation necessary to restore normal blood pH and acid-base balance.

Erythropoietin

Erythropoietin (EPO) is a hormone that is mainly produced by the kidney (see chapter 9). It is produced in response to hypoxia, and anemia that may result from increased blood loss (e.g., hemorrhage). EPO functions by stimulating the

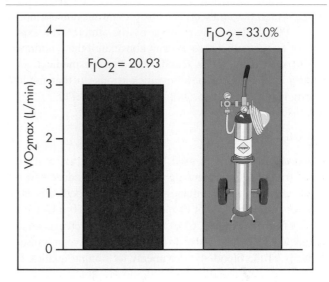

FIGURE 12.4

When pure oxygen is inhaled during intense exercise, oxygen consumption increases more rapidly, causing a lower oxygen deficit, and intense exercise can be tolerated for longer periods prior to fatigue.

bone marrow to specifically increase the differentiation of stem cells to erythrocytes. EPO is used clinically for patients with anemic conditions that often result from kidney damage. For example, there is a growing body of research on the effects of EPO administration on the exercise tolerance and hematology of renal dialysis patients.

As with most of the pharmacological ergogenic aids, the fact that EPO works (26) has led to its exploitation in the athletic and sports arenas. In late 1980s several Dutch cyclists attempted to use EPO to increase their blood oxygen transport capacities. Unfortunately, the EPO worked too well, causing large increases in red blood cell production, increased blood

sodium bicarbonate the molecule in blood that provides the greatest buffer power of acid

dichloroacetate (DCA) (di-klor'o-ass'e-tate) an artificial chlorinated derivative of acetyl CoA that stimulates the activity of pyruvate dehydrogenase, reduces lactate accumulation in the blood, and decreases peripheral vascular resistance

creatine (cre-a'tin) the amino acid "backbone" structure of creatine phosphate in skeletal muscle

branched-chain amino acids a subgroup of the large side chain and neutral amino acids that compete with the movement of tryptophan across the blood-brain barrier

central fatigue the term used for the increased perceptions of fatigue during prolonged exercise

erythropoietin (EPO) (e'rith-ro-poy'e-tin) a hormone released from the kidney that is responsible for stimulating red blood cell production (erythropoiesis)

viscosity, large increases in blood pressure, pulmonary embolism, and eventual death. Hopefully, the death of these athletes will divert attention away from EPO use.

In the 1998 Tour deFrance, EPO abuse by elite cyclists was shown to still occur. The race was characterized by raids on team facilities and searches for illicit drugs and hormones (i.e., EPO), followed by protests by the athletes, the expulsion of one team because of drug abuse, and the withdrawal of six other teams. This scandal has had the medical community searching for new testing options so that random testing can identify those athletes who abuse EPO.

Blood Doping

Blood doping is a term used for the procedure of removing blood from the body, allowing the body to reproduce new red blood cells, and then reinfusing the removed blood cells. Usually between 1 to 4 units of blood (1 unit = 450 mL) are removed from the body (2, 62). One unit is removed every 4 to 8 weeks to prevent excessive lowering of the oxygen transport capacity of the blood and detriments to training quality. The plasma from the blood is reinfused into the athlete, and the remaining blood cells are processed to isolate the erythrocytes and then stored in a special preserving and storage solution. Approximately 1 week prior to an event, the stored erythrocytes are reinfused back into the athlete. This process is termed an **autologous transfusion** because the blood cells are from the same person. When blood from another person is infused, the process is termed **homologous transfusion.**

Blood doping can double the hemoglobin concentration and hematocrit. However, because of the increased viscosity of the blood, the potential increase in oxygen transport capacity is compromised by the increased demand on the cardiovascular system. Thus, athletes usually wait at least 1 week after reinfusion to allow for the natural removal of some of the excess blood cells prior to competition. If the hemoglobin concentration has been increased from 140 g/L to 200 g/L, when 98% saturated, this extra oxygen transport capacity will transport an added 79 mL O_2/L, and circulate an added 1.58 L O_2/min at a cardiac output of 20 L/min. This provides athletes the potential to exercise at steady-state at higher-than-normal intensities, increase their maximal steady-state exercise intensity, and improve endurance performance.

$$140 \text{ g/L} \times 1.34 \text{ mL/g} \times 0.98 = 184 \text{ mL/L}$$
$$200 \text{ g/L} \times 1.34 \text{ mL/g} \times 0.98 = 263 \text{ mL/L}$$
$$263 - 184 = 79 \text{ mL}$$
$$79 \text{ mL/L} \times 20 \text{ L/min} = 1580 \text{ mL}$$
$$= 1.58 \text{ L/min}$$

Research on the effects of blood transfusions on exercise performance has been evaluated since the 1970s (25, 31, 61). Most of this work stemmed from the known improvements in erythrocyte mass in blood following prolonged altitude exposure, a process termed **polycythemia.** These early studies revealed that artificially raising the erythrocyte content of

the blood had potential to improve endurance exercise tolerance. The artificial increase in blood erythrocyte content has been termed **erythrocythemia** to emphasize its difference from the natural increases that occur with polycythemia. Spriet and associates (61) conducted a classic study of the effects of erythrocythemia on oxygen transport and VO_{2max}. The autologous infusion of 1 unit of blood did not increase oxygen transport or exercise capacities. However, the infusion of 2 and 3 units improved oxygen transport and exercise capacities, with 3 units providing the greatest improvement.

Growth Hormone

Growth hormone is a natural glucoregulatory and anabolic hormone of the body. It has been and continues to be used as a prescription to combat disorders that result in limited growth (e.g., dwarfism) or increased wasting of the body (e.g., AIDS infection). The obvious use of growth hormone to increase muscle hypertrophy made it attractive to athletes who could perform better with increased muscle mass. Additional perceived benefits of growth hormone administration by athletes include increased use of the body's free fatty acids, which caused a decrease in body fat content, increased bone growth in immature long bones and flat bones, and increased healing of musculoskeletal injury.

Research has shown that growth hormone administration in the elderly (61 to 81 years) increased lean body mass, reduced fat mass, and caused minor increases in bone mineral density (37). For younger men who performed resistance training with or without growth hormone, those who received the growth hormone demonstrated the largest increases in lean body mass.

Anabolic-Androgenic Steroids

Anabolic steroids are a family of steroid hormones that are similar to natural steroid hormones (e.g., testosterone) that increase protein synthesis and resultant muscle hypertrophy (*anabolic*), as well as develop male secondary sex characteristics (*androgenic*) such as hirsutism, deepening of the voice, and aggressive behavior. Because of these characteristics, these drugs are termed **anabolic-androgenic steroids.**

The natural increase in anabolic steroids in males increases lean body mass and develops the secondary sex characteristics. Additional use of anabolic-androgenic steroids is known to further increase lean body mass, decrease fat mass, and result in greater increases in training-related improvements in muscle strength (1).

The dose of steroids used is important because research has shown that large gains in hypertrophy and strength occur only with very high doses (29). It is unclear what the optimal amount of protein is that fosters maximal gains in hypertrophy when anabolic steroids are used in conjunction with resistance training; however, an intake of at least three times the current recommended daily allowance may be required. The same concerns are also true for growth hormone.

FOCUS BOX 12.2

Medical Problems Associated with Abuse of Anabolic-Androgenic Steroids

- Early calcification of epiphyseal plates of long bones, causing stunted growth
- Prolonged suppression of gonadal hormone secretion
- Testicular atrophy in males
- Menstrual irregularities in females
- Reduced sperm count
- Prostate gland enlargement in males

- Liver damage because of exaggerated needs for metabolic removal of the steroids
- Cardiomyopathy
- Decreased HDL cholesterol
- Increased risk for atherosclerotic cardiovascular disease
- Increased risk for cancer

Other potential benefits of steroid use have been their proposed ability to increase maximal oxygen uptake and improve tolerance to and recovery from intense training. Research does not clarify the accuracy of these claims because results are contradictory on VO_{2max} improvement; also, the influence of anabolic steroids on muscle repair and recovery has not been adequately researched.

The need to use large doses of anabolic-androgenic steroids is potentially dangerous because these steroids provide the potential for health risks. Regardless of this dilemma, athletes are often forced to decide on whether to use anabolic steroids in order to remain competitive in an event that is associated with steroid abuse. For example, estimations of steroid use by athletes involved in power events such as the throwing events of discus, shot put, and javelin; pure strength sports such as weight lifting; and body building exceeds 50% of participants (73). This incidence of use is problematic when there are well-documented medical risks associated with the abuse of steroids.

The potential medical problems associated with steroid abuse are listed in focus box 12.2.

The health-related side effects of anabolic steroid use by females is unclear. Anabolic steroids result in similar developmental effects in females as in males, with the added occurrences of increased sebaceous glands and incidence of acne, and enlargement of the clitoris. The long-term consequences of a disrupted menstrual cycle in the female because of steroid abuse is unknown, and it is also unclear whether the increased weight bearing activity performed by females who use anabolic steroids offsets the known potential for bone mineral losses because of chronically low estradiol concentrations.

Amphetamines

Amphetamines are a group of stimulants to the central nervous system, and are far more potent than caffeine. They are reported to have the effects of heightened arousal, euphoria, and increased alertness (13, 42). As with other potentially harmful ergogenic agents, minimally controlled scientific research has been completed on the use of amphetamines. However, studies that have been completed

(11) indicate that athletes may be able to increase their tolerance to fatigue, as indicated by increased muscular strength and time to fatigue. In addition, amphetamines overcome central nervous system inhibition to movement, as indicated by increased acceleration and decreased response times. It is unknown whether these proven benefits improve actual athletic performance, or whether larger doses of amphetamines induce greater changes in these or other parameters.

The dangers of amphetamines lie in their excessive stimulation to the cardiovascular system. Individuals can experience cardiac arrhythmias, and excessive blood pressure responses to exercise. Exercise participation beyond the normal limits posed by fatigue symptoms is also inherently dangerous for the musculoskeletal system, increasing the risk for orthopedic injury. In addition, symptoms of amphetamine abuse include dizziness, irritability, and headache for mild dosages, to addiction, paranoid delusions, and neuropathy for habitual abuse (73).

blood doping the term used for the removal of blood from the body, and its eventual reinfusion at a later date for the purpose of increasing hematocrit and blood oxygen–carrying capacity

autologous transfusion the reinfusion of red blood cells that were removed from the same individual

homologous transfusion the reinfusion of red blood cells that were removed from a different individual

polycythemia (pol′i-si-the′mi-ah) increased red blood cell concentrations in the blood

erythrocythemia (e-rith′ro-si-the′mi-ah) artificially increased red blood cell concetrations in the blood

growth hormone a hormone that functions to primarily regulate blood glucose and to secondarily function in concert with somatomedins to stimulate bone and muscle growth

anabolic-androgenic steroids hormones that stimulate growth and the development of secondary sex characteristics

amphetamines (am′fet-a′meens) drugs that overcome the discomfort and some of the neuromuscular recruitment limitations experienced during intense exercise

WEBSITE BOX

Chapter 12: Ergogenic Aids

The newest information regarding exercise physiology can be viewed at the following sites.[*]
brainmac.demon.co.uk/whatsnew.htm
Excellent site intended for coaches to have access to exercise-related information, including field tests of physical fitness, training strategies, nutritional ergogenics, and coaching strategies.
http://137.142.42.95/Students/Bio380/Flinton/Seminar/seminar2.html
Slide format lecture material about caffeine as an ergogenic aid.
musculardevelopment.com/oct/andro1.html
Excellent overview of testosterone and androstanedione, including the biochemical pathway of steroid synthesis.

vcurtin.edu.au/curtin/dept/physio/pt/edres/exphys/e552_96/
Index of brief reviews of exercise physiology by students from Curtin University, Australia. Topics include nutrition, ergogenic aids, environmental physiology, training, and clinical applications.

_____
[*]Unless indicated, all URLs preceded by http://www.

Note: These URLs were valid at the time of publication, but could have changed or been deleted from Internet access since that time.

SUMMARY

- The term **ergogenic aid** refers to, ". . . a physical, mechanical, nutritional, psychological, or pharmacological substance or treatment that either directly improves physiological variables associated with exercise performance or removes subjective restraints which may limit physiological capacity."

- The benefits of **warm-up** are related to increases in muscle temperature and energy metabolism, increased tissue elasticity, increases in cardiac output and peripheral blood flow, improved function of the central nervous system and neuromuscular recruitment of motor units, and a decreased risk for unusual heart beats and rhythms.

- Warm-up should be active, not too intense, and use the muscles that will be the prime movers in the exercise bout. General warm-ups, such as muscle stretching and total body exercise can provide some benefits, but are not as effective in stimulating increased blood flow and muscle mitochondrial respiration as a specific warm-up.

- **Caffeine** functions as a central nervous system stimulant, a stimulator of adipocyte lipolysis, a mild diuretic, and a potentiator of muscle contraction. The International Olympic Committee (IOC) has classified caffeine as a banned substance if urinary caffeine concentrations exceed 12 mg/L. This level of urinary caffeine would require the ingestion of approximately 13 cups of coffee.

- **Glycerol** is a natural metabolite of the body. When glycerol is ingested with large volumes of water prior to exercise it can increase the retention of water in the body by up to 700 mL over a 2-h period—a process termed *glycerol hyperhydration*. Glycerol hyperhydration has been shown to improve cardiovascular function and thermoregulation during exercise, especially in a hot or humid environment.

- **Carnitine** is a molecule that is essential for the transportation of acylated free fatty acids into mitochondria. It has been proposed that the limiting step for continued fatty acid entry into mitochondria and its subsequent degradation in β-oxidation is the availability of carnitine. However, research that has evaluated this hypothesis has shown no ergogenic benefit to the ingestion of carnitine.

- It has been hypothesized that if added phosphate (**phosphate loading**) can be provided to the muscles during intense exercise, it would take longer to exhaust creatine phosphate stores, and intense exercise could be performed for longer periods prior to fatigue. Despite evidence of no benefit of phosphate loading during intense isokinetic resistance exercise and treadmill running to exhaustion, phosphate ingestion has significantly improved VO_{2max} and the ventilation threshold, and may improve 5-mi run performance.

- A common method of increasing blood HCO_3^- is to ingest **sodium bicarbonate** (baking soda). However, the ingestion of baking soda can be accompanied by an increased likelihood for gastrointestinal distress. When intense exercise is performed for between 1 and 7 min, and when the exercise is intermittent, definite improvements in performance have been documented following the ingestion of sodium bicarbonate.

- **Dichloroacetate (DCA)** is an artificial derivative of a substrate the occurs in the body (acetate) during lipid catabolism in the liver. DCA does not have approval from the Food and Drug Administration (FDA); however, it has been used in research and is known to decrease peripheral vascular resistance and thereby increase muscle blood flow and stimulate pyruvate dehydrogenase, which increases pyruvate oxidation and decreases lactate production.

■ **Creatine** is an amino acid that forms the main component of CrP. Supplementing the diet with at least 15 g/day of creatine (creatine monohydrate) for between 2 to 7 days elevates skeletal muscle total creatine by between 10 and 20%, with up to 40% of the increased creatine present in the form of CrP. Creatine ingestion has been shown to improve high-intensity exercise performance during a variety of activities including rowing, running, cycling, swimming, and weight lifting. In addition, creatine ingestion has been associated with rapid increases in body mass, which have been interpreted to be due to fluid retention. Longer durations of creatine ingestion (up to 28 days) have caused increases in lean body mass in athletes involved in intense resistance and power training.

■ The inhalation of pure oxygen will raise the partial pressure of arterial oxygen from approximately 98 mmHg to over 600 mmHg, depending on the barometric pressure and extent of mixing that occurs with atmospheric air during inhalation. This increase results in an increase in the oxygen dissolved in plasma, and amounts to 14.9 mL/L. Use of pure oxygen during exercise has resulted in significant increases in VO_{2max}, VO_2 during the initial minutes of intense exercise, and time to exhaustion. There is no experimental support for a benefit of pure oxygen during the recovery from intense exercise.

■ **Erythropoietin (EPO)** functions by stimulating the bone marrow to specifically increase the differentiation of stem cells to erythrocytes. However, abuse of EPO can cause excessive increases in blood hematocrit and viscosity, and has resulted in the death of several elite cyclists.

■ **Blood doping** is a term used for the procedure of removing blood from the body, allowing the body to reproduce new red blood cells, and then reinfusing the removed blood cells. **Autologous transfusion** refers to the reinfusion of the blood cells from the same person. When blood from another person is infused, the process is termed a **homologous transfusion.**

■ **Growth hormone** is a natural glucoregulatory and anabolic hormone of the body. It has been and continues to be used as a prescription to combat disorders that result in limited growth (e.g., dwarfism) or increased wasting of the body (e.g., AIDS infection). The obvious use of growth hormone to increase muscle hypertrophy made it attractive to athletes who could perform better with increased muscle mass. The same benefits occur from abuse of **anabolic-androgenic steroids,** which are also known to further increase lean body mass, decrease fat mass, and result in greater increases in training-related improvements in muscle strength. There are numerous risks to the abuse of steroids, including testicular atrophy in men, menstrual irregularities in women, liver damage, cardiomyopathy, and increased risk of atherosclerotic cardiovascular diseases.

■ **Amphetamines** are a group of stimulants to the central nervous system, and are far more potent than caffeine. They are reported to have the effects of heightened arousal, euphoria, and increased alertness. The dangers of amphetamines lie in their excessive stimulation to the cardiovascular system. Individuals can experience cardiac arrhythmias and excessive blood pressure responses to exercise. Exercise participation beyond the normal limits posed by fatigue symptoms is also inherently dangerous for the musculoskeletal system, increasing the risk for orthopedic injury. In addition, symptoms of amphetamine abuse include dizziness, irritability, and headache for mild dosages, to addiction, paranoid delusions, and neuropathy for habitual abuse.

STUDY QUESTIONS

1. What are the benefits a warm-up can have for both intense and prolonged submaximal exercise?

2. For what types of exercise does the ingestion of sodium bicarbonate provide an ergogenic affect?

3. Does improving the oxygen transported in the blood improve VO_{2max} and endurance exercise performance?

4. What ergogenic aids exist that increase blood oxygen content?

5. Why would an increase in blood viscosity be detrimental to exercise performance?

6. What are the exercise performance benefits and health risks of the abuse of growth hormone, anabolic steroids, and amphetamines?

7. Provide a summary of ergogenic aids that would apply to either short-term intense exercise or prolonged submaximal exercise.

APPLICATIONS

1. Although they were not covered in this chapter, several prescription drugs are known to have a positive effect on exercise performance; others are known to diminish it. Try to name some drugs in either category (or both), and explain the mechanism or mechanisms by which they would affect exercise performance.

2. Detail the cardiorespiratory complications inherent in blood doping.

REFERENCES

1. American College of Sports Medicine. Position stand on the use of anabolic-androgenic steroids in sports. *Med. Sci. Sports Exerc.* 19:534–539, 1987.

2. American College of Sports Medicine. Position stand on blood doping as an ergogenic aid. *Med. Sci. Sports Exerc.* 19(5):540–543, 1984.

3. Balsom, P. D., B. Ekblom, K. Soderland, B. Sjodin, and E. Hultman. Creatine supplementation and dynamic high-intensity intermittent exercise. *Scand. J. Med. Sci. Sports* 3:143–149, 1993.

4. Balsom, P. D., K. Soderlund, and B. Ekblom. Creatine in humans with special reference to creatine supplementation. *Sports Medicine* 18(4):268–280, 1994.

5. Balsom, P. D., K. Soderland, B. Sjodin, and B. Ekblom. Skeletal muscle metabolism during short duration, high-intensity exercise: Influence of creatine supplementation. *Acta Physiol. Scand.* 1154:303–310, 1995.

6. Barnard, R. J. Ischemic response to sudden strenuous exercise in healthy men. *Circulation* 48:936–942, 1973.

7. Basuttil, C. P., and R. O. Ruhling. Warm-up and circulo-respiratory adaptations. *J. Sports Med.* 17:69–74, 1977.

8. Burke, L. M., D. B. Pyne, and R. D. Telford. Effect of oral creatine supplementation on single effort sprint performance in elite swimmers. *Int. J. Sports Nutr.* 6:222–233, 1996.

9. Cadarette, B. S., L. Levine, and C. L. Berube. Effects of varied dosages of caffeine on endurance exercise to fatigue. *Biochem. Exerc.* 13:871–877, 1983.

10. Carraro, F., S. Klein, J. I. Rosenblatt, and R. R. Wolfe. Effect of dichloroacetate on lactate concentration in exercising humans. *J. Appl. Physiol.* 66(2):591–597, 1989.

11. Chandler, J. V., and S. N. Blair. The effect of amphetamines on selected physiological components related to athletic success. *Med. Sci. Sports Exerc.* 12:65–69, 1980.

12. Clarkson, P. M. Nutrition for improved sports performance: Current issues on ergogenic aids. *Sports Medicine* 21(6):393–401, 1996.

13. Conlee, R. K. Amphetamine, caffeine, and cocaine. In D. R. Lamb and M. H. Williams (eds.), *Ergogenics-enhancement of performance in exercise and sport*. Brown & Benchmark, Dubuque, IA, 1991, pp. 285–325.

14. Costill, D. L., G. P. Dalsky, and W. J. Fink. Effects of caffeine ingestion on metabolism and exercise performance. *Med. Sci. Sports Exerc.* 10:155–158, 1978.

15. Costill, D. L., F. Verstappen, H. Kuipers, E. Janssen, and W. J. Fink. Acid-base balance during repeated bouts of exercise: Influence of HCO_3. *Int. J. Sports Med.* 5:228–231, 1984.

16. Davis, J. M. Carbohydrates, branched chain amino acids and endurance: The central fatigue hypothesis. *Gatorade Sports Science Exchange* 9(2)(SSE No. 61):1–10, 1996.

17. Dawson, B., M. Cutler, A. Moody, S. Lawrence, C. Goodman, and N. Randall. Effects of oral creatine loading on single and repeated maximal short sprints. *Aust. J. Sci. Med. Sport.* 27:56–61, 1995.

18. De Bruyn-Prevost, P. The effects of varying warming up intensities and durations upon some physiological variables during an exercise corresponding to the WC170. *Eur. J. Appl. Physiol.* 43:93–100, 1980.

19. Delehanty, J. M., M. Naoaki, and L. Chang-Seng. Effects of dichloroacetate on hemodynamic responses to dynamic exercise in dogs. *J. Appl. Physiol.* 72(2):515–520, 1992.

20. Dodd, S. L., R. A. Herb, and S. K. Powers. Caffeine and exercise performance: An update. *Sports Med.* 15:14–23, 1993.

21. Duffy, D. J., and R. K. Conlee. Effects of phosphate loading on leg power and high-intensity treadmill exercise. *Med. Sci. Sports Exerc.* 18(6):674–677, 1986.

22. Duthel, J. M., J. J. Vallon, G. Martin, J. M. Ferret, R. Mathieu, and R. Videman. Caffeine and sport: Role of physical exercise upon elimination. *Med. Sci. Sports Exerc.* 23(8):980–985, 1991.

23. Earnest, C. P., P. G. Snell, R. Rodriguez, A. L. Almada, and T. L. Mitchell. The effect of creatine monohydrate ingestion on anaerobic power indices, muscular strength, and body composition. *Acta Physiol. Scand.* 153:207–209, 1995.

24. Edwards, H. T., R. C. Harris, E. Hultman, L. Kaijser, D. Koh, and L. O. Norsdesjo. Effect of temperature on muscle energy metabolism and endurance during successive isometric contractions, sustained to fatigue, of the quadriceps muscle in man. *J. Physiol.* 220:335–352, 1972.

25. Ekblom, B., A. N. Goldbarg, and B. Gullbring. Response to exercise after blood loss and reinfusion. *J. Appl. Physiol.* 33:175–180, 1972.

26. Ekblom, B., and B. Berglund. Effect of erythropoeitin administration on maximal aerobic power. *Scand. J. Med. Sci. Sports* 1:88–93, 1991.

27. Erikson, M. A., R. J. Schwartzkopf, and R. D. McKenzie. Effects of caffeine, fructose, and glucose ingestion on muscle glycogen utilization during exercise. *Med. Sci. Sports Exerc.* 19:579–583, 1987.

28. Essig, D., D. L. Costill, and P. J. Van Handel. Effects of caffeine ingestion on utilization of muscle glycogen and lipid during the ergometer cycling. *Int. J. Sports Med.* 1:86–90, 1980.

29. Forbes, G. B. The effect of anabolic steroids on lean body mass: The dose response curve. *Metabolism* 34:571–573, 1985.

30. Freund, B. J., et al. Glycerol hyperhydration: Hormonal, renal, and vascular fluid responses. *J. Appl. Physiol.* 79(6):2069–2077, 1995.

31. Gledhill, N. The influence of altered blood volume and oxygen transport capacity on arobic performance. *Exerc. Sport Sci. Rev.* 13:75–93, 1985.

32. Graham, T. E., and L. L. Spriet. Performance and metabolic responses to a high caffeine dose during prolonged exercise. *J. Appl. Physiol.* 71:2292–2298, 1991.

33. Greenhaff, P. L., A. Casey, A. H. Short, R. C. Harris, K. Soderlund, and E. Hultman. Effect of oral creatine supplementation on muscle torque during repeated bouts of maximal voluntary exercise in man. *Clin. Sci.* 84:565–571, 1993.

34. Greenhaff, P. L., K. Bodin, K. Soderlund, and E. Hultman. Effect of oral creatine supplementation on skeletal muscle phosphocreatine resynthesis. *Am. J. Physiol.* 266:E725–E730, 1994.

35. Harris, R. C., K. Soderlund, and E. Hultman. Elevation of creatine in resting and exercised muscle of normal subjects by creatine supplementation. *Clin. Sci.* 83:367–374, 1992.

36. Heinonen, O. J. Carnitine and physical exercise. *Sports Medicine* 22(2):109–132, 1996.

37. Hervey, G. R., et al. Effects of methandienone on the performance and body composition of men undergoing athletic training. *Clin. Sci.* 60:457–461, 1981.

38. Hetzler, R. K., R. G. Knowlton, L. A. Kaminsky, and G. H. Kamimori. Effect of warm-up on plasma free fatty acid responses and substrate utilization during submaximal exercise. *Res. Quart.* 57:223–228, 1986.

39. Horswill, C. A., et al. Influence of sodium bicarbonate on sprint performance: Relationship to dosage. *Med. Sci. Sports Exerc.* 20(6):566–569, 1988.

40. Hultman, E., and K. Sahlin. Acid-base balance during exercise. *Exerc. Sport Sci. Rev.* 7:41–128, 1980.

41. Ingjer, F., and S. B. Stromme. Effects of active, passive, or no warm-up on the physiological responses to heavy exercise. *Eur. J. Appl. Physiol.* 40:273–282, 1979.

42. Ivy, J. L. Amphetamines. In M. H. Williams (ed.), *Ergogenic aids in sport.* Human Kinetics, Champaign, IL, 1983, pp. 101–127.

43. Karlsson, J., F. Bonde-Petersen, J. Henriksson, and H. G. Knuttgen. Effects of previous exercise with arms or legs on metabolism and performance in exhaustive exercise. *J. Appl. Physiol.* 38:763–767, 1975.

44. Kreider, R. B., G. W. Miller, M. H. Williams, C. Thomas Somma, and T. A. Nasser. Effects of phosphate loading on oxygen uptake, ventilatory anaerobic threshold, and run performance. *Med. Sci. Sports Exerc.* 22(2):250–256, 1990.

45. Kreider, R.B., et al. Effects of creatine supplementation on body composition, strength, and sprint performance. *Med. Sci. Sports Exerc.* 30(1):73–82, 1998.

46. Kreider, R. B. Creatine supplementation: Analysis of ergogenic value, medical safety, and concerns. *J. Exerc. Physiol.* online: http://www.css.edu/users/tboone2/asep/toc.htm., 1998.

47. Kruhoffer, P., and O. H. Nissan. Handling of glycerol in the kidney. *Acta Physiol. Scand.* 59:284–294, 1963.

48. Linderman, J., and T. D. Fahey. Sodium bicarbonate ingestion and exercise performance: An update. *Sports Med.* 11:71–77, 1991.

49. Linderman, J. K., and K. L. Gosselink. The effects of sodium bicarbonate ingestion on exercise performance. *Sports Medicine* 18(2):75–80, 1994.

50. Ludvik, B., G. Peer, and A. Berzlanovich. Effects of dichloracetate and bicarbonate on hemodynamic parameters in healthy volunteers. *Clin. Sci.* 80(1):47–51, 1991.

51. Lyons, T. P., M. L. Riedesel, L. E. Meuli, and T. W. Chick. Effects of glycerol-induced hyperhydration prior to exercise in the heat on sweating and core temperature. *Med. Sci. Sports Exerc.* 22(4):477–483, 1990.

52. McNaughton, L. R., B. Dalton, J. Tarr, and D. Buck. Neutralize acid to enhance performance. *Training and Technology* online: http://www.sportsci.org., 1997.

53. Malareck, I. Investigation on physiological justification of so called "warming up." *Acta Physiol. Pol.* 4:543–546, 1954.

54. Montner, P., et al. Preexercise glycerol hydration improves cycling endurance time. *Int. J. Sports Med.* 17(1):27–33, 1996.

55. Riedesel, M. L., D. Y. Allen, G. T. Peake, and K. Al-Qattan. Hyperhydration with glycerol solutions. *J. Appl. Physiol.* 63(6):2262–2268, 1987.

56. Robergs, R. A., et al. Effects of warm-up on blood gases, lactate and acid-base status during sprint swimming. *Int. J. Sports Med.* 11(4):273–278, 1990.

57. Robergs, R. A., et al. Effects of warm-up on muscle glycogenolysis during intense exercise. *Med. Sci. Sports Exerc.* 23(1):37–43, 1991.

58. Robergs, R. A. Glycerol hyperhydration to beat the heat. *Sportscience Training and Technology* section online: http://www.sportsci.org., 1998.

59. Robergs, R. A., and S. E. Griffin. Glycerol, biochemistry, pharmacokinetics, clinical and applied applications. *Sports Medicine* 26(3):145–167, 1998.

60. Rossiter, H. B., E. R. Cannell, and P. M. Jakeman. The effect of oral creatine supplementation on the 1000-m performance of competitive rowers. *J. Sports Sci.* 14:175–179, 1996.

61. Spriet, L. L., M. I. Lindinger, G. J. F. Heigenhauser, and N. L. Jones. Effects of alkalosis on skeletal muscle metabolism and performance during exercise. *Am. J. Physiol.* 251(20):R833–R839, 1986.

62. Spriet, L. L., N. Gledhill, A. B. Froese, and D. L. Wilkes. Effect of graded erythrocythemia on cardiovascular and metabolic responses to exercise. *J. Appl. Physiol.* 61(5):1942–1948, 1986.

63. Spriet, L. L., D. A. MacLean, D. J. Dyck, E. Hultman, G. Cederblad, and T. E. Graham. Caffeine ingestion and muscle metabolism during prolonged exercise in humans. *Am. J. Physiol.* 262(25):E891–E898, 1992.

64. Stacpoole, P. W. The pharmacology of dichloracetate. *Metabolism* 38(11):1124–1144, 1989.

65. Tarnopolsky, M. A., S. A. Atkinson, J. D. MacDougall, D. G. Sale, and J. R. Sutton. Physiologic response to caffeine during endurance running in habitual caffeine users. *Med. Sci. Sports Exerc.* 21:418–424, 1989.

66. Tarnopolsky, M. A. Caffeine and endurance performance. *Sports Medicine* 18(2):109–125, 1994.

67. Vukovich, M. D., D. L. Costill, and W. J. Fink. L-carnitine supplementation: Effect on muscle carnitine content and glycogen utilization during exercise. *Med. Sci. Sports Exerc.* 26(5)(Abstract 44):S8, 1994.

68. Webster, M. J., M. N. Webster, R. E. Crawford, and L. B. Gladden. Effects of sodium bicarbonate ingestion on exhaustive resistance exercise performance. *Med. Sci. Sports Exerc.* 25(8):960–965, 1993.

69. Weir, J., T. D. Noakes, K. Myburgh, and B. Adams. A high carbohydrate diet negates the metabolic effects of caffeine during exercise. *Med. Sci. Sports Exerc.* 12:100–105, 1987.

70. Williams, J. H. Caffeine, neuromuscular function and high-intensity exercise performance. *J. Sports Med. Phys. Fit.* 31:481–489, 1991.

REFERENCES

71. Williams, M. H. Bicarbonate loading. *Sports Science Exchange* 4(36):1–4, 1992.

72. Winter, F. D., P. G. Snell, and J. Stray-Gundersen. Effects of 100% oxygen on performance of professional soccer players. *JAMA*. 262:227–229, 1989.

73. Yesalis, C. E., J. E. Wright, and M. S. Bahrke. Epidemiological and policy issues in the measurement of the long-term health effects of anabolic-androgenic steroids. *Sports Med.* 8:129–138, 1989.

74. Ziegenfuss, T. N., L. M. Lowry, and P. W. R. Lemon. Acute fluid volume changes in men during three days of creatine supplementation. *J. Exerc. Physiol.* online: http://www.css.edu/users/tboone2/asep/toc.htm., 1998.

RECOMMENDED READINGS

American College of Sports Medicine. Position stand on the use of anabolic-androgenic steroids in sports. *Med. Sci. Sports Exerc.* 19:534–539, 1987.

American College of Sports Medicine. Position stand on blood doping as an ergogenic aid. *Med. Sci. Sports Exerc.* 19(5):540–543, 1984.

Balsom, P. D., K. Soderlund, and B. Ekblom. Creatine in humans with special reference to creatine supplementation. *Sports Medicine* 18(4):268–280, 1994.

Carraro, F., S. Klein, J. I. Rosenblatt, and R. R. Wolfe. Effect of dichloroacetate on lactate concentration in exercising humans. *J. Appl. Physiol.* 66(2):591–597, 1989.

Davis, J. M. Carbohydrates, branched chain amino acids and endurance: The central fatigue hypothesis. *Gatorade Sports Science Exchange* 9(2):(SSE no.61):1–10, 1996.

Freund, B. J., et al. Glycerol hyperhydration: Hormonal, renal, and vascular fluid responses. *J. Appl. Physiol.* 79(6):2069–2077, 1995.

Heinonen, O. J. Carnitine and physical exercise. *Sports Medicine* 22(20):109–132, 1996.

Robergs, R. A., and S. E. Griffin. Glycerol, biochemistry, pharmacokinetics, clinical, and applied applications. *Sports Medicine* 26(3):145–167, 1998.

Spriet, L. L., N. Gledhill, A. B. Froese, and D. L. Wilkes. Effect of graded erythrocythemia on cardiovascular and metabolic responses to exercise. *J. Appl. Physiol.* 61(5):1942–1948, 1986.

Tarnopolsky, M. A. Caffeine, and endurance performance. *Sports Medicine* 18(2):109–125, 1994.

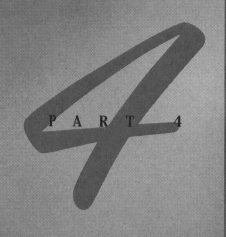

oxygen

$$Q = SV \times HR$$

$$HRmax = 220 - age$$

RQ

fatigue   RER

stress

mmHg

VO_2max

Measurements of Fitness and Exercise Performance

CHAPTER 13

13

Measuring Endurance, Anaerobic Capacity, and Strength

he exercise physiologist often tries to measure variables in a laboratory that reflect a person's abilities to excel in competitive sports and athletics. There is no better example of this than the scientifically based training centers of the Olympic organizations of most developed countries. In these facilities, athletes are tested routinely for data on their specific cardiorespiratory, neuromuscular, and strength capacities, as well as additional factors such as body composition, biomechanics, and sport psychology. Such tests provide data of these capacities and measurements for the coaches and athletes, and are used to monitor progress in training and to fine-tune the training program for individual athletes. These tests can be applied to the less-elite athlete for the same purposes and can assess suitability for the demands of specific vocations (e.g., fire fighting, the military, police). Laboratory testing is also useful in disease prevention, or rehabilitation from disease or injury (e.g., cardiac and/or pulmonary rehabilitation, physical therapy). Periodic physiological testing can help evaluate an exercise training program, or provide motivation for behavioral change. The purposes of this chapter are to explain how to conduct and interpret the different tests available to measure or estimate cardiorespiratory endurance and related metabolic capacities, and muscular power and strength. In addition, where appropriate, normal scores on these tests for specific populations will be provided.

OBJECTIVES

After studying this chapter, you should be able to:

- List and describe the protocol requirements for a valid test of VO_{2max}.
- Interpret data from a test of VO_{2max}.
- Identify the ventilation and lactate thresholds from appropriate data.
- Interpret data of VO_{2max}, heart rate, the lactate threshold/ventilation thresholds, and laboratory exercise performance for assessments of race performance for different prolonged-endurance events.
- Explain the different methods available for assessing maximal muscular power and anaerobic capacity.
- Explain the different methods available for maximal and submaximal muscular strength.

KEY TERMS

VO_{2max}	muscle power	muscular strength
VO_{2peak}	Wingate test	dynamometer
Åstrand-Rhyming nomogram	anaerobic capacity accumulated oxygen deficit	1 repetition maximum (1 RM)
running economy		

Metabolic Determinants of Physiological Capacities

*M*any of the tests that quantify physiological capacity are heavily reliant on the metabolic processes that support exercise for the intensity and duration at question. As explained in chapter 3, the duration of exercise (and therefore the intensity) will determine the predominance of creatine phosphate hydrolysis, glycolysis, or mitochondrial respiration to the regeneration of muscle ATP (adenine triphosphate). In a very simple sense, if a given activity is reliant on one or a combination of multiple metabolic pathways, a laboratory test can be developed to test as much of the maximal capacity of that pathway(s) as possible. The greater the maximal capacity, and the more specific that metabolic pathway is to success in a given event/activity, the better the test is for assessing potential for success in that event/activity. The fundamental knowledge base for an exercise physiologist is therefore to *know the metabolic demands and related physiological support functions of specific events/activities.*

Figure 13.1 is a flow diagram that identifies the different broad categories of events/activities and connects them to the metabolic and physiological capacities that contribute to them. These capacities are then connected to the laboratory tests that can be used to estimate the capacities. The remainder of the chapter is structured on the basis of the laboratory tests that are identified in figure 13.1.

Measuring Cardiorespiratory and Muscular Endurance

Maximal Oxygen Consumption (VO_2)

Traditionally, the test used to measure cardiorespiratory and muscular endurance has been that of the maximal rate of oxygen consumption (VO_{2max}) (3, 5, 10, 13, 25, 47). However, research evidence indicates that VO_{2max} alone may not be an accurate assessment of the cardiorespiratory demands of submaximal exercise (16, 40, 52, 55). For example, research since the 1970s has shown that although VO_{2max} predicts endurance exercise performance in a large group of individuals with a large range of VO_{2max} values ($r > 0.85$) (40), it has less importance in determining exercise performance in a group of individuals with a similar VO_{2max} (40). Obviously, other factors are involved in determining how well a person can perform in endurance exercise.

Direct measurement of VO_2 requires the measurement of expired gas fractions and ventilation during exercise. A variety of gas-analyzing systems have been developed over the years, ranging from expired gas collection in Douglas bags with the chemical analysis of expired air for oxygen and carbon dioxide content, to today's sophisticated computer-driven

> **VO_{2max}** the maximal rate of oxygen consumption for a given individual

---

FIGURE 13.1

Schematics of how certain laboratory tests relate to the physiological capacities that combine to influence each of *(a)* prolonged endurance, and *(b)* short-term intense exercise. Note that other (nonphysiological) factors also exist that influence the two types of exercise conditions and it is naïve to think that the physiological capacities identified are the only factors that influence exercise/sports performance.

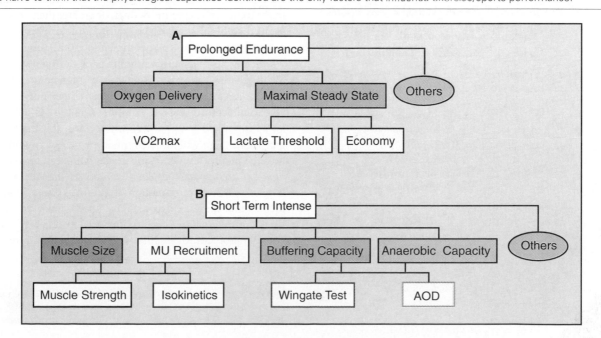

equipment with electronic analyzers that compute data for each breath (see chapter 4).

The decision over whether a time-averaged or breath-by-breath system is to be used depends on the purpose of the test. If the purpose is to simply measure VO_{2max}, than either method is suitable. However, there is arguably a greater ability to detect a plateau in VO_2 with breath-by-breath systems. If additional data of the rate of change (kinetics) of VO_2, or end-tidal gas fractions are required, then a breath-by-breath system should be used (60).

The test of VO_{2max} must meet several requirements in order for the peak VO_2 attained to be VO_{2max}. Any measure of VO_{2max} that is questionable, thereby increasing the risk for underestimating VO_{2max}, is typically denoted as $\mathbf{VO_{2peak}}$. These test criteria for VO_{2max} measurement have been excellently reviewed by Howley and colleagues (31), and are presented in table 13.1. The duration and increment magnitude of the test can influence the VO_{2max} (11, 49). A total test duration in excess of 16 min can lower VO_{2max}. Conversely, test durations less than 8 min involve large increments in intensity, and lead to premature fatigue and a low VO_{2max}. Buchfuher (11) recommends that test durations should be between 8 and 12 min to obtain a true VO_{2max}.

In addition to test duration, criteria of a plateau in VO_2 with increasing exercise intensity, an RER greater than 1.1, and the attainment of age-predicted maximal heart rate (220 − age) have also been used as criteria to validate VO_{2peak} as VO_{2max} (31). However, of these additional criteria, a plateau in VO_{2max} has not been conclusively demonstrated as valid because of the difficulty more than 50% of healthy individuals have in demonstrating a plateau in VO_2 during a maximal test (3, 4, 47). Furthermore, individuals with cardiovascular diseases or chronic obstructive pulmonary disease will prematurely termi-

nate a maximal test because of clinical symptoms of exercise intolerance, such as angina, abnormal ECG, dyspnea (breathlessness), or leg fatigue because of claudication. For the more clinically determined maximal VO_2 values, the expressions *symptom-limited VO_{2max}* and *VO_{2peak}* are more appropriate.

Finally, a decision on the exercise mode used to conduct the test needs to be made. As explained in chapter 6, sedentary and moderately trained individuals attain a higher VO_{2max} during treadmill protocols. However, highly trained individuals on exercise modes that differ from running may have the same or a higher VO_{2max} than during treadmill running. In addition, if a treadmill protocol is chosen, there is evidence that individuals who train on hilly terrain will do better on a protocol involving an inclination than do runners who train on level ground (1, 24).

Testing Protocols

The need to maintain a test duration of 12 min would mean that increments in intensity would be different for individuals of differing cardiorespiratory fitness. This fact stresses the need *to tailor a protocol to suit a given individual.* Therefore, estimations of a person's cardiorespiratory fitness and training history are important first steps in determining a protocol for a test of VO_{2max}. This estimation can then be applied to cycling or running using the equations of the American College of Sports Medicine (2), Wasserman and Whipp (59), or the others listed in table 13.2. For example, when estimating a VO_{2max} of 4.0 L/min during cycle ergometry, the maximal power output would approximate 390 W. When using 400 W as an estimated maximal intensity, a warm-up ending at 100 W would leave 300 W of increment to VO_{2max}. When dividing 300 by 12, the result is an increment of 25 W/min.

For the same person running on a treadmill, VO_2 needs to be estimated in mL/kg/min (4000/75 = 53.3 mL/kg/min), and a running pace that is comfortable needs to be estimated. This is difficult, because it could be less than 7 km/h (4.4 mi/h) for an untrained individual, or greater than 16 km/h (10 mi/h) for a highly endurance-trained athlete. This pace is important, because it is recommended that the subject be warmed up to sustain this running pace during level running, and thereafter have exercise intensity augmented by increasing the grade of the treadmill. Thus if the individual were able to run comfortably at 12 km/h (7.5 mi/h), which requires an approximate VO_2 of 43.8 mL/kg/min (tables 13.2, 13.3 and 13.4), there would be a remaining 9.5 mL/kg/min which must be met by an increasing grade. Although *the energy demand of an increase in grade increases with increasing running speed,* an approximation of 1.5 mL/kg/min/% grade indicates that the maximal exercise speed and grade required by this individual will approximate 12 km/h at 7% grade. A suitable protocol for this individual would therefore involve

---

TABLE 13.1

Criteria for a valid protocol and data evaluation to measure VO_{2max}

CRITERIA	DESCRIPTION
Protocol	
Test duration	8–12 min
Stage duration	Ramp, or 1–3 min
Intensity increment	Based on stage duration and cardiorespiratory fitness of the subject
Mode	Subject specific on the basis of training, disease states, and musculoskeletal concerns
Data Interpretation	
Criteria to establish VO_{2max} vs. VO_{2peak}	Plateau in VO_2 RER > 1.1 HR_{max}* < 10 b/min from predicted

*HR_{max} is maximal or peak heart rate attained during the test.

Source: Adapted from Howley et al. (31).

VO_{2peak} the largest VO_2 during an incremental exercise test where all criteria of VO_{2max} have not been met

TABLE 13.2

Summary of VO_2 prediction equations

EXERCISE MODE	STUDY	N	POPULATION AGES	POPULATION GENDER/HEALTH	EQUATION	R	SEE
Submaximal VO_2 *							
Treadmill walking (mL/kg/min)	ACSM[2]			M,F healthy	[0.1(m/min)] + [(grade;fraction) (m/min)(1.8)] = 3.5		
Treadmill running (mL/kg/min)	ACSM[2]			M,F healthy	[0.2(m/min)] + [(grade,fraction) (m)/min)(1.8)(0.5) + 3.5]		
Cycle ergometry (mL/min)	ACSM[2]			M,F healthy	[2.0(kg/min)] + [3.5(wt,kg)]		
(L/min)	ACSM[2]			M,F healthy	[0.012(W)] + 0.3		
(mL/min)	Latin[45]	110	18–38	M healthy	[kg/min(1.9)] + [3.5(wt,kg)] + 260	0.96	154.0
	Legge[46]	15	20–29	M trained	[0.034(ΔHR)] + 1.03		0.39
		10		M untrained	[0.023(ΔHR)] + 1.09		0.32
(mL/min)	Wasserman[70]				[10(W)] + 500		
Arm ergometry (mL/min)	ACSM[2]			M,F healthy	[3(kg/min)] + [3.5(body weight,kg)]		
Bench stepping (mL/kg/min)	ACSM[2]			M,F healthy	[0.35(steps/min)] + [(height,m) (steps/min)(1.33)(1.8)]		
Maximal VO_2 (VO_{2max})							
Maximal tests							
Treadmill (mL/kg/min)							
Bruce protocol	Bruce[11]	44		M active	3.778(time) + 0.19	0.906	
		94		M sedentary	3.298(time) + 4.07	0.906	
		97		M cardiac	2.327(time) + 9.48	0.865	
		295		M,F healthy	6.70 − [2.82(gender)] + [0.056(time)]	0.920	
	Foster[27]	230		M varied	14.76 − [1.38(time)] + [0.451($time^2$)] − [0.12($time^3$)]	0.977	3.35
Balke protocol	Froelicher[30]	1025	20–53	M healthy	11.12 + [1.51(time)]	0.72	4.26
Cycle ergometry (mL/min)	Patton[56]	15		M healthy	[(0.012)W] − 0.099	0.89	
		12		F healthy	[(0.008)W] + 0.732	0.88	
(mL/min)	Storer[67]	115	20–70	M healthy	[10.51(W,max)] + [6.35(wt,kg)] − [10.49(age,yr)] + 519.3	0.94	212.0
		116		F healthy	[9.39(W,max)] + [7.7(wt,kg)] − [5.88(age,yr)] + 136.7	0.93	147.0
Bench stepping None							
Submaximal tests							
Treadmill (mL/kg/min)	Ebbeling[22]	67	20–59	M	15.1 + [p21.8(walk speed,mph)] − [0.327(HR)] − [0.263(speed) (age)] + [0.00504(HR)(age)] + [5.989(gender,F = 0,M = 1)]	0.96	5.0
		72		F			
	Widrick[72]	145	20–59	M healthy F healthy	see Kline[40]	0.91	5.26
	Wilmore[74]	42	18–30	M healthy		0.76	5.0
Cycle ergometry (mL/min)	Fox[28]	87	17–27	M	6,300 − [19.26(HR-at 5th min at 150 − W)]	0.76	246.0
(L/min)	Åstrand[3]	27	18–30	M healthy	Nomogram		0.28
		31		F healthy	Nomogram		0.27

*Assumes steady-state conditions.

TABLE 13.2

Summary of VO₂ prediction equations—cont'd

| EXERCISE MODE | STUDY | N | POPULATION | | EQUATION | R | SEE |
			AGES	GENDER/HEALTH			
Submaximal tests (Cont'd)							
(L/min)	Siconolfi[64]	25	20–70	M healthy	$[0.348(VO_2, \text{Åstrand})] -$ $[0.035(\text{age}) + 3.011]$	0.86	0.36
		28		F healthy	$[0.302(VO_2, \text{Åstrand})] -$ $[0.019(\text{age}) + 1.593]$	0.97	0.20
	Legge[46]	25	2–29	M healthy	Nomogram using ΔHR ($_{max}HR$ = zero loadHR)	0.98	0.17
Bench stepping (mL/kg/min)	McArdle[50]	41	18–22 18–22	F healthy M healthy	$65.81 - [0.1847(\text{recovery HR})]$ $111.33 + [0.42(\text{recovery HR})]$	0.92	2.9
Field tests	Cooper[15]	115	17–52	M	$35.97(\text{miles after 12 min}) - 11.29$	0.90	
	Kline[40]	343	18–23	M,F healthy	$6.9652 + [0.0091(\text{weight,kg})] -$ $[0.02579(\text{age})] + [0.5955$ $(\text{gender} = F = 0, M = 1)] -$ $[0.224(\text{time,1-mi walk})] -$ $0.0115(HR)$	0.93	0.325
	Coleman[16]	90	20–29	M,F healthy	see Kline[40]	0.79	5.68

TABLE 13.3

Estimated oxygen consumption* for jogging/running on a level surface and uphill

% GRADE		5.0	6.0	7.0	7.5	8	9	10
	mi/h	5.0	6.0	7.0	7.5	8	9	10
	km/h	8.0	9.7	11.3	12.1	12.9	14.5	16.1
	m/min	134	161	188	201	215	241	268
a. Outdoor Terrain								
0		30.1	35.7	41.0	43.8	48.6	51.8	57.1
2.5		36.1	43.1	49.4	52.9	56.4	62.7	69.0
5.0		42.0	50.1	57.8	62.0	65.8		
7.5		48.3	57.4	66.2				
10.0		54.3	64.8					
b. Treadmill								
0		30.1	35.7	41.0	43.8	46.6	51.8	57.1
2.5		33.3	39.2	45.2	48.3	51.5	57.1	63.0
5.0		36.1	43.1	49.4	52.9	56.4	62.7	69.0
7.5		39.2	46.6	53.6	57.4	60.9	67.9	
10.0		42.0	50.1	57.8	62.0	66.5		
12.5		45.2	53.9	62.0	66.5			
15.0		48.3	57.4	66.2				

* Assumes steady-state conditions.

Source: Adapted from ACSM (2).

1-min stage durations requiring 1 km/h increments from 8 to 12 km/h, followed by 1% grade increments to exhaustion. After the warm-up to 8 km/h, the test would take 11 min.

The need to tailor a protocol to the fitness and health status of an individual indicates that use of predetermined protocols is inappropriate. In testing healthy or highly trained athletes, this is true. However, the exercise testing of diseased individuals has been performed using standard protocols that allow comparison of data within and between populations. For example, during treadmill testing of individuals with cardiovascular diseases, the Bruce protocol is used routinely, even despite the bias of this protocol to an increasing grade and the increased likelihood for leg fatigue limiting exercise duration. However, a walking protocol has advantages in that it decreases electrical artifact during electrocardiogram evaluation of heart function and allows more accurate monitoring of

TABLE 13.4

Estimated oxygen consumption* for walking on a level surface and uphill

% GRADE	mi/h km/h m/min	1.7 2.7 45.6	2.0 3.2 53.7	2.5 4.0 67.0	3.0 4.8 80.5	3.4 5.5 91.2	3.75 6.00 100.5
0		8.0	8.8	10.2	11.6	12.6	13.7
2.5		10.2	11.2	13.3	15.1	16.8	18.2
5.0		12.3	13.7	16.1	18.9	20.7	22.8
7.5		14.4	16.1	19.3	22.4	24.9	27.3
10.0		16.1	18.6	22.1	25.9	29.1	31.9
12.5		18.2	21.0	25.2	29.8	33.3	36.4
15.0		20.3	23.1	28.4	33.3	37.1	41.0
17.5		22.4	25.6	31.2	36.8	41.3	45.2
20.0		24.5	28.0	34.3	40.6	45.5	49.7
22.5		26.6	30.5	37.1	44.1	49.7	54.3
25.0		28.7	32.9	40.3	47.6	53.6	58.8

* Assumes steady-state conditions.

Source: Adapted from ACSM (2).

blood pressure. Other commonly used treadmill protocols for the exercise evaluation of "high risk" individuals are those of Naughton and associates (46) and Balke and Ware (5).

Predicting Cardiorespiratory and Muscular Endurance

Submaximal VO_2

Typically the ACSM equations have been used to calculate submaximal VO_2 during treadmill, cycle ergometry, arm ergometry, and stepping. Recently, the accuracy of the ACSM equation for cycle ergomety has been questioned. Lang and colleagues (37) revealed that the ACSM equation underestimated VO_2 by approximately 260 mL/min across a range of VO_2 from 0.5 to 2.5 L/min. A new equation was subsequently validated (38) and shown to have better accuracy of prediction with a similar correlation and standard error of estimate (table 13.2). It is recommended that this new equation be used to estimate submaximal steady-state VO_2 during cycle ergometry.

Variables Used to Predict VO_{2max}   The methods used to estimate VO_{2max} can be divided into those involving either maximal or submaximal exercise. The reasons for the presence of prediction equations based on maximal and submaximal exercise is that for many individuals the risks inherent in maximal exercise testing may be avoided when using a submaximal test. However, as indicated in table 13.2, many of the submaximal prediction equations were formulated from apparently healthy and young individuals. It is unclear how this fact influences the generalizability of the equations to more elderly individuals, or individuals with degenerative diseases.

Prediction of VO_{2max} is dependent on measuring variables that are known to change proportionally with VO_2.

Thus, heart rate, change in heart rate, and exercise duration for a given protocol have been used widely by different researchers (table 13.2). The heart rate response to exercise is an important variable for predicting VO_{2max}, because individuals with increased cardiorespiratory endurance have a lower heart rate for a given exercise intensity. However, because other variables other than VO_2 are known to influence heart rate (e.g., dehydration, arousal, the type of exercise) and because there is individual variability in the profile of the heart rate versus the VO_2 curve (see chapter 7), prediction of VO_{2max} on the basis of heart rate alone is associated with considerable prediction error. Error of prediction is also associated with maximal exercise times that are due to differences among individuals in tolerance to intense exercise because of motivation, muscle strength and power, and anaerobic capacity.

Maximal Tests

Treadmill Protocols VO_{2max} can be predicted from maximal exercise duration during the Bruce or Balke treadmill protocols for specific populations (10, 23), and generally have moderate to high correlations among tests that measure VO_2 directly (see table 13.2); however, the standard error of estimate is typically high. For example, figure 13.2 presents data for measured and estimated VO_{2max} versus exercise duration during the Bruce protocol. The resulting curve is sigmoidal, and reveals that data were equally distributed above and below the line of identity throughout the range of exercise duration studied. However, the variation in data around the line of identity reveal that for individuals who exercised for 12 min, actual VO_{2max} values ranged from 36 to 50 mL/kg/min, a potential maximal error of ±7 mL/kg/min (± 16%).

FIGURE 13.2

The relationship between predicted VO_{2max} from exercise duration during the Bruce protocol versus measured VO_{2max}.

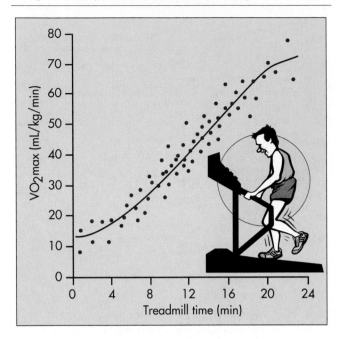

Cycle Ergometer Protocols   The maximal cycle ergometer protocol by Storer and associates (56) is the most accurate method and equation for estimating VO_{2max} during cycle ergometry. After a warm-up of 4 min with zero load, subjects perform an incremental exercise test with a 15 W/min increment until volitional fatigue. The maximal watts attained during the exercise are used in gender-specific equations that also involve body weight and age (table 13.2).

Submaximal Tests

Treadmill Protocols VO_{2max} can also be estimated by equations that use the heart rate response to exercise at different submaximal intensities, accompanied by the ACSM equations for steady-state VO_2. For example, if a 35-year-old female completed a steady-state treadmill running exercise at 6.7 km/h at 0% grade at a heart rate of 125 b/min (test A), and 12.1 km/h at 2.5% grade at a heart rate of 155 b/min (test B), VO_2 would be calculated by estimating VO_2 at each intensity from the ACSM equations, and completing the following calculations:

13.1
$$AVO_2 = 35.7\,mL/kg/min$$
$$BVO_2 = 48.3\ mL/kg/min$$
$$\mathbf{b} = (BVO_2 - AVO_2)\,/\,(BHR - AHR)$$
$$= (48.3 - 35.7)/(155 - 125)$$
$$= 12.6\,/\,30$$
$$= 0.42$$

13.2
$$VO_{2max} = BVO_2 + [\mathbf{b}(HR_{max} - BHR)]$$
$$= 48.3 + \{0.42[(220 - 35) - 155)]\}$$
$$= 48.3 + [0.42(185 - 155)]$$
$$= 48.3 + 12.6$$

$$= 60.9\ mL/kg/min$$
$\mathbf{b}$ = slope of the VO_2/HR relationship

Other protocols exist for estimating VO_{2max} from treadmill walking protocols. Widrick and associates (61) applied the Rockport walk test to a treadmill situation, where subjects had to walk 1.61 km (1 mi) as fast as possible. Walk time, heart rate during the last 2 min of walking, body mass, gender, and age were used to estimate VO_{2max} from gender-specific and general equations. Results indicated that predicted VO_{2max} was accurate for unfit to moderately fit individuals of both genders, but VO_{2max} was underpredicted in highly fit males ($VO_{2max} > 55$ mL/kg/min).

Ebbeling and colleagues (20) also developed a walking test on the treadmill, but unlike the Rockport walk test, this test was based on an estimation of VO_{2max} from a single submaximal stage. The test is conducted by having subjects perform a warm-up of 4 min of walking at a self-selected speed between 4.0 and 7.2 km/h (2.0 − 4.5 mi/h) at 0% grade, causing heart rate to be between 50 and 70% of age-predicted maximum. The grade is then increased to 5% for another 4 min, where heart rate is recorded during the final 30 s. Treadmill speed, final heart rate, age, and gender were used to estimate VO_{2max} expressed as mL/kg/min.

Cycle Ergometer Protocols   Bicycle ergometer tests are commonly used to measure and predict oxygen uptake. One of the most common submaximal cycle ergometer protocols used to predict VO_{2max} was developed by the YMCA (27). This protocol uses 3-min stages. In order to calculate functional capacity, 2 HR and power output data points need to be obtained within a 110 to 150 b/min HR range. Functional capacity can be predicted by plotting the last two heart rate–power output values obtained on a calibrated chart (fig. 13.3).

Another widely used protocol is that of the Åstrand-Rhyming (3) test and nomogram (fig. 13.4a). The original nomogram did not have an age adjustment, which decreased accuracy of the prediction because of the known reduction in maximal heart rate with increasing age. The age-corrected factors were validated by Åstrand (4) on 144 subjects. However, because of the limited number of subjects in these early validation studies, research has produced varied results on the accuracy of the **Åstrand-Rhyming nomogram** and exercise protocol. Legge and Bannister (39) modified the Åstrand-Rhyming nomogram (fig. 13.4b) by using the change in heart rate after zero-loaded cycling rather than absolute heart rate during exercise. Such a change decreased the error of prediction and improved the accuracy of prediction of VO_{2max} in a small sample of trained and untrained males.

Because of the small numbers of subjects and limited populations used by Legge and Bannister (39), it is difficult to recommend this modified nomogram for widespread use in the prediction of VO_{2max}. However, the modified nomogram does seem to have improved accuracy that needs to be validated on differing populations and larger numbers of subjects.

FIGURE 13.3

The chart developed for use with the YMCA submaximal exercise prediction of VO_{2max}.

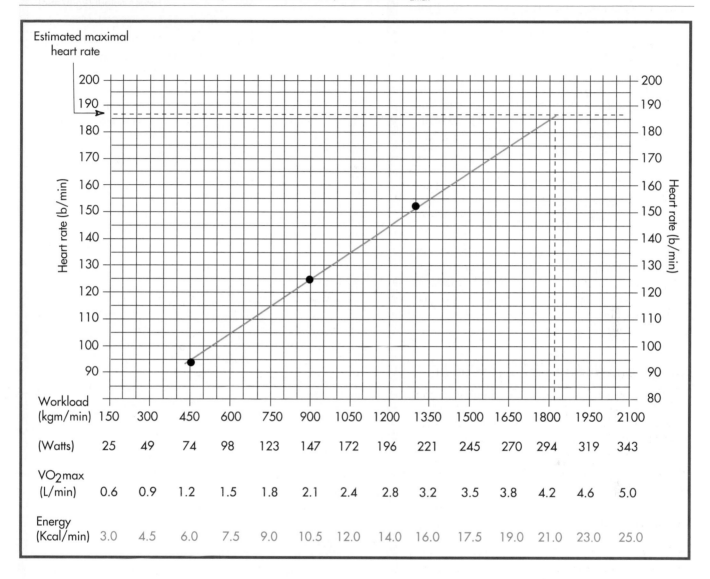

To perform the exercise suited for either nomogram, subjects perform cycle ergometry at 75, 100, or 125 W depending on their endurance training status. Heart rates are recorded at 5 and 6 min. If these heart rates do not differ by more than 5 b/min, they are averaged and their value determines the progression of exercise. If the average heart rate is less than 150, the intensity should be increased by 50 W and exercise should be continued. This is repeated until the average heart rate exceeds 130 b/min after 6 min. Data used in the Åstrand-Rhyming nomogram are the final power output (Watts), and final exercise heart rate. A line is drawn connecting the inner axis of the exercise intensity scale to the exercise heart rate. The intercept of the line across the VO_{2max} axis indicates the VO_{2max}.

Siconolfi and associates (53) modified the YMCA and Åstrand-Rhyming procedures. Exercise is performed similar to the YMCA procedure. An estimated VO_2 from the Åstrand-Rhyming nomogram is obtained (not age-corrected), and used with age in a gender-specific regression equation. This test had good accuracy and low error of prediction across a wide range of VO_2 (1.0 to 3.0 L/min), for individuals between the ages of 20 to 70 years.

Field Tests

Cooper's 1.5-mi Run   The 1.5-mi test, originally developed by Kenneth Cooper, is a popular test used to predict cardiovascular fitness (13). This test is conducted on a quarter-mi

Åstrand-Rhyming nomogram the nomogram for estimating VO_{2max} from a single bout of cycle ergometry

track. After subjects have warmed up, they walk, jog, or run as fast as they can 6 times around the track. Oxygen uptake is predicted by formula (table 13.2).

Rockport Walk Test   The Rockport walk test is an excellent test to predict cardiovascular fitness, especially for sedentary individuals. Individuals are instructed to "walk" as fast as they can for 1 mi and then record their heart rate at the end of the walk. VO_{2max} is predicted by using a multiple regression equation developed by Kline and colleagues (34).

Step Tests   The 3-min step test predicts oxygen uptake from the recovery heart rate following 3 min of stepping (42). The test is conducted using a bench 16¼ in high. A metronome should be set to 88 counts, or 22 steps/min for women, and 96 counts or 24 steps/min for men. At the signal to start, subjects step to a four-step cadence (up-up-down-down). At the end of 3 min, the subject remains standing and a 15-s pulse rate is recorded between 5 to 20 s into recovery.

Lactate and Ventilatory Thresholds

The best measure of success in running events longer than 1500 m for running, and also in long-distance road cycling is the pace or VO_2 at the lactate threshold (LT) (16, 22, 32, 36, 40, 50, 54, 57). As previously explained, it is generally accepted that the *intensity at the LT reflects an individual's maximal steady-state intensity* (see chapter 6). Research has continually revealed very high correlations (> 0.9) between the pace at the LT and some expression of race performance (time, average pace, etc) (16, 22, 32, 36, 40, 50, 54, 57). Similar results have resulted from use of the ventilatory threshold (40, 52). Furthermore, for individuals with a similar VO_{2max}, differences in the LT among the individuals provide a better measure of race performance than VO_{2max} alone.

Despite the evidence for and general interpretation of the LT representing the maximal steady-state intensity, there is also a large body of research which indicates that individuals can race for durations of less than 60 min at intensities above the LT (16, 22, 36, 48). Thus, for relatively short-duration events, the LT underestimates the maximal steady-state intensity, and should be used to reflect a greater capacity to sustain higher-intensity exercise.

As people function in daily activities and compete in endurance events at intensities that are well below VO_{2max}, the LT may be a more valid measure of cardiorespiratory endurance than is VO_{2max}. However, it should be noted that to have a high LT, an individual needs to also have a moderate

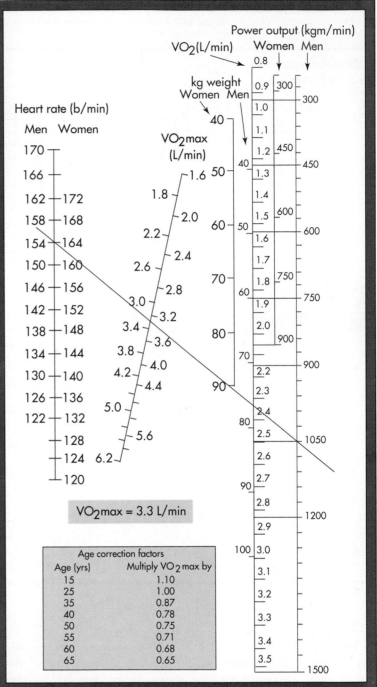

A

to high VO_{2max}. Thus, *the measures of VO_{2max} and the LT combine to provide an accurate indication of cardiorespiratory and muscular endurance,* as well as the potential for success in prolonged endurance events.

The LT is typically measured during a test of VO_{2max} by sampling blood from one of several possible sites. As such, the LT is used to represent whole-body lactate kinetics, and either central venous or central arterial blood is sampled for this purpose. However, because of the invasiveness, potential risk for complications that are due to the procedure and need for medical supervision, arterial and central venous

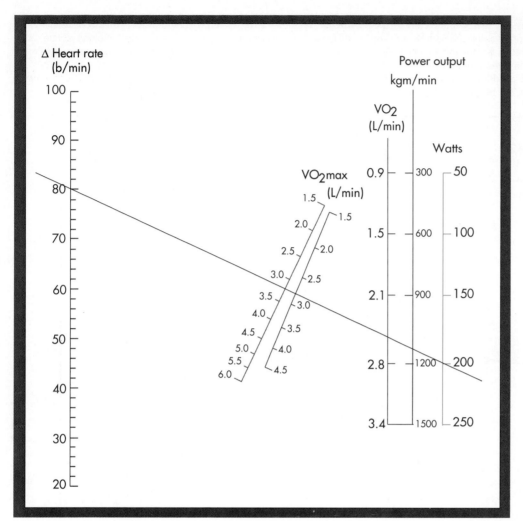

FIGURE 13.4

Two nomograms used to predict VO$_{2max}$ from submaximal steady-state cycle ergometer exercise. *(a)* The Åstrand-Rhyming nomogram. *(b)* The Bannister-Legge nomogram. The Åstrand-Rhyming nomogram has been the most validated of the two nomograms; however, research done in the development of the Bannister-Legge nomogram indicates that it may have significantly better accuracy in predicting VO$_{2max}$ for untrained to moderately trained males.

blood samples are difficult to justify for the purpose of determining the LT. Alternative, more accessible sites for blood sampling are an antecubital vein, dorsal hand vein, finger capillary, or ear lobe. The choice of a sampling site is dependent on the exercise mode. For example, during arm exercise, the blood from the antecubital vein, dorsal hand vein, or finger tip would have an increased lactate concentration because of the altered blood flow and increased lactate release from the working musculature. Furthermore, depending on the method used to detect the LT, venous, arterial, and capillary blood samples will have different lactate concentrations for a given exercise condition, and may in turn cause different estimations of the LT (51). Of course, the best way to avoid the complications of these issues is to *always sample blood for a given exercise mode from the same site*.

The detection of the LT is based on graphing blood lactate concentration (*y*-axis) versus some measure of exercise intensity (VO$_2$, watts, running velocity, etc) (*x*-axis) (fig. 13.5*a* and *b*). Thus, *there is increased precision in detecting the LT with more data points*. Therefore it is recommended that at least eight blood samples be obtained during an incremental exercise test. As previously described, if the test of VO$_{2max}$

is to be based on 1-min stage durations, lasting a total of 12 min, this requires a blood sample every minute. Unless a catheter is being used, this is a demanding task for both the subject and researcher. A compromise is to make stage durations 2 min, and include a warm-up in the protocol. Thus, if the first three stages of the protocol are the warm-up totaling six min, then a 12-min test would provide six additional 2-min stages, and provide a total of nine blood samples.

Methods for Detecting the LT

The concept of an LT has received criticism because of the subjective methods for detecting the intensity at the LT and the fact that blood lactate may not increase in a threshold manner, but rather as an exponential function of exercise intensity (7). Consequently, *visual detection is no longer an acceptable method for detecting the LT*.

Figure 13.5*b* presents an increasingly used method for decreasing the error of subjective detection of the LT. Both axes, or just the lactate axis, can be converted into logarithm values. A purely exponential increase in lactate would then result in a straight line. Conversely, an increase in lactate that has two or more exponential components would reveal the same number of linear segments. Simple

FIGURE 13.5

Examples of blood lactate data graphed as *(a)* absolute data as well as *(b)* log transformed data. In each case, two different blood lactate profiles are shown. For subject 1, blood lactate accumulation proceeds as a two-function relationship with increasing exercise intensity. For subject 2, blood lactate increases as three functions. When log transformed, the increases in blood lactate more clearly appear as two or more functions that can be treated individually using regression to identify an intercept of the lines. For subject 1, the intersection of the two lines represents the LT. For subject 2, it remains unclear which of the thresholds should be used as the LT.

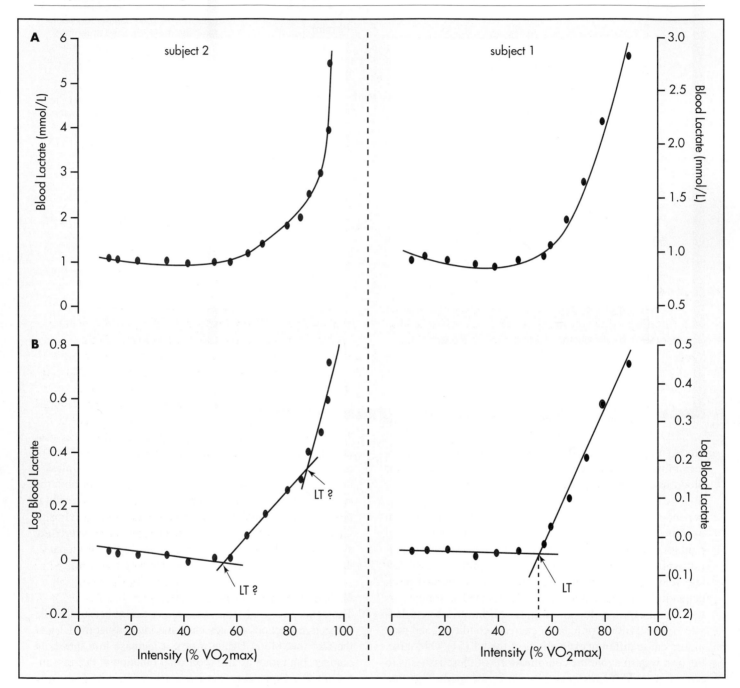

linear regression of two segments of the data set that results in the least error reveals that the LT is the intensity at which the two lines intersect (7). However, for some individuals, more than two functions of the lactate-VO$_2$ plot can be seen. Davis and associates (18) have termed the second inflection as the "lactate turn point" and argue that the second inflection represents the LT (fig. 13.5). It remains unclear

why some individuals have this second inflection, and others do not.

There are numerous other methods for detecting the LT. Fixed blood lactate concentrations have been used, with 2 mmol/L referred to as the aerobic threshold and 4 mmol/L termed the anaerobic threshold (16, 17), or onset of blood lactate accumulation (OBLA) (40, 51, 54, 55). These additional versions of the LT are also accurate predictors of endurance performance; however, the running pace at the LT best resembles the average race pace during prolonged (> 1 h) endurance events.

The Ventilatory Threshold

The LT can be noninvasively determined by plotting ventilation and other respiratory data obtained from an incremental exercise test to VO_{2max}. Caiozzeo and associates (12) have determined that the most accurate variables to use are minute ventilation (V_E), the ventilatory equivalent for oxygen (V_E/VO_2), and the ventilatory equivalent for carbon dioxide (V_E/VCO_2) (see chapter 8).

The exercise intensity at the LT is very similar to the intensity where there is a rate of increase in V_E that exceeds the rate of increase in VO_2. For this reason, the V_E/VO_2 data set is usually most sensitive to detecting the change in ventilation and metabolism. Thus the ventilatory threshold (VT) is detected as the first increase in V_E/VO_2 that corresponds to an abrupt increased rate of ventilation without a change in V_E/VCO_2. Depending on the protocol used, V_E/VCO_2 increases between 1 and 2 min after the increase in V_E/VO_2. The delayed increase in V_E/VCO_2 is a secondary criterion for detecting the VT.

The physiological explanation for an increase in ventilation to correspond to an increase in blood lactate accumulation has been based on the acidosis and increased venous blood PCO_2 that accompanies lactate production (see chapters 6 and 8). However, the exact mechanisms that cause the increase in ventilation are unclear as P_aCO_2 actually decreases during incremental exercise at intensities above the LT because of hyperventilation (see chapter 8), and threshold increases in ventilation have been demonstrated in individuals who were not acidotic. Nevertheless, as previously explained, LT and VT are known to be very accurate predictors of success in prolonged endurance exercise.

Running Economy

Several studies that have evaluated the contribution of multiple variables to prolonged endurance running performance have shown that **running economy** is an additional independent factor that is important (32, 40). As explained in chapters 4 and 6, good running economy involves a low submaximal VO_2, and therefore the ability to run faster at a given percent of the LT or VO_{2max}.

Running economy is determined by having the subject complete at least thee exercise intensities known to be below the LT. The duration of each stage should be at least 4 min, and data of VO_2 should be obtained continuously during the testing. The steady-state VO_2 values (*y*-axis) are graphed against intensity on the *x*-axis, and the linear regression line of best fit represents the change in VO_2 for a change in power output (*efficiency*) of the subject (fig. 13.6).

This test sequence is also useful in research when specific running paces or cycle ergometer intensities (Watts) need to

FIGURE 13.6

A subject's economy and efficiency during cycling can be determined by graphing at least three submaximal steady-state VO_2 data points with exercise intensity (watts). A linear fit of this data can be used to determine the VO_2 for a given intensity, as well as intensities that correspond to certain percentages of VO_{2max}.

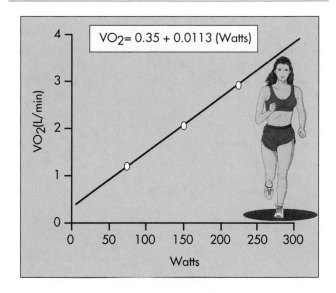

$$VO_2 = 0.35 + 0.0113 \text{ (Watts)}$$

be determined. For this purpose, the regression equation is used to calculate the intensity at a given VO_2. Thus, if a protocol was required to demand an exercise intensity of 60% VO_{2max}, the VO_{2max} could be determined from an incremental exercise test to VO_{2max}, and the steady-state VO_2 versus exercise intensity relationship would need to be obtained from additional testing. A regression equation would be determined from the steady-state VO_2 data, and the exercise intensity at 60% VO_{2max} could be calculated.

VO₂ Kinetics

Another test to evaluate the cardiorespiratory condition of a subject is to measure the rate of change in VO_2 for a given increase in exercise intensity. The more rapid the increase in VO_2, the greater the cardiorespiratory and muscular endurance. This test requires the use of a breath-by-breath indirect calorimetry system, as detailed and illustrated in chapter 4. The rate of increase in VO_2 is typically expressed as a time constant (tVO_2) from a single exponential equation such as $VO_2 = A(1 - e^{-Bx}) + E$ (60), where A = magnitude of change in VO_2; B = rate constant; e = natural log base = 2.7183; E = beginning VO_2; x = time. Such an equation is derived from a computer curve-fitting program. However, care should be taken when statistically comparing rate

running economy a contributor to prolonged endurance running performance involving a low submaximal VO_2

constants due to their susceptibility for change from erroneous noise in data rather than from changes of a physiological cause.

Heart Rate Threshold

During incremental exercise, heart rate has been shown to increase in a linear manner until a given submaximal exercise intensity (denoted fc) that corresponds to the LT (14). However, results from different studies have produced conflicting findings over the similarity/dissimilarity between the LT and fc (29, 30, 33, 35, 52, 58), and reports indicate that an fc can be detected only in less than 50% of individuals (28). Furthermore, Parker and colleagues (48) have shown no relationship between the fc and conventional indices of cardiorespiratory endurance (VO_{2max} or LT) in 24 subjects. Clearly, more research needs to be done on this topic, as a noninvasive and inexpensive method to estimate the LT would have considerable application to sports and athletics.

Measuring Maximal Muscle Power and Anaerobic Capacity

During high-intensity exercise, muscle ATP regeneration must be provided at a high rate in order to prevent fatigue and continue muscle contraction. In many daily, sports, and athletic activities, intense muscle contraction is required and often completed before significant increases in mitochondrial respiration. For these activities, a large capacity for ATP regeneration despite low oxygen consumption is essential for optimal performance. Research has had difficulty in measuring the capacity of nonmitochondrial ATP regeneration, or *anaerobic capacity;* however, several methods are available to estimate this component of fitness.

Maximal muscle power and anaerobic capacity are largely dependent on age, gender, morphological characteristics, and training (8), all of which need to be taken into account during testing and in interpreting the results of a test. Tests of maximal muscle power can be conducted in the field and in the laboratory. Simple tests of muscle power involve quantifying and comparing an athlete's performance during bouts of high-intensity exercise (e.g., stair climbing), whereas more sophisticated laboratory tests can involve isokinetic testing equipment or computer-integrated cycle ergometers.

Measuring Maximal Muscle Power

The tests of **muscle power** are categorized according to the length of the test. Short-term tests last 10 s or less, the intermediate-term anaerobic tests last between 20 and 60 s, and long-term anaerobic tests last 60 to 120 s. Each type of test indirectly reflects a measure of the subject's ability to regenerate ATP during that interval. As will be explained,

additional factors such as muscle fiber type proportions and muscle buffer capacity also influence ATP regeneration.

Short-Term Tests of Muscle Power

Sargent's Jump and Reach   The Sargent's jump and reach test measures the difference between standing reach height and the maximum jumping reach height. Although Sargent's jump and reach test has been used for decades to evaluate leg power, its ability to assess an individual's anaerobic capacity or true muscle power is questionable. The test can produce erroneous results because of the brevity of the test and because the skills involved in performing the test are not factored into the nomogram equation. Muscle power is calculated from the vertical height as follows:

13.3
$$Power(W) = 21.67 \times mass(kg) \times vertical\ displacement(m)^{0.5}$$

Bosco and associates (9) developed a 60-s vertical jump test protocol. The test consists of performing consecutive maximal vertical jumps during a 60-s period. The time in contact with the platform and time in the air are measured via a force plate and electrical timing device. Bosco and associates (9) reported a test-retest reliability of 0.95. Power is calculated as:

13.4
$$W = (9.8 \times Tf \times 60) / 4N (60 - Tf)$$

where W =   mechanical power (W/ kg)

Tf =   sum of total flight time of all jumps
N =   number of jumps during 60 s
9.8 =   acceleration of gravity (m/s^2)

Margaria Power Test   The Margaria test was developed in the early 1960s (41), and was modified by Kalamen (33). The Margaria-Kalamen protocol has subjects start 6 m from a flight of stairs, and run up the stairs taking two or three steps at a time for a total vertical distance of 1.75 m. Because this distance can be spanned in less than 1 s, electronic timing mats are recommended at the first and last step.

Power is calculated from the following equation:

13.5
$$Power\ (W) = [(mass, kg)(vertical\ displacement, m)(9.8)] / (time, s)$$

Intermediate-Term Tests of Muscle Power

Wingate Test   The **Wingate test** (WT), developed in the early 1970s at the Wingate Institute in Israel, has become one of the most widely used protocols for determining peak muscle power, and indirectly reflecting anaerobic capacity (6). The WT involves pedaling or arm cranking at maximal effort for 30 s against a constant load. Performance is expressed as *mean power* (mean work output over 30 s), *peak power* (highest power output during any one 5-s period), or *fatigue index* (difference between the peak power and the lowest 5-s power output divided by peak power).

The resistance setting equations for leg cycling for women is equal to (kp/kg BW = 0.075) and for men (kp/kg BW = 0.083 to 0.092), where kg BW = body weight in kg and kp = kg load (19, 21).

Isokinetic Tests   Isokinetic testing protocols for determining intermediate anaerobic power are popular because they can be designed to test specific muscle groups (fig. 13.7). The ability to generate peak force is indicative of an individual's anaerobic power, and this premise is supported by research documenting significant relationships between peak power and muscle fiber type proportions (chapter 5). Furthermore, isokinetic testing can be used to profile a subject's muscle groups for changes in torque production at different velocities. Presumably, the greater the torque at faster velocities, the greater the likelihood for a bias in fast-twitch motor unit proportions, and the greater potential for high muscle power.

Anaerobic Capacity

The **anaerobic capacity** of an individual represents the ability to regenerate ATP from nonmitochondrial sources. Although the name reflects a capacity, and therefore a given amount of energy, such a capacity is difficult to measure, as will be discussed below.

Muscle Metabolite Accumulation   The rate of ATP regeneration cannot be measured directly, but is often estimated by sampling muscle tissue and assaying for key intermediates of glycogenolysis and glycolysis (see chapters 3 and 6). It is assumed that during intense muscle contractions there is minimal muscle blood flow resulting from high-intramuscular pressures. Consequently, muscle contraction occurs in a closed system where the accumulation of glycolytic intermediates (including lactate) reflects glucose-6-phosphate flux though glycolysis, from which ATP regeneration can be

estimated (e.g., 3 ATP from one glucose-6-phosphate flux to lactate when muscle glycogen is the carbohydrate source).

Accumulated Oxygen Deficit   An indirect and noninvasive method for determining anaerobic capacity is to estimate the total energy requirements of exercise by calculating the theoretical VO_2 required for the exercise intensity and subtracting from this value the measured VO_2. Exercise is usually performed on a cycle ergometer or treadmill. The difference between these two integrated values has been termed the **accumulated oxygen deficit** (aO_2D) and has been argued to reflect anaerobic capacity (43–45) (fig. 13.8).

The aO_2D is maximal after intense exercise is performed that causes fatigue between 2 and 5 min (43–45). Figure 13.9 illustrates values for aO_2D for different athletes and different testing conditions.

Strength

Defining Muscular Strength

Muscular strength is defined as the maximal force exerted by a muscle or muscle group at a specific velocity. Measurement of strength has application to the monitoring of improvement during a resistance-training program. Given that resistance-training programs are used by individuals of all ages and health status, correct evaluation of strength is a

TABLE 13.5				
Norms for grip strength				
	LEFT GRIP (kg)		**RIGHT GRIP (kg)**	
RATING	**M**	**F**	**M**	**F**
Excellent	> 68	> 37	> 70	> 41
Good	56–67	34–36	62–69	38–40
Average	43–55	22–33	48–61	25–37
Poor	39–42	18–21	41–47	22–24
Very poor	< 39	< 18	< 41	< 22

Source: From Corbin, et al. (15).

FIGURE 13.7

A Cybex isokinetic muscle testing system.

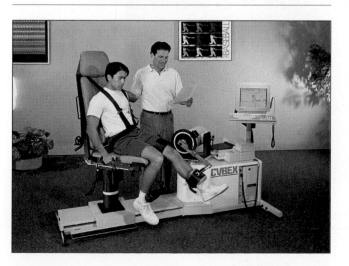

muscle power the mechanical power during dynamic exercise by muscle contractions

Wingate test a 30-s all-out cycle ergometer test that is used to measure maximal power generation as an indirect reflection of a person's anaerobic capacity

anaerobic capacity the capacity of skeletal muscle to regenerate ATP from nonmitochondrial respiration pathways

accumulated oxygen deficit the amount of energy able to be generated by contracting skeletal muscle that did not involve mitochondrial respiration

muscular strength the maximal force generated by contracting skeletal muscle for a given contractile velocity

FIGURE 13.8

The procedure for estimating the aO$_2$D. *(a)* The quantified VO$_2$-watts data points from multiple submaximal exercise tests are fit to a linear regression. This line is extrapolated (dashed line) to the estimated oxygen cost of the power output used for the 2- to 3-min test. *(b)* When the VO$_2$ is measured during the intense exercise bout, the difference between the integration of the measured and estimated oxygen cost represents the aO$_2$D. The accuracy of the aO$_2$D test is dependent on the accuracy of the submaximal steady-state VO$_2$-watts linear regression, and the assumption that the efficiency of the subject during cycling remains consistent during steady-state and non-steady-state exercise.

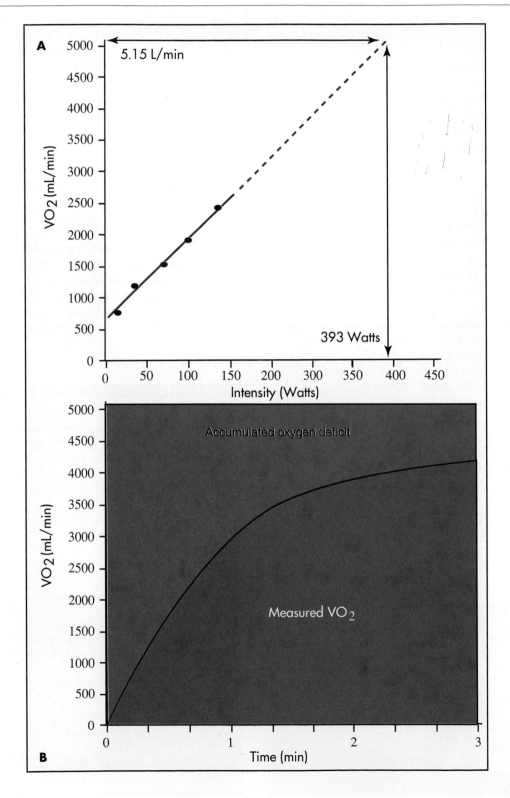

FIGURE 13.9

The accumulated oxygen deficit (aO₂D) of differently trained athletes. The fact that the aO₂D is larger in power-trained individuals provides some degree of validation of the measure and method.

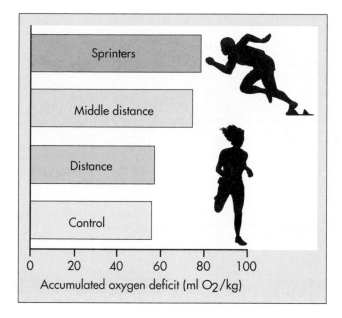

an inexpensive device used to measure static strength. Dynamometers typically have an adjustable handle to fit varying hand sizes. A common dynamometer measures forces between 0 and 100 kg (table 13.5). Larger dynamometers are also available to measure back and leg strength. *Cable tensiometers* are used in conjunction with special tables to also measure static strength of up to 38 different muscle groups.

Strength can also be tested with free weights, variable resistance weight lifting machines, and isokinetic systems. Isotonic or dynamic strength is typically measured by the maximum amount of weight that can be lifted in one repetition (**1 repetition maximum—1 RM**), or in a given number of repetitions (e.g., 10 RM) using either free weights or a resistance machine. As multiple joints and muscles are involved in muscle strength testing with free weights, free weight testing may be better suited to specific sports or athletic movements. Conversely, resistance machines better isolate specific muscles, and therefore can evaluate how specific muscles or muscle groups are responding to a given intervention.

Isokinetic measurements of strength can be performed at different contraction velocities, with the velocity of contraction determining the time for force application, and therefore muscular strength. Thus contractile velocity must be known before comparisons on strength can be made from isokinetic machines.

necessity. Muscular strength can be measured during each type of muscle contraction: isotonic, isometric, eccentric, and isokinetic; however, tests of dynamic muscle strength using isotonic contractions are most common.

Muscular Strength Testing Equipment

Strength testing equipment can vary in price from several hundred dollars to thousands of dollars. A **dynamometer** is

Interpreting Results of Muscular Strength Tests

Muscular strength and endurance are specific to the muscle group being tested, and thus there is no single test available to assess total body muscular strength and endurance. It is recommended that a variety of muscular strength tests be performed so that a fair assessment of upper- and lower-body strength is determined (table 13.6). As with all previous comments on measuring physiological capacities, the evaluation of strength changes requires that the same test be performed in as identical a manner as possible as the previous test.

TABLE 13.6

Strength* norms expressed relative to body weight for 1 RM bench press

RATING	20–29	30–39	40–49	50–59	60+
Men					
Excellent	> 1.26	> 1.08	> 0.97	> 0.86	> 0.78
Good	1.17–1.25	1.01–1.07	0.91–0.96	0.81–0.85	0.74–0.77
Average	0.97–1.16	0.86–1.00	0.78–0.90	0.70–0.80	0.64–0.73
Fair	0.88–0.96	0.79–0.85	0.72–0.77	0.65–0.69	0.60–0.63
Poor	< 0.87	< 0.78	< 0.71	< 0.64	< 0.59
Women					
Excellent	> 0.78	> 0.66	> 0.61	> 0.54	> 0.55
Good	0.72–0.77	0.62–0.65	0.57–0.60	0.51–0.53	0.51–0.54
Average	0.59–0.71	0.53–0.61	0.48–0.56	0.43–0.50	0.41–0.50
Fair	0.53–0.58	0.49–0.52	0.44–0.47	0.40–0.42	0.37–0.40
Poor	< 0.52	< 0.48	< 0.43	< 0.39	< 0.36

* Strength data = strength(lb)/body weight (lb).

Source: Adapted from Gettman (26).

dynamometer (di-na-mom'e-ter) an instrument for the measurement of muscle force application

1 repetition maximum (1 RM) the maximum strength from one contraction; typically, the 1 RM obtained during dynamic contractions [When the contraction is isometric, this strength measure is termed the maximal voluntary contraction (MVC)]

WEBSITE BOX

Chapter 13: Measuring Endurance, Anaerobic Capacity, and Strength

The newest information regarding exercise physiology can be viewed at the following sites.*

af.mil/news/may1996/n19960520_960473.html
   Brooks Airforce Base descriptions of how they use cycle ergometry in fitness testing.

krs.hia.no/~stephens/vo2max.htm
   Detailed description of the rationale and meaning of the test of VO_{2max}.

vertimax.com/
   Commercial site that presents a novel method for quantifying muscle jumping power, and training for an explosive vertical jump.

tees.ac.uk/sportscience/PDA_PDRS/lect6/sld001.htm
   PowerPoint slide presentation on the use of knowledge of muscle metabolism for improved exercise training.

brainmac.demon.co.uk/whatsnew.htm
   Excellent site intended for coaches to have access to exercise-related information, including field tests of physical fitness, training strategies, nutrition, and coaching strategies.

http://fitnesslink.com/nutri.htm
   Information-packed site on exercise and the mind and body, nutrition, fitness programs, how to train, and more.

*Unless indicated, all URLs preceded by http://www.

Note: These URLs were valid at the time of publication, but could have changed or been deleted from Internet access since that time.

SUMMARY

- Many of the tests that quantify a physiological capacity are heavily reliant on the metabolic processes that support exercise for the intensity and duration at question. In a very simple sense, for a given activity that is reliant on one or a combination of multiple metabolic pathways, a laboratory test can be developed to test as much of the maximal capacity of that pathway(s) as possible. The fundamental knowledge base for an exercise physiologist is therefore to *know the metabolic demands and related physiological support functions of specific events/activities.*

- Traditionally, the test used to measure cardiorespiratory and muscular endurance has been that of the maximal rate of oxygen consumption (**VO_{2max}**). However, research indicates that VO_{2max} alone may not be an accurate assessment of the cardiorespiratory demands of submaximal exercise.

- The test of VO_{2max} must meet several requirements in order for the peak VO_2 attained to be VO_{2max}, and these include a test duration between 8 and 12 min, a plateau in VO_{2max}, an RER > 1.1, and HR_{max} < 10 b/min from estimated HR_{max}. Any measure of VO_{2max} that is questionable, thereby increasing the risk for underestimating VO_{2max}, is typically denoted as **VO_{2peak}**.

- The need to tailor a protocol to the fitness and health status of an individual indicates that using predetermined protocols is inappropriate. When testing healthy or highly trained athletes, this is true. However, the exercise testing of diseased individuals has been performed using standard protocols that allow comparison of data within and among populations.

- VO_{2max} can also be estimated by equations that use the heart rate response to exercise at different submaximal intensities, accompanied by the ACSM equations for steady-state VO_2.

- One of the most common submaximal cycle ergometer protocols used to predict VO_{2max} was developed by the YMCA. Another widely used protocol is that of the **Åstrand-Rhyming nomogram.** The original nomogram did not have an age adjustment, which decreased accuracy of the prediction because of the known reduction in maximal heart rate with increasing age. The age-corrected factors were validated on 144 subjects.

- The best measure of success in running events longer than 1,500 m, and also in long-distance road cycling is the pace or VO_2 at the lactate threshold. As previously explained, it is generally accepted that *the intensity at the LT reflects an individual's maximal steady-state intensity.*

- The concept of an LT has received criticism because of the subjective methods for detecting the intensity at the LT, and the fact that blood lactate may not increase in a threshold manner but rather as an exponential function of exercise intensity. Consequently, *visual detection is no longer an acceptable method for detecting the LT.*

- Several studies that have evaluated the contribution of multiple variables to prolonged endurance running performance have shown that **running economy** is an additional independent factor that is important. Good running economy involves a low submaximal VO_2, and therefore the ability to run faster at a given percent of the LT or VO_{2max}.

- Another test to evaluate the cardiorespiratory condition of a subject is to measure the rate of change in VO_2 for a given increase in exercise intensity. The more rapid the increase in VO_2, the greater the cardiorespiratory and muscular endurance. The rate of increase in VO_2 is typically expressed as a time constant (tVO^2) from a single exponential equation such as $VO_2 = A(1 - e^{-Boc}) + E$.

- During incremental exercise, heart rate has been shown to increase in a linear manner until a given submaximal exercise intensity (denoted fc) that corresponds to the LT. However, results from different studies have produced conflicting findings over the similarity/dissimilarity between the LT and fc, and reports indicate that an fc can be detected only in less than 50% of individuals.

- Maximal **muscle power** and *anaerobic capacity* are largely dependent on age, gender, morphological characteristics, and training, all of which need to be taken into account during testing and in interpreting the results of a test.

- Tests of muscle power are categorized according to the length of the test. Short-term tests last 10 seconds or less, the intermediate-term anaerobic tests last between 20 to 60 s, and long-term anaerobic tests last 60 to 120 s.

- Short-term tests of muscle power are the Sargent's jump, and the Margaria tests. A popular intermediate duration test is the **Wingate test** (WT), developed in the early 1970s at the Wingate Institute in Israel. Isokinetic testing protocols for determining intermediate anaerobic power are also popular because they can be designed to test specific muscle groups.

- The **anaerobic capacity** of an individual represents the ability to regenerate ATP from nonmitochondrial sources. The rate of anaerobic ATP regeneration cannot be measured directly, but is often estimated by sampling muscle tissue and assaying for key intermediates of glycogenolysis and glycolysis. An indirect and noninvasive method for determining anaerobic capacity is to estimate the total energy requirements of exercise by calculating the theoretical VO_2 required for the exercise intensity and subtracting from this value the measured VO_2. Exercise is usually performed on a cycle ergometer or treadmill. The difference between these two integrated values has been termed the **accumulated oxygen deficit** (aO_2D) and has been argued to reflect anaerobic capacity.

- **Muscular strength** is defined as the maximal force exerted by a muscle or muscle group at a specific velocity. Measurement of strength has application to the monitoring of improvement during a resistance-training program. A **dynamometer** is an inexpensive device used to measure static strength.

- Strength can also be tested with free weights, variable resistance weight lifting machines, and isokinetic systems. Isotonic or dynamic strength is typically measured by the maximum amount of weight that can be lifted in one repetition (**1 repetition maximum—1 RM**), or in a given number of repetitions (e.g., 10 RM) using either free weights or a resistance machine.

STUDY QUESTIONS

1. Explain the laboratory-based tests you would use to evaluate each of the following: (a) 100-m sprint performance potential, (b) the ability to sustain intense exercise for durations as long as 2 min, (c) the 10,000-m running event.

2. What is a better test of cardiorespiratory endurance, VO_{2max} or the LT? Explain your answer.

3. Why are good running economy and rapid VO_2 kinetics important for optimizing distance running performance?

4. Explain the concept of the accumulated oxygen deficit. What are some potential problems that might exist for its accurate measurement?

5. What are some typical assessment activities that are used to measure muscular strength?

APPLICATIONS

1. Given your increased understanding of exercise physiology, and the fact that there is considerable error in the use of variables from submaximal exercise to estimate VO_{2max}, how would you devise a study to decrease this error and generate an improved prediction equation?

2. Isokinetic testing has been criticized for being too localized to certain muscle groups, and involving a type of contraction that is unnatural and therefore not specific to actual athletic performance. Given these facts, do you think isokinetic testing has merit to assessing muscular power and strength? If so, how should isokinetic testing versus free-weight testing be used?

3. As most athletic performance involves bouts of intense exercise, shouldn't there be more interest in quantifying the anaerobic capacity of skeletal muscle, even for endurance-related events? Explain.

REFERENCES

1. Allen, G., B. J. Freund, and J. H. Wilmore. Interaction of test protocol and horizontal run training on maximal oxygen uptake. *Med. Sci. Sports Exerc.* 18(5):581–587, 1986.

2. American College of Sports Medicine. *Guidelines for exercise testing and prescription,* 4th ed. Williams & Wilkins, Baltimore, 1991.

3. Åstrand, P. O., and I. Rhyming. A nomogram for calculation of aerobic capacity (physical fitness) from pulse rate during submaximal work. *J. Appl. Physiol.* 7:218–221, 1954.

4. Åstrand, P. O. Aerobic work capacity in men and women with special reference to age. *Acta Physiol. Scand.* 49(Suppl. 169):1–92, 1960.

5. Balke, B., and R. Ware. An experimental study of Air Force personnel. *U.S. Armed Forces Med. J.* 10:675–688, 1959.

6. Bar-Or, O. The Wingate anaerobic test: An update on methodology, reliability and validity. *Sports Med.* 4:381–394, 1987.

7. Beaver, W. L., K. Wasserman, and B. J. Whipp. Improved detection of the lactate threshold during exercise using a log-log transformation. *J. Appl. Physiol.* 59:1936–1940, 1985.

8. Bouchard, C., F. T. Dionne, J.-A. Simoneau, and M. R. Boulay. Genetics of aerobic and anaerobic performances. In J. Holloszy (ed.), *Exercise and sport sciences reviews,* Vol. 20, Williams & Wilkins, Baltimore, 1992, pp. 27–58.

9. Bosco, C., P. Luhtanen, and P. V. Komi. A simple method for measurement of mechanical power in jumping. *Eur. J. Appl. Physiol.* 50:273–282, 1983.

10. Bruce, R. L., F. Kusumi, and D. Hosmer. Maximal oxygen intake and nomographic assessment of functional aerobic impairment in cardiovascular disease. *Am. Heart J.* 85:545–562, 1973.

11. Buchfuhrer, M. J., J. E. Hansen, T. E. Robinson, D. Y. Sue, K. Wasserman, and B. J. Whipp. Optimizing the exercise protocol for cardiopulmonary assessment. *J. Appl. Physiol.* 55(5):1558–1564, 1983.

12. Caiozzeo, V. J., et al. A comparison of gas exchange indices used to detect the anaerobic threshold. *J. Appl. Physiol.* 53:1184–1189, 1982.

13. Cooper, K. H. A means of assessing maximal oxygen intake. *J. Am. Med. Assoc.* 203:201–204, 1968.

14. Conconi, F., M. Ferrari, P. G. Ziglio, P. Droghetti, and L. Codeca. Determination of the anaerobic threshold by a non-invasive field test in runners. *J. Appl. Physiol.* 52(4):869–873, 1982.

15. Corbin, C. B., L. J. Dowell, R. Lindsey, and H. Tolson. Concepts in physical education. Brown, Dubuque, IA, 1978.

16. Coyle, E. F., A. R. Coggan, M. K. Hopper, and T. J. Walters. Determinants of endurance in well trained cyclists. *J. Appl. Physiol.* 64(6):2622–2630, 1988.

17. Davis, J. A., et al. Does the gas exchange anaerobic threshold occur at a fixed blood lactate concentration of 2 or 4 mM? *Int. J. Sports Med.* 4:89–93, 1983.

18. Davis, H. A., J. Bassett, P. Hughes, and G. C. Gass. Anaerobic threshold and lactate turnpoint. *Eur. J. Appl. Physiol* 50: 383–392, 1983.

19. Dotan, R., and O. Bar-Or. Load optimization from the Wingate anaerobic test. *Eur. J. Appl. Physiol.* 51:409–417, 1983.

20. Ebbling, C. B., A. Ward, E. M. Puleo, J. Widrick, and J. M. Rippe. Development of single stage submaximal walking test. *Med. Sci. Sports Exerc.* 23(8):966–973, 1991.

21. Evans, J. A., and H. A. Quinney. Determination of resistance settings for anaerobic power testing. *Can. J. Appl. Sports Sci.* 6:53–56, 1981.

22. Farrell, P., J. H. Wilmore, E. Coyle, J. Billing, and D. L. Costill. Plasma lactate accumulation and distance running performance. *Med. Sci. Sports Exerc.* 11(4):338–344, 1979.

23. Foster, C., et al. Generalized equations for predicting functional capacity from treadmill performance. *Am. Heart J.* 107:1229–1234, 1984.

24. Freund, B. J., D. Allen, and J. H. Wilmore. Interaction of test protocol and inclined run training on maximal oxygen uptake. *Med. Sci. Sports Exerc.* 18(5):588–592, 1986.

25. Froelicher, V. F., and M. C. Lancaster. The prediction of maximal oxygen consumption from a continuous graded exercise protocol. *Am. Heart J.* 87:445–450, 1974.

26. Gettman, L. R. Fitness testing. In S. Blair, P. Painter, R. Pate, L. Smith, and C. Taylor (eds.), *Resource manual for guidelines for exercise testing and prescription.* Lea & Febiger, Philadelphia, 1988.

27. Golding, L. A., C. R. Meyers, and W. E. Shinning. *Y's way to physical fitness: The complete guide to fitness testing and instruction,* 3rd ed. Human Kinetics, Champaign, IL, 1989.

28. Heck, H., K. Beckers, W. Lammerschmidt, E. Purin, G. Hess, and W. Hollman. Identification, objectivity, and validity of

Conconi threshold by cycle stress tests. *Dtsch. Z. Sportmed.* 40:388–412, 1989.

29. Hofmann, P., V. Bunc, H. Leitner, R. Pokan, and G. Gaisl. Heart rate threshold related to lactate turn point and steady-state exercise on a cycle ergometer. *Eur. J. Appl. Physiol.* 69:132–139, 1994.

30. Hofmann, P., et al. Relationship between heart rate threshold, lactate turn point, and myocardial function. *Int. J. Sports Med.* 15:232–237, 1994.

31. Howley, E. T., D. R. Bassett, and H. G. Welch. Criteria for maximal oxygen uptake: Review and commentary. *Med. Sci. Sports Exerc.* 27(9):1292–1301, 1995.

32. Joyner, M. J. Modeling: Optimal marathon performance on the basis of physiological factors. *J. Appl. Physiol.* 70(2):683–687, 1991.

33. Kalamen, J. *Measurement of maximum muscular power in man.* Doctoral dissertation, Ohio State University, 1968.

34. Kline, G. M., et al. Estimation of VO_{2max} from a one-mile track walk, gender, age, and body weight. *Med. Sci. Sports Exerc.* 19:253–259, 1987.

35. Kuipers, H., H. A. Keizer, T. deVries, P. van Rijthoven, and M. Wijts. Comparison of heart rate as a noninvasive determinant of the anaerobic threshold with the lactate threshold when cycling. *Eur. J. Appl. Physiol.* 58:303–306, 1988.

36. Kumagai, S., K. Tanaka, V. Matsuura, A. Matsuzaka, and K. Hirakoba. Relationships of the anaerobic threshold with the 5 km, 10 km, and 20 mile races. *Eur. J. Appl. Physiol.* 49:13–23, 1982.

37. Lang, P. B., R. W. Latin, K. E. Berg, and M. B. Mellion. The accuracy of the ACSM cycle ergometry equation. *Med. Sci. Sports Exerc.* 24(2):272–276, 1992.

38. Latin, R. W., K. E. Berg, P. Smith, R. Tolle, and S. Woodby-Brown. Vaildation of a cycle ergometry equation for predicting steady-rate VO_2. *Med. Sci. Sports Exerc.* 25(8):970–974, 1993.

39. Legge, B. J., and E. W. Bannister. The Åstrand-Rhyming nomogram revisited. *J. Appl. Physiol.* 61(3):1203–1209, 1986.

40. Londeree, B. R. The use of laboratory tests with long distance runners. *Sports Med.* 3:201–213, 1986.

41. Margaria, R. Measurement of muscular power in man. *J. Appl. Physiol.* 21:1662–1664, 1966.

42. McArdle, W. D., F. I. Katch, G. S. Pechar, L. Jacobson, and S. Ruck. Reliability and interrelationships between maximal oxygen intake, physical work capacity, and step-test scores in college women. *Med. Sci. Sports Exerc.* 4(4):182–186, 1972.

43. Medbo, J. I., A. C. Mohm, I. Tabata, R. Bah, O. Vaage, and O. M. Sejersted. Anaerobic capacity determined by the accumulated O_2 deficit. *J. Appl. Physiol.* 64(1):50–60, 1988.

44. Medbo, J. I., and I. Tabata. Relative importance of aerobic and anaerobic energy release during short lasting, exhausting bicycle exercise. *J. Appl. Physiol.* 67(5):1881–1886, 1989.

45. Medbo, J. I., and S. Burgers. Effect of training on the anaerobic capacity. *Med. Sci. Sports Exerc.* 22(4):501–507, 1990.

46. Naughton, J., B. Balke, and F. Nagle. Refinement in methods of evaluation and physical conditioning before and after myocardial infarction. *Am. J. Cardiol.* 14:837, 1964.

47. Noakes, T. D. Implications of exercise testing for prediction of athletic performance: A contemporary perspective. *Med. Sci. Sports Exerc.* 20:319–330, 1988.

48. Parker, D., R. Quintana, C. C. Frankel, and R. A. Robergs. Relationships between isokinetic cycling performance and each of VO_{2max} and thresholds for heart rate and blood lactate. *J. Exerc. Physiol.* online 2(4), 1999.

49. Pollock, M. L., C. Foster, D. Schmidt, C. Hellman, A. C. Linnerud, and A. Ward. Comparative anaysis of physiological responses to three different maximal graded exercise protocols in healthy women. *Am. Heart J.* 103:363–373, 1982.

50. Rhodes, E. C., and D. C. McKenzie. Prediciting marathon time from anaerobic threshold measurements. *Phys. Sports Med.* 12:95–98, 1984.

51. Robergs, R. A., D. L. Costill, W. J. Fink, J. Chwalbinska-Moneta, and D. D. Pascoe. Blood lactate differences between arterialized and venous blood. *Int. J. Sports Med.* 11(6):446–451, 1990.

52. Robergs, R. A. Predictors of marathon running performance. In S. Wood and R. Roach (eds.), *Sports and exercise medicine, Vol. 76: Lung biology in health and disease.* Marcel Dekker, New York, 1994.

53. Siconolfi, S. F., E. M. Cullinane, R. A. Careton, and P. D. Thompson. Assessing VO_{2max} in epidemiologic studies: Modification of the Åstrand-Rhyming test. *Med. Sci. Sports Exerc.* 14(5):335–338, 1982.

54. Sjodin, B., and J. Svedenhag. Applied physiology of marathon running. *Sports Med.* 2:83–99, 1985.

55. Stegman, H., W. Kinderman, and A. Schnabel. Lactate kinetics and individual anaerobic threshold. *Int. J. Sports Med.* 3:105–110, 1982.

56. Storer, T. W., J. A. Davis, and V. J. Caiozzeo. Accurate prediction of VO_{2max} in cycle ergometry. *Med. Sci. Sports Exerc.* 22(5):704–712, 1990.

57. Tanaka, K., and Y. Matsuura. Marathon performance, anaerobic threshold, and onset of blood lactate accumulation. *J. Appl. Physiol.* 57(3):640–643, 1984.

58. Tokmakidis, S. P., and L. A. Leger. Comparison of mathematically determined blood lactate and heart rate "threshold" points and relationship with performance. *Eur. J. Appl. Physiol.* 64:309–317, 1992.

59. Wasserman, K., and B. J. Whipp. Exercise physiology in health and disease. *Am. Rev. Resp. Dis.* 112:219–249, 1975.

60. Whipp, B. J., S. A. Ward, N. Lamarra, J. A. Davis, and K. Wasserman. Parameters of ventilatory and gas exchange dynamics during exercise. *J. Appl. Physiol.* 52(6):1506–1513, 1982.

61. Widrick, J., A. Ward, C. Ebbeling, E. Clemente, and J. M. Rippe. Treadmill validation of an overground walking test to predict peak oxygen consumption. *Eur. J. Appl. Physiol.* 64:304–308, 1992.

RECOMMENDED READINGS

American College of Sports Medicine. *Guidelines for exercise testing and prescription,* 5th ed. Williams & Wilkins, Baltimore, 1995.

Beaver, W. L., K. Wasserman, and B. J. Whipp. Improved detection of the lactate threshold during exercise using a log-log transformation. *J. Appl. Physiol.* 59:1936–1940, 1985.

Caiozzeo, V. J., et al. A comparison of gas exchange indices used to detect the anaerobic threshold. *J. Appl. Physiol.* 53:1184–1189, 1982.

Coyle, E. F., A. R. Coggan, M. K. Hopper, and T. J. Walters. Determinants of endurance in well trained cyclists. *J. Appl. Physiol.* 64(6):2622–2630, 1988.

Howley, E. T., D. R. Bassett, and H. G. Welch. Criteria for maximal oxygen uptake: Review and commentary. *Med. Sci. Sports Exerc.* 27(9):1292–1301, 1995.

Kline, G. M., et al. Estimation of VO_{2max} from a one-mile track walk, gender, age, and body weight. *Med. Sci. Sports Exer.* 19:253–259, 1987.

Londeree, B. R. The use of laboratory tests with long distance runners. *Sports Med.* 3:201–213, 1986.

Parker, D., R. Quintana, C. C. Frankel, and R. A. Robergs. Relationships between isokinetic cycling performance and each of VO_{2max} and thresholds for heart rate and blood lactate. *J. Exerc. Physiol.* online 2(3), 1999.

Sjodin, B., and J. Svedenhag. Applied physiology of marathon running. *Sports Med.* 2:83–99, 1985.

Storer, T. W., J. A. Davis, and V. J. Caiozzeo. Accurate prediction of VO_{2max} in cycle ergometry. *Med. Sci. Sports Exerc.* 22(5):704–712, 1990.

Tokmakidis, S. P., and L. A. Leger. Comparison of mathematically determined blood lactate and heart rate "threshold" points and relationship with performance. *Eur. J. Appl. Physiol.* 64:309–317, 1992.

CHAPTER 14

Measuring Pulmonary Function

ormal pulmonary function enables the body to adequately support oxygen delivery and carbon dioxide removal from the body. However, in many individuals pulmonary function is impaired, resulting in disturbances to blood oxygen transport and limitations to exercise tolerance. An impaired pulmonary function may be caused by asthma, allergies, exercise-induced bronchoconstriction, or the structural damage caused by tobacco smoke. In any case, knowledge of the severity of the impairment in quantifiable terms is valuable for monitoring the condition to assess further degeneration or improvement because of changes in lifestyle or medications. The purpose of this chapter is to introduce the principles of specific pulmonary function testing by describing the equipment that is used, detailing the variables that can be measured, and indicating how to interpret changes in these measures.

OBJECTIVES

After studying this chapter, you should be able to:

- Identify the terms used for the different components of the total lung volume.
- Provide estimates of the volumes for the components of the total lung volume.
- Explain the procedures involved in spirometry testing.
- Calculate lung volumes from a spirometry tracing.
- Identify and describe the different instruments and methods used in pulmonary function testing.

KEY TERMS

spirometry	oximetry	residual volume
kymograph	minute ventilation	helium dilution
spirometer	alveolar ventilation	nitrogen washout
vital capacity	anatomical dead	
pneumotachometer	space	

Overview of Pulmonary Function Testing

*T*able 14.1 lists some of the different pulmonary function tests and the criteria they measure. Pulmonary function testing is performed in a variety of settings and for many different reasons. For example, tests performed in hospitals and physician's offices are done to evaluate lung damage from cigarette smoke or other pollutants, or the severity of asthma or the effects of medications. Tests conducted in exercise physiology laboratories may be a part of a total fitness and health series of tests, which in part are to evaluate the function of the lungs relative to possible lung damage (e.g., emphysema) or to form a body composition assessment in the measurement of residual volume. It is also important to conduct pulmonary function tests when performing research of oxygen transport during exercise or exercise performance; Dempsey and colleagues (6) have reported the incidence of exercise-induced bronchoconstriction in unsymptomatic (undiagnosed) patients to be as high as 30% within a population of young recreational- to elite-level athletes.

Pulmonary Function Testing: Equipment and Methods

Pulmonary function testing equipment has become quite sophisticated in the last century. Equipment used to test pulmonary function can cost less than $100 for portable instruments that measure flow rates, to more than $20,000 for whole-body plethysmographs or computerized lung volume and airflow systems. In this chapter, several important instruments that are used in the testing of athletes, as well as the routine clinical testing of patients, will be presented and their measurements explained.

Volume-Displaced Spirometer

In the early 1800s, John Hutchinson (10) discovered that lung volumes could be accurately measured by having subjects breathe into a system that records volume displacements on paper. John Hutchinson's early experiments led to the development of the technique which we now call **spirometry.** Even today, the spirometer remains one of the basic tools for evaluating pulmonary function.

A spirometer (fig. 14.1) consists of (1) an upright metal cylinder that is open at the top, (2) a second cylinder approximately $\frac{1}{2}$ in smaller in diameter which is closed at the top except for two holes (which are exit holes for the tubes that run from the inside of the spirometer to the outside), and (3) a plastic cylinder (often called a bell) which is open at the bottom. The first and second cylinders create a space which is filled with water. The bell sits in the water between the first and second cylinders. When the bell

TABLE 14.1

Examples of specific pulmonary function tests and the purpose(s) for which they are performed

TESTS	PURPOSES
Lung Volumes and Capacities	
Vital capacity	Functional lung volume
Residual lung volume	Body composition assessment
	Evaluation of lung damage
Lung Mechanics	
Lung and chest compliance	Evaluation of airway damage
Airway closure	Evaluation of airway damage
Lung Dynamics	
Flow rates	Evaluation of lung damage
	Evaluation of ventilatory muscle power
Airway closure	Evaluation of integrity of small airways
Gas Exchange	
Ventilation - perfusion	Assessment of regional distributions of lung ventilation and perfusion
	Estimation of physiological dead space
Gas diffusion	Assessment of edema, lung damage
Blood gas measurement	Evaluation of functional gas exchange
Pulse oximetry (hemoglobin saturation)	Evaluation of alveolar to arterial oxygen diffusion

Source: Adapted from Chusid (3).

rests in the water, an airtight seal is made between the bell and the water, and when air is forced into or out of the spirometer, the bell will either move upward or downward.

When a subject breathes into the spirometer (exhales), the bell moves up because air is forced into the closed system. The air exhaled into the system is mixed throughout by a fan and CO_2 is absorbed by soda lime contained in a canister inside the bell. During inhalation, air is removed from the closed system, which causes a vacuum-like effect because of the airtight seal, and the bell moves downward. The oxygen removed from the air in the system by the body is added by an inflow of pure oxygen at a rate that equals VO_2. Thus spirometry is also a means to measure VO_2, and this method is termed *closed-circuit spirometry*. However, as CO_2 is removed and not measured, VCO_2 is not known and therefore RER (respiratory exchange ratio) and an accurate estimate of energy expenditure can not be calculated.

The movement of the bell upward and downward represents the volume of air entering and exiting the lungs. When the bell is connected to a pen, the movements of the bell can be recorded on a rotating drum called a **kymograph.** Once the volume conversion of the bell is known (mL/mm), volume (ATPS) can be calculated. The various lung volumes and capacities at rest are illustrated in figure

FIGURE 14.1

A Collins™ spirometer used for quantifying lung volumes and capacities. Air is directed into and from the spirometer by pipes and low-resistance tubing that connect the system to the outside air or to the subject. Vertical displacement of the floating bell during inspiration and expiration is marked on paper on the kymograph (rotating bell). Each mm rise or fall of the bell represents a given volume of gas, which depends on the volume conversion factor for the bell expressed in ATPS conditions.

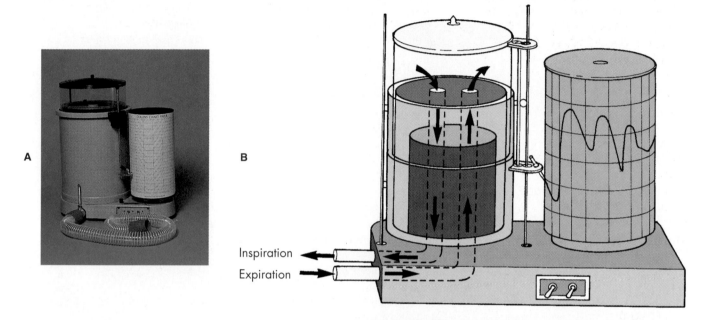

14.2, and table 14.2 indicates which lung volumes change during exercise.

Bellows-Type Spirometer

Another type of volume-displacement system for measuring lung volumes is the bellows-type **spirometer**, often termed a *spirograph* or *vitalograph*. The bellows-type spirometer consists of collapsible bellows that fold and unfold in response to inhalation and exhalation. When a subject exhales into the spirometer, the bellows expand and record the volume of air on paper. Thus the displacement of the bellows by a volume of air is transferred to either a mechanical recording or an electrical recording on a computer (fig. 14.3). Typically, an individual will exhale as hard and as fast as possible into a vitalograph, and **vital capacity** and expired flow rates can be computed from the calibrated paper used on the instrument.

Flow-Sensing Spirometers

A more sophisticated type of spirometer calculates lung volumes by directly measuring the flow of air (fig. 14.4). A **pneumotachometer** measures the rate of flow of air during inhalation and exhalation (fig. 14.4). Airflow during exhalation is based on the difference between the pressure of air entering the pneumotach against resistance (usually a small mesh screen) (P_1), and the pressure of air on the other side of the resistance (P_2). The greater the flow of air into the pneumotach, the greater the resistance, and the greater the pres-

FIGURE 14.2

A standard trace from a spirometer showing lung volumes. A standard spirometer can also be used to measure lung capacities and flow rates by increasing the speed of the paper and recording forced maximal inspiratory and expiratory efforts.

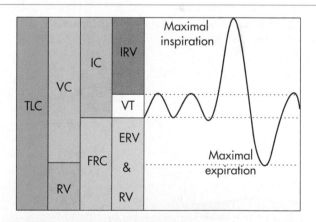

spirometry (spi-rom′e-tri) the measurement of human lung volumes and functional capacities with a spirometer

kymograph (ki′mo-graf) the rotating drum component of an instrument (e.g., spirometer) that is used to record wave-like modulations (e.g., ventilation)

spirometer (spi-rom′e-ter) a device used to measure lung volumes

vital capacity the maximal volume of air that can be exhaled from the lungs in one expiratory effort

pneumotachometer (nu′mo-ta-kom′e-ter) an instrument for measuring the instantaneous flow during ventilation

TABLE 14.2

Pulmonary lung volumes and capacities measured by spirometry and their changes during exercise

VOLUME CAPACITY	ABBREVIATION	DESCRIPTION	CHANGE DURING EXERCISE
Residual volume	RV	Volume of air remaining in the lungs after maximum exhalation; cannot be determined with spirometry	Slight increase
Expiratory reserve volume	ERV	Maximum volume of air exhaled from end-expiratory level	Slight decrease
Functional residual capacity	FRC	Sum of RV and ERV; cannot be determined with spirometry	Slight increase
Tidal volume	V_T	Volume of air inhaled and exhaled with each breath during quiet breathing	Increase
Inspiratory reserve volume	IRV	Maximum volume of air inhaled from end-inspiratory level	Decrease
Inspiratory capacity	IC	Sum of IRV and V_T	Increase
Vital capacity	VC	Maximum volume of air exhaled from the point of maximum inspiration	Slight decrease
Total lung capacity	TLC	Sum of all volume compartments of the lung	Slight decrease
Forced vital capacity	FVC	Forced vital capacity performed with maximally forced expiratory effort	Decrease
Forced expiratory volume in 1 sec	FEV_1	Volume of air expired in 1 s	
Maximum voluntary ventilation	MVV	Volume of air expired in a specified period during repetitive maximum respiratory effort	Slight decrease

FIGURE 14.3

A bellows-type spirometer. The version illustrated has a bellow that expands during expiration and can be used to measure vital capacity.

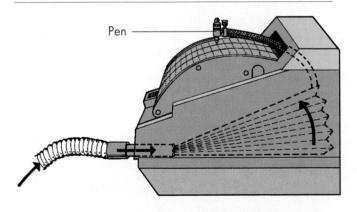

Pen

sure difference, and thus the greater the volume of air moving through the pneumotach.

The pressure difference ($P_1 - P_2$) is measured continuously with a special pressure-sensing transducer, and the signal is then transmitted to a computer which then integrates the signal and transforms flow rates into volumes per unit time. Volumes can be calculated from the flow measure-

ments because volume (mL) = flow (mL/s) × time (s). Pneumotach spirometers are becoming increasingly used when conducting cardiopulmonary testing because of their small size and high sensitivity and accuracy.

Breathing Valves

There are two types of breathing valves commonly used in pulmonary function testing: free-breathing and multiple one-way directional valves (fig. 14.5). A free-breathing valve is commonly seen on a volume-displacement spirometer, because it allows the subject to be switched from breathing room air (open-circuit) to breathing gas contained in a spirometer (closed-circuit). The most common directional valve apparatus used in exercise testing is the Daniel's valve. This valve apparatus actually contains two one-way valves that direct inspired air into the mouth and expired air to a sampling hose.

The difficulty with a valve apparatus for placement in the mouth is the stimulus this gives to increase ventilation. Thus, when testing ventilation using a mouthpiece valve apparatus, subjects need to be given a familiarization period (usually 2 to 3 min of quiet breathing through the mouthpiece) before actual data collection is begun. To minimize hyperventilation, face masks are also available that have multiple one-way valves to direct inspired and expired air.

FIGURE 14.4

Advances in electronics has developed the pneumotach, which measures flow rates by sensing pressure differences between air before and after crossing a resistance membrane. Devices like the pneumotach can record airflow changes during inspiration and expiration. Computer processing of the signal can convert flow rates into ventilation volumes per unit time.

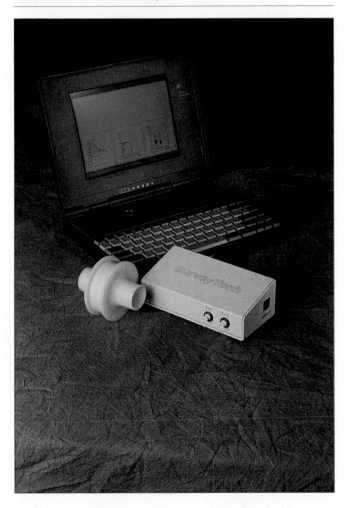

Pulse Oximetry

Oximetry involves the indirect determination of the percent of hemoglobin that is bound with oxygen (S_aO_2). Oximetry is a commonly used (noninvasive) method in hospitals and also during exercise testing to assess blood oxygenation. One of the newest methods of oximetry during exercise testing is the pulse oximeter (8, 16, 17). Pulse oximeters measure the change in infra-red light transmission through a finger or the earlobe to calculate arterial saturation. Such a principle is based on the color change in oxy-hemoglobin at different oxygen saturations. The pulse oximeter has been shown to be fairly accurate in exercise testing (8, 16, 17). A drop in arterial oxygenation under normal barometric pressure conditions is an indication of respiratory failure or, as discussed in chapter 12, when used during exercise it is able to detect an inadequate pulmonary function indicated by exercise-induced hypoxemia.

Gas Analyzers and Metabolic Carts

The need and use for oxygen and carbon dioxide analyzers during exercise was discussed in chapter 4. However, it needs to be stressed that expired gas concentrations also have application to pulmonary function. Concentrations of oxygen and carbon dioxide in expired air differ depending on the phase of tidal volume. At end-tidal volume, air represents alveolar air and, therefore, is very similar to true alveolar fractions of oxygen and carbon dioxide. Of course, rapidly responding analyzers are needed for these purposes, and models can be purchased that operate on the basis of standard electronic principles. In addition, gas mass spectrometers have a response time measured in milliseconds, and such instruments are being applied to both pulmonary function and exercise cardiorespiratory measurement conditions.

Pretest Scheduling Instructions

There are a few important conditions that must be met for pulmonary function tests to be valid. Research has shown that prior submaximal and maximal exercise reduces vital capacity and FEV_1 within 30 min of recovery (12, 14, 16), and increases residual volume (2, 7). It has been recommended that exercise should not be performed for up to 12 h prior to pulmonary function measurements (3, 5). A patient's medical history should also be taken prior to each test to ascertain the presence of upper respiratory tract infections, asthma, or allergies. Finally, although no difference in lung volumes and functional capacities has been detected between the standing and seated position, the posture used during testing should be recorded and used consistently.

Table 14.3 lists the normal values for lung volumes, and table 14.4 provides equations suitable for estimating dynamic lung capacities. These values and equations should be used to compare measured results so that abnormalities can be detected.

Minute Ventilation

The amount of air inspired and expired in 1 min is referred to as **minute ventilation** (V_E). At rest, the normal minute ventilation is equal to approximately 6 L of air.

14.1   Minute ventilation $(V_E) = 12\ (f) \times 0.5\ (V_T) = 6$ L/min

oximetry (ok'sim'e-tri) indirect measurement of the oxygen saturation of hemoglobin in blood

minute ventilation the volume of air ventilated in and from the lungs in 1 min

FIGURE 14.5

A typical Daniel's valve, with two one-way valves that direct inspired air into the mouth via one valve, and expired air away from the subject via a second valve. Typically, expired air is collected and analyzed for expired gas fractions and volume.

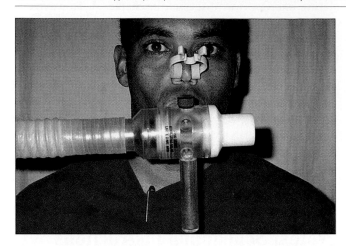 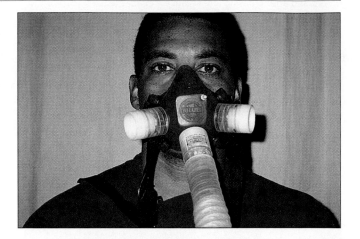

During exercise, V_E increases as a result of a combination of an increase in breathing frequency (f) and tidal volume (V_T). During strenuous exercise in well-conditioned endurance athletes, minute ventilation can increase 27 times above the resting value (20) (table 14.5).

Alveolar Ventilation

It is important to remember that not all of the air inspired reaches the alveoli (the site of gas exchange). **Alveolar ventilation** (V_A) is the portion of inspired air that reaches the alveoli, and thus takes place in gas exchange. There is also a portion of inspired air which remains in the upper respiratory tract, and thus does not take place in gas exchange; it is referred to as **anatomical dead space** (V_D). Dead space averages approximately 30% of resting tidal volume.

Alveolar ventilation can be estimated from spirometry by multiplying the difference of tidal volume (V_T) and dead space (V_D) times breathing frequency (f).

14.2
$$\begin{aligned} V_A &= (V_T - V_D) \times (br/min) \\ &= (0.5 - 0.15) \times 12 \\ &= 4.2 \ L/min \end{aligned}$$

Changes in breathing patterns can affect alveolar ventilation, and thus the amount of air available for gas exchange (table 14.6). An increase in breathing frequency (rapid shallow breathing) causes a decrease in V_T and V_A, which also

TABLE 14.3

Values for lung volumes* for healthy men and women

MEASURE	MALES	FEMALES
V_T	400–500	350–450
IRV	3100	1900
ERV	1200	900
RV	1200	1000
	[Age (yrs) × 0.0115] + [height (cm) × 0.019] − 2.24	[Age (yrs) × 0.03] + [height (cm) × 0.0387] − [body surface area (mm²) × 0.73] − 2.24
TLC	6000	4200

*Lung volumes (mL, BTPS); VT = tidal volume; IRV = inspiratory reserve volume; ERV = expiratory reserve volume; RV = residual volume; TLC = total lung capacity.

Sources: RV equations are from Boren et al. (1) for men and O'Brien and Drizd (15) for women.

TABLE 14.3

Equations to predict pulmonary capacities

PULMONARY CAPACITIES	MEN	WOMEN
	< 25 years	**< 20 years**
FVC	(0.05 × H) + (0.078 × A) − 5.508	(0.033 × H) + (0.092 × A) − 3.469
FEV$_1$	(0.046 × H) + (0.045 × A) − 4.808	(0.027 × H) − (0.085 × A) − 2.703
FEV$_1$%	103.64 − (0.087 × H) − (0.14 × A)	107.38 − (0.111 × H) − (0.109 × A)
	> 20 years	**> 25 years**
FVC	(0.065 × H) + (0.029 × A) − 5.459	(0.037 × H) + (0.022 × A) − 1.774
FEV$_1$	(0.052 × H) + (0.027 × A) − 4.203	(0.027 × H) − (0.021 × A) − 0.794
FEV$_1$%	103.64 − (0.087 × H) − (0.14 × A)	107.38 − (0.111 × H) − (0.109 × A)
MVV	(1.15 × H) − (1.27 × A) + 14	(0.55 × H) − (0.72 × A) + 50

Sources: Adapted from Comroe et al. (4), Knudson et al. (11) and Taylor et al. (19). FVC = forced vital capacity; FEV$_1$ = forced expired volume in 1 S; FEV$_1$% = FEV$_1$ expressed as percent of FVC; MVV = maximal voluntary ventilation; H = height (cm); A = age (yr).

causes V_A to be less than V_E. Slow deep breathing causes V_T and V_A to both increase. During exercise V_A is maintained by both an increase in tidal volume and breathing frequency. At the start of exercise, V_A is maintained more by increases in V_T, with only a slight increase in breathing frequency. During intense exercise, V_T plateaus and further increases in ventilation occur as a result of increased breathing frequency. Anatomical dead space also increase slightly during exercise.

Residual Lung Volume

Residual volume (RV) is the volume of air remaining in the lungs after a maximal exhalation. RV represents the difference between TLC and VC. RV, which is a subdivision of FRC (functional residual capacity), must be measured, and is important for the accurate calculation of body density measured by hydrostatic weighing. In addition, for individuals with chronic obstructive lung disease, residual volume is increased because of premature airway closure (9, 13, 18). There are a variety of methods used to indi-

rectly measure RV. Most researchers use either a closed-circuit **helium dilution** or open-circuit **nitrogen washout** method.

TABLE 14.6
Effect of changes in breathing patterns on alveolar ventilation

BREATHING	V_T (L/min)	f (br/min)	V_E (L/min)	V_A (L/min)
Shallow and rapid	0.24	25	6	2.25
Normal resting	0.5	12	6	4.2
Slow and deep	1.0	6	6.0	5.1

Ventilatory volumes in BTPS and assuming a constant DS (0.15 L).

alveolar ventilation the volume of air per unit time that reaches the respiratory zone of the lung (where gas exchange occurs)

anatomical dead space the volume of air within the conducting zone of the lung (it is not involved in gas exchange)

residual volume the volume remaining in the lungs after a forced maximal exhalation

helium dilution the method used to measure the functional residual capacity (FRC) of the lung that is based on the dilution of a known amount of helium

nitrogen washout an alternative method for measuring the residual volume of the lung

TABLE 14.5
Pulmonary ventilation at rest and during exercise

CONDITION	V_E (L/min)	= f (br/min)	× V_T (L/br)
Rest	6	12	0.5
Mild exercise	72	32	2.25
Maximal exercise	160	48	3.33

Volumes in BTPS conditions.

WEBSITE BOX

Chapter 14: Measuring Pulmonary Function

The newest information regarding exercise physiology can be viewed at the following sites.*
lungusa.org/
   Homepage of the American Lung Association, including links to numerous topics such as asthma, tobacco control, lung diseases, smoking cessation, etc.
mdnet.de/asthma/
   Information-packed site with links to all topics on asthma, including a module to help calculate reference lung function values for children.
mediconsult.com/
   Information source for any medical condition, including asthma.
nimbus.ocis.temple.edu/~dnowosie/
   Information about asthma and exercise-induced bronchoconstriction.

pedi.resp-pulmonary-com/
   Informative and educational site on pediatric issues, especially pulmonary care and lung function testing.
njc.org/MFhtml/SPI_MF.html
   Explanation of spirometry testing.
thoracic.org/
   Homepage of the American Thoracic Society. This is an extensive site that contains medical, research, educational, and professional information.

*Unless indicated, all URLs preceded by http://www.

Note: These URLs were valid at the time of publication, but could have changed or been deleted from Internet access since that time.

SUMMARY

■ In the early 1800s, John Hutchinson discovered that lung volumes could be accurately measured by having subjects breathe into a system that could record volume displacements on paper. John Hutchinson's early experiments lead to the development of the technique we now call **spirometry**.

■ The movement of the spirometry bell upward and downward represents the volume of air entering and exiting the lungs. When the bell is connected to a pen, the movements of the bell can be recorded on a rotating drum called a **kymograph**. Once the volume conversion of the bell is known (mL/mm), volume (ATPS) can be calculated.

■ Another type of volume-displacement system for measuring lung volumes is the bellows-type **spirometer**, often termed a *spirograph* or *vitalograph*. The bellows-type spirometer consists of collapsible bellows that fold and unfold in response to inhalation and exhalation. Typically, an individual will exhale as hard and as fast as possible into a vitalograph, and **vital capacity** and expired flow rates can be computed from the calibrated paper used on the instrument.

■ A more sophisticated type of spirometer calculates lung volumes by directly measuring the flow of air. A **pneumotachometer** measures the rate of flow of air during inhalation and exhalation. Pneumotach spirometers are becoming increasingly used when conducting cardiopulmonary testing because of their small size, and high sensitivity and accuracy.

■ There are two types of breathing valves commonly used in pulmonary function testing: free-breathing and multiple one-way directional valves. The difficulty with a valve apparatus for placement in the mouth is the stimulus this gives to increase ventilation. Thus, when testing ventilation using a mouthpiece valve apparatus, subjects need to be given a familiarization period (usually 2 to 3 min of quiet breathing through the mouthpiece) before actual data collection is begun. To avoid hyperventilation, face masks are also available that have multiple one-way valves to direct inspired and expired air.

■ **Oximetry** involves the indirect determination of the percent of hemoglobin that is combined with oxygen. Oximetry is a commonly used (noninvasive) method in hospitals and also during exercise testing to assess blood oxygenation. One of the newest methods of oximetry during exercise testing is the pulse oximeter.

■ Research has shown that prior submaximal and maximal exercise reduces vital capacity and FEV_1 within 30 min of recovery, and increases residual volume. It has been recommended that exercise should not be performed for up to 12 h prior to pulmonary function measurements.

■ The amount of air inspired and expired in 1 min is referred to as **minute ventilation** (V_E). At rest, the normal minute ventilation is equal to approximately 6 L of air. During exercise, V_E increases as a result of a combination of an increase in breathing frequency (f) and tidal volume (V_T). During strenuous exercise in well-conditioned endurance athletes, minute ventilation can increase 27 times above the resting value.

■ It is important to remember that not all of the air inspired reaches the alveoli (the site of gas exchange). **Alveolar ventilation** (V_A) is the portion of inspired air that reaches the alveoli, and thus takes place in gas exchange. There is also a portion of inspired air which remains in the upper respiratory tract, and thus does not take place in gas exchange, and it is referred to as **anatomical dead space** (V_D). Dead space averages approximately 30% of resting tidal volume.

■ **Residual volume** (RV) is the volume of air remaining in the lungs after a maximal exhalation. RV represents the difference between TLC and VC. RV, which is a subdivision of FRC, must be measured, and is important for the accurate calculation of body density measured by hydrostatic weighing. In addition, for individuals with chronic obstructive lung disease, residual volume is increased because of premature airway closure. Most researchers use either a closed-circuit **helium dilution** or open-circuit **nitrogen washout** method.

STUDY QUESTIONS

1. From a spirogram tracing, calculate IRV, TV, VC (vital capacity), ERV, and TLC.

2. If the FVC of a subject is 5.75L (ATPS), the room and water temperature is 21.50°C and PB is 715 mm Hg, convert FVC (ATPS) to a BTPS volume (see app. B).

3. Why are lung volumes reported in BTPS conditions?

4. What are typical resting values for a normal, healthy subject for:

a. Lung volumes (BTPS)—IC, ERV, VC, RV, FRC and TLC

b. Ventilation (BTPS)—V_T, f, and V_E

c. Pulmonary dynamics—FVC, FEV_1, and MVV

5. The following are values for pulmonary measurements (volume$_{ATPS}$):

Dead space = 165 mL; vital capacity = 5.4 L

Resting V_E = 6 L/min, breathing frequency = 12/min

Exercise V_E = 76 L/min, breathing frequency = 45/min

Maximal exercise V_E = 185 L/min

For rest and exercise, calculate V_T. For maximal exercise, calculate what the V_T and breathing frequency would probably be if a person used only 60% of the vital capacity per breath during maximal exercise.

6. What are the limitations placed on the conducting and respiratory zones of the lungs during exercise to VO_{2max}?

APPLICATIONS

1. Why would lung damage (e.g., emphysema) increase residual volume?

2. Refer to chapter 8. Individuals who suffer from exercise-induced bronchospasm have a reduced FEV_1 during recovery from exercise. Explain how FEV_1 is measured. What other pulmonary function tests would detect increased airway resistance?

3. Tests that measure lung compliance and elasticity were not covered in this chapter. Nevertheless, how would conditions of lung damage (e.g., emphysema) affect lung compliance, and what would be the functional consequences of this condition?

REFERENCES

1. Boren, H. G., R. C. Kory, and J. C. Synder. The Veteran's Administration Army cooperative study of pulmonary function. II: The lung volume and its subdivisions in normal men. *Am. J. Med.* 41:96–114, 1966.

2. Buono, M. J., S. H. Constable, A. R. Morton, T. C. Rotkis, P. R. Stanforth, and J. H. Wilmore. The effect of an acute bout of exercise on selected pulmonary function measurements. *Med. Sci. Sports Exerc.* 13(5):290–293, 1981.

3. Chusid, E. L. Pulmonary function testing: An overview. In E. L. Chusid, (ed.), *The selective and comprehensive testing of adult pulmonary function.* Futra, Mount Kisco, NY, 1983.

4. Comroe, J. H., R. E. Foster, A. B. Dubois, W. A. Briscoe, and E. Carlsen. *The lung.* Year Book Medical Publishers, Chicago, 1962.

5. Cordain, L., A. Tucker, D. Moon, and J. M. Stager. Lung volumes and maximal respiratory pressures in collegiate swimmers and runners. *Res. Quart. Exerc. Sport.* 61(1):70–74, 1990.

6. Dempsey, J. A., B. D. Johnson, and K.W. Saupe. Adaptations and limitations in the pulmonary system during exercise. *Chest* 97(Suppl. 3):81S–87S, 1990.

7. Girandola, R., R. Wiswell, J. Mohler, G. Romero, and W. Barnes. Effects of water immersion on lung volumes: Implications for body compositional analysis. *J. Appl. Physiol.* 43(2):276–279, 1977.

8. Hansen, J. E. and R. Casaburi. Validity of ear oximetry in clinical exercise testing. *Chest* 91:333–337, 1987.

9. Hickman, J. B., E. Blair and R. Frayser. An open circuit helium method for measuring functional residual capacity and defective intrapulmonary gas mixing. *J. Clin. Invest.* 33: 1277–1282, /1954.

10. Hutchinson, J. Lecture on vital statistics, embracing an account of a new instrument for detecting the presence of disease in the system. *Lancet* 1:567, 594, 1844.

11. Knudsen, R. J., R. C. Slatin, M. D. Lebowitz, and B. Burrows. The maximal expiratory flow-volume curve. Normal standards, variability, and effects of age. *Am. Rev. Resp. Dis.* 113:587–600, 1976.

12. Mahler, D. A. Exercise-induced asthma. *Med. Sci. Sports Exerc.* 25(5):554–561, 1993.

13. Meneely, G. R., C. O. T. Ball, and R. C. Kory. A simplified closed circuit helium dilution method for the determination of the residual volume in the lungs. *Am. J. Med.* 28:824–831, 1960.

14. Morris, J. F. Spirometry in the evaluation of pulmonary function. *West. J. Med.* 125(2):110–118, 1976.

15. O'Brien, R. J., and T.A. Drizd. Roentgenographic determination of total lung capacity: Normal values from a national population survey. *Am. Rev. Resp. Dis.* 128:949–952, 1983.

16. O'Krory, J. A., R. A. Loy, and J. R. Coast. Pulmonary function changes following exercise. *Med. Sci. Sports Exerc.* 24(12):1359–1364, 1992.

17. Rebuk, A. S., K. R. Chapman, and A. D'Urzo. The accuracy and response characteristics of a simplified ear oximeter. *Chest* 83:860–864, 1983.

18. Ruegg, W. R., and G. P. Reynolds. A procedure for the measurement of lung volumes by helium dilution. *Analyzer* 10:18–22, 1980.

19. Taylor, A. E., K. Rehder, R. E. Hyatt, and J. C. Parker. *Clinical respiratory physiology.* Saunders, Philadelphia, 1989.

20. West, J. B. *Respiratory physiology: The essentials,* 3rd ed. Williams & Wilkins, Philadelphia, 1985.

RECOMMENDED READINGS

Dempsey, J. A., B. D. Johnson, and K.W. Saupe. Adaptations and limitations in the pulmonary system during exercise. *Chest* 97(Suppl. 3):81S–87S, 1990.

Mahler, D. A. Exercise-induced asthma. *Med. Sci. Sports Exerc.* 25(5):554–561, 1993.

O'Brien, R. J., and T. A. Drizd. Roentgenographic determination of total lung capacity: Normal values from a national population survey. *Am.Rev. Resp. Dis.* 128:949–952, 1983.

O'Krory, J. A., R. A. Loy, and J. R. Coast. Pulmonary function changes following exercise. *Med. Sci. Sports Exerc.* 24(12):1359–1364, 1992.

West, J. B. *Respiratory physiology: The essentials*, 3rd ed. Williams & Wilkins, Philadelphia, 1985.

Body Composition Assessment

he body is composed of different components. Chemists study body composition at the level of atoms, whereas biochemists study body composition in terms of molecules and their reactions. When you take a holistic and applied approach to body composition, it is apparent that the body's composition can also be quantified by more major components such as that of fat and nonfat. Such a two-component classification scheme for body composition assessment has proved very effective for improving understanding of sports performance, weight loss and gain, and risk for cardiovascular diseases and diabetes. There are many methods available for the quantification of body fat, yet they are not all equal in their accuracy. The purposes of this chapter are to identify and explain the different methods available to determine the fat and fat-free composition of the body, and comment on the accuracy and recommended conditions for the use of each method.

OBJECTIVES

After studying this chapter, you should be able to:

- Understand the importance of accurate body composition assessment.
- Demonstrate a basic understanding of the two-component model of body composition.
- Define the terms *ideal body weight, overweight,* and *overfat.*
- Discuss the drawbacks and benefits of the different laboratory methods for body composition assessment.
- Discuss the drawbacks and benefits of the different field methods for body composition assessment.

KEY TERMS

body composition
overweight
overfat
body mass index (BMI)
essential fat
storage fat
ideal body weight

lean body mass (LBM)
fat-free body mass (FFBM)
two-component model
body density
hydrodensitometry

air-displacement plethysmography
skinfold
dual x-ray absorptiometry (DEXA)
bioelectrical impedance (BIA)

What Is Body Composition?

Body composition refers to the relative amounts of the different compounds in the body. Typically, researchers have focused on the proportion of the body mass that is water, protein, mineral, and fat. However, the majority of techniques for body composition assessment simply provide an estimate of lean ("nonfat" or "fat free") and fat body masses. Excellent textbooks have been written on body composition assessment (18, 30), and the material presented in this chapter functions as an overview of the fundamental knowledge and skills that a student should acquire during undergraduate preparation toward any exercise science, exercise physiology, or health-related degree.

Why Study Body Composition?

The assessment of body composition is generally performed in order to determine and monitor one's health and fitness status, and to aid in planning training programs for athletes. It has been well established that a high percentage of body fat (low lean body mass) is associated with a higher risk of heart disease, diabetes, hypertension, cancer, hyperlipidemia, and a variety of other health problems (30, 41). On the other hand, a high percentage of lean body mass and low-fat mass is associated with athletic prowess and good health (43, 44).

Overweight is defined as body weight in excess of a reference standard, generally a mean weight for a given height and skeletal frame size grouped by sex (table 15.1). However, research has clearly shown the inadequacy of this approach to defining overweight (44), because individuals with a large muscle mass and minimal fat can be classified as overweight, yet be less fat and more healthy than individuals of similar stature with minimal muscle mass. Consequently, height-weight tables should be avoided (33), and the concept of overweight should be replaced with the condition of being **overfat** (20).

Despite the aforementioned recommendation, an important measure in research on the health status of large populations continues to be a modification of body mass and height—the **body mass index (BMI)**. The BMI is the ratio of weight to height squared.

15.1 $BMI = body\ mass\ (kg)/body\ height\ (m)^2$

For example, a 80-kg person who is 1.7 m tall has the following BMI:

$$BMI = 80/1.7^2 = 27.68\ kg/m^2$$

Note: 1 kg = 2.22 lb, and 1 m = 3.28 ft = 39.37 in.

A BMI score less than 20.0 is considered underweight, 20.0 to 24.9 is desirable, 25.0 to 30 is overweight, and greater than 30 is considered obese (table 15.2). A high BMI is associated with a high prevalence of mortality from heart disease, cancer, and diabetes (fig. 15.1). However, BMI is not a sensitive measure that reflects actual body fat content, and the relationships between BMI and disease risk and mortality may be due to the fact that they are associated with, but not identical to, total and regional body fat content (8).

Understanding Body Fat

Being overfat indicates an excess accumulation of body fat. Thus the prediction of body fat from body composition analysis is required before this term can be used. The details of how to assess body fat content will be presented later in this chapter.

Body composition is often expressed as the relative amounts of fat mass to fat-free mass. Fat mass (FM) includes both essential and storage fat. **Essential fat** is found in bone marrow, brain, spinal cord, muscles, and other internal organs, and is "essential" to normal physiological and biological functioning. The minimum level below which essential fat should never go is believed to be approximately 3% of the total body weight for men and 12% of total body weight for women. Women have a higher essential fat storage requirement because of sex-specific fat deposits in breast tissue and surrounding the uterus. When essential fat drops below these critical values, normal physiological and biological functioning may be impaired.

Storage fat is comprised of two types of fat, yellow fat which is approximately 99% of all storage fat, and brown fat, which is rich in mitochondria and can increase heat production because of a slightly lowered biochemical efficiency of ATP (aderosine triphosphate) synthesis. Yellow fat is found in adipose tissue and serves three basic functions: (1) as an insulator to retain body heat, (2) as an energy substrate, and (3) as padding against trauma. The majority of adipose tissue is found directly beneath the skin. Subcutaneous fat distribution can vary between sexes and with age (27). Men tend to store more fat around the waist (android obesity), whereas women tend to store more fat around their hips and thighs (gynoid obesity). Older individuals tend to have less subcutaneous fat than younger subjects, but have greater fat deposits within and between skeletal muscles.

Fat-free body mass (FFBM), often referred to as lean tissue or lean body mass (LBM), includes muscle, bone, organs, fluid, and any other tissues excluding lipid and fat tissue. There is often argument between the use of the term LBM and FFBM. One of the first definitions of LBM included a small amount of essential fat, approximately 2 to 3% (3, 24, 36). Lohman (30) has suggested that researchers and clinicians use the term LBM in most applications, and FFBM when conducting body composition validation studies.

TABLE 15.1

1983 Metropolitan height and weight tables for men and women between the ages of 25 and 59

HEIGHT		WEIGHT					
		SMALL FRAME		MEDIUM FRAME		LARGE FRAME	
(ft:in)	(cm)	(lb)	(kg)	(lb)	(kg)	(lb)	(kg)
*Men**							
5:2	157.5	128–134	57.6–60.3	131–141	59.0–63.5	138–150	62.1–67.5
5:3	160.0	130–136	58.5–61.2	133–143	59.9–64.4	140–153	63.0–68.9
5:4	162.6	132–138	59.4–62.1	135–145	60.8–65.3	142–156	63.9–70.2
5:5	165.1	134–140	60.3–63.0	137–148	61.7–66.6	144–160	64.8–72.0
5:6	167.6	136–142	61.2–63.9	139–151	62.6–68.0	146–164	65.7–73.8
5:7	170.2	138–145	62.1–65.3	142–154	63.9–69.3	149–168	67.1–75.6
5:8	172.7	140–148	63.0–66.6	145–157	65.3–70.7	152–172	68.4–77.4
5:9	175.3	142–151	63.9–68.0	148–160	66.6–72.0	155–176	69.8–79.2
5:10	177.8	144–154	64.8–69.3	151–163	68.0–73.4	158–180	71.1–81.0
5:11	180.3	146–157	65.7–70.7	154–166	69.3–74.7	161–184	72.5–82.8
6:0	182.9	149–160	67.1–72.0	157–170	70.7–76.5	164–188	73.8–84.6
6:1	185.4	152–164	68.4–73.8	160–174	72.0–78.3	168–192	75.6–86.4
6:2	188.0	155–168	69.8–75.6	164–178	73.8–80.1	172–197	77.4–88.7
6:3	190.5	158–172	75.6–77.4	167–182	75.2–81.9	176–202	79.2–90.9
6:4	193.0	162–176	72.9–79.2	171–187	77.0–84.2	182–207	81.9–93.2
Women†							
4:10	147.3	102–111	45.9–50.0	109–121	49.1–54.5	118–131	53.1–59.0
4:11	149.8	103–113	46.4–50.9	111–123	50.0–55.4	120–134	54.0–60.3
5:0	152.4	104–115	46.8–51.8	113–126	50.9–56.7	122–137	54.9–61.7
5:1	154.9	106–118	47.7–53.1	115–129	51.8–58.1	125–140	56.3–63.0
5:2	157.5	108–121	48.6–54.5	118–132	53.1–59.4	128–143	57.6–64.4
5:3	160.0	111–124	50.0–55.8	121–135	54.5–60.8	131–147	59.0–66.2
5:4	162.6	114–127	51.3–57.2	124–138	55.8–62.1	134–151	60.3–68.0
5:5	165.1	117–130	52.7–58.5	127–141	57.2–63.5	137–155	61.7–69.8
5:6	167.6	120–133	54.0–59.9	130–144	58.5–64.8	130–159	63.0–71.6
5:7	170.2	123–136	55.4–61.2	133–147	59.9–66.2	143–163	64.4–73.4
5:8	172.7	126–139	56.7–62.6	136–150	61.2–67.5	146–167	65.7–75.2
5:9	175.3	129–142	58.1–63.9	139–153	62.6–68.9	149–170	67.1–76.5
5:10	177.8	132–145	59.4–65.3	142–156	63.9–70.2	152–173	68.4–77.9
5:11	180.3	135–148	60.8–66.6	145–159	65.3–71.6	155–176	69.8–79.2
6:0	182.9	138–151	62.1–68.0	148–162	66.6–72.9	158–179	71.1–80.6

*Indoor clothing weighing 2.3 kg.
†Indoor clothing weighing 1.4 kg.

Adult Norms for Body Fatness and Health and Fitness

Desirable body weight and percentage of body fat are important for three reasons: (1) health, (2) athletic performance, and (3) aesthetics. From a health perspective, excessive weight and body fat is a major concern in the United States.

Table 15.3 lists standard values for % body fat for health and fitness considerations.

Some athletic events are associated with individuals who have extremely low percentages of body fat. For example,

body composition the science of determining the absolute and relative contributions of specific components of the body

overweight a condition of excess weight based on a height-weight relationship or computed from body composition analysis

overfat a condition of excess body fat, as determined from body composition analysis

body mass index (BMI) the ratio of body weight/height^2

essential fat fat and lipid component of the body that comprises cell membranes, bone marrow, intramuscular fat, etc.

storage fat fat and lipid stored in adipose tissue

TABLE 15.2

Values for BMI that are related to different levels of being "overfat" and at risk for certain diseases

BMI (KG/M)	DESCRIPTION
20–24.9	Desirable range for adult men and women
25–29.9	Grade I obesity
30–40	Grade II obesity
> 40	Grade III obesity

Source: Adapted from ACSM (1).

FIGURE 15.1

The increase in mortality with increases in body mass index.

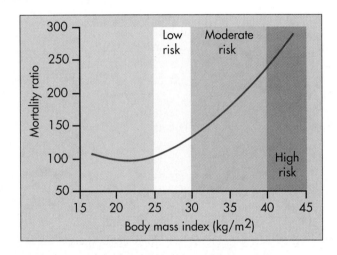

TABLE 15.3

Standard values for % body fat

RATING	AGE (yr)	20–29	30–39	40–49	50–59	60+
Men						
Excellent		< 11	< 12	< 14	< 15	< 16
Good		11–13	12–14	14–16	15–17	16–18
Average		14–20	15–21	17–23	18–24	19–25
Fair		21–23	22–24	24–26	25–27	26–28
Poor		> 23	> 24	> 26	> 27	> 28
Women						
Excellent		< 16	< 17	< 18	< 19	< 20
Good		16–19	17–20	18–21	19–22	20–23
Average		20–28	21–29	22–30	23–31	24–32
Fair		29–31	30–32	31–33	32–34	33–35
Poor		> 31	> 32	> 33	> 34	> 35

Sources: Adapted from Jackson and Pollock (21) and Jackson et al. (22).

15.4   Ideal weight = LBM/[1 − (% fat desired/100)]

15.5   Desirable fat loss = present weight − desirable body weight

For example, a person who weighs 90 kg, with a % fat = 28%, an ideal % fat of 15%, and who wants to retain the current LBM,

Fat weight = 90 × (28/100) = 98 × 0.28 = 27.44 kg

LBM = 90 − 27.44 = 62.56 kg

Ideal weight = 62.56*/[1 − (15/100)] = 62.56/(1 − 0.15) = 62.56/0.85   = 72.6 kg

Desirable fat loss = 90 − 72.6 = 17.4 kg

some elite marathon runners have body fat percentages as low as 3 to 5%. Other sports allow for high percentages of body fat (table 15.4). Nevertheless, success in any athletic event or sport is due to multiple factors, and an overemphasis on the importance of specific body fat "ideals" is not supported by scientific research, and is therefore misleading and can be potentially detrimental to health (42).

Using Body Fat to Determine Ideal Weight

Once an individual's body composition has been obtained, an **ideal body weight** can be determined. An individual's ideal weight should be carefully chosen. Generally, most people have an unrealistic expectation of their "ideal" weight. Ideal or desirable weight calculations should be used as a tool/goal to help promote weight loss for good health, and can be estimated as follows:

15.2   Fat weight = current weight x (% fat/100)

15.3   Lean body mass (LBM) = current weight − fat weight

The Two-Component System of Body Composition Assessment

The body can be divided into components that differ in composition. In the original body component system described by Benke and associates (2) (fig. 15.2), the body was divided into two simple components: lean and fat body mass. Since this time, **lean body mass (LBM)** has been identified as not being completely fat free, because it contained lipid within muscle, cell membranes, bone marrow, and so forth. The term **fat-free body mass (FFBM)** therefore represents a large component of LBM (7, 35).

Despite the growing complexity of body composition assessment, the two-component system remains a widely used approach in research, clinical practice, health assessment, and physical fitness evaluation. Such acceptance is based on the applied interest in knowing the absolute and relative

---

*Some individuals may want to increase LBM and decrease % fat. For these individuals, simply use a realistically increased LBM.

TABLE 15.4

Body composition characteristics of athletes grouped by sports type

ATHLETIC/SPORT GROUP	GENDER	AGE	HEIGHT (cm)	WEIGHT (kg)	% FAT
Baseball	M	20.8	182.7	83.3	14.2
Basketball	M	26.8	193.6	91.2	9.7
	F	19.2	168.0	79.0	24.0
Gymnastics	M	20.3	178.5	69.2	4.6
	F	20.0	158.5	51.1	15.5
	F	19.4	163.0	57.9	23.8
Ice hockey	M	26.3	180.3	86.7	15.1
Horse riding (jockeys)	M	30.9	158.2	50.3	14.1
Swimming	M	21.8	182.3	79.1	8.5
	F	19.4	168.0	63.8	26.3
Track and field	M	21.3	180.6	71.6	3.7
Distance running	M	22–26	176.0	64.5	7.0
	M	40–59	180.7	71.6	11.2
	M	> 60	175.5	67.0	13.0
	F	20.0	161.3	52.9	19.2
	F	32.4	169.4	57.2	15.2
Jumpers and hurdlers	M	20.3	165.9	59.0	20.7
Volleyball	M	19.4	266.0	59.8	25.3
Wrestling	M	15–18	172.3	66.3	6.9
	M	20–25	176.0	80.0	9.5
Weight lifting	M	24.9	166.4	59.8	25.3
Body builders	M	29.0	172.4	83.1	8.4

Sources: Adapted from Wilmore and Bergfeld (43) and Wilmore and Haskell (44).

FIGURE 15.2

The compartmental models of body composition. The original two-compartment model has been further subdivided on the basis of the chemical divisions of the body that are able to be quantified, either directly or indirectly. These multiple-compartment models are used to modify the equation of Siri (1961) to provide a more accurate conversion of body density to % body fat.

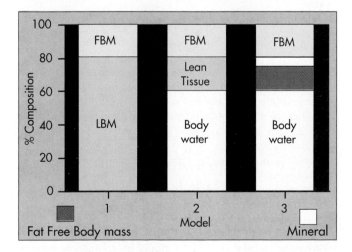

Brozek and colleagues (7), Siri (35), and Behnke and associates (2) developed the two-component system of body composition based on the following assumptions:

1. The density of fat is 0.900 g/mL at 37°C.
2. The density of lean body mass is 1.100 g/mL at 37°C.
3. All individuals have the previously stated densities for fat and lean body mass.
4. The body's LBM is 73.8% water, 19.4% protein, and 6.8% mineral.

Of the assumptions 1 to 4 listed above, assumptions 2 to 4 can be invalid, depending on the person being studied (37). For example, the density of the lean body mass is variable because of differences in bone mineral density between individuals of different races, ages, and certain disease states. In addition, the proportion of the LBM that is water also can vary between individuals of different age, sex, and ethnicity. As will be discussed below, researchers have and continue to

ideal body weight the projected weight of a person that would exist with appropriate changes in one or both of lean body mass and fat body mass

lean body mass (LBM) the component of the body that is not storage fat

fat-free body mass (FFBM) the component of the body that is not storage and essential fat

amounts of body fat, and the fact that a two-component approach can provide a very accurate estimate of fat and fat-free body composition, and often by a simple method.

improve on simple methods for estimating body composition for individuals. They do this by researching the actual bone mineral and body water of subjects of different populations, and when needed adjust the fat, lean body mass, and water content assumptions. This enables researchers to develop more specific and accurate equations to estimate body fat content for individuals of given populations or groups.

Methods for Estimating Body Fat Content Using the Two-Component Model

Laboratory Methods

There are numerous methods to assess body composition that require expensive and/or large pieces of equipment, typically found in a laboratory facility. The laboratory methods that rely on the **two-component model** covered in this chapter are hydrodensitometry and air-displacement plethysmography.

Densitometry

Densitometry (*density* = mass per unit volume; *ometry* = measurement) is the study of the measurement of human **body density.** Body density has long been measured using the procedure of *hydrodensitometry.* More recently, a body density method based on air-displacement has been developed (11, 31), which overcomes the methodological difficulties associated with water submersion.

Hydrodensitometry **Hydrodensitometry,** or *hydrostatic weighing,* has been the "gold standard" by which all other methods of body composition assessment have been validated. However, as early as 1961 Siri (35) reported that differences among individuals in the density of the FFBM would cause errors in % fat as large as ± 4%.

Hydrostatic weighing is based on Archimedes' principle, which states that when an object is placed in water it is buoyed up by a counterforce equal to the water it displaces. Thus there are two ways to measure body density: (1) by measuring the displaced water volume, or (2) by measuring the change in body weight underwater. The latter method is widely used, and is the method discussed in focus box 15.1.

Obtaining an accurate underwater weight is crucial to hydrodensitometry. Given the need for subjects to submerge themselves and maintain a still posture at residual volume, the accurate measurement of underwater weight is not a simple task. Early research indicated that *there is a learning curve to the measurement of underwater weight,* involving both the subject and technician (23). Based on this fact, it was recom-

---

two-component model a model of body composition that divides the body into fat and fat-free (lean) components

body density the density of the body when submerged in water, expressed in g/mL

hydrodensitometry (hi'dro-den'si-tom'e-tri) the method of determining body density by underwater weighing

---

FOCUS BOX 15.1

The Principles and Pretest Requirements of Hydrostatic Weighing

On the basis of Archimedes' principle, body density can be calculated as follows:

15.6 $D_b = mass_b/volume_b$

15.7 $D_b = W_a/\{[(W_a - W_w)/D_w] - (RV + 100\ mL)\}$

where D_b = body density (g/mL)
  W_a = body weight out of water (kg)
  W_w = weight in water (kg)
  D_w = density of water (g/mL)
  RV = residual volume (mL)

The major disadvantages of hydrostatic weighing are:

1. The cost and time to conduct a test
2. The need for subjects to tolerate water submersion at a residual lung volume
3. The constraints by limited population-specific equations that convert body density to a % body fat

The pretest requirements for underwater weighing include:

1. A normal diet and fluid intake but with no ingestion of food or liquids 3 h prior to the test
2. Avoidance of foods that cause increased intestinal gas
3. Because of the need to expel lung air to residual volume, subjects should not have smoked for 2 h prior to the test
4. Avoidance of any condition that would alter the hydration of the body, such as physical activity, saunas, inadequate or overhydration, etc.
5. Avoid testing females for 3 days prior, during, and 3 days after menstruation
6. Minimal swim clothing to decrease the risk for air trapping in the swim suit
7. A soap shower to remove excess body oils
8. Emptying of the bowel and bladder prior to testing
9. When in the tank, the body should be completely submerged and the skin and hair rubbed to remove air bubbles

mended that up to 10 recordings of underwater weight were required for acceptable accuracy (23). However, subsequent research has shown that *averaging three underwater weights that are within 100g* is equally accurate (5), and therefore saves time and prevents undue stress on the subject.

The determination of residual volume of the subject can be conducted before, during, or after the test. There is no significant difference in the estimation of % body fat so long as residual volume measured outside the tank is done in a similar posture to the residual volume maneuver underwater

---

FOCUS BOX 15.2

Estimating Body Composition from Hydrodensitometry

Once whole-body density (D_b) is determined, a decision must be made on which equation to use to convert body density to % body fat. As previously explained, the original equations of Brozek and associates (1963) (7) and Siri (1961) (35) were based on a sample of male cadavers and violate known differences in the FFBM among individuals of different gender, age, race, and specific illnesses.

(15.8)   Siri   % Body Fat = $[(4.95/D_b) - 4.50] \times 100$

(15.9)   Brozek   % Body Fat = $[(4.57/D_b) - 4.142] \times 100$

Table 15.5 presents other equations that can be used, and the populations which they represent.

TABLE 15.5

Alternative equations to that of Siri (1961) and Brozek (1963) for estimating % body fat

AGE	GENDER	% BODY FAT	D_{FFB}
15–16	M	$[(5.03/D_b) - 4.59] \times 100$	1.096
	F	$[(5.07/D_b) - 4.64] \times 100$	1.094
17–19	M	$[(4.98/D_b) - 4.53] \times 100$	1.0985
	F	$[(5.05/D_b) - 4.62] \times 100$	1.095
20–50	M	$[(4.95/D_b) - 4.50] \times 100$	1.100
	F	$[(5.03/D_b) - 4.59] \times 100$	1.096

For African-Americans, subtract 1.9% (males) and 1% (females) from each % body fat calculation.

Source: Adapted from Lohman (29).

Procedure for Measuring Underwater Weight

Underwater weight can be measured from either suspension from an autopsy scale, or by using a submerged seat/support that is connected to strain gauges (fig. 15.3).

Step 1: Complete pretesting requirements and the measurement of RV (see text).
Step 2: Obtain a dry onland body weight (kg).
Step 3: Determine tare weight of the weighing apparatus.
Step 4: Record the temperature of the water (°C).
Step 5: Record D_w from table 15.6.
Step 6: Determine the underwater weight of the subject (W_{uw}).
Step 7: Compute body density using equations (15.6) and (15.7).
Step 8: Convert body density to % body fat using an appropriate formula (Siri, Brozek, or those in table 15.5).

TABLE 15.6

Determining the density of water

WATER TEMP (°C)	WATER DENSITY (G/ML)
23	0.997569
24	0.997327
25	0.997075
26	0.996814
27	0.996544
28	0.996264
29	0.995976
30	0.995678
31	0.995372
32	0.995057
33	0.994734
34	0.994403
35	0.994063
36	0.993716
37	0.993360

For example, for a healthy male who weighs 68 kg, and has a residual lung volume of 1.60 L, and obtains the following underwater weights in water at a density of 0.9937 g/mL:

Trial 1—3.98
Trial 2—4.05
Trial 3—4.08
Trial 4—3.92
Trial 5—4.08

Average weight = (4.05 + 4.08 + 4.08)/3   = 4.07 kg

Tare weight = 2.0 kg

Underwater weight = 4.07 − 2.0   = 2.07 kg

$$D_b = 68.0/\{[(68.0 - 2.07)/0.9937] - (1.60 + 0.10)\}$$

$$= [68/(66.3480 - 1.70)]$$

$$= 68/79.8863$$

$$= 1.0518$$

Using the Siri equation, % body fat calculates to be:

% fat = $[(4.95/1.0518) - 4.5] \times 100$

= 20.62

FOCUS BOX 15.2

Estimating Body Composition from Hydrodensitometry

FIGURE 15.3

A photograph of two underwater systems. One can measure underwater weight by the traditional autopsy scale method, and the other uses the more modern strain gauge method that is interfaced to a computer. All components are labeled on the photograph.

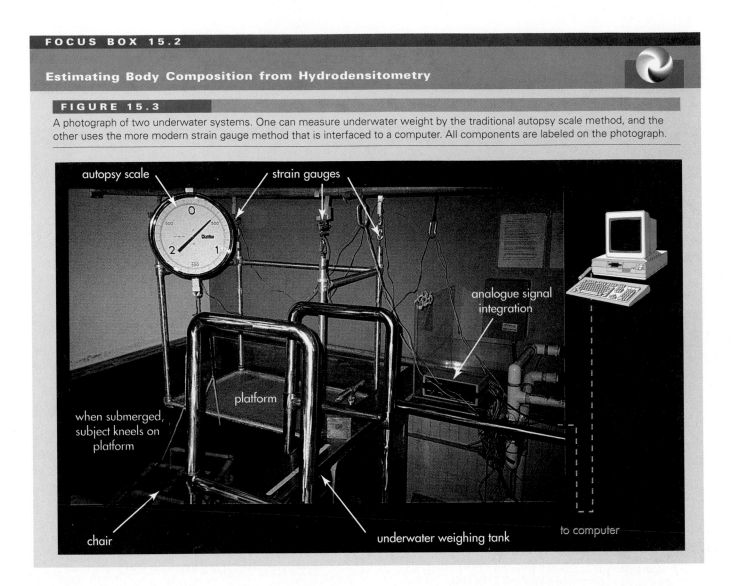

(4, 6, 10). Because of the added expense and equipment needs for RV determination while underwater, most laboratories perform the RV measurement either before or after the underwater weighing (38). If RV is estimated (see chapter 14), errors of estimation of % body fat can increase by as much as 3% body fat (34). Consequently, the accuracy of hydrodensitometry is decreased to the extent that body fat estimation could be done with equal accuracy by less sophisticated and time-consuming methods (e.g., skinfold analysis).

The procedures for conducting a test of hydrodensitometry are provided in focus box 15.2.

Air-Displacement Plethysmography Scientists have recently developed another densitometry method for body composition assessment. Rather than being submerged in water, subjects sit inside a precisely calibrated device and displace air rather than water (fig. 15.4). **Air-displacement plethysmography** has produced % fat results similar to those obtained from hydrodensitometry, with a mean % fat difference compared to hydrodensitometry of only − 0.3%,

a correlation coefficient = 0.96, and a standard error of the estimate = 1.81 % fat (11, 31). Air densitometry appears to be an accurate alternative to hydrodensitometry, especially for subjects who are unable to be submerged in water at residual lung volume for long enough to allow stable readings of underwater weight (e.g., children, individuals with disabilities or disease). Furthermore, because of the recent introduction of the technology, future models of devices based on air-displacement plethysmography and accompanied software, should yield even more accurate results.

Field Methods

Skinfold Measurements

It is possible to measure the subcutaneous fat at selected sites with skinfold calipers and predict the percentage of body fat by using various regression equations. Assessing body composition by measuring the thickness of selected **skinfold** sites is probably the most common and widely available technique in use today (fig. 15.5). It is important

FIGURE 15.4

A subject prepared for air densitometry measurement using the BodPod body composition system.

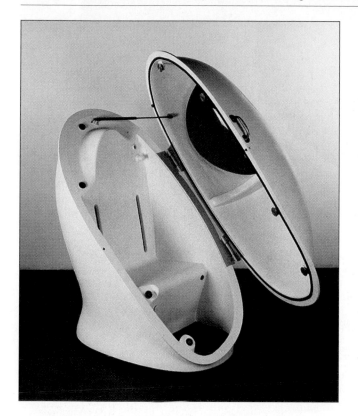

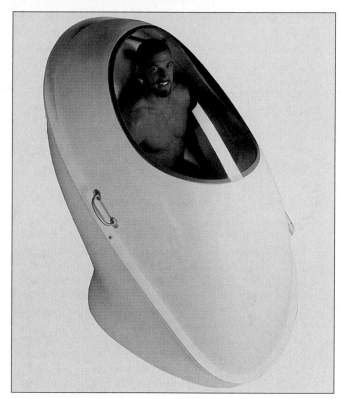

that fitness instructors and exercise physiology students become proficient in this technique.

There are a variety of skinfold calipers on the market. There are expensive research calipers including the Harpenden, Lange, and Lafayette calipers, which generally cost in excess of $200. Conversely, the less expensive (not necessarily less accurate) calipers include the Slimguide, the Fat-O-Meter, and the Adipometer, which range in price from $10 to $50. The more expensive calipers maintain a constant jaw pressure of 10 g per square millimeter of surface area. Such precision is required for the accurate use of the skinfold technique to estimate % body fat. Furthermore, evidence exists to indicate that the same skinfold calipers should be used that were used in the formulation of specific equations (28), because a given skinfold thickness can differ even between the expensive calipers.

Before taking any skinfold measurements, it is important to follow the guidelines listed in focus box 15.3.

Once the necessary final skinfold measurements (table 15.7) have been recorded, the percentage of body fat can be obtained by using a variety of tables or formulas. For the highest reliability and validity, it is important to choose the right regression equation and/or prediction table based on the population being tested. Regression equations, such as those listed in table 15.8, estimate whole-body density which can then be used to predict the percentage of body

FIGURE 15.5

A subject prepared for skinfold assessment.

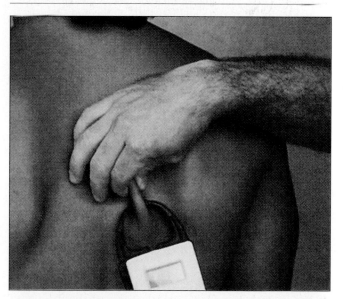

air-displacement plethysmography the method of determining body density by the displacement of air within an enclosed device

skinfold the fold of skin and fat that is measured for thickness at selected sites of the body

FOCUS BOX 15.3

Measurement of Skinfolds for Body Fat Percentage Estimation

Research has provided many validated equations for estimating body fat from skinfolds. Some of these equations were developed from cadaver analysis, but the majority were validated against underwatering weighing as the so-called gold standard.

1. It is important that the technician explain the following points to the subject:
   a. Why the test is being performed
   b. The technique involved
   c. Any risks or discomforts the subject might experience
   d. What the subject has to do to get prepared
   e. How the data will be used to predict the subject's percentage of body fat
   The equation used should be predetermined on the basis of the subject's personal demographics and health history.
2. Once the test and procedures have been thoroughly explained to the subject, and all questions have been answered, the subject should be taken to a location where the subject's privacy is protected.
3. All sites to be measured should be first marked with a water-soluble felt-tip pen (table 15.9). All measurements should be taken on the right side of the body (fig. 15.5).
4. After all the sites have been marked, measure each fold by grasping (drawing up) a layer of skin (skinfold) with the thumb and forefinger of the nondominant hand. For example, if you are right-handed, hold the caliper in your right hand, and grasp the skin with your left hand. Avoid "pinching" the subject. The proper technique is to pull the skin together and slightly away from the body, but not so hard that the skinfold gets compressed (see fig. 15.5).
5. With the skinfold site isolated, place the calipers perpendicular to the fold, approximately 1/2 in below the index finger and thumb of the left hand. Release the pressure on the calipers completely, and the skinfold grasp of your left hand.
6. The caliper should have a chance to settle for 2 to 3 s, after which a reading should be recorded in millimeters, and the caliper opened and removed completely.

7. Three measurements should be recorded to the nearest 0.1 to 0.5 mm. The average of the two closest readings should be recorded for the final value. All recordings should be taken as quickly as possible to avoid excessive compression of the skin.
8. For good reliability and validity, all repeat measurements should be taken at the same time of the day, preferably in the morning.

TABLE 15.7

Skinfold sites.

1. **Abdominal fold:** A vertical fold taken at a distance of 2 cm to the right of the umbilicus.
2. **Biceps fold:** A vertical fold (taken 1 cm above the level used to mark the triceps) on the anterior aspect of the arm over the belly of the biceps muscle.
3. **Chest/pectoral fold:** A diagonal fold taken one-half the distance between the anterior axillary line and the nipple for men and one-third the distance between the anterior axillary line and the nipple for women.
4. **Medial calf fold:** A vertical fold at a level of the maximum circumference of the calf on the midline of the medial border.
5. **Midaxillary fold:** A vertical fold taken on the midaxillary line at the level of the xyphoid process of the sternum.
6. **Subscapular fold:** An angular fold taken at a 45-degree angle 1 to 2 cm below the inferior angle of the scapula.
7. **Suprailium fold:** An oblique fold in line with the natural angle of the iliac crest taken in the anterior axillary line immediately superior to the iliac crest.
8. **Thigh fold:** A vertical fold on the anterior midline of the thigh, midway between the border of the patella and the inguinal crease (knee joint and the hip). The midpoint should be marked while the subject is seated.
9. **Tricep fold:** A vertical fold on the posterior midline of the upper right arm, halfway between the acromion and the olecranon process (tip of the shoulder to the tip of the elbow). The arm should be relaxed and fully extended.

---

fat (table 15.5, focus box 15.2). The percentage of body fat can also be predicted from charts such as that of tables 15.9 and 15.10.

Multiple Compartment Methods of Body Composition

As previously explained, the lean body mass consists of water, protein, and mineral. However, because of the gender, age, population, and ethnicity specific differences that exit in either the density of these components or the proportion of LBM they represent, use of assumed refer-

ence values can cause considerable error in densitometry methods of body composition assessment. To decrease the error of using densitometry on different populations known to violate the assumptions of the *reference body*, researchers have attempted to specifically measure body mineral or total body water to better determine the average density of the LBM. When body composition assessment includes measures of the subcomponents of the LBM, it is termed a *multicompartment model* of body composition assessment.

Researchers typically conduct multicompartment research of body composition to derive a more accurate formula for

TABLE 15.8

Regression equations to predict body density from skinfold measurements

EQUATION	r*	SE*	REFERENCE
Nonspecific			
$D_b = 1.0982 - 0.000815(\text{sum of 3}) + 0.00000084^2(\text{sum of 3})^2$			46
Where (sum of 3) = triceps, subscapula, and abdomen			
Males			
18–61 years			
$D_b = 1.1093800 - 0.0008267(\text{sum of 3}) + 0.0000016\,(\text{sum of 3})^2 -$	0.91	0.0077	35
$0.0002574(\text{age})$			
Where (sum of 3) = chest, abdomen, and thigh			
College athletes			
$D_b = 1.10647 - 0.00162(\text{subscapular}) - 0.00144(\text{abdominal}) -$	0.84	0.006	24
$0.00077(\text{triceps}) + 0.00071(\text{midaxillary})$			
Females			
18–55 years			
$D_b = 1.0994921 - 0.0009929(\text{sum of 3}) + 0.0000023(\text{sum of 3})^2 -$	0.84	0.0086	36
$0.001392(\text{age})$			
Where (sum of 3) = triceps, suprailiac, and thigh			
College athletes			
$D_b = 1.096095 - 0.0006952(\text{sum of 4}) - 0.0000011(\text{sum of 4})^2 -$	0.85	0.0084	36
$0.0000714(\text{age})$			

Source: Data modified from Jackson and Pollock (21), Jackson et al. (22), and Lohman (30).

*r = correlation coefficient; SE = standard error of estimate.

FIGURE 15.6

(a) A photograph of a subject being scanned by dual energy x-ray absorptiometry (DEXA). (b) The data obtained from DEXA provides a measure of bone mineral, as well as lean body mass and estimated body fat.

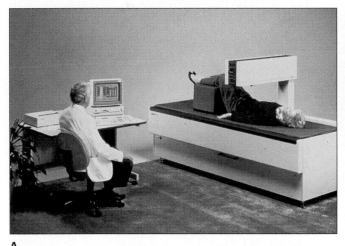

A

B

converting body density to % fat using standard two-component densitometry. Age- and gender-specific equations for converting body density to % fat were presented in Table 15.5.

Other Laboratory or Field Methods

Dual X-Ray Absorptiometry

Dual X-ray absorptiometry (DEXA) is a method of body composition assessment that has been developed from bone mineral measurement (fig. 15.6). DEXA actually measures the mass of the body that is mineral, lean soft tissue, or fat. Because data are used to calculate a fat and fat-free body mass from a procedure that does not depend on densitometry, DEXA is not a two-component method. Similarly, because bone mineral content is not used to adjust a density of the LBM, it is also

dual x-ray absorptiometry (DEXA) the method of body composition assessment that involves scanning the body to differentiate among soft lean tissue, bone mineral, and fat

TABLE 15.9

Percent fat estimate for women: sum of triceps, abdomen, and suprailium skinfolds

SUM OF SKINFOLDS (mm)	PERCENT FAT AGE TO LAST YEAR								
	18–22	23–27	28–32	33–37	38–42	43–47	48–52	53–57	OVER 57
8–12	8.8	9.0	9.2	9.4	9.5	9.7	9.9	10.1	10.3
13–17	10.8	10.9	11.1	11.3	11.5	11.7	11.8	12.0	12.2
18–22	12.6	12.8	13.0	13.2	13.4	13.5	13.7	13.9	14.1
23–27	14.5	14.6	14.8	15.0	15.2	15.4	15.6	15.7	15.9
28–32	16.2	16.4	16.6	16.8	17.0	17.1	17.3	17.5	17.7
33–37	17.9	18.1	18.3	18.5	18.7	18.9	19.0	19.2	19.4
38–42	19.6	19.8	20.0	20.2	20.3	20.5	20.7	20.9	21.2
43–47	21.2	21.4	21.6	21.8	21.9	22.1	22.3	22.5	22.7
48–52	22.8	22.9	23.1	23.3	23.5	23.7	23.8	24.0	24.2
53–57	24.2	24.4	24.6	24.8	25.0	25.2	25.3	25.5	25.7
58–62	25.7	25.9	26.0	26.2	26.4	26.6	26.8	27.0	27.1
63–67	27.1	27.2	27.4	27.6	27.8	28.0	28.2	28.3	28.5
68–72	28.4	28.6	28.7	28.9	29.1	29.3	29.5	29.7	29.8
73–77	29.6	29.8	30.0	30.2	30.4	30.6	30.7	30.9	31.1
78–82	30.9	31.0	31.2	31.4	31.6	31.8	31.9	32.1	32.3
83–87	32.0	32.2	32.4	32.6	32.7	32.9	33.1	33.3	33.5
88–92	33.1	33.3	33.5	33.7	33.8	34.0	34.2	34.4	34.6
93–97	34.1	34.3	34.5	34.7	34.9	35.1	35.2	35.4	35.6
98–102	35.1	35.3	35.5	35.7	35.9	36.0	36.2	36.4	36.6
103–107	36.1	36.2	36.4	36.6	36.8	37.0	37.2	37.3	37.5
108–112	36.9	37.1	37.3	37.5	37.7	37.9	38.0	38.2	38.4
113–117	37.8	37.9	38.1	38.3	39.2	39.4	39.6	39.8	39.2
118–122	38.5	38.7	38.9	39.1	39.4	39.6	39.8	40.0	40.0
123–127	39.2	39.4	39.6	39.8	40.0	40.1	40.3	40.5	40.7
128–132	39.9	40.1	40.2	40.4	40.6	40.8	41.0	41.2	41.3
133–137	40.5	40.7	40.8	41.0	41.2	41.4	41.6	41.7	41.9
138–142	41.0	41.2	41.4	41.6	41.7	41.9	42.1	42.3	42.5
143–147	41.5	41.7	41.9	42.0	42.2	42.4	42.6	42.8	43.0
148–152	41.9	42.1	42.3	42.8	42.6	42.8	43.0	43.2	43.4
153–157	42.3	42.5	42.6	42.8	43.0	43.2	43.4	43.6	43.7
158–162	42.6	42.8	43.0	43.1	43.3	43.5	43.7	43.9	44.1
163–167	42.9	43.0	43.2	43.4	43.6	43.8	44.0	44.1	44.3
168–172	43.1	43.2	43.4	43.6	43.8	44.0	44.2	44.3	44.5
173–177	43.2	43.4	43.6	43.8	43.9	44.1	44.3	44.5	44.7
178–182	43.3	43.5	43.7	43.8	44.0	44.2	44.4	44.6	44.8

not a multicomponent method. Nevertheless, the data from DEXA for % fat have been shown to have high agreement to that obtained from multicompartment densitometry (18, 40). Because of the ease of measurement, safety, minimal need for subject pretest and during-test cooperation, direct adjustment for bone mineral content and apparent accuracy, DEXA is gaining support for becoming the new "gold standard" for body composition assessment. Unfortunately, the only drawback for the widespread use of DEXA is the cost (> $50,000 per unit). Consequently, body composition researchers continue to use multicompartment and DEXA models of assessment to improve on existing equations for use in densitometry.

Bioelectrical Impedance

Bioelectrical impedance (BIA) is a relatively new body composition assessment technique based on Hoffer and associates' (19) research, which demonstrates a high correlation between whole-body electrical impedance and total body water (TBW). Hoffer further demonstrated that TBW and LBM were strongly correlated with $height^2$/resistance, where body resistance or impedance was measured with a tetrapolar electrode configuration (fig. 15.7). The principle of BIA is based on electrical conductance and on the fact that fat-free body mass, with its richer electrolyte content, has a much greater conductivity than does fat, thus allowing the

TABLE 15.10

Percent fat estimate for men: sum of triceps, chest, and subscapular skinfolds

SUM OF SKINFOLDS (mm)	PERCENT FAT AGE TO LAST YEAR								
	UNDER 22	23–27	28–32	33–37	38–42	43–47	48–52	53–57	OVER 57
8–10	1.5	2.0	2.5	3.1	3.6	4.1	4.6	5.1	5.6
11–13	3.0	3.5	4.0	4.5	5.1	5.6	6.1	6.6	7.1
14–16	4.5	5.0	5.5	6.0	6.5	7.0	7.6	8.1	8.6
17–19	5.9	6.4	6.9	7.4	8.0	8.5	9.0	9.5	10.0
20–22	7.3	7.8	8.3	8.8	9.4	9.9	10.4	10.9	11.4
23–25	8.6	9.2	9.7	10.2	10.7	11.2	11.8	12.3	12.8
26–28	10.0	10.5	11.0	11.5	12.1	12.6	13.1	13.6	14.2
29–31	11.2	11.8	12.3	12.8	13.4	13.9	14.4	14.9	15.5
32–34	12.5	13.0	13.5	14.1	14.6	15.1	15.7	16.2	16.7
35–37	13.7	14.2	14.8	15.3	15.8	16.4	16.9	17.4	18.0
38–40	14.9	15.4	15.9	16.5	17.0	17.6	18.1	18.6	19.2
41–43	16.0	16.6	17.1	17.6	18.2	18.7	19.3	19.8	20.3
44–46	17.1	17.7	18.2	18.7	19.3	19.8	20.4	20.9	21.5
47–49	18.2	18.7	19.3	19.8	20.4	20.9	21.4	22.0	22.5
50–52	19.2	19.7	20.3	20.8	21.4	21.9	22.5	23.0	23.6
53–55	20.2	20.7	21.3	21.8	22.4	22.9	23.5	24.0	24.6
56–58	21.1	21.7	22.2	22.8	23.3	23.9	24.4	25.0	25.5
59–61	22.0	22.6	23.1	23.7	24.2	24.8	25.3	25.9	26.5
62–64	22.9	23.4	24.0	24.5	25.1	25.7	26.2	26.8	27.3
65–67	23.7	24.3	24.8	25.4	25.9	26.5	27.1	27.6	28.2
68–70	24.5	25.0	25.6	26.2	26.7	27.3	27.8	28.4	29.0
71–73	25.2	25.8	26.3	26.9	27.5	28.0	28.6	29.1	29.7
74–76	25.9	26.5	27.0	27.6	28.2	28.7	29.3	29.9	30.4
77–79	26.6	27.1	27.7	28.2	28.8	29.4	29.9	30.5	31.1
80–82	27.2	27.7	28.3	28.9	29.4	30.0	30.6	31.1	31.7
83–85	27.7	28.3	28.8	29.4	30.0	30.5	31.1	31.7	32.3
86–88	28.2	28.8	29.4	29.9	30.5	31.1	31.6	32.2	32.8
89–91	28.7	29.3	29.8	30.4	31.0	31.5	32.1	32.7	33.3
92–94	29.1	29.7	30.3	30.8	31.4	32.0	32.6	33.1	33.4
95–97	29.5	30.1	30.6	31.2	31.8	32.4	32.9	33.5	34.1
98–100	29.8	30.4	31.0	31.6	32.1	32.7	33.3	33.9	34.4
101–103	30.1	30.7	31.3	31.8	32.4	33.0	33.6	34.1	34.7
104–106	30.4	30.9	31.5	32.1	32.7	33.2	33.8	34.4	35.0
107–109	30.6	31.1	31.7	32.3	32.9	33.4	34.0	34.6	35.2
110–112	30.7	31.3	31.9	32.4	33.0	33.6	34.2	34.7	35.3
113–115	30.8	31.4	32.0	32.5	33.1	33.7	34.3	34.9	35.4
116–118	30.9	31.5	32.0	32.6	33.2	33.8	34.3	34.9	35.5

establishment of a relationship between conductance and fat-free mass. Once the electrical resistance has been determined, body composition estimates can be extrapolated from generalized prediction equations (table 15.11) (14, 15).

Changes in electrolyte status of the body will dramatically affect BIA measurements, which is one of the main limitations of the BIA technique. In addition, when BIA was first developed for body composition analysis, the prediction equations supplied by the manufacturers of BIA testing equipment often overestimated LMB in obese subjects. However, recent cross-validation studies have suggested that prediction of LBM can be enhanced by sex- and fatness-specific equations (16).

bioelectrical impedance (BIA) the method of determining body fat, fat-free body mass, and total body water by measuring the resistance to current passed through the body

FIGURE 15.7

A subject prepared for body composition analysis by bioelectrical impedance (BIA).

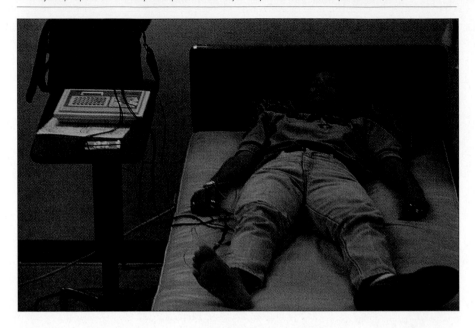

TABLE 15.11

Regression equations to predict fat-free body mass (kg) from bioelectrical impedance measurements

EQUATION*	r*	SE*	REFERENCE
Male			
$[0.485(L^2/R)] +$		2.9	46
$[0.338(\text{weight,kg})] + 5.32$			
Female			
$[0.475(L^2/R)] +$		2.9	46
$[0.295(\text{weight,kg})] + 5.49$			

*r = correlation coefficient; SE = standard error of estimate.

Equations derived from combined data from multiple research studies; L^2/R = resistive index = height²/resistance.

Source: Modified from Lohman (30).

Although BIA testing is a rapid, safe, and noninvasive method of estimating body composition, its accuracy can be questioned. Liang and Norris (26) revealed that % body fat from BIA analysis was overestimated by approximately 3% and Eckerson and colleagues (13) reported that BIA equations did not improve body fat prediction better than body weight alone, and % body fat in lean males has been reported to be better predicted from visual observation than by BIA analysis (12). Nevertheless, reports of the accuracy of BIA analysis exist, and Kushner (25) and Van Loan and Mayclin (39) have written excellent reviews on the use of BIA in body composition analysis.

To improve the accuracy of BIA testing, it is important that subjects strictly follow guidelines prior to testing:

1. Urinate within 30 min of the test
2. Consume no alcohol 48 h prior to the test
3. Do not exercise within 12 h of the test
4. Consume no food or fluid within 4 h of the test

These guidelines exist to avoid alterations in hydration of the body. As far as exercise is concerned, the recommendation of no prior exercise is not entirely supported by research; Liang and Norris (26) performed BIA analysis before and immediately after 30 min of exercise at 83% of maximal heart rate and found that BIA analysis were unchanged.

Near-Infrared Interactance

Near-infrared interactance (NIR) is a relatively recent technique that involves the transmission of electromagnetic radiation through a probe into subcutaneous tissue and analysis of the reflected and scattered energy from the electromagnetic radiation to estimate tissue composition. The commercially available (NIR) testing device (Futrex-5000) has been cross-validated with other techniques (9, 17, 32). It appears that NIR overestimates body fat in lean subjects < 8% and underestimates it in subjects with > 30% body fat. As with the BIA method, many equations have been developed using this methodology; however, compared to the accuracy of underwater weighing or skinfold techniques, it is not a method of choice in the laboratory or in the field.

WEBSITE BOX

Chapter 15: Body Composition Assessment

The newest information regarding exercise physiology can be viewed at the following sites.*

brainmac.demon.co.uk/whatsnew.htm

    Excellent site intended for coaches to have access to exercise-related information, including field tests of physical fitness, training strategies, nutrition, and coaching strategies.

http://acs6.bu.edu:8001/~jinhwa/

    Nice site that explains the principle of buoyancy, and concludes with applications to underwater weighing and body composition.

vig.com.au/updates.html

    Provides a technical update on the use of DEXA in bone mineral density assessment.

*Unless indicated, all URLs preceded by http://www.

Note: These URLs were valid at the time of publication, but could have changed or been deleted from Internet access since that time.

SUMMARY

■ **Body composition** refers to the relative amounts of the different compounds in the body. Typically, researchers have focused on the proportion of the body mass that is lean ("nonfat" or "fat free") and fat.

■ **Overweight** is defined as body weight in excess of a reference standard, generally a mean weight for a given height and skeletal frame size grouped by sex. However, research has clearly shown the inadequacy of this approach to defining overweight. Consequently, height-weight tables should be avoided, and the concept of overweight should be replaced with the condition of being **overfat.**

■ An important measure in research on the health status of large populations continues to be a modification of body mass and height—the **body mass index (BMI).** The BMI is the ratio of weight to height squared.

BMI = body mass (kg)/body height (m)^2

■ Body composition is often expressed as the relative amounts of fat mass to fat-free mass. Fat mass (FM) includes both essential and storage fat. **Essential fat** is found in bone marrow, brain, spinal cord, muscles, and other internal organs, and is "essential" to normal physiological and biological functioning. The minimum level below which essential fat should never go is believed to be approximately 3% of the total body weight for men and 12% of total body weight for women.

■ **Storage fat** is comprised of two types of fat, yellow fat which is approximately 99% of all storage fat, and brown fat, which is rich in mitochondria and can increase heat production because of a slightly lowered biochemical efficiency of ATP synthesis. Men tend to store more fat around the waist (android obesity), whereas women tend to store more fat around their hips and thighs (gynoid obesity). Older individuals tend to have less subcutaneous fat than younger subjects, but have greater fat deposits within and between skeletal muscles.

■ Once an individual's body composition has been obtained, an **ideal body weight** can be determined. An individual's ideal body weight should be carefully chosen. Generally, most people have an unrealistic expectation of their "desirable" weight.

■ The body can be divided into components that differ in composition. In the original body component system, the body was divided into two simple components: lean and fat body mass. Since that time, **lean body mass (LBM)** has been identified as not being completely fat-free, because it contains lipid within muscle, cell membranes, bone marrow, and so on. The term **fat-free body mass (FFBM)** therefore represents a large component of LBM.

SUMMARY

■ Despite the growing complexity of body composition assessment, the two-component system remains a widely used approach in research, clinical practice, health assessment, and physical fitness evaluation. Such acceptance is based on the applied interest in knowing the absolute and relative amounts of body fat, and the fact that a two-component approach can provide a very accurate estimate of fat and fat-free body composition, and often by a simple method.

■ The **two-component model** of body composition is based on the following assumptions: (1) the density of fat is 0.900 g/mL at 37° C; (2) the density of lean body mass is 1.100 g/mL at 37° C; (3) that all individuals have the previously stated densities for fat and lean body mass; (4) that the body's LBM is 73.8% water, 19.4% protein, and 6.8% mineral. However, each of the aforementioned assumptions can be invalid, depending on the person being studied.

■ *Densitometry* is the study of the measurement of human **body density. Hydrodensitometry,** or *hydrostatic weighing,* has been the "gold standard" by which all other methods of body composition assessment have validated. Recently, **air-displacement plethysmography** has been developed as another method of measuring body density, and has been shown to produce similar results to hydrodensitometry and DEXA.

■ It is possible to measure the subcutaneous fat at selected sites with skinfold calipers and predict the percentage of body fat by using various regression equations. Assessing body composition by measuring the thickness of selected **skinfolds** is probably the most common and widely available technique in use today. It is important that fitness instructors and exercise physiology students become proficient in this technique.

■ When body composition assessment includes measures of the subcomponents of the LBM, it is termed a *multicompartment model* of body composition assessment.

■ **Dual x-ray absorptiometry (DEXA)** is a method of body composition assessment that has been developed from bone mineral measurement. DEXA actually measures the mass of the body that is mineral, lean soft tissue, or fat. Because data are used to calculate a fat and fat-free body mass from a procedure that does not depend on densitometry, DEXA is not a two-component method.

■ **Bioelectrical impedance (BIA)** is a relatively new body composition assessment technique based on electrical conductance and on the fact that fat-free mass, with its richer electrolyte content, has a much greater conductivity than does fat, thus allowing for the establishment of a relationship between conductance and fat-free mass. Once the electrical resistance has been determined, body composition estimates can be extrapolated from generalized prediction equations.

■ Near-infrared interactance (NIR) involves the transmission of electromagnetic radiation through a probe into subcutaneous tissue and analysis of the reflected and scattered energy from the electromagnetic radiation to estimate tissue composition. NIR overestimates body fat in lean subjects < 8% and underestimates it in subjects with > 30% body fat.

STUDY QUESTIONS

1. What are the limitations of body composition assessment when using the standard height and weight table and the calculation of body mass index?

2. Explain the differences among the terms, essential fat, storage fat, fat-free body mass, lean body mass, and ideal body weight.

3. Define the two-component densitometry system of body composition. What are some of the weaknesses of the model?

4. How were the Siri and Brozek equations derived?

5. Is measurement of residual volume necessary for optimal accuracy of body composition determined by hydrodensitometry? Explain.

6. How do researchers currently validate new equations for skinfold assessment of body composition?

7. What methods of body composition assessment are viewed as "gold standards" to validate body composition methods? Is there really a gold standard? Explain.

8. Know the standard values of % body fat for different age ranges and genders.

9. Sally is a 20-year-old female, with a body fat of 34.5%, and her weight is 68 kg. Determine her desirable weight if her goal is to be 18% body fat with the same LBM.

10. Calculate a BMI score with a weight of 95 kg and a height of 181 cm. Remember, BMI = kg/m^2.

11. With the data listed below, calculate the percentage of body fat for a male using the appropriate regression equations of table 15.8.
    Age = 27
    Gender = male
    Race = Caucasian
    Fitness = endurance-trained athlete
    Chest skinfolds = 12.20, 13.5, 13.5, 13.5, and 13.5
    Abdomen skinfolds = 18.5, 18.25, 19.0, 18.5, and 18.4
    Thigh skinfolds = 13.5, 14.0, 13.5, 13.8, 14.0, and 14.0

12. Calculate the percentage of body fat based on the following data obtained during a hydrostatic weighing test.
    Age = 53
    Gender = female
    Subject height = 158 cm
    Subject weight = 69 kg
    Suit weight = 13.5 g
    RV = 1.48 L
    Weight of scale underwater = 2.95 kg
    Water temperature = 36.5°C
    Underwater weights = 4.71, 4.68, 4.70, 4.69, 4.71, 4.70

APPLICATIONS

1. Measurement of the body composition of clinically ill individuals in a hospital setting presents several obstacles for the application of hydrodensitometry. What are some patient populations that should not be submerged in water? What alternative methods would you use for each population and why?

2. How accurate should body composition analysis be? For example, is an error greater than ± 3% body fat really unacceptable for application to clinical and general use? Explain.

REFERENCES

1. American College of Sports Medicine. *ACSM's guidelines for exercise testing and prescription*, 5th ed., Williams & Wilkins, Baltimore, 1995.

2. Behnke, A. R., B. G. Feen, and W. C. Welman. The specific gravity of healthy men: Body weight/volume as an index of obesity. *J. Am. Med. Assoc.* 118:495–498, 1942.

3. Behnke, A. R. The estimation of lean body weight from skeletal measurement. *Human Biol.* 31:295–315, 1959.

4. Behnke, A. R., and J. H. Wilmore. *Evaluation and regulation of body build and composition.* Prentice Hall, Englewood Cliffs, NJ, 1974.

5. Bonge, D., and J. E. Donnelly. Trials to criteria for hydrostatic weighing at residual volume. *Res. Quart. Exerc. Sport.* 60(2):176–179, 1989.

6. Bosch, P. R., and C. L. Wells. Effect of immersion on residual lung volume of able-bodied and spinal cord injured males. *Med. Sci. Sports Exerc.* 23(3):384–388, 1991.

7. Brozek, J., F. Grande, J. T. Anderson, and A. Keys. Densiometric analysis of body composition: Revision of some quantitative assumptions. *Ann. N.Y. Acad. Sci.* 110:113–140, 1963.

8. Casey, V. A., J. T. Dwyer, K. A. Coleman, and I. Valadian. Body mass index from childhood to middle age: A 50-yr follow-up. *Am. J. Clin. Nutr.* 56:14–18, 1992.

9. Cassady, S. L., D. H. Nielsen, K. F. Janz. Y. Wu, J. S. Cook, and J. R. Hansen. Validity of near infrared body composition analysis in children and adolescents. *Med. Sci. Sports Med.* 25(10):1185–1191, 1993.

10. Craig, A. B., and L. H. Kyle. Effect of immersion in water on vital capacity and residual volume of lungs. *J. Appl. Physiol.* 23(4):423–425, 1967.

11. Dempster, P., and S. Aitkens. A new air-displacement method for the determination of human body composition. *Med. Sci. Sports Exerc.* 27(12):1692–1697, 1995.

12. Eckerson, J. M., T. J. Housh, and G. O. Johnson. The validity of visual estimations of percent body fat in lean males. *Med. Sci. Sports Exerc.* 24(5):615–618, 1992.

13. Eckerson, J. M., T. J. Housh, and G. O. Johnson. Validity of bioelectrical impedance equations for estimating fat-free weight in lean males. *Med. Sci. Sports Exerc.* 24(11):1298–1302, 1992.

14. Forbes, G. B., W. Simon, and J. M. Amatruda. Is bioimpedance a good predictor of body-composition change? *Am. J. Clin. Nutr.* 56:4–6, 1992.

15. Fuller, N. J., and M. Elia. Potential use of bioelectrical impedance of the whole body and of body segments for the assessment of body composition: Comparison with densitometry and anthropometry. *Eur. J. Clin. Nutr.* 43:779–791, 1988.

16. Gray, D. S., G. A. Brag, N. Gemayel, and K. Kaplan. Effect of obesity on bioelectrical impedance. *Am. J. Clin. Nutr.* 50:255–260, 1989.

REFERENCES

17. Heyward, V. H., et al. Validity of single site and multi-site models for estimating body composition of women using near-infrared interactance. *Am. J. Human Biol.* 4:579–593, 1992.

18. Heyward, V., and L. Stolarczyk. *Applied body composition assessment.* Human Kinetics, Champaign, IL, 1996.

19. Hoffer, E. C., C. K. Meador, and D. C. Simpson. Correlation of whole-body impedance with total body water volume. *J. Appl. Physiol.* 27:531–534, 1969.

20. Jackson, A. S., and M. L. Pollock. Factor analysis and multivariate scaling of anthropometric variables for the assessment of body composition. *Med. Sci. Sports Exerc.* 8(3):196–203, 1976.

21. Jackson, A. S., and M. L. Pollock. Generalized equations for predicting body density of men. *Brit. J. Nutr.* 40:497–504, (1978).

22. Jackson, A. S., M. L. Pollock, and A. Ward. Generalized equations for predicting body density of women. *Med. Sci. Sport Exerc.* 12:175–182, 1980.

23. Katch, F. I. Practice curves and errors of measurement in estimating underwater weight by hydrostatic weighing. *Med. Sci. Sports Exerc.* 1(4):212–216, 1969.

24. Keys, A., and J. Brozek. Body fat in adult men. *Physiol. Rev.* 33:245–325, 1953.

25. Kushner, R. F. Bioelectrical impedance analysis: A review of principles and applications. *J. Am. Coll. Nutr.* 11(2):199–209, 1992.

26. Liang, M.T., and S. Norris. Effects of skin blood flow and temperature on bioelectrical impedance after exercise. *Med. Sci. Sports Exerc.* 25(11):1231–1239, 1993.

27. Lohman, T. G. Skinfolds and body density and their relation to body fatness: A review. *Human Biol.* 53:181–225, 1981.

28. Lohman, T. G. Research progress in validation of laboratory methods of assessing body composition. *Med. Sci. Sport Exerc.* 16:596–603, 1984.

29. Lohman, T. G. Applicability of body composition techniques and constants for children and youths. *Exerc. Sports Sci. Rev.* 14:325–357, 1986.

30. Lohman, T. G. *Advances in body composition assessment.* Current issues in Exercise Science Series: Monograph No. 3. Human Kinetics, Champaign, IL, 1992.

31. McCrory, M. A., T. D. Gomez, E. M. Bernauer, and P. A. Mole. Evaluation of a new air-displacement plethysmograph for measuring human body composition. *Med. Sci. Sports Exerc.* 27(12):1686–1691, 1995.

32. McLean, K. P., and J. S. Skinner. Validity of Futrex-5000 for body composition determination. *Med. Sci. Sports Exerc.* 24(2):253–258, 1992.

33. Metropolitan Life Insurance Company. *1983 height and weight tables.* Metropolitan Life Insurance Company, New York, 1983.

34. Morrow, J. R., A. S. Jackson, P. W. Bradely, and G. Harley Hartung. Accuracy of measured and predicted residual lung volume on body density measurement. *Med. Sci. Sports Exerc.* 18(6):647–652, 1986.

35. Siri, W. E. Body composition from fluid space and density. In J. Brozek and A. Hanschel (eds.), *Techniques for measuring body composition.* National Academy of Science, Washington, DC, 1961.

36. Sloan, A. W. Estimation of body fat in young men. *J. Appl. Physiol.* 23:311–315, 1967.

37. Snyder, W. S., M. J. Cook, E. S. Nasset, L. R. Karhausen, G. P. Howells, and I. H. Tipton. *Report on the task group on reference man.* Pergamon Press, Oxford, 1984.

38. Timson, B. F., and J. L. Coffman. Body composition by hydrostatic weighing at total lung capacity and residual volume. *Med. Sci. Sports Exerc.* 16(4):411–414, 1984.

39. Van Loan, M. D. Bioelectrical impedance analysis to determine fat-free mass, total body water and body fat. *Sports Med.* 10(4):205–217, 1990.

40. Van Loan, M. D., and P. L. Mayclin. Body composition assessment: Dual-energy x-ray absorptiometry (DEXA) compared to other methods. *Eur. J. Clin. Nutr.* 46:125–130, 1992.

41. Wang, Z. M., R. N. Pierson, and S. B. Heymsfield. The five-level model: A new approach to organizing body-composition research. *Am. J. Clin. Nutr.* 56:19–28, 1992.

42. Ward, D. S., and O. Bar-Or. Role of the physician and physical education teacher in the treatment of obesity at school. *Pediatrician* 13:44–51, 1986.

43. Wilmore, J. H., and J. A. Bergfeld. A comparison of sports: Physiological and medical aspects. In R. J. Strauss (ed.), *Sports medicine and physiology.* Saunders, Philadelphia, 1979.

44. Wilmore, J. H., and W. L. Haskell. Body composition and endurance capacity of professional football players. *J. Appl. Physiol.* 33(5):564–567, 1972.

RECOMMENDED READINGS

Brozek, J., F. Grande, J. T. Anderson, and A. Keys. Densitometric analysis of body composition: Revision of some quantitative assumptions. *Ann. N.Y. Acad. Sci.* 110:113–140, 1963.

Eckerson, J. M., T. J. Housh, and G. O. Johnson. The validity of visual estimations of percent body fat in lean males. *Med. Sci. Sports Exerc.* 24(5):615–618, 1992.

Heyward, V., and L. Stolarczyk. *Body composition assessment.* Human Kinetics, Champaign, IL, 1996.

Jackson, A. S., and M. L. Pollock. Generalized equations for predicting body density of men. *Brit. J. Nutr.* 40:497–504, 1978.

Jackson, A. S., M. L. Pollock, and A. Ward. Generalized equations for predicting body density of women. *Med. Sci. Sports Exer.* 12, 175–182, 1980.

Kushner, R. F. Bioelectrical impedance analysis: A review of principles and applications. *J. Am. Coll. Nutr.* 11(2):199–209, 1992.

Lohman, T. G. *Advances in body composition assessment.* Current issues in Exercise Science Series: Monograph No. 3, Human Kinetics, Champaign, IL, 1992.

Van Loan, M. D. Bioelectrical impedance analysis to determine fat-free mass, total body water and body fat. *Sports Med.* 10(4):205–217, 1990.

Wang, Z. M., R.N. Pierson, and S.B. Heymsfield. The five-level model: A new approach to organizing body-composition research. *Am. J. Clin. Nutr.* 56:19–28, 1992.

Clinical Exercise Testing

his chapter introduces the student to the fundamental principles of clinical exercise testing. The term "clinical" implies that the exercise test is "medically" oriented. Earlier chapters discussed the principles of exercise testing to measure and estimate VO_{2max} and cardiorespiratory function. How then does clinical exercise testing differ from fitness or performance exercise testing? First, unlike general fitness tests, which are conducted to measure or predict aerobic or anaerobic power in apparently healthy individuals, clinical exercise tests are typically ordered by physicians to screen for coronary heart disease, to diagnosis the severity of coronary heart disease, and to assess the status of the cardiovascular system following a myocardial infarction or medical procedure, such as coronary bypass surgery. Second, clinical exercise testing generally requires that personnel conducting the test have advanced training in emergency procedures, electrocardiography, stress testing principles, and basic and advanced principles of cardiovascular medicine. Third, clinical exercise testing has different equipment needs, including emergency equipment, an electrocardiogram machine, and so forth. And fourth, clinical exercise tests are generally performed in a hospital or physician's office, whereas fitness tests are commonly performed in health clubs, YMCAs, or exercise physiology laboratories at colleges and universities. The purpose of this chapter is to introduce the student to the fundamental principles of clinical exercise testing, and to help provide the foundation for more advanced training and education.

OBJECTIVES

After studying this chapter, you should be able to:

- Describe the indications, contraindications and uses of clinical exercise testing.
- List the guidelines for testing healthy and high-risk individuals and individuals with known disease(s).
- Identify the basic elements of electrocardiography.
- Explain normal and abnormal responses to clinical exercise testing.
- Describe the predictive value (Bayes's theorem) of clinical exercise testing.
- Explain the procedures involved in conducting an exercise test.
- Describe the procedures for interpreting the results of an exercise test.

KEY TERMS

diagnostic test
functional capacity test
electrocardiogram
arrhythmia
ST-segment depression

myocardial infarction
informed consent
myocardial ischemia
predictive value
Bayes's theorem

sensitivity
specificity
cardiac catheterization

Indications and Uses of Clinical Exercise Testing

C linical exercise testing has three main uses: (1) to diagnose the presence or severity of disease, (2) to establish the functional capacity of an individual, and (3) to evaluate medical therapy. Diagnostic and prognostic evaluation of suspected or established cardiovascular disease is perhaps the most common clinical application of clinical exercise testing. The exercise test is probably the best test of the heart because it is the most common everyday stress that humans undertake. Table 16.1 lists common uses of clinical exercise testing.

Before a clinical exercise test is ordered by a physician, sufficient evidence must be present and documented on the patient to justify ordering the test. *With any kind of exercise testing or exercise prescription, the benefits must outweigh the potential risks!*

One of the most common reasons for ordering a clinical exercise test is to diagnose and evaluate the status of suspected or known cardiovascular disease. An example of when clinical exercise testing is indicated is when a patient comes to a physician's office for a regular check-up so he/she can start an exercise program. The physician discovers that the patient is sedentary, overweight, smokes a pack of cigarettes per day, has high cholesterol, and has recently complained of several episodes of chest pain during physical exertion. Because the patient in question is at high risk for coronary artery disease, the physician should order a clinical exercise evaluation before allowing the patient to exercise. See table 16.2 for cardiovascular disease risk factors.

Clinical exercise testing is an effective way to evaluate an individual's cardiovascular system's response to controlled physiological stress (exercise). Regardless of whether the patient passes or fails the test, both the physician and patient can be better assured of the patient's ability or inability to

participate in an exercise program. Thus, clinical exercise testing is useful in **diagnostic testing** or quantifying heart and/or other chronic disease conditions.

Clinical exercise testing is also commonly used to determine the **functional capacity** of healthy, sedentary, and/or asymptomatic individuals. For example, after an individual has suffered a heart attack or is recovering from a coronary

---

TABLE 16.1

Uses of clinical exercise testing

Exercise Testing Apparently Healthy Individuals
Determine functional capacity

Screen for disease

Motivation

Develop an exercise prescription

Exercise Testing High-Risk Individuals
Diagnostic tool

Evaluation of suspected heart disease

Evaluation of asymptomatic individuals with risk of coronary heart disease

After myocardial infarction

After coronary angioplasty

Evaluate dysrhythmias

Evaluate peripheral vascular disease

Evaluate medical therapy

Exercise Testing Individuals with a Known Disease
Determine functional capacity

After myocardial infarction

After heart surgery

After repair of heart valves or defects

Chronic pulmonary disease

Chronic renal disease

Diabetes

Evaluate medical therapy

TABLE 16.2

Cardiovascular risk factors

Age	Men > 45 years; women > 55 or premature menopause without estrogen replacement therapy
Family history	MI or sudden death before 55 years of age in father or other male first-degree relative, or before 65 years of age in mother or other female first-degree relative
Current cigarette smoking	
Hypertension	Blood pressure > 140/90 mmHg, confirmed by measurement on at least two separate occasions, or on antihypertensive medication
Hypercholesterolemia	Total serum cholesterol > 200 mg/dL or HDL < 35 mg/dL
Diabetes mellitus	Persons with insulin-dependent diabetes mellitus (IDDM) who are > 30 years of age, or have had IDDM for > 15 years, and persons with noninsulin-dependent diabetes mellitus (NIDDM) who are > 35 years of age classified as patients with disease
Sedentary lifestyle	Persons comprising the least active 25% of the population, as defined by the combination of sedentary jobs involving sitting for a large part of the day and no regular exercise or active recreational pursuits

FOCUS BOX 16.1

Absolute Contraindications to Exercise Testing

1. A recent significant change in the resting ECG
2. Recent complicated myocardial infarction
3. Unstable angina (angina which is not controlled by medication)
4. Uncontrolled ventricular arrhythmias
5. Uncontrolled atrial arrhythmias that compromise cardiac function
6. Third-degree AV block without a pacemaker
7. Acute congestive heart failure (CHR is a condition characterized by extreme weakness, edema (water retention) in the lower extremities, and breathlessness because of poor or reduced pumping ability of the heart)
8. Severe aortic stenosis (aortic stenosis is a narrowing of the aorta or aortic valve)
9. Suspected or known dissecting aneurysm (a dissecting aneurysm is one in which the blood makes its way between the layers of a blood vessel wall, separating them in the process)
10. Active or suspected myocarditis (myocarditis is an inflammation of the myocardium)
11. Thrombophlebitis or intercardiac thrombi (thrombophlebitis is an inflammation of a vein in conjunction with the formation of a thrombus [blood clot])
12. Recent systemic or pulmonary embolus (an embolus is a mass of undissolved matter [solid, liquid, or gaseous] in the blood)
13. Acute infection
14. Significant emotional distress

ACSM's Guidelines for Exercise Testing and Prescription, 5th Edition.

bypass operation, clinical exercise testing is useful in developing an exercise prescription. Exercise testing can be used to develop a safe and effective level of exercise for individuals with or without disease. The results of an exercise test can be used to set the initial intensity, duration, and frequency of exercise. Follow-up testing can be used to modify an earlier exercise prescription.

Risk Stratification

Several medical organizations have developed categories that stratify individuals according to their medical and/or health conditions and their potential risks for injury during exercise testing or training (ACSM). In essence, risk stratification before exercise testing or training is one tool that helps establish whether or not *the benefits outweigh the potential risks!* There are situations in which exercise testing or training may not be appropriate at a particular time, or further tests may need to be performed before proceeding. The American College of Sports Medicine has established three categories of risk stratification (apparently healthy, increased risk, and known disease) (ACSM).

Individuals who fall into the apparently healthy category are at the least risk for problems during exercise. Routine testing for coronary artery disease in asymptomatic low-risk individuals remains controversial because of the limited ability to detect disease in this group (1, 3, 4). Individuals who are at increased risk have symptoms suggestive of possible cardiopulmonary or metabolic disease (i.e., chest pain, diabetes) and/or have two or more major coronary risk factors and thus are at greater risk during exercise. A physician may need to be present when testing high-risk individuals, depending on the medical history of the individual. Individuals with documented evidence of cardiovascular, pulmonary, or metabolic disease are at the greatest risk during exercise. A physician always needs to be present when testing an individual with known disease, or who is at high risk for heart disease.

Contraindications of Clinical Exercise Testing

A variety of benefits can be derived from exercise testing; however, the procedure is not without risks. The fatal risk of an exercise test is approximately 0.5 per 10,000 tests (6). Based on data from several different studies (6) it has been determined that the risk of death following exercise testing is 1 per 10,000 tests, myocardial infarction 4 per 10,000 tests, and approximately five hospital admissions (including infarctions) per 10,000 tests (7). Thus, the test is extremely safe, as long as the personnel administering the test follow the recommended safety procedures and the patient is properly screened for potential contraindications prior to testing. Focus box 16.1 lists the absolute contraindications to exercise testing. For individuals with absolute contraindications, the risks of the test may outweigh the potential benefits. Other forms of diagnostic testing may be more appropriate in these situations (see other cardiovascular tests). An understanding of these contraindications is increased by knowing the arterial vasculature of the heart (See focus box 16.2).

diagnostic test exercise test performed to diagnose or detect a medical condition

functional capacity test exercise test performed to assess the functional capacity of an individual

FIGURE 16.1
ECG of normal sinus rhythm.

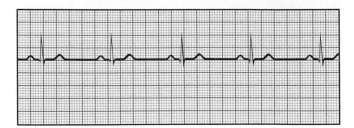

Electrocardiography

One of the essential tools used in clinical exercise testing is the **electrocardiogram**. There are two common abbreviations for electrocardiogram, EKG and ECG. EKG is used more frequently and comes from the German language where cardiogram is written as kardiogram. Both abbreviations are correct. The ECG is a recording of the electrical activity of the heart, whereas the mechanical activity of the heart is assessed by *echocardiography*. An ECG machine is able to pick up and record small amounts of electrical activity that originates in the heart, some of which reaches the body surface. When electrodes are placed on the body and hooked up to an ECG machine, a reproducible tracing of the electrical activity of the heart can be recorded (fig. 16 .1). One complete cardiac cycle (heartbeat) record on the ECG represents the spread of electrical activity from the SA node all the way to the Purkinje fibers (fig. 16.2). It is important to realize that the ECG records the differences in voltage between positive and negative electrodes. As a wave of electricity or depolarization reaches a positive electrode, an upward deflection occurs on the ECG paper. As a wave of depolarization moves away from the positive electrode, a downward deflection occurs.

Basic Characteristics of the ECG

There are five key waves and intervals that make up the ECG. Each wave or interval represents a particular function of the heart. A wave represents depolarization or repolarization, whereas an interval represents time during which the electrical signal is traveling away from the SA node. The height, width, and shape of the wave and the length and shape of the interval can indicate a variety of pathological and/or medical conditions. Figure 16.4 identifies the ECG waves and intervals.

The Standard 12-Lead Electrocardiogram

The standard 12-lead electrocardiogram is composed of three limb leads—I, II, III; three augmented limb leads—aV_R, aV_L, aV_F; and six chest leads—V_{1-6}. The limb leads all lie in a plane which can be visualized over the chest (frontal plane or top to bottom) (fig. 16.5). The chest leads circle the

FIGURE 16.2
Top: The standard electrocardiograph showing repeated waves and segments. *Bottom:* The electrical changes during the cardiac cycle cause the changes seen on a standard electrocardiograph. Depolarization of the atrium causes the P wave, depolarization of the ventricular myocardium causes the QRS complex, and repolarization of the ventricular myocardium causes the T wave.

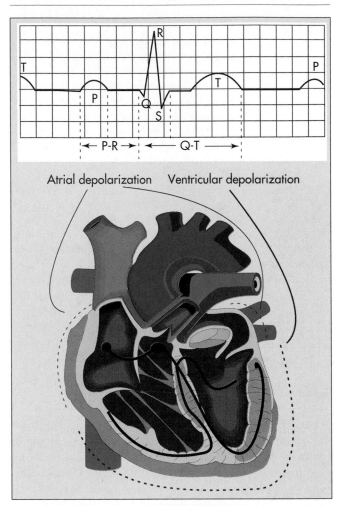

heart and form the horizontal plane or front to back. Each lead provides a different angle or picture of the heart. It is possible to obtain a picture of the anterior part of the heart by looking at leads V_1 through V_4, a lateral view of the heart by looking at leads I, aV_L, V_5 and V_6, an inferior view of the heart by looking at leads II, III, and aV_F. Figure 16.6 is an actual example of a resting 12-lead report.

Interpretation of the 12-Lead Electrocardiogram

The basic rule in ECG interpretation is to use the same approach or system every time you evaluate an ECG. There are three key steps to follow when evaluating any ECG. These steps include determining the rate, rhythm, and axis. Eventu-

FOCUS BOX 16.2

The Coronary Circulation

Because one of the main purposes of exercise testing is to identify poor circulation in the coronary arteries, a brief review of the coronary circulation is helpful. Remember that the heart has its own blood supply. The coronary arteries originate from the aorta at two main sites, the right and left coronary arteries. The left main artery divides into two major divisions, the left anterior descending and the left circumflex. The coronary arteries can be thought of as branches of a tree. Consider the aorta as the trunk, the right and left main coronary arteries, the posterior descending , anterior descending, and the circumflex as the main branches, and the other arteries as smaller branches. When new branches form be-cause of ischemia, they are referred to as *collaterals*. Coronary collateral circulation becomes an important supply of blood to the heart muscle following a myocardial infarction. Because the heart muscle cells are highly aerobic (a – vO₂ = 70 to 80%), the only way the heart can get additional oxygen during periods of increased demand is by an increase in coronary blood supply. When coronary arteries become blocked because of coronary heart disease or if they have a spasm, coronary artery blood supply is compromised, resulting in a mismatch between supply and demand. This mismatch in supply and demand, if severe enough, can be detected on the ECG as ST-segment depression (fig. 16.11).

FIGURE 16.3

Coronary circulation from an *(a)* anterior (arteries) and *(b)* posterior perspective (veins). From an anterior perspective, the major coronary arteries seen are the left and right coronary arteries, circumflex artery, and left anterior descending artery. From the posterior perspective, the major arteries seen are the circumflex artery, right coronary artery, posterior descending artery, and the nodal artery. The majority of coronary venors blood drains into the right atrium.

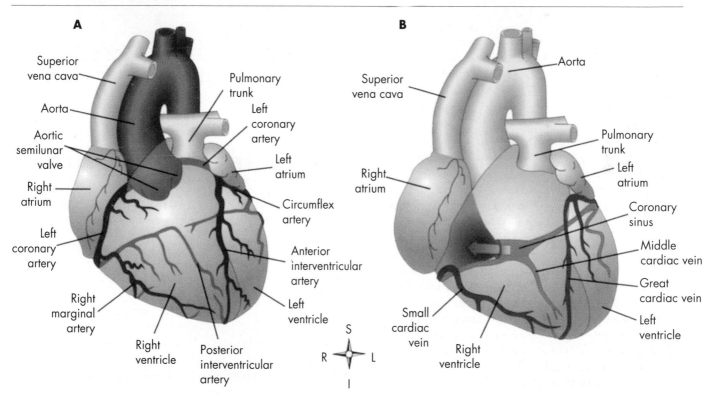

ally you will learn to analyze all of the different waves, segments, and intervals in order to determine any abnormalities in the ECG. Because many exercise physiology students are finding employment opportunities in clinical settings, such as working in a hospital as an exercise technologist, it is highly recommended that students take a basic and advanced electrocardiography class. These classes are held at local hospitals and, often, students are welcome to attend.

Rate

The first measurement to calculate when looking at the electrocardiogram is the heart rate. The rate is measured as cycles per minute or beats per minute (b/min). The PQRST

electrocardiogram recording from an electrocardiograph

FIGURE 16.4

ECG waves, intervals, and forms.

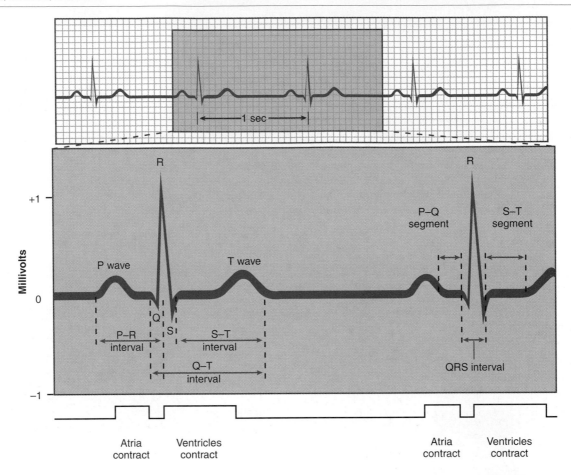

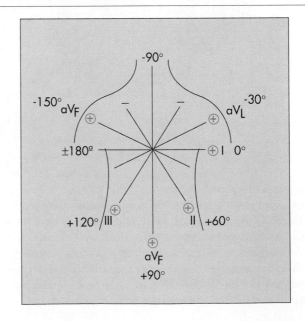

FIGURE 16.5

The limb leads of the 12-lead electrocardiograph (ECG) can be viewed radially, so that each passes through an identical central location. Such a hexaxial arrangement of the leads allows the 12-lead ECG to evaluate electrical axes and assist in relating one lead to another.

waves represent one complete cardiac cycle. The first way to determine heart rate from the ECG is to find an R wave that falls on a heavy black line, next count off 300, 150, 100, 75, 60 for each heavy black line that follows. Where the next R wave falls determines the rate. It is important to accurately and quickly determine heart rate in order to assess whether or not there are any abnormalities present.

Figure 16.7 provides an example of how to determine HR from the ECG.

Abnormalities in Heart Rate

A heart rate over 100 beats per minute is referred to as tachycardia (*tachy* means fast). A heart rate below 60 beats per minute is referred to as bradycardia (*brady* means slow). A variety of factors affect heart rate including age (declines with age), gender (females generally have higher resting heart rates), physical stature (small animals have higher heart rates), emotion (stress can elevate heart rate), type of food consumed (caffeine stimulates heart rate), body temperature (as body temp rises, so does heart rate),

FIGURE 16.6

12-lead ECG.

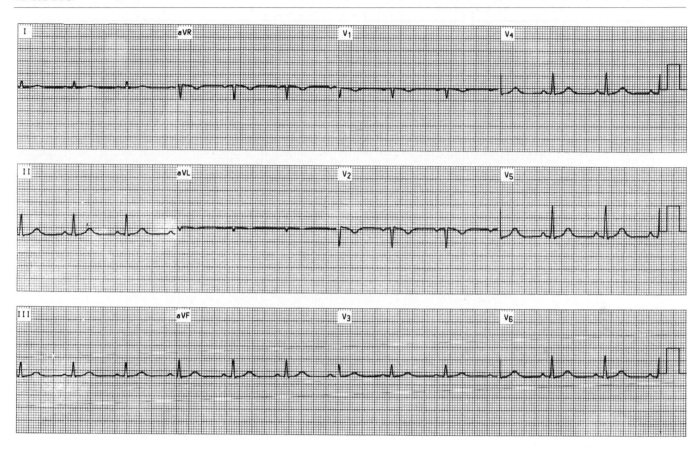

Abnormalities in Rhythm

Remember that any variation from the normal rhythm and normal electrical conduction pattern of the heart is referred to as an arrhythmia. Arrhythmias are generally categorized on the basis of the location of the ECG problem in relation to the electrical conduction system. Some common arrhythmias are described below.

Normal sinus rhythm (NSR) (see figs. 16.1 and 16.6)

> Rate—60–100 b/min
> Rhythm—regular
> P waves—upright in leads I, II, aV_F

Atrial fibrillation (A-FIB)—A-FIB results from multiple sites of depolarization within the atria (fig. 16.9a).

> Rate—atrial rate is 400 to 700 b/min, but cannot be counted with accuracy; the ventricle rate is 160 to 180 b/min.
> Rhythm—Irregular

arrhythmia abnormal cardiac rhythm

environmental factors (smoking), medication, and exercise. Highly trained endurance athletes tend to have extremely low resting rates (< 40 b/min) as a result of greater parasympathetic tone at rest. It is important to recognize that some abnormalities in heart rate are naturally caused (exercise) and may be perfectly fine for an individual, whereas other abnormalities may be pathogenic in nature (sick sinus syndrome and bundle branch block) and may require medical therapy to correct. Other causes may not be natural (taking stimulants) and may lead to medical problems, especially during exercise.

Rhythm

Rhythm is the most difficult part of the ECG to interpret. The normal cardiac rhythm is such that there is a constant distance between similar waves (R wave to R wave or P wave to P wave). **Arrhythmias** are abnormal (inconsistent) cardiac rhythms. Rhythm is determined by looking at a continuous ECG strip versus a static 12-lead ECG. To determine rhythm, measure the R-R intervals across the entire strip. A constant R-R interval would mean that the rhythm is regular, or sinus, meaning that the rhythm originates in the SA node. Figure 16.8 shows an example of how to assess cardiac rhythm.

FIGURE 16.7
Determining heart rate.

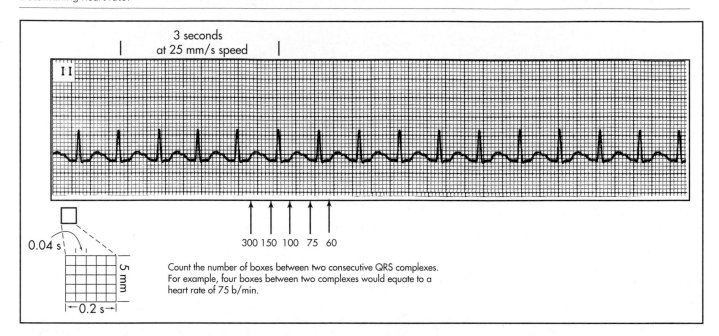

3 seconds at 25 mm/s speed

0.04 s

5 mm

←0.2 s→

300 150 100 75 60

Count the number of boxes between two consecutive QRS complexes. For example, four boxes between two complexes would equate to a heart rate of 75 b/min.

FIGURE 16.8
Determining heart rhythm.

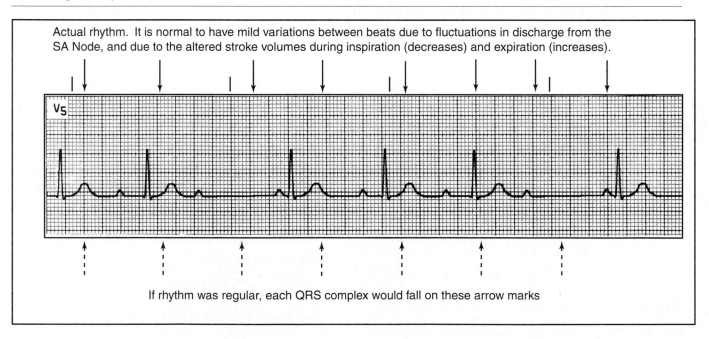

Actual rhythm. It is normal to have mild variations between beats due to fluctuations in discharge from the SA Node, and due to the altered stroke volumes during inspiration (decreases) and expiration (increases).

If rhythm was regular, each QRS complex would fall on these arrow marks

P waves—organized atrial activity absent; rhythm can be described as chaotic.

Premature ventricular contraction (PVC)—PVCs are caused by depolarization that arises in either ventricle prior to the next expected beat. (fig. 16.9c and d).

Rate—varies
Rhythm—irregular

P waves—may be obscured by the QRS, ST segment, or T wave of the PVC

Axis

Axis refers to the direction of depolarization throughout the heart to stimulate the muscle fibers to contract. The electrical axis is referred to as the *mean QRS vector* and

FIGURE 16.9

Examples of *(a)* atrial fibrillation; *(b)* nonsinus premature atrial contraction (PAC); *(c)* single premature ventricular contraction (PVC); *(d)* multifocal premature ventricular contractions (PVCs).

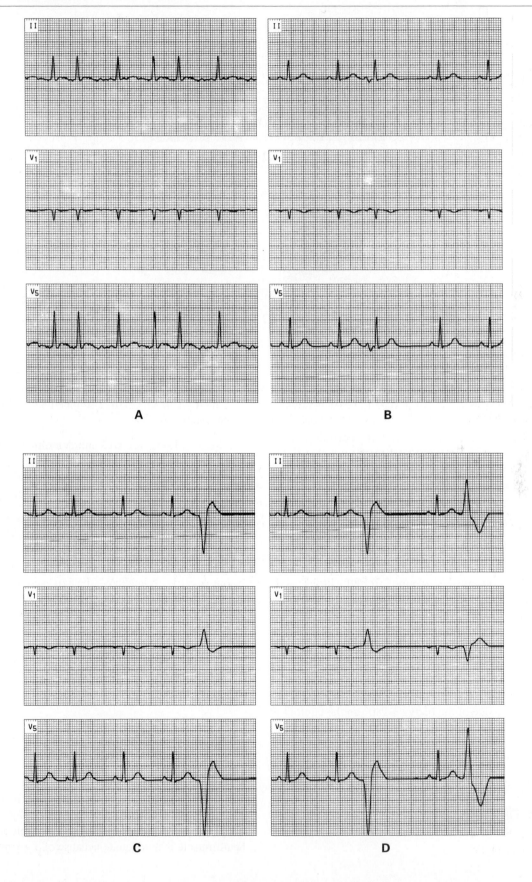

FIGURE 16.10
Quadrant determination.

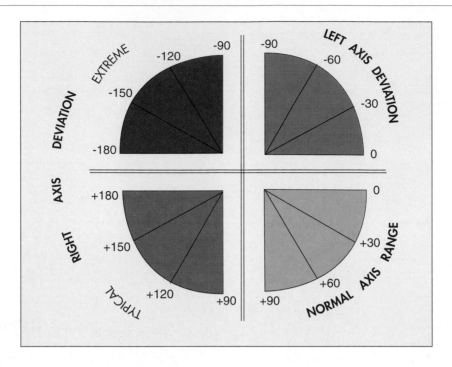

represents the mean direction of depolarization throughout the heart, which begins at the SA node and spreads downward and to the left. The normal QRS vector is located between 0 and +90 degrees. When the left ventricle is hypertrophied (either from exercise or disease) the electrical axis shifts toward it. In cases on necrosis caused by a heart attack, the electrical axis shifts away from the left ventricle. Determining axis assists in the overall interpretation of the ECG.

Determining Axis

The electrical axis system is determined from the limb leads. The electrical activity of the heart originates in the SA node and spreads throughout the heart down and leftward toward the left ventricle. If an imaginary circle is drawn over the chest, the center of the circle would lie over the AV node. The circle is divided into a vertical plane and a horizontal plane. The vertical plane runs from the head ($-90°$ on the circle), to the feet ($+90°$ on the circle). The horizontal plane runs from the right side of the body ($+180°$ on the circle) to the left side of the body is ($0°$ on the circle). The normal axis of the heart is between 0 and $+90°$ (see fig. 16.5).

> Positive QRS deflection: occurs when the height of the R wave exceeds the combined deflection of the Q and S waves.
> Negative QRS deflection: occurs when the combined deflection of the Q and S waves exceeds the height of the R wave.

Zero mean QRS deflection: occurs when the height of the R wave equals the combined deflection of the Q and S waves.

Step 1: Look at lead I and determine if the mean QRS deflection is positive or negative.
Step 2: Look at lead aV_F and determine if the mean QRS deflection is positive or negative.

1. If the mean QRS deflection activity is upright in both leads, the axis is in the normal quadrant ($0°$ to $+90°$) (see fig. 16.10).
2. If the mean QRS deflection activity is positive in lead I but negative in lead aV_F, the axis is in the left-axis quadrant ($0°$ to $-90°$) (see fig. 16.10).
3. If the mean QRS deflection activity is positive in lead aV_F but negative in lead I the axis is in the right-axis quadrant ($+90°$ to $+180°$) (see fig. 16.10).
4. If the mean QRS deflection activity is negative in both leads then the axis is in the extreme right-axis quadrant ($-90°$ to $-180°$) (see fig. 16.10).

ST-Segment Depression

ST depression on the ECG is the hallmark of myocardial ischemia. **ST-segment depression** is the principal abnormality during exercise that should concern individuals supervising a treadmill test. When the delivery of blood supply to the heart muscle is inadequate because of a mismatch in supply

FIGURE 16.11

The three types of ST-segment depression: *(a)* Downsloping; *(b)* horizontal; and *(c)* upsloping.

Downsloping

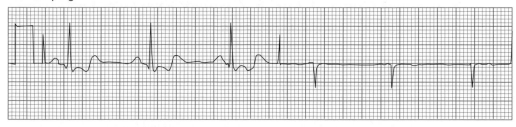

Horizontal

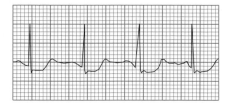

Upsloping

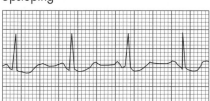

versus demand, the inner lining of the heart (subendocardium) suffers first. At the onset of ischemia, the reduction of blood supply alters the normal cellular actions causing the ST segment to be displaced below the baseline. ST-segment depression resulting from exercise is usually subendocardial ischemia. Analysis of the ST segment provides the best evidence for the presence of *myocardial ischemia* (see fig. 16.11).

Myocardial Infarction

When the delivery of blood supply to the heart muscle is compromised for an extended period of time because of a spasm or a blood clot, the inner lining of the heart *(subendocardial)* or the entire thickness of the heart *(transmural)* can be affected. ST-segment elevation represents transmural ischemia, whereas ST-segment depression represents subendocardial ischemia. If the ischemia is severe or prolonged, the tissue being affected is injured, cell functions cease, and irreversible cell death occurs. The majority of **myocardial infarctions** (> 87%) result from a portion of a plaque in the coronary arteries breaking loose and lodging at a site of narrowing further down the artery forming a clot. The affected muscle tissue is no longer able to contract.

Conducting the Clinical Exercise Test

Pretest Data Collection

Before an exercise test is administered for diagnostic purposes, certain medical information needs to be obtained from the patient.

The following data should be obtained before conducting the test:

Recent medical history.
Coronary heart disease risk factor assessment.
A brief physical examination should be conducted by a trained medical professional.
Laboratory tests should include: total cholesterol and HDL cholesterol. Other lab tests might include triglycerides and blood glucose.

When all these data are collected, the physician or technician can determine if there are any absolute or relative contraindications to testing.

Patient Instructions

Pretest instructions should always be given to patients before the day of the test. General pretest patient instructions include:

Abstain from food, tobacco, alcohol, and caffeine for at least 3 h before the test.
Wear comfortable clothing, including a sport or athletic shoe.
Women patients should wear a sports bra if they have one.
Continue to take prescribed medications, unless the physician has instructed otherwise.

ST-segment depression lowering of the ST segment, usually because of myocardial ischemia

myocardial infarction lack of blood flow long enough to cause injury to the heart

FIGURE 16.12
A typical informed consent used for graded exercise testing.

Informed Consent For A Graded Exercise Test
Center For Exercise and Applied Human Physiology
The University of New Mexico

I agree to voluntarily engage in the following test for the evaluation of cardiovascular function and the prescription of an exercise training program.

Prior to exercise, I will be asked to complete a questionnaire that evaluates my medical history. I will then be asked several questions about my health and the answers I provided. Assuming I am able to perform exercise to exhaustion, I will then be prepared for the test. In order to evaluate heart function, I will have electrodes placed on several sites on my upper body. To improve the ability of the electrodes to detect electrical signals from my heart, my skin will first be cleaned with alcohol and rubbed with an abrasive material. This may cause some minor discomfort to me. If I have hair on the upper body locations that require electrodes, this hair will be shaved off. I will then have wires placed on the electrodes, with the wires then being connected to a machine that records the electrical activity of my heart (electrocardiogram, or ECG). Various recordings from the ECG will be made while I am lying and in the position I exercise in, and my blood pressure will also be taken when I am in these positions.

After the previous pre-test procedures are complete, I will perform a graded exercise test (GXT). A GXT involves exercise for a period of time between 10 to 15 minutes, characterized by a progressive increase in intensity. The exercise I will perform could be on a treadmill, indoor cycle, or arm ergometer (similar to a cycle but using the arms) depending on my preference, functional limitations, or health requirements.

If I so desire, I may have expired air collected during the exercise for measurements and calculations that provide values for the rate of oxygen consumption and carbon dioxide production by my body. Such added procedures require that I have a mouthpiece in my mouth (similar to a snorkel mouthpiece) that is connected to tubing that goes to a computerized gas analysis system. To ensure that I only breathe through my mouth, a nose clip is placed on my nose. I understand that these additional items do not interfere with my abilities to breathe hard and at higher rates during exercise, although I might find them to be initially uncomfortable.

During the GXT I will experience increasing perceptions of fatigue in my muscles, and there may be increased difficulty in being able to breathe air into and from my lungs. These are normal responses to the demands of a GXT. I understand that the test will be terminated if I decide to stop, the ECG does not work properly, or if events that indicate there are increased risks to my health or life occur. However, the longer I exercise so that I reach true maximal exertion the better the test will be as an evaluation of my abilities to tolerate exercise, reflect the health of my cardiovascular system, and provide a sound assessment from which to prescribe exercise training guidelines.

Completion of a GXT is not without risk. Nevertheless, every effort is made to minimize these risks through adequate pre-test questions and evaluations, the use of appropriately trained and qualified personnel, and the presence of emergency equipment and procedures. For example, I could experience abnormally large increases in blood pressure which could damage blood vessels. I could also experience abnormal heart function that could lead to dizziness, chest pain, and even sudden death. However, the likelihood for these events is extremely rare (< 1 death in 10,000 tests for individuals who have or are at increased risk for heart disease), and the pre-test procedures and ECG evaluation during exercise aid in detecting events so that exercise can be stopped prior to events that can progress to more serious conditions.

To aid the technicians conducting the GXT, I understand that I should provide feedback to them about how I feel during the exercise, and I should answer their questions as honestly and accurately as possible.

I understand that my completion of these test procedures is voluntary. I am free to deny consent if I so desire. I may terminate the testing at any time without fear of consequence. I understand that any emergency medical care I need will be given to me. However, any emergency transportation and medical care costs will be incurred by myself through my own health insurance.

I hereby consent to participate in the procedures detailed above for the completion of a graded exercise test.

_____
Signature of Subject

_____
Signature of Witness

_____
Signature of Parent

_____
Signature of Test Supervisor

Date: _____

Once the patient arrives in the clinic, the patient should be made as comfortable as possible. Patients are often very anxious prior to a diagnostic exercise test. To help make the patient feel more relaxed, the exercise test technologist should:

Explain the purpose of the test and the various procedures they are to follow.

Explain each procedure before starting.

Ensure that the patient's privacy is protected at all times.

Explain what types and how often different measurements will be taken.

Explain the Borg RPE scale.

Informed Consent

Before a patient is allowed to exercise, he/she must sign an informed consent. An **informed consent** is used to "inform" the patient of the benefits and potential risks of the test. If a patient refuses to sign the informed consent form, the pretest procedures should be stopped and the physician notified.

Preparing Patient

After all the preliminary data have been collected, the informed consent has been signed, all the procedures have been obtained, and all the patient's questions have been answered, the exercise test technologist can start preparing the patient for the test. Obtain the patient's weight (kg) and height (cm). Disposable electrodes with gel-filled caps and a silver chloride element are recommended to decrease motion artifact and to improve the accuracy of the recording. The importance of skin preparation prior to electrode placement cannot be overemphasized. All the sophisticated computerized equipment in use today is of little value if a clear recording with minimal artifact is not maintained during the stress test. Good electrode contact is the key to a high-quality recording. Skin oils should be removed with alcohol or acetone at the sites of electrode placement. Male patients may have to have hair shaved off in the appropriate locations. This is followed by removal of a superficial layer of skin with light abrasion with a fine-grained emery paper or other abrasive pad. Dead skin cells act as an insulator, increasing the skin resistance. After placement, each electrode should be tapped with a finger to ensure that there is a minimum of "noise" on the recorder with this maneuver. A well-prepared electrode should display no artifacts.

The electrode sites should first be identified and marked with a felt pen.

If the subject has a great deal of hair, the hair should be dry shaved around the marked sites.

The electrode sites should then be scrubbed with alcohol and a gauze abrasive pad (3 × 3) until the skin is slightly red.

An abrasive device, such as an emery board or a small piece of fine sandpaper can also be used to remove superficial layers of skin.

The electrodes should be checked to make sure there is sufficient gel present.

Peel the protective cover off the electrode and place it on the desired location.

Press firmly around the edges of the electrode, paying careful attention not to press directly on the center of the electrode.

Electrode Sites for Exercise Testing

RA—right intraclavicular fossa

LA—left intraclavicular fossa

LL—anterolateral surface of the left external oblique muscle

RL—anterolateral surface of the right external oblique muscle

V_1—right of the sternal border in the 4th intercostal space

V_2—left of the sternal border in the 4th intercostal space

V_3—equally spaced between V_2 and V_4

V_4—along the midclavicular line in the 5th intercostal space

V_5—along the anterior axillary line in the 5th intercostal space

V_6—along the midaxillary line in the 5th intercostal space

Lead Systems

During electrocardiographic analysis of exercise, the use of multiple lead systems has been shown to be more sensitive than single lead systems in accurately detecting evidence of coronary artery disease (2). Optimal lead systems are those that include 12 leads. During exercise, because of significant limb movement, a 12-lead ECG cannot be obtained accurately if electrodes are placed on wrists and ankles during exercise. Mason and Likar developed a system with 12 leads where limb leads were placed at the base of the limbs on the torso, thereby avoiding placement of electrodes on exercising limbs (5). The Mason-Likar arrangement is the most commonly used electrode system in use today for exercise testing (see fig. 16.13).

Choosing the Test Protocol

There are a variety of graded exercise test protocols available to choose from. The exercise testing protocol should be individually selected on the basis of the clinical and functional status of the patient. All protocols should have a gradual warm-up period, and a progressive increase in workload. The

informed consent written explanation of the risks and benefits of an exercise test

FIGURE 16.13

The Mason-Likar system.

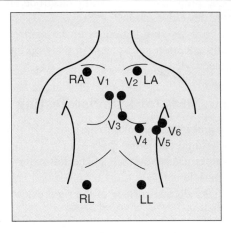

Bruce protocol is a popular protocol in clinical settings. Most deconditioned patients can complete only 1 to 3 stages of the Bruce protocol, and thus the test ends quickly. Cardiac patients and extremely deconditioned individuals request to stop because of musculoskeletal pain and fatigue because of the abrupt workload changes; thus the Bruce protocol is generally not recommended for these individuals. Other protocols such as the Naughton-Balke or the Modified Balke protocols are more appropriate for cardiac and extremely sedentary individuals. Bicycle exercise protocols can also be used in the clinical setting. Table 16.3 lists several common treadmill protocols.

Exercise Test Sequence

Pretest Sequence

After the patient has been hooked up to the ECG machine, a "standard" 12-lead ECG should be obtained while the patient is in the supine position. A standard 12-lead ECG is obtained by placing the limb leads on the inside of the wrists and the inside of the ankles. After the standard 12-lead ECG is obtained, the ECG limb lead cables are placed in the modified position. A 12-lead with the modified hook-up should then be obtained. All ECGs should be clearly marked (standard supine, or modified supine). A resting supine blood pressure should be recorded. Next, have the patient stand and record a standing ECG and blood pressure (on the arm to be used during the exercise test) (see focus box 16.3).

Test Sequence

After a detailed explanation of the testing procedures, the test is ready to start. A blood pressure recording should be obtained once every stage, or additionally when necessary. The ECG should be continually monitored at all times dur-

TABLE 16.3

Common treadmill protocols

BRUCE				
STAGE	DURATION	SPEED (MI/H)	GRADE (%)	METS
Rest/Recovery		1.2	0.0	
1	3:00	1.7	10.0	4.6
2	3:00	2.5	12.0	7.0
3	3:00	3.4	14.0	10.1
4	3:00	4.2	16.0	12.9
5	3:00	5.0	18.0	15.0
6	3:00	5.5	20.0	16.9
7	3:00	6.0	22.0	19.1

NAUGHTON-BALKE				
STAGE	DURATION	SPEED (MI/H)	GRADE (%)	METS
Rest/Recovery		1.2	0.0	
1	2:00	1.0	0.0	1.8
2	2:00	2.0	0.0	2.5
3	2:00	2.0	3.5	3.4
4	2:00	2.0	7.0	4.4
5	2:00	2.0	10.5	5.3
6	2:00	2.0	14.0	6.3
7	2:00	2.0	17.5	7.3

MODIFIED BALKE				
STAGE	DURATION	SPEED (MI/H)	GRADE (%)	METS
Rest/Recovery		1.2	0.0	
1	1:00	3.4	0.0	3.6
2	1:00	3.4	1.0	4.1
3	1:00	3.4	2.0	4.5
4	1:00	3.4	3.0	5.0
5	1:00	3.4	4.0	5.5
6	1:00	3.4	5.0	5.9
7	1:00	3.4	6.0	6.4
8	1:00	3.4	7.0	6.9
9	1:00	3.4	8.0	7.3
10	1:00	3.4	9.0	7.8
11	1:00	3.4	10.0	8.3
12	1:00	3.4	11.0	8.7
13	1:00	3.4	12.0	9.2
14	1:00	3.4	13.0	9.7
15	1:00	3.4	14.0	10.1
16	1:00	3.4	15.0	10.6
17	1:00	3.4	16.0	11.1
18	1:00	3.4	17.0	11.5
19	1:00	3.4	18.0	12.0
20	1:00	3.4	19.0	12.4
21	1:00	3.4	20.0	12.9
22	1:00	3.4	21.0	13.4
23	1:00	3.4	22.0	13.8
24	1:00	3.4	23.0	14.3
25	1:00	3.4	24.0	14.8
26	1:00	3.4	25.0	15.2

FOCUS BOX 16.3

How to Accurately Measure Blood Pressure

1. The subject should be seated in a comfortable position, with the right arm at approximately heart level. Note: the right arm is the universal arm used to measure resting blood pressure.
2. The subject should be rested, relaxed, and free of distractions.
3. A loose-fitting short-sleeve shirt or blouse should be worn. If a shirt sleeve needs to be rolled or pushed up to access the arm, that garment should be taken off.
4. The proper cuff size should be determined ahead of time. Proper cuff size can be determined by measuring arm circumference and then looking at the table below. Most blood pressure cuffs today have index lines marked on the cuff that tell you if the cuff is the proper size (index lines should fall in-between the two range lines). Note: If the blood pressure cuff is too small, blood pressure will be overestimated, and if the cuff is too big, blood pressure will be underestimated (see table 16.4).
5. The subject's arm should be rotated outward (anatomical position) and the arm straight. The cuff should be placed on the arm so that the lower lip of the cuff is approximately 1 in above the antecubital space (the crease in the arm at the elbow joint).
6. The brachial artery should be located by palpating for it. Once the brachial artery is located, the head (or diaphragm) of the stethoscope should be firmly placed over the brachial artery.
7. The cuff should be inflated to approximately 160 mm Hg or 20 to 30 mm Hg above the expected or known pressure.

8. With the manometer (blood pressure gauge) in good view, the air-release screw should be adjusted so that the cuff pressure is reduced by 2 to 5 mm Hg per second. Note: Low readings may occur if the rate is too fast, and slow deflation may cause erroneously high values.
9. Blood pressure is recorded as the first sound heard (systolic blood pressure) and the last sound heard or transition from clear to muffled sound (diastolic blood pressure).
10. The cuff should be completely deflated between measurements.
11. Resting blood pressure should be obtained in the supine, sitting, and standing positions. Any large differences between the supine and standing blood pressures should be reported to the client's physician. Some individuals have a condition called *orthostatic hypotension,* which may cause lightheadedness or fainting, especially during exercise.

TABLE 16.4

Guidelines for type of blood pressure cuff

Size (cm)	Type of Cuff	Bladder Size (cm) (Upper Arm Circumference)
33–47	Large adult	33 or 42 x 15
25–35	Adult	24 x 12.5
18–26	Child	21.5 x 10

ing the test, and recordings should be obtained every minute. An RPE reading should be obtained once each stage.

Recovery Sequence

Once the test has stopped, blood pressure and ECG recordings should continue for 4 to 6 min, or until the HR and BP are close to resting values. Some physicians like to have patients lie down immediately following the end of the test (stat-supine protocol). A stat-supine protocol may help in detecting ischemic ECG changes. Unless a stat-supine protocol is requested, the patient should continue to walk or cycle at a low intensity to cool down.

Test End Points

Either the patient or physician will decide when to stop the test. The patient may decide to stop because of pain, fatigue, or other symptoms, or the physician or the *exercise test technologist (ETT)* may choose to stop the test because of some abnormal findings, or a predetermined end point was

reached (patient reached 85% of the age-adjusted heart rate). Table 16.5 lists test termination end points.

Interpretation of Exercise Test Results
Normal Physiological Responses

Heart rate increases linearly with work.
Oxygen consumption increases.
Systolic blood pressure increases linearly with work.
Diastolic blood pressure stays the same, slightly increases, or decreases (within 10 mm Hg).
No significant ST changes.
No significant arrhythmias.

Abnormal Responses to Dynamic Exercise

The normal response to exercise is an increase in cardiac output and a decrease in total peripheral resistance. When the heart muscle is damaged (due to an infection or

TABLE 16.5

Indications for stopping an exercise test

Absolute

1. Acute MI or suspicion of one.

2. Progressive angina during the exercise test.

   On a scale of 1 to 4 with 1 being barely noticeable and 4 being the most severe pain ever experienced, a test should be stopped at a rating of 3 or greater.

3. Ventricular tachycardia (VT).

   VT is defined as three or more successive PVCs in a row. Sustained VT is a medical emergency.

4. Any significant drop (20 mm Hg) of systolic blood pressure or a failure of the systolic blood pressure to rise with an increase in exercise load.

5. Lightheadedness, confusion, a loss of muscular coordination, nausea, or change of skin color to a pale complexion.

6. Central nervous system symptoms (ataxia, vertigo, or visual problems).

7. Onset of second- or third-degree heart block.

8. Subject requests to stop.

9. Failure of the monitoring system.

10. Unusual or severe shortness of breath.

Relative

1. Pronounced ECG changes from baseline (> 2 mm of horizontal or downsloping ST-segment depression, or > 2 mm of ST-segment elevation (except in aVR)

2. Chest pain that increases during the test

3. Physical or verbal manifestations of severe fatigue or SOB

4. Wheezing

5. Leg cramps or intermittent claudication

6. Hypertension response (SBP > 260 or DBP > 115 mm Hg)

7. Arrhythmias such as supraventricular tachycardia

8. Exercise-induced left bundle branch block

Source: ACSM Guidelines Book.

myocardial infarction) the ability to respond to the increased demands of exercise may be reduced. The diseased heart has less reserve to respond to an increased demand, thus cardiac output and stroke volume may not increase in a normal fashion. Another sign of heart failure is a drop, or failure, of HR to increase during exercise. A drop in SBP, or a failure of SBP to rise, during incremental exercise is also a sign of a failing heart. ST-segment depression below the baseline is the classic ECG response to coronary insufficiency, or **myocardial ischemia.** Myocardial ischemia results from an imbalance between myocardial oxygen supply and demand. The cause of this imbalance is almost always the result of atherosclerotic plaques that narrow and sometimes completely block the blood supply to the heart.

FIGURE 16.14

Normal hemodynamic responses to exercise.

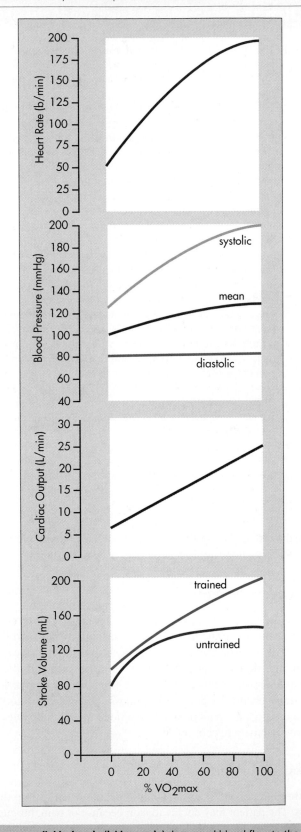

myocardial ischemia (is' ke–me 'a) decreased blood flow to the heart

FOCUS BOX 16.4

Interpreting Graded Exercise Test Summary Sheets

Below you will find an example of a typical summary sheet from a graded exercise test (GXT). Let's go through this summary sheet and identify some key points. An asterisk * *identifies a key point.*

1. You should be familiar with this term by now. The reason for the test is one of the most important items to consider when looking at these reports. Think about normal and abnormal responses for this person.
2. You need to know what effect these drugs have on the exercise test and your exercise prescription.
3. Nonspecific ST changes at rest means that the ST changes were not clinically significant.
4. The Bruce protocol is the most common GXT protocol.
5. Do you think just under 5 min is good for a 65-year-old male?
6. Normal BP and HR response.
7. This confirms a maximum effort for this individual.
8. Double product is maximum heart rate × maximum blood pressure. The double product is a good indication of overall myocardial oxygen demand.
9. It looks like this patient did not exercise to his predicted time for his age. What does this tell you (sedentary)?
10. This is a positive treadmill test (abnormal). This person may have serious CAD.

Sample Summary Sheet

DOB: 10/3/33
SEX: M
*(1) REASON FOR REFERRAL: Angina
*(2) CURRENT MEDICATIONS: Propranolol and Aspirin
*(3) BASELINE ECG: Nonspecific ST changes in inferior leads and V_6.
    RESTING HR: 86
    RESTING BP: 120/80
*(4) TESTING PROTOCOL: Bruce

STAGE	STAGE TIME	HR(B/MIN)	BP
Supine		84	120/80
Standing		109	
I	1:00	125	
	2:00	142	
	3:00	137	125/70
II	4:00	159	
	4:47	172	140/85
			termination
Recovery	1:00	123	
	2:00	91	130/85
	3:00	104	
	4:00	103	120/80
	5:00	100	114/80
	6:00	93	

TREADMILL RESULTS:
* (5) TOTAL EXERCISE TIME: 4:45 min. TOTAL METS: 6.7
* (6) MAX HR: 182   MAX BP: 140/85
* (7) MAX HR ACHIEVED/
     MAX HR PREDICTED: 101%
     PREDICTED MAX HR/
     TARGET HR: 180/153
* (8) DOUBLE PRODUCT:
     23.6 (thousands)
* (9) PREDICTED AGE/
     SEX EXERCISE DURATION
     (minutes): 8.5

MET = Metabolic Equivalent = 3.5 mL O_2/kg/min
PHYSIOLOGICAL RESPONSE TO EXERCISE:
Normal heart rate and blood pressure response.
TEST STOPPED FOR:
* (10) ST depression > 2 mm
ARRHYTHMIAS:
None
ST-SEGMENT RESPONSE:
    RESTING ECG: Nonspecific ST change(s). ST changes in inferior leads and V_6.
    EXERCISE ECG: Horizontal ST depression 2 to 3 mm in inferior leads and V_3 to V_6. ST elevation 2 mm AVR. ST segment returns to baseline in recovery within 1 to 5 min.
IMPRESSION:
    TMT:
    Positive for ischemia.
    Specificity reduced because of resting ECG changes.
OTHER COMMENTS:
A stress echo was performed as well and found hypokineses of a small inferior segment during exercise, with normal increases in ejection fraction during exercise. Resting ejection fraction was in the 50s and postexercise in the 60s.
POSTTEST LIKELIHOOD OF CAD: 98.2%
ESTIMATED 5-YEAR SURVIVAL RATE: 80%
Overall Summary:
This was a positive treadmill test. This person more than likely would not be cleared to exercise until the source of the ischemia (ST-segment depression) was determined.

Normal Electrocardiographic Responses to Dynamic Exercise

During dynamic exercise in the healthy, normal, or nondiseased heart, the following electrocardiographic responses are considered normal during exercise.

P wave—increases in amplitude above resting level

PR interval—becomes shorter

QT interval—becomes shorter

J point—depression below the baseline

ST segment—depression of the early part of the segment, turning into upsloping ST segment

T wave—amplitude decreases above resting level

R wave—amplitude decreases above resting level

Q wave—increases in amplitude above resting level

Axis—may shift to the right

Arrhythmias—ectopic beats are common, especially at peak exercise

Predictive Value of Clinical Exercise Testing

The **predictive value** of exercise testing is a measure of how accurately an exercise test correctly identifies an individual with coronary artery disease (positive test), or without coronary artery disease (negative test). Establishing the predictive value of exercise testing is based on Bayes's theorem, which is a mathematical rule relating the interpretation of present observations in light of past experience. The **Bayes's theorem** helps increase the accuracy of predicting coronary artery disease *(pretest probability)* before the test is performed and the probability of disease after the test *(posttest probability)*. The accuracy of diagnosing coronary artery disease based on ischemic ST changes during treadmill testing comes from studies that compared exercise electrocardiography data with coronary angiography findings, because coronary artery angiography is the gold standard of detecting the extent and severity of coronary artery disease.

With Bayes's theorem it is easy to understand that the ability of a given test result to predict the presence or absence of disease is related to the presence of disease in that population of subjects being tested. For example, a teenage female with a positive ST-segment depression during a stress test has a low posttest likelihood of coronary disease compared to a 65-year-old male with typical chest pain and multiple risk factors who would have a very high posttest likelihood of coronary artery disease. This is due to the significant difference in the pretest likelihood of disease in these two

different populations, in spite of similar ST-segment displacement during exercise.

Sensitivity

The predictive accuracy of exercise testing is determined by the sensitivity and specificity of the test and the prevalence of coronary artery disease in the population tested. **Sensitivity** refers to the percentage of individuals being tested who will have an abnormal test. The sensitivity of clinical exercise testing varies from 50 to 90%, or approximately 71%. The sensitivity of exercise testing can be enhanced (increase in the likelihood of a true positive test) by (1) administering a true maximal exercise test, (2) using multiple-lead ECG monitoring, and (3) monitoring additional data, such as abnormal blood pressure responses. It can also be decreased (increase in the likelihood of a false negative test) by (1) administering a submaximal exercise test, (2) insufficient ECG monitoring, and (3) certain cardiac drugs (beta blockers and nitrates).

Specificity

Specificity refers to the percentage of individuals being tested who will have a normal exercise stress test. Thus a true negative stress test correctly identifies a person without coronary artery disease. Specificity of exercise stress testing varies from 60 to 98%, or approximately 73%. The specificity of exercise testing is reduced (increase in the likelihood of a false-positive test) by (1) preexisting abnormal resting ECG abnormalities, (2) hypertrophy of the left ventricle, (3) certain medications (e.g., digitalis), (4) mitral valve prolapse, and (5) anemia.

---

predictive value measure of how accurately an exercise test correctly identifies an individual with coronary artery disease (positive test), or without it (negative test)

Bayes's theorem mathematical theorem used to increase the accuracy of predicting coronary artery disease by comparing the pretest probability before a test is performed and the probability of disease after the test

sensitivity the percentage of individuals being tested who will have an abnormal test; the sensitivity of clinical exercise testing varies from 50 to 90%

specificity the percentage of individuals being tested who will have a normal exercise test; specificity varies from 60 to 90%

cardiac catheterization an invasive procedure where a catheter is advanced to the heart via the femoral artery; performed to evaluate the heart's overall function and to determine the presence and severity of blockages

FOCUS BOX 16.5

Other Diagnostic Cardiovascular Testing Procedures

Echocardiography

An echocardiogram is a safe and painless diagnostic procedure that uses high-frequency sound waves (ultrasound) to take dynamic pictures of the heart. Sound waves emitted from a transducer penetrate the patient's chest wall so that various cardiac structures can be observed. From the echocardiogram recordings, it is possible to measure the size of the chambers of the heart, how well the heart valves are working, and how forceful the heart muscle is contracting. Doppler echocardiography is another form of echocardiography that uses sound waves to measure the speed, amount, and direction of blood flow. With Doppler echocardiography, accurate measurements of cardiac output and stroke volume can be obtained.

Thallium-201 Stress Testing

The thallium-201 stress test is a diagnostic exam used to evaluate the adequacy of blood supply to the heart. Prior to the start of an exercise test, an intravenous (IV) line is inserted into the patient's arm. At peak exercise, thallium-201 radioisotope is injected into the IV line. The radioisotope is then carried to the heart via the blood. Immediately after the patient stops exercise, a special camera that can detect radiation visualizes the thallium-201 as it flows to the heart. If the coronary arteries are clear, thallium-201 is absorbed evenly throughout the myocardium within a matter of minutes. The first set of pictures taken immediately following exercise determines the adequacy of blood supply to the heart during stress. If the coronary arteries are normal, the myocardium will receive approximately the same amount of radioactive isotope and the pictures taken will have a uniform appearance. If one or more of the coronary arteries is blocked, then a portion of the myocardium will not receive the isotope and the pictures will show a spot of nonabsorption, sometimes referred to as a "cold spot". After a period of time, the iso-

tope eventually gets absorbed into the tissue, and the cold spot disappears. The second set of pictures taken several hours later after exercise, helps differentiate between exercise-induced ischemia and an area of nonabsorbing tissue (usually resulting from a heart attack). Old heart attacks will leave a scar on the heart muscle, and these scars or injuries will not absorb the isotope at all. If the cold spot was caused by exercise-induced ischemia (temporarily reduced isotope absorption), the second set of pictures will be normal. If the cold spot was caused by scar tissue, then the second set of pictures will be abnormal as well. The location of the absorption defects can be used to predict which coronary artery is blocked.

Cardiac Catheterization

Cardiac catheterization is an invasive procedure, meaning that the body is entered in some way. Cardiac catheterization is the most accurate method of measuring a patient's heart performance and is the only way to determine which coronary arteries are blocked, and to what degree. The entire procedure lasts less than an hour. During the procedure, a narrow, flexible tube (catheter) is inserted through the brachial or femoral artery. After the catheter has been inserted into the artery, it is slowly advanced toward the heart while the physician watches its progress on a television screen. During a *left ventricular angiogram* the catheter is advanced into the left ventricle. Dye is then injected and a series of pictures is obtained during contraction. During a *coronary angiogram* a catheter is inserted into the opening of the left and then the right main coronary artery. Dye is injected through the catheter into each coronary artery, and an x-ray camera takes a series of pictures of the coronary arteries. These pictures will detect areas of narrowing (blockages) and assess their severity.

Predictive Value

The *predictive value* of exercise stress testing is a measure of how accurately the results from an exercise stress test identifies the presence or absence of coronary artery disease in individuals being tested (positive test = disease; negative test = no disease). When an individual comes to a physician's office to have an exercise stress test and has the factors and symptoms discussed earlier, the pretest likelihood of disease is high (predictive value for a positive test is high). On the other hand, if a young, active, healthy individ-

ual with maybe only one or two CAD risk factors has an exercise stress test, the pretest likelihood of disease is low (predictive value for a positive test is low). In addition to ECG recordings, the predictive value of exercise stress testing is enhanced by recording additional data such as the total exercise time; maximal MET level obtained; blood pressure responses before, during, and following exercise; and symptoms of angina or shortness of breath.

Focus box 16.5 describes other diagnostic cardiovascular testing procedures.

WEBSITE BOX

Chapter 16: Clinical Exercise Testing

The newest information regarding exercise physiology can be viewed at the following sites.*

cardiology.org
Diverse information on clinical exercise physiology, including several slide shows.

amhrt.org/
Homepage of the American Heart Association, providing information on all matters of the prevention, diagnosis, and rehabilitation from cardiovascular diseases.

alexian.org/heartcare/heartx.html
Explanation of how exercise influences heart function and should be used by individuals with documented heart disease.

mediconsult.com/
Information source for any medical condition, including exercise and health.

http://software2.bu.edu/cohis/cardvasc/risks/
Provides links to detailed explanations of the risk factors for heart disease. Provides good educational content, at a basic level, on exercise and the heart.

arfa.org/index.htm
Excellent site providing comprehensive information on many topics within exercise physiology.

curtin.edu.au/curtin/dept/physio/pt/edres/exphys/e552_96/
Index of brief reviews of exercise physiology by students from Curtin University, Australia. Topics include nutrition, ergogenic aids, environmental physiology, training, and clinical applications.

---

*Unless indicated, all URLs preceded by http://www.

Note: These URLs were valid at the time of publication, but could have changed or been deleted from Internet access since that time.

SUMMARY

▪ This chapter introduces the student to the fundamental principles of clinical exercise testing. The term "clinical" implies that the exercise test is "medically" oriented. The exercise test is probably the best test of the heart because it is the most common everyday stress that humans undertake.

▪ The most common reasons for ordering a clinical exercise test is for **diagnostic testing** and for evaluating the status of suspected or known cardiovascular disease.

▪ Clinical exercise testing is also commonly used to determine the **functional capacity** of healthy, sedentary, and/or asymptomatic individuals.

▪ A variety of benefits can be derived from exercise testing; however, the procedure is not without risks. Ideally, the benefits of the test, and the subsequent results obtained, should outweigh the potential risks of performing the test.

▪ The ECG is a recording of the electrical activity of the heart, whereas the mechanical activity of the heart is assessed by echocardiography.

▪ There are five key waves and intervals that make up the ECG. Each wave or interval represents a particular function of the heart. A wave represents depolarization or repolarization, whereas an interval represents time during which the electrical signal is traveling away from the SA node.

▪ The standard 12-lead **electrocardiogram** is composed of three limb leads—I, II, III; three augmented limb leads—aV_R, aV_L, aV_F; and six chest leads—V_{1-6}.

▪ The basic rule in ECG interpretation is to use the same approach or system every time you evaluate an ECG. There are three key steps to follow when evaluating any

ECG. These steps include determining the rate, rhythm, and axis.

▪ Any variation from the normal rhythm and normal electrical conduction pattern of the heart is referred to as an **arrhythmia**.

▪ ST depression on the ECG is the hallmark of myocardial ischemia. **ST-segment depression** is the principal abnormality during exercise that should concern individuals supervising a treadmill test.

▪ When the delivery of blood supply to the heart muscle is compromised for an extended period of time because of a spasm or or blood clot, the inner lining of the heart (*subendocardial*) or the entire thickness of the heart (*transmural*) can be affected.

▪ The majority of **myocardial infarctions** (> 87%) result from a portion of plaque in the coronary arteries breaking loose and lodging at a site of narrowing further down the artery forming a clot. The affected muscle tissue is no longer able to contract.

▪ Before a patient is allowed to exercise, he or she must sign an informed consent. An **informed consent** is used to "inform" the patient of the benefits and potential risks of the test.

▪ The Mason-Likar arrangement is the most commonly used electrode system in use today for exercise testing.

▪ Standing and hyperventilation can change the configuration of the baseline ECG. Axis shifts, Q-wave formation, and ST- and T-wave changes may occur as a result of these maneuvers.

■ There are a variety of graded exercise test protocols available to choose from. The exercise testing protocol should be individually selected on the basis of the clinical and functional status of the patient.

■ **Myocardial ischemia** results from an imbalance between myocardial oxygen supply and demand. The cause of this imbalance is almost always the result of atherosclerotic plaques that narrow and sometimes completely block the blood supply to the heart.

■ The **predictive value** of exercise stress testing is a measure of how accurately the results from an exercise stress test correctly identifies the presence or absence of coronary artery disease in individuals being tested (*positive test* = disease; *negative test* = no disease). The **Bayes's theorem** helps increase the accuracy of predicting coronary artery disease (*pretest probability*) before the test is performed to the probability of disease after the test (*posttest probability*).

■ An echocardiogram is a safe and painless diagnostic procedure which uses high-frequency sound waves (ultrasound) to take dynamic pictures of the heart. The thallium-201 stress test is a diagnostic exam used to evaluate the adequacy of blood supply to the heart.

■ **Sensitivity** refers to the percentage of individuals being tested who will have an abnormal test. The sensitivity of clinical exercise testing varies from 50 to 90%, or approximately 71%.

■ **Specificity** refers to the percentage of individuals being tested who will have a normal exercise stress test. Thus a true negative stress test correctly identifies a person without coronary artery disease. Specificity of exercise stress testing varies from 60 to 98%, or approximately 73%.

■ **Cardiac catheterization** is the most accurate method of measuring a patient's heart performance and is the only way to determine which coronary arteries are blocked, and to what degree.

■ The primary responsibility of the exercise test technologist is to administer exercise tests safely to individuals in various states of illness and health in order to obtain reliable and valid data.

STUDY QUESTIONS

1. List five indications and contraindications to clinical exercise testing.

2. Describe the difference between a diagnostic and a functional capacity exercise test.

3. Explain the importance of safety, as it applies to testing someone who is apparently healthy and someone who is at high risk.

4. Discuss how the heart receives its blood supply.

5. What is the clinical significance of ST-segment depression?

6. Explain what happens during a myocardial infarction.

7. What information has to be obtained before an exercise test is performed?

8. List the correct anatomical locations for electrode placement during exercise testing.

9. What are some normal and abnormal hemodynamic and ECG responses to exercise testing?

10. Define sensitivity, specificity, and predictive value.

APPLICATIONS

1. Call a local hospital or physician's office and make an appointment to observe a clinical exercise test. Before the test begins or after it is completed, ask the physician or the exercise test technologist the following questions. Note: Please be sensitive to the ETT and/or physician's time spent with you. Make sure you stress how interested you are in learning more about this field. If you show interest in their professions, they will generally be willing to spend time with you.

   a. What was the reason(s) for the test?

   b. What protocol was used?

   c. What medications was the patient taking and what effects might the medications have on the results of the test?

   d. Was there anything unusual about the resting patient data?

   e. What was the patient's physiological response to the exercise?

   f. Were the heart rate and blood pressure responses appropriate?

   g. Why was the test stopped? Were there any arrhythmias?

APPLICATIONS

   h. Did the ST segment change during or after the test?

   i. What were the physician's impressions?

2. Review the ECGs in this chapter, and try to determine the following:

   a. What the heart rate is.

   b. Whether the rhythm is normal or abnormal.

   c. The quadrant the axis falls into, and the specific degree of axis.

   d. Whether any ST-segment depression is present.

RECOMMENDED READINGS

Kenney, W. L. *American college of sports medicine guidelines for exercise testing and prescription,* 5th ed. Williams & Wilkins, Philadephia, 1995.

American College of Sports Medicine. *Resource manual for guidelines for exercise testing and prescription,* 3rd ed. Williams & Wilkins, Philadelphia, 1998.

Roberts, S. O., R. A. Robergs, and P. Hanson. *Clinical exercise testing and prescription: Theory and application.* CRC Press, Boca Raton, FL, 1997.

Durstine, J. L., et al. (eds). *ACSM's exercise management for persons with chronic diseases and disabilities.* Human Kinetics, Champaign, IL, 1997.

Conover, M. B. *Understanding electrocardiography: Arrhythmias and the 12-lead ECG.* Mosby-Year Book, St. Louis, 1992.

Froelicher, V. F. *Manual of exercise testing,* 2nd ed. Mosby-Year Book, St. Louis, 1994.

REFERENCES

1. Allen, W. H., et al. Five-year follow-up of maximal treadmill stress test in asymptomatic men and women. *Circulation* 62:522–531, 1980.

2. Chung, E. K. *Principles of cardiac arrythmias,* Williams & Wilkins, Baltimore, 1989.

3. Cumming, G. R., et al. Electrocardiographic changes during exercise in asymptomatic men: 3-year follow-up. *Can. Med. Assoc. J.* 112:578–595, 1975.

4. Froelicher, V. F., et al. An epidemiological study of asymptomatic men screened with exercise testing for latent coronary heart disease. *Am. J. Cardiol.* 34:770–779. 1975.

5. Mason, R. E., and I. Likar. A new system of multiple-lead exercise electrocardiography. *Am Heart J.* 71:196–205, 1966.

6. Rochmis, P., and H. Blackburn. Exercise tests: A survey of procedures, safety, and litigation experience in approximately 170,000 tests. *J. Am. Med. Assoc.* 217:1061–1070, 1971.

7. Thompson, P. D. The safety of exercise testing and participation. In S. N. Blair, P. Painter, R. R. Pate, L. K. Smith, and C. B. Taylor (eds.), *American College of Sports Medicine: Resource manual for guidelines for exercise testing and prescription.* Lea & Febiger, Philadephia, p. 361, 1993.

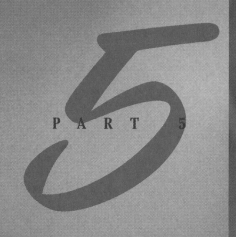

PART 5

oxygen

$Q = SV \times HR$

$HRmax = 220 - age$

RQ

fatigue   RER

stress

mmHg

VO_2max

Special Topics

CHAPTER 17

Growth, Development, and Exercise

t has been said many times, and in many ways, that the children of today are the future of tomorrow. It is because of the general acceptance of this fact that our society strives to be more environmentally friendly, conservation conscious, and focused to prevent war and self-destruction. Our society does these things to provide a functional and "healthy" planet for tomorrow's children. However, what are we doing to provide a functional and "healthy" human being for tomorrow's earth? There is an underlying disease that is currently reducing the quality of life of today's children and tomorrow's adults: physical inactivity. Just as physical inactivity is devastating to the life span and quality of adult life, a lack of regular exercise and physical activity by today's youth merely exacerbates the disease incidence and severity of tomorrow's adults. A vicious cycle has developed, reinforcing the negative health consequences of physical inactivity in today's society. It seems that now, more than ever before, there is a need to promote lifestyle patterns in children that can track into adulthood. This need has further emphasized the importance of studying how children respond to exercise in order to identify any special needs or concerns that exist for children. The purpose of this chapter is to explain the consequences of childhood physical inactivity and how children of different ages respond acutely and chronically to exercise and training, and to identify areas of concern regarding children's participation in specific exercise conditions.

OBJECTIVES

After studying this chapter, you should be able to:

- Describe the present status of childhood fitness and physical activity in many countries of the world.
- List the immediate benefits of an active lifestyle in children, and discuss whether these benefits are more likely to be retained through adulthood.
- Identify and explain the unique ways children and youth respond and adapt to exercise when compared to adults.
- Describe the normal growth and development of children, and how exercise affects growth and development.

KEY TERMS

criterion-referenced fitness standards

puberty

pubertal growth spurt

peak height velocity (PHV)

maturation

Exercise and Children

For the most part, children respond to exercise in very much the same way as adults. Usually with little encouragement, most children in good health are willing to be physically active. National attention continues to focus on the health and fitness of American children, which has sparked a great deal of debate over topics such as (1) how much exercise should children and adolescents be getting, and at what age; (2) who is responsible for making sure children get enough exercise; and (3) what kind of exercise is important, and at what age? Many of these issues have yet to be resolved. Except for the alarming increase in childhood obesity, children are healthier today than ever before. (see focus box 17.1)

Health and Fitness of Children

Several large youth fitness surveys have been conducted, and the results provide much of the evidence that is used to judge the past and current health and fitness status of American children and youth. The first youth fitness tests focused on "skill-related" fitness, whereas more recent surveys have focused on "health-related" fitness. Test items such as the softball throw, long jump, and 50-yd dash have been deleted and replaced with test items such as body composition, flexibility, muscular strength, and endurance (table 17.1). The initiative to change youth fitness tests to include more health-related variables has been based on the available literature linking improved cardiovascular fitness, muscle strength, flexibility, and body composition to reduced disease and disability.

Beginning in the late 1950s and early 1960s several organizations began surveying youth fitness in the United States. In 1957 AAHPER developed a youth fitness test and established national fitness norms (3). Since the first AAHPER test, numerous other organizations, including AAHPER, have conducted youth fitness tests (1, 4, 17, 28, 53, 54). How best to interpret the results of these tests

---

FOCUS BOX 17.1

Summary of the Surgeon General's Report on Exercise

Adolescents and young adults, both male and female, benefit from physical activity. Physical activity need not be strenuous to be beneficial. Moderate amounts of daily physical activity are recommended for people of all ages. This amount can be obtained in longer sessions of moderate activities, such as brisk walking for 30 min, or in shorter sessions of more intense activities, such as jogging or playing basketball for 15 to 20 min. Greater amounts of physical activity are even more beneficial, up to a point. Excessive amounts of physical activity can lead to injuries, menstrual abnormalities, and bone weakening.

Facts

Nearly half of American youths aged 12 to 21 years are not vigorously active on a regular basis.

- About 14% of young people report no recent physical activity. Inactivity is more common among females (14%) than males (7%) and among black females (21%) than white females (12%).
- Participation in all types of physical activity declines strikingly as age or grade in school increases.
- Only 19% of all high school students are physically active for 20 min or more, 5 days a week, in physical education classes.
- Daily enrollment in physical education classes dropped from 42 to 25% among high school students between 1991 and 1995.
- Well-designed school-based interventions directed at increasing physical activity in physical education classes have been shown to be effective.
- Social support from family and friends has been consistently and positively related to regular physical activity.

Benefits of Physical Activity

- Helps build and maintain healthy bones, muscles, and joints.
- Helps control weight, build lean muscle, and reduce fat.
- Prevents or delays the development of high blood pressure and helps reduce blood pressure in some adolescents with hypertension.

What Communities Can Do

- Provide quality, preferably daily, K–12 physical education classes and hire physical education specialists to teach the children.
- Create opportunities for physical activities that are enjoyable, that promote adolescents' and young adults' confidence in their ability to be physically active, and that involve friends, peers, and parents.
- Provide appropriate physically active role models for youths.
- Provide access to school buildings and community facilities that enable safe participation in physical activity.
- Provide a range of extracurricular programs in schools and community recreation centers to meet the needs and interests of specific adolescent and young adult populations, such as racial and ethnic minority groups, females, persons with disabilities, and low-income groups.
- Encourage health care providers to talk routinely to adolescents and young adults about the importance of incorporating physical activity into their lives.

FOCUS BOX 17.2

Body Composition Skinfold Equations for Children

Males

FFB, kg = 0.87(wt,kg) − 0.36(triceps) −
0.40(subscapular) + 3.7

SEE = 1.8 kg

A male with a 7-mm tricep score and a 6-mm subscapular score and a body weight of 28 kg would have an estimated body fat of 17.2%.

Females

FFB, kg = 0.65(wt,kg) − 0.17(triceps) −
0.19(subscapular) + 6.8

SEE = 2.0 kg

A female weighing 28 kg with a 10-mm tricep score and a 6-mm subscapular score would be 20.9 % body fat.

Note: FFB 5 fat free body mass   SEE 5 standard errors of estimate

TABLE 17.1

Description of different youth fitness tests (1958 through 1988)

FITNESS COMPONENT	AAHPER YOUTH FITNESS TEST (1958)	AAHPER YOUTH FITNESS TEST (1965)	AAHPER YOUTH FITNESS TEST (1975)	AAHPERD HEALTH-RELATED PHYSICAL FITNESS TEST (1980)	AAHPERD PHYSICAL BEST (1988)
Cardiorespiratory endurance	600-yd (550-m) walk/run	600-yd (550-m) walk/run	600-yd (550-m) walk/run Options: 1-mile (1.6-km) or 9-min run (ages 10–12); 1.5-mile (2.4-km) or 12-min run (ages > 13)	1-mile (1.6-km) or 9-min run Option: 1.5-mile (2.4-km) or 12-min run	1-mile (1.6-k) run/walk
Body composition	None	None	None	Sum of skinfolds (triceps and subscapular)	Sum of skinfolds (triceps and calf) Options: Sum of triceps and subscapular Triceps only Body mass index
Flexibility	None	None	None	Sit-and-reach	Sit-and-reach
Muscular strength and endurance; abdominal	Sit-ups (straight leg, hands behind head; elbow touches opposite knee; maximum number)	Sit-ups (same as 1958)	Sit-ups (bent knee; arms across chest; number in 1 min)	Sit-ups (arms across chest; curl up to sitting position; elbows touch thighs; number in 1 min)	Situps (same as 1980)
Upper body	Pull-ups	Pull-ups (boys) Flexed arm hang (girls)	Pull-ups (boys) Flexed arm hang (girls)	None	Pull-ups
Anaerobic power	Standing long jump	Standing long jump	Standing long jump	None	None
Speed	50-yd (45.9-m) dash	50-yd (45.9-m) dash	50-yd (45.9-m) dash	None	None
Agility	Shuttle run	Shuttle run	Shuttle run	None	None
Motor skill	Softball throw for distance	Softball throw	None	None	None

continues to be a highly debatable topic among physical educators and exercise physiologists.

Many fitness experts believe the use of criterion-referenced fitness standards that are based on established fitness and health relationships are the most appropriate model to use. **Criterion-referenced fitness standards** set a minimal level score for selected variables that meet acceptable standards for good health (18). Criterion-referenced standards for children have been developed by the Institute for Aerobic Research (38) (table 17.2). On the basis of criterion-referenced

TABLE 17.2

The Prudential FITNESSGRAM: Standards for healthy fitness zone*

GIRLS

AGE	1-MILE (min:s)		PACER (# LAPS)		VO2MAX (mL/kg/min)		% FAT		BODY MASS INDEX		CURL-UP (# COMPLETED)	
5	Completion of distance. Time standards not recommended.		Participate in run Lap count standards not recommended.				32	17	21	16.2	2	10
6							32	17	21	16.2	2	10
7							32	17	22	16.2	4	14
8							32	17	22	16.2	6	20
9							32	17	23	16.2	9	22
10	12:30	9:30	7	35	39	47	32	17	23.5	16.6	12	26
11	12:00	9:00	9	37	38	46	32	17	24	16.9	15	29
12	12:00	9:00	13	40	37	45	32	17	24.5	16.9	18	32
13	11:30	9:00	15	42	36	44	32	17	24.5	17.5	18	32
14	11:00	8:30	18	44	35	43	32	17	25	17.5	18	32
15	10:30	8:00	23	50	35	43	32	17	25	17.5	18	35
16	10:00	8:00	28	56	35	43	32	17	25	17.5	18	35
17	10:00	8:00	34	61	35	43	32	17	26	17.5	18	35
17+	10:00	8:00	34	61	35	43	32	17	27.3	18.0	18	35

AGE	TRUNK LIFT (in)		PUSH-UP (# COMPLETED)		MODIFIED PULL-UP (# COMPLETED)		PULL-UP (# COMPLETED)		FLEXED ARM HANG (s)		BACK SAVER AND SIT AND REACH† (in)	SHOULDER STRETCH
5	6	12	3	8	2	7	1	2	2	8	9	
6	6	12	3	8	2	7	1	2	2	8	9	
7	6	12	4	10	3	9	1	2	3	8	9	
8	6	12	5	13	4	11	1	2	3	10	9	
9	6	12	6	15	4	11	1	2	4	10	9	
10	9	12	7	15	4	13	1	2	4	10	9	Passing = touching the fingertips together behind the back.
11	9	12	7	15	4	13	1	2	6	12	10	
12	9	12	7	15	4	13	1	2	7	12	10	
13	9	12	7	15	4	13	1	2	8	12	10	
14	9	12	7	15	4	13	1	2	8	12	10	
15	9	12	7	15	4	13	1	2	8	12	12	
16	9	12	7	15	4	13	1	2	8	12	12	
17	9	12	7	15	4	13	1	2	8	12	12	
17+	9	12	7	15	4	13	1	2	8	12	12	

*Number on left is lower end of HFZ; number on right is upper end of HFZ.

†Test scored pass/fail; must reach this distance to pass.

fitness standards, U.S. children appear to be reasonably fit (table 17.3). The only area where children appear to have below-average fitness level is in upper-body strength.

Body Fat

The only secular trends in youth fitness that have been analyzed with a high degree of accuracy is skinfold data (see focus box 17.2). Skinfold data collected in the 1960s to the 1970s have been compared to data collected in the National Children and Youth Fitness Survey II (55) (fig. 17.1). There appears to be a systematic increase in skinfold thickness among 6- to 9-year-old boys and girls from the 1960s and 1970s to the 1980s. Gortmaker and colleagues (22) investigated the prevalence of obesity in children ages 6 to 17 using skinfold data obtained in the National Health Examination Survey (NHES) (1963–1970) and the National Health and Nutrition Examination Survey (1971–1974 and 1976–1980). Obesity was defined as being above the 85th percentile for

criterion-referenced fitness standards fitness standards that are based on an established fitness and health relationship

TABLE 17.3

The Prudential FITNESSGRAM: Standards for healthy fitness zone[*]

			BOYS			
AGE	1-MILE (min:s)	PACER (# LAPS)	VO$_2$MAX (mL/kg/min)	% FAT	BODY MASS INDEX	CURL-UP (# COMPLETED)
5	Completion of distance. Time standards not recommended.	Participate in run. Lap count standards not recommended.		25 10	20 14.7	2 10
6				25 10	20 14.7	2 10
7				25 10	20 14.9	4 14
8				25 10	20 15.1	6 20
9				25 10	20 15.2	9 24
10	11:30 9:00	17 55	42 52	25 10	21 15.3	12 24
11	11:00 8:30	23 61	42 52	25 10	21 15.8	15 28
12	10:30 8:00	29 68	42 52	25 10	22 16.0	18 36
13	10:00 7:30	35 74	42 52	25 10	23 16.6	21 40
14	9:30 7:00	41 80	42 52	25 10	24.5 17.5	24 45
15	9:00 7:00	46 85	42 52	25 10	25 18.1	24 47
16	8:30 7:00	52 90	42 52	25 10	26.5 18.5	24 47
17	8:30 7:00	57 94	42 52	25 10	27 18.8	24 47
17+	8:30 7:00	57 94	42 52	25 10	27.8 19.0	24 47

AGE	TRUNK LIFT (in)	PUSH-UP (# COMPLETED)	MODIFIED PULL-UP (# COMPLETED)	PULL-UP (# COMPLETED)	FLEXED ARM HANG (s)	BACK SAVER AND SIT AND REACH[†] (in)	SHOULDER STRETCH
5	6 12	3 8	2 7	1 2	2 8	8	
6	6 12	3 8	2 7	1 2	2 8	8	
7	6 12	4 10	3 9	1 2	3 8	8	
8	6 12	5 13	4 11	1 2	3 10	8	Passing = touching the fingertips together behind the back.
9	6 12	6 15	5 11	1 2	4 10	8	
10	9 12	7 20	5 15	1 2	4 10	8	
11	9 12	8 20	6 17	1 3	6 13	8	
12	9 12	10 20	7 20	1 3	10 15	8	
13	9 12	12 25	8 22	1 4	12 17	8	
14	9 12	14 30	9 25	2 5	15 20	8	
15	9 12	16 35	10 27	3 7	15 20	8	
16	9 12	18 35	12 30	5 8	15 20	8	
17	9 12	18 35	14 30	5 8	15 20	8	
17+	9 12	18 35	14 30	5 8	15 20	8	

[*]Number on left is lower end of HFZ; number on right is upper end of HFZ.

[†]Test scored pass/fail; must reach this distance to pass.

triceps skinfolds. Gortmaker and colleagues estimated that obesity had increased from 17.6% in the 6 to 11 age group between 1963 and 1965 and 27.1% between 1976 and 1980. Lohman and colleagues (32) compared NHES skinfold data from the 1960s with the National Children Youth Fitness Study (NCYFS) skinfold data from the mid-1980s. Lohman's analysis revealed that obesity has increased during this time period when using 25% body fat for males and 32% body fat for females as the criterion. The cause of the increase in body fat over the years has been related to decreased habitual physical activity (22, 43, 44) and increased television viewing (52).

Strength

Another particularly alarming statistic is the poor levels of strength in American children, particularly upper-body strength (59). Field tests for upper-body strength included pull-up for boys, and flexed arm hang for girls. Although upper-body strength for both boys and girls has long been a fitness concern, the validity of such field tests as the pull-up and flexed arm hang have never been well validated. Furthermore, the relationship between muscular strength and endurance field tests and poor health has not been clearly established in children.

FIGURE 17.1

Comparison of the sum of median triceps and subscapular skinfold measurements taken during the 1960s, compared to data collected in the National Children and Youth Fitness Survey II of the 1980s.

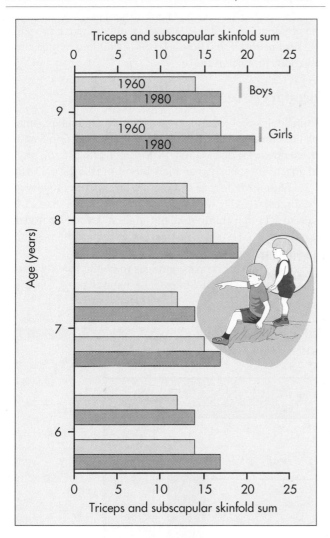

17 could not perform one pull-up. The mean number of pull-ups for boys did not exceed 10 for any age group, 6 to 17.

In 1986, part II of the NCYFS study (54), upper-body strength was tested in 4678 children from ages 6 to 9 using a modified pull-up test (fig. 17.2). The rationale for the use of the modified pull-up test was that the traditional pull-up or flexed arm hang test has traditionally provided poor measurement sensitivity for the range of children tested (44). The median score for girls ranged from 6 to 9, and for the boys 6 to 10. Although there was an improvement in upper-body strength compared to part I of the study, NCYFS II was the first large-scale test to use the modified pull-up and further studies are needed to validate the results of NCYFS II.

Recently Pate and colleagues (47) determined the concurrent and constructive validity of three common field tests of upper-body muscular strength/endurance in children aged 9 to 10. The field tests included the pull-up, flexed arm hang, and the push-up. In addition, two modified pull-up tests were examined, the Vermont modified pull-up (VMPU), and the New York modified pull-up (NYMPU). The authors concluded that the most commonly used field tests for upper-body strength and endurance do not significantly correlate well with laboratory measures of absolute muscular strength and endurance. The authors state, "these field tests are, at best, moderately valid measures of weight-relative muscular strength."

As discussed earlier, the rationale for the use of the modified pull-up test was that the traditional pull-up or flexed arm hang tests have traditionally provided poor measurement sensitivity for the range of children tested (54). Pate and colleagues (47) found that the pull-up, push-up, and NYMPU tests had the highest percentage of zero scores, meaning a large number of children could not even record one score. Although the flexed arm hang yielded no zero scores in their study, many of the subjects could only perform the test for 1 to 2 s. By far, the VMPU produced the best results. Only 7% of the subjects tested with the VMPU scored zero, and it also correlated highest with

The result of several large-scale fitness tests have reported that upper-body strength among American children is poor. In Part I of the National Children and Youth Fitness Study (53), it was reported that over 30% of 10- to 11-year-old boys and 60% of 10- to 18-year-old girls were unable to perform one chin-up. In a 1985 study conducted by the President's Council on Physical Fitness and Sports (50), 18,857 American school children ages 6 through 17 were tested. The results of the strength tests included the following:

- 40% of the boys ages 6 to 12 could not do more than one pull-up. One in four could not do any.
- 70% of all girls tested could not do more than one pull-up and 55% could not do any.
- 45% of the boys 6 to 14 and 55% of all the girls tested could not hold their chins over a raised bar for more than 10 s.

A 1981–1982 test conducted by the Amateur Athletic Union (1) found that 60% of the girls tested from ages 6 to

FIGURE 17.2

A modified pull-up test for the assessment of upper-body strength.

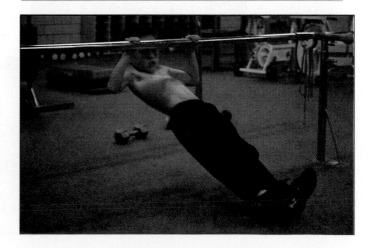

weight-relative strength. The authors concluded, "the VMPU is the most valid and appropriate test for application with 9 to 10 year old children." Nevertheless, the fact remains that U.S. children perform poorly in field tests that require upper-body strength, and changing the test and/or lowering the standard of test scores does not change this fact.

Aerobic Capacity

Exercise capacity and maximal oxygen uptake (VO_{2max}) increase throughout childhood. The increase in endurance capacity is due to enhanced oxygen transport and enhanced metabolic capacities. In addition, as running economy improves, children are able to run at a lower percentage of VO_{2max}. The health-related reference standards for boys and girls for the 1-mi run/walk were listed in tables 17.2 and 17.3. One-mile run times for boys and girls have been compared from data collected in the Health-Related Physical Fitness Test (HRPFT) conducted in 1980 and the NCYFS (53) published in 1985. In comparing the 50th percentile scores for the 1-mi run for boys and girls from data collected in

1980 and 1985, the 1980 results were superior to the 1985 results. When American children are compared to children from other countries (Europe, Great Britain, Australia, Canada), foreign children appear to have better cardiovascular endurance. The reason for the discrepancy is not clear. One group of researchers (31) reported that there has been a 10% decline in aerobic fitness levels of children as measured by various distance runs.

Coronary Artery Disease

Serum cholesterol levels and obesity rates are high in American children. As many as 40% of children ages 5 to 8 show at least one heart disease risk factor (high cholesterol, physical inactivity, obesity, or high blood pressure) (21) (fig. 17.3). With the evidence linking the origins of coronary artery disease (CAD) to childhood years, efforts should be made to identify children at the highest level of coronary heart disease (CHD) risk in an effort to reduce the potential for children maturing into high-risk adults.

Cardiovascular disease continues to be the leading cause of death in the United States. The natural progression of

---

FIGURE 17.3

The prevalence of risk factors for atherosclerotic coronary artery disease in children aged 7 to 12 years.

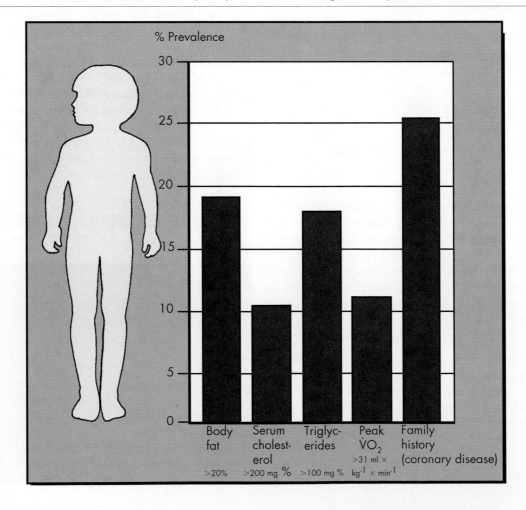

CAD is believed to be strongly correlated with the presence of the classic risk factors; hypertension, cigarette smoking, high serum cholesterol, and physical inactivity. Coronary artery disease is now recognized as a pediatric disease (29); there are three basic periods of disease development (36). The first stage, the incubation period, occurs between infancy and adolescence. During this period, mesenchymal cushions form on the inner layer of the arterial wall. In the second phase of this period, fatty streaks begin to appear. Fatty streaks are found in the aorta in the first years of life and almost universally by the age of 3 years (36). The second phase, or the latent period, occurs between adolescence and early adulthood. During this period, the fatty streaks are found in the coronary arteries. The final period is referred to as the clinical period, in which the clinical manifestations of the disease become apparent.

Several large-scale epidemiological studies have been conducted to assess cardiovascular disease risk factors and children. From a total of 5000 children examined, 24% had total cholesterol levels > 220 mg/dL, 20% were > 110% relative body weight, and after the age of 9, 19% had diastolic blood pressures > 94 mmHg. Wilmore and McNamara (66) and Gilliam and associates (21) also noted that > 50% of the children they tested had one or more risk factors (elevated blood pressure, elevated total cholesterol, elevated triglycerides, or elevated body fat). Khoury and colleagues (30) found the children they examined to be at high risk for CHD by virtue of their low-density lipoprotein cholesterol levels and low-density lipoprotein cholesterol. It appears, at least with lipoproteins (70) and blood pressure (67), that children who have risk factors at an early age remain at risk as they age.

Parents, teachers, and physicians need to be aware that healthy children face heart disease at a very early age. Heart disease is often thought of as a disease of the elderly but, in fact, the beginning stages of heart disease occur at a very young age. Lifestyle behaviors and habits are established early and continue throughout adulthood. If all health trends remain the same, 35 million of today's 83 million children will eventually die of cardiovascular disease. Early education about heart disease risk factors may help reverse this startling trend. Some of the reasons why we should be concerned about the health of children today are listed below:

- Heart disease takes more than 20 years to develop.
- Children are heavier and less fit than 20 years ago.
- 30 to 35% of school-age children are at risk for heart disease.
- 50% of children are overweight.
- 42% of children have high blood cholesterol.
- 28% of children have high blood pressure.
- The average 2- to 5-year-old watches 22 h of television a week.
- The average 6- to 11-year-old watches 20 h of television a week.
- 11 million children in the U.S. are considered obese.

Growth and Development

Children do not grow at a uniform rate throughout the course of their development. There is a rapid increase in height, followed (particularly in boys) by a rapid increase in body mass over the period of **puberty** (the **pubertal growth spurt**). Further, there are substantial interindividual differences in biological age at any given calendar age, with corresponding variations in the timing and magnitude of the pubertal growth spurt. These factors have implications for the fitness professional in terms of appropriate procedures for the standardization of fitness testing and programming.

Phases of Growth

There are four main phases of growth in humans (61). Growth is rapid in infancy and early childhood, remains relatively steady during middle childhood, then again increases

FIGURE 17.4

The average growth (distance) curves for stature and body weight for American children from birth to 18 years of age.

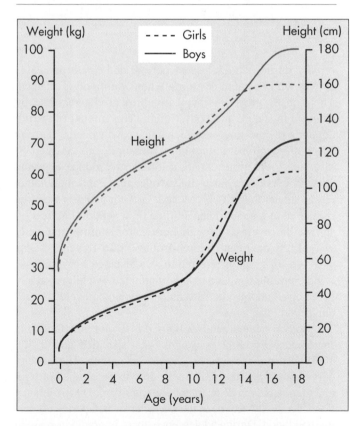

puberty the period of a child's development when androgen hormones are released and secondary sex characteristics develop

pubertal growth spurt the rapid growth of a child associated with puberty

FIGURE 17.5

The velocity growth curves for British males and females from birth to maturity.

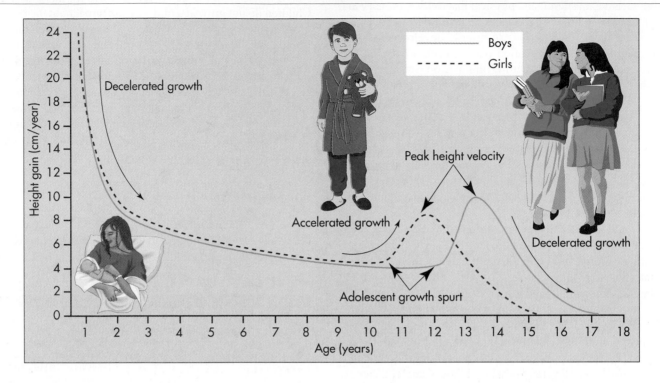

rapidly during the adolescent period, and finally increases slowly with eventual cessation when adulthood is attained. The rate of growth is typically measured over time by changes in stature and body weight. The amount of growth depends on the time at which the growth occurs and the speed of growth per unit of time. Measurements taken on individuals over time can be plotted to produce a graph. Growth curves are fairly linear over time, and then flatten out as sexual maturity is reached. Growth patterns are often measured at a pediatrician's office or at school. Figure 17.4 shows the average growth curves for stature and body weight for American children from birth to 18 years of age. This type of graph is referred to as a distance curve because it indicates the weight and height attained by children at any given age, and thus the "distance" they have traveled toward adulthood (34).

Another method commonly used is to plot growth in time increments of height or weight for a specified period (fig. 17.5). Velocity curves show the rate of growth. The velocity curve shows that the most rapid growth occurs before birth and then begins to decelerate before delivery. During infancy there is a steady decline in the rate of growth, tapering off during childhood. During adolescence, there is a rapid increase in both height and weight. This rapid increase in growth has been termed "the adolescent growth spurt." Girls reach their peak height velocity by age 12, whereas boys reach this event around the age of 14. Following the rapid spurt, growth dramatically slows. Girls reach 98% of their final height by the age of 16.5; boys at about 17.75 years (61).

Figures 17.6 and 17.7 are referred to as reference growth charts. These reference charts are used to assess children's growth status over time. The National Center for Health Statistics has compiled these growth curves based on a very large sample of children. Pediatricians use these reference charts to plot growth patterns over time. Pediatricians will often reference children's height and weight based on percentages of population norm (i.e., 75th percentile for age and weight, and 95th percentile for height). Plotting growth over time can identify anomalies in growth and development that, if detected early, can often be corrected with medical therapy.

Age and Gender Variation in Growth

A variety of biological processes change with age. In addition, there are tremendous gender-related differences during growth. There is a rapid rate of growth during the adolescent years, referred to as the **peak height velocity (PHV).** PHV usually occurs 2 years earlier for girls than boys. Girls tend to be slightly bigger and heavier than boys from 2 years to 10 years of age. Strength and body proportions of boys and girls are essentially equal until the beginning of the

peak height velocity (PHV) the period of rapid growth during the adolescent period, usually occurring 2 years earlier for girls than boys

FIGURE 17.6

Reference growth chart for boys, ages 2 to 18 years.

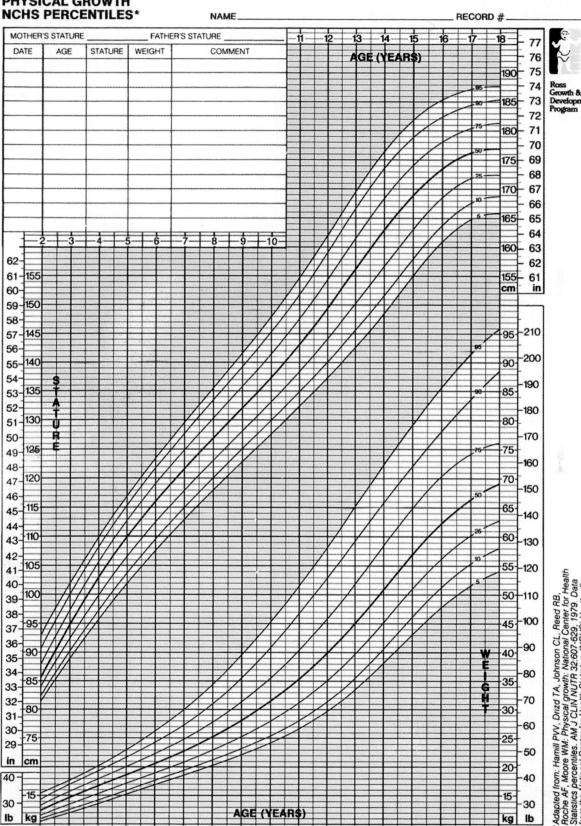

BOYS: 2 TO 18 YEARS
PHYSICAL GROWTH
NCHS PERCENTILES*

*Adapted from: Hamill PVV, Drizd TA, Johnson CL, Reed RB, Roche AF, Moore WM: Physical growth: National Center for Health Statistics percentiles. AM J CLIN NUTR 32:607-629, 1979. Data from the National Center for Health Statistics (NCHS), Hyattsville, Maryland.

© 1982 ROSS LABORATORIES

Ross
Growth &
Development
Program

FIGURE 17.7

Reference growth chart for girls, ages 2 to 18 years.

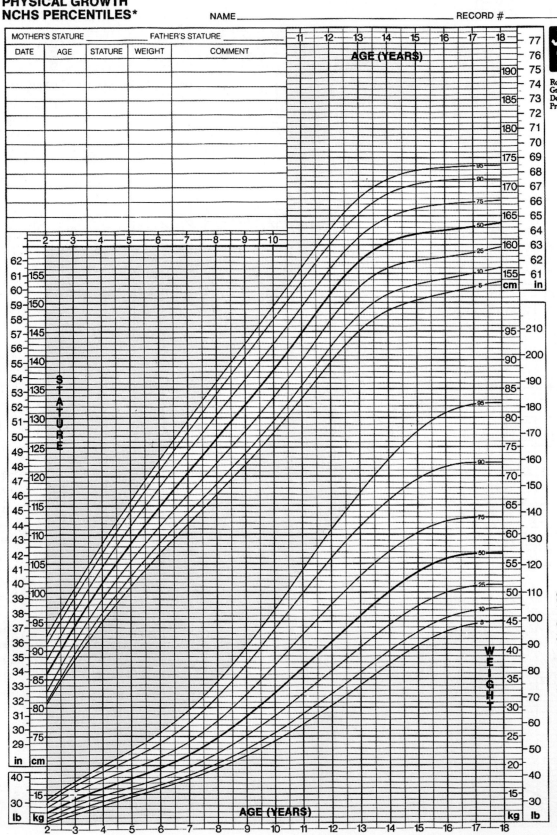

**GIRLS: 2 TO 18 YEARS
PHYSICAL GROWTH
NCHS PERCENTILES***

NAME _____ RECORD # _____

* Adapted from: Hamill PVV, Drizd T.A, Johnson CL, Reed RB,
Roche AF, Moore WM: Physical growth: National Center for Health
Statistics percentiles. AM J CLIN NUTR 32:607-629, 1979. Data
from the National Center for Health Statistics (NCHS) Hyattsville,
Maryland.

© 1982 ROSS LABORATORIES

adolescent period. During puberty, hormonal changes begin to cause significant variation between the sexes. Increased testosterone release in boys causes an increase in lean body mass, whereas in females an increase in estrogen causes an increase in body fat deposition, breast development, and a widening of the hips.

Assessment of Maturation

The assessment of **maturation** is important for a variety of reasons. First, maturity assessment is important in the research process. Pediatric researchers try to match young subjects based on their maturity status. Even if two children are the same age, height, and weight, they may be at different stages of development, and thus the more mature child could be at an advantage. Second, maturity assessment is frequently used by pediatricians to evaluate growth and development patterns. Third, maturation assessment can help assure that children are evenly matched for athletic competition. A variety of maturity assessment techniques exist, including skeletal age, sexual maturation, somatic maturation, and dental maturation. The pubertal stages of sexual maturity are outlined in table 17.4. Sexual maturation is typically defined in a preparticipation physical examination.

The simplest method of adjusting data for individual differences in body size is to express findings as a ratio to body mass. For example, a subject's maximal aerobic power may be expressed in units of (mL/kg/min). If a test score is to be used to assess a child's performance potential, this may be quite an effective tactic because most vigorous athletic activities involve the displacement of body mass against gravity, and the oxygen cost of a sustained physical task is usually roughly proportional to the individual's body mass. If the intent is to compare fitness scores from one age category to another, the choice of units becomes more controversial.

When aerobic power is expressed per kilogram of body mass, scores commonly decrease over much of childhood, with the rate of loss accelerating at puberty; this has led to the inference that because of insufficient or inadequate school programs of physical education, aerobic fitness deteriorates once a child sits behind a classroom desk. However, there is no fundamental biological reason why maximal oxygen intake should develop as a constant linear function of a child's body mass. When a $height^2$ comparison is made, aerobic power remains relatively stable throughout childhood; therefore schools should no longer stand accused of causing a decrease in fitness among their pupils.

Team competitions such as football are commonly classified by age group. However, this is not a good approach, given the substantial interindividual differences in body size at any given calendar age. Particularly around the time of puberty, children may find they are playing against others who are much larger, stronger, and heavier than themselves. In consequence, small and late-maturing children are at a substantially increased risk of physical injury if they partici-pate in contact sports. A combination of such hazards with the discouragement of unequal competition leads to a high drop-out rate from age-category sports leagues, with selective retention of a minority of tall, heavy, early maturers. An alternative option is to base the classification of players on their body mass, as is already done for some individual contests such as wrestling.

Laboratory Measures of Physical Fitness in Children

Aerobic Capacity

In absolute terms, the maximal oxygen uptake of children is much lower than that of adults, but when corrected for body weight, the VO_{2max} of boys is similar to that found in young men. Young girls have a greater VO_{2max} per kilogram body weight than young women, but when adjusted for $height^2$, they have lower capacities. However, peak oxygen uptake may be a better expression of aerobic power in children than VO_{2max}, because children have a difficult time reaching a true maximal effort because of (1) local muscular fatigue, (2) a limited attention span during testing, and (3) a low threshold for discomfort (12).

The accuracy of VO_{2max} to predict cardiorespiratory fitness and endurance performance in children is not well established (56). Maximal oxygen uptake is directly related to the maturity level of the individual (i.e., lean body mass, height, and weight). As children mature, maximal oxygen uptake levels increase. Until maturity is reached, a relative rather than an absolute expression should be used to compare peak aerobic power in children (fig. 17.8). Values for VO_{2max} increase at about the same rate in both sexes until age 12. After age 12, boys continue to increase their maximal oxygen uptake until the age of 18, whereas girls show little improvement after age 14.

Exercise capacity and maximal oxygen uptake increase throughout childhood. The increase in endurance capacity is due to enhanced oxygen transport and enhanced metabolic capacities. Several excellent reviews have been written looking at the effects of physical activity on the trainability of prepubescent children (12, 46, 57, 63). Some of the physiological effects of training, growth, and maturation in children are listed in table 17.5. In addition, numerous researchers have demonstrated improvements in VO_{2max} following endurance training (19, 56), with changes ranging from 5 to 18%, depending on the mode of training, the intensity of the exercise, and the length of study.

---

maturation (mat-u'ra-shun) the biological and/or behavioral development of a person; maturation is not necessarily associated with age

TABLE 17.4

Tanner Stage of Sexual Maturation

STAGE	DESCRIPTION
1	Prepubertal stage of development. Absence of development of any secondary sexual characteristics.
2	Indicates the initial development of each secondary sexual characteristic. Initial elevation of breasts in girls and enlargement of the genitals in boys. For both sexes, pubic hair begins to appear.
3 & 4	Continued maturation of each secondary sexual characteristic. Pubic hair becomes coarser and begins to curl. Relative enlargement of larynx in boys. Increase in pelvic diameter begins in girls.
5	Indicates adult maturation. Mature spermatozoa are present in males. Full reproductivity in women. Axially hair is present and sweat and sebaceous glands are very active in both sexes.

Modified from: Tanner, J.M.: *Growth at adolescence*. Blackwell Scientific, Oxford, 1962.

Payne and Morrow (48) have performed a metanalysis on exercise and VO_{2max} in children. Payne and Morrow found 69 training studies using children, and used 28 of them in their analysis. In their review, Payne and Morrow found that the typical child in the studies they reviewed would expect to improve (pre- to post-training) their VO_{2max} by only 2.07 mL/kg/min as a result of training. The researchers concluded by stating, "our work suggests the aerobic benefit of training is small-to-moderate for children and is a function of the experimental design."

Training Considerations

Sufficient evidence exists that children do physiologically adapt to endurance training. However, a general consensus is lacking on the quality and quantity of exercise required to improve and maintain a minimum level of aerobic fitness in children. Recommendations for adults have been published by the American College of Sports Medicine in their position, first published in 1978 (5), and recently revised in 1990 (7). In 1988 the American College of Sports Medicine published an opinion statement on physical fitness in children and youth (6). ACSM states:

The amount of exercise required for optimal functional capacity and health at various ages has not been precisely defined. Until more definitive evidence is available, current recommendations are that children and youth obtain 20–30 minutes of

FIGURE 17.8

The relationships between VO_{2max} and chronological age. *(a)* VO_{2max} is expressed absolutely (L/min) and *(b)* relative to body mass.

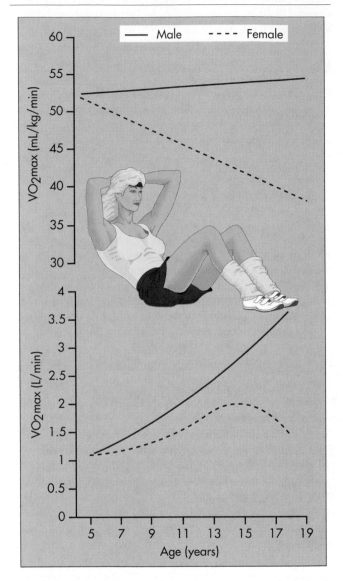

vigorous exercise each day. Physical education classes typically devote instructional time to physical fitness.

Several investigators have recommended that adult standards be used when establishing the intensity of exercise, as well as the frequency and duration of children's fitness programs (11, 57). These recommendations are supported by Rowland (57), in which he found that of the eight studies he reviewed, six that used adult standards of aerobic training produced significant improvements in aerobic power; whereas no significant improvements were noted in the other two studies.

TABLE 17.5

Physiologic changes in children resulting from training and physical growth and maturation

CHARACTERISTIC	CHANGE
Heart rate, resting and submaximal	Decrease
Arterial blood pressure, maximal	Increase
Minute ventilation, submaximal	Decrease
Minute ventilation, maximal	Increase
Respiratory frequency, submaximal and maximal	Decrease
Ventilatory equivalent, submaximal and maximal	Decrease
Oxygen uptake, submaximal (per kilogram of body weight)	Decrease
Oxygen uptake, maximal (L/min)	Increase
Blood lactate, maximal	Increase
Muscle lactate, maximal	Increase
Lowest blood pH	Decrease
Muscle strength	Increase
Anaerobic power (in watts and per kilogram of body weight)	Increase
Muscle endurance* (in Watts and per kilogram of body weight)	Increase

From Bar-Or O: The O_2 cost of child's movement in health and disease. In Russo P, Gass G, editors: *Exercise, nutrition and performances,* Sydney, Australia, 1985, Cumberland College.

*Represented by mean power in the Wingate Anaerobic Test.

Anaerobic Capacity

Anaerobic capacity is defined as the energy (ATP) production during exercise that occurs from reactions other than mitochondrial respiration. Anaerobic activities are those that are high in intensity and short in duration. Several tests are commonly used to assess anaerobic power; one of the most frequently used is the Wingate test. The Wingate test is designed to determine both peak anaerobic power and mean power output during a 30-s test. The Wingate test has been used extensively in assessing the anaerobic capacity of children (13, 33).

Young children have a distinctly lower anaerobic capacity when compared to adolescents and adults (11). Some of the reasons for these differences may be related to (1) low levels of male hormones, (2) a lower glycolytic capacity, (3) lower lactate production during exercise, (4) a decreased capacity to buffer acidosis during exercise, (5) lower rates of glycogenolysis during exercise, and (6) a lower lactate threshold (11, 33). As children mature, their ability to increase anaerobic capacity improves (11, 19, 23).

The responses to training improve with maturity. Maximal oxygen uptake is strongly related to lean body mass, which increases throughout childhood. In addition, oxygen delivery to the working muscles and oxygen extraction and utilization all improve with age and growth. Peak anaerobic power also increases with age and growth (fig. 17.9).

Muscular Strength and Endurance

Adequate strength is considered an important part of health-related fitness and optimal physiological function for both children and adults. It is also recognized as an important contribution to improved motor performance, self-image, and athletic performance for both children and adults. In support of these facts, the National Strength and Conditioning Association, the American Orthopaedic Society for Sports Medicine, and the American Physical Therapy Association support supervised resistance training in children in an effort to help reduce the chances of injury.

Despite the importance of the development of muscular strength, there remains a lingering concern that resistance exercises performed by prepubescent children are potentially dangerous and should be avoided. For example, early investigators concluded that strength gains were not possible in prepubertal children (62), and that strength training could cause irreversible injury to the developing growth plates in bones (65). In the late 1970s and early 1980s, several scientific reports recommended that children not participate in weight training because the developing bones and musculature of young children are more susceptible to injuries compared to adults (2, 65). These

FIGURE 17.9

The increase in maximal anaerobic power in children as they age.

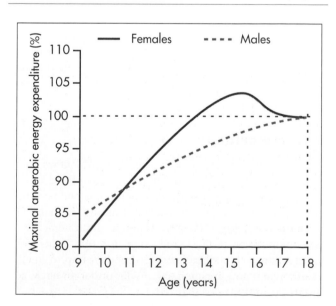

recommendations were primarily based on the published report about growth plate injuries that occurred in adolescent weight lifters (24, 58). The type of injury reported in the earlier reports were injuries to the wrist that occurred during "excessive" overhead lifts (24, 58). Growth plate injuries do occur in young children. Some of the more prevalent causes of growth plate injuries in children are common accidents and participation in sports such as baseball, skiing, football, gymnastics, and long-distance running (16). There is, however, little if any evidence to support the belief that "supervised" resistance training causes harm to the musculoskeletal system in children (51) (see focus boxes 17.3 and 17.4).

Weltman and colleagues (64) studied the safety and effectiveness of resistance training in 26 prepubescent children. Weltman and his colleagues found no evidence of damage to the epiphysis, bone, or muscle following a 14-week supervised strength-training program. Dr. Weltman concluded that "supervised strength training using hydraulic strength training equipment is safe and effective in prepubertal boys." Blimkie and associates (14) at McMaster University in Ontario, Canada, also evaluated the safety and effectiveness of resistance training using prepubescent boys. Safety was monitored via physician evaluation before, during, and following training. The results of this research found no evidence of damage to the musculoskeletal system following resistance training, and found significant strength gains and improved sports performance.

There have been several studies published that have evaluated the effects of resistance training on athletic performance (42, 49, 64). Following 14 weeks of supervised hydraulic resistance training, improvements in the vertical jump performance improved by 10.4% in the trained group versus a 3.0% decrease in performance in the control group from pretest values (64). Following isometric strength training, improvement in vertical jump scores for girls 7 to 19 years old was demonstrated (42). Significant improvements in strength and performance have been demonstrated in prepubescent female gymnasts following 4 weeks of supervised resistance training (49). Further research is needed to examine the effects of resistance training on performance in different sports.

Health Benefits

Numerous health-related benefits following resistance training have been reported in the literature. In addition to improvements in muscular strength, other fitness and performance-related effects of resistance training include (1) increased flexibility (60), (2) favorable improvements in body composition (60), (3) reduction in serum lipids (50), (4) reductions in blood pressures (26), and (5) improvements in cardiorespiratory function (64). With further research, additional benefits may be realized.

Injury Prevention

Recent studies have shown that a strength development program may help with injury prevention. A report by the American Physical Therapy Association concluded that the poor physical conditioning of children participating in youth sports may be the leading cause of injury in youth sports. Other data suggest that resistance training may have a protective value against injury prevention in young children (15, 26, 39). All sports place demands on the musculoskeletal system, and there is general agreement among medical and sports medicine experts that increasing the strength of the athlete will enhance performance and decrease the chance of injury in adults. Because it has been demonstrated that children can increase both muscle and bone growth following resistance training, encouraging children to participate in well-structured and supervised resistance training appears justified.

Thermoregulation During Exercise

In normal or moderate climates, children are able to exercise and dissipate heat quite effectively. However, in very hot environments, children are limited in their ability to dissipate heat. Children are not as efficient in dissipating heat as adults because (1) they produce a greater amount of heat relative to their body mass, (2) they have a lower sweat rate at rest and during exercise, (3) they have greater energy expenditure during exercise, (4) they have a lower cardiac output at any given metabolic level (12, 27), and (5) they rely on greater cutaneous blood flow during exercise for convective heat loss during exercise. Children can acclimatize to hot conditions, but the process takes considerably more time (repeated exposure) than with adults (27). Special precautions should always be taken when children are exercising in extreme environmental conditions. Because of children's limited thermoregulatory capacities, the risk of thermal injury is much greater in children than in adults.

Safety Guidelines for Resistance Training

Although there are fewer resistance training studies involving children than adults, the evidence demonstrating increases in strength following structured resistance training in children is mounting. The increases reported in the literature are similar to those observed in older age groups. Furthermore, the safety and efficacy of resistance training programs for prepubescent children have been well documented. The risk of injuries to children participating in resistance training programs is low. However, injuries can occur in any sport or strenuous physical activity. To minimize the risk of injury

FOCUS BOX 17.3

Professional Guidelines and Recommendations for Strength Training by Prepubescent Children

Three professional organizations have published position stands on prepubescent strength training: the American Academy of Pediatrics (AAP), the National Strength and Conditioning Association (NSCA), and the American Orthopaedeic Society for Sports Medicine (AOSSM).

In 1990 the American Academy of Pediatrics released an updated version of their 1983 report (2). In this report, the AAP recommended the following:

Strength training programs for prepubescent, pubescent, and postpubescent athletes should be permitted only if conducted by well-trained adults. The adults should be qualified to plan programs appropriate to the athlete's stage of maturation, which should be assessed by medical personnel.

Unless good medical data become available that demonstrate safety, children and adolescents should avoid the practice of weight lifting, power lifting, and body building, as well as the repetitive use of maximal amounts of weight in strength training programs, until they have reached Tanner stage 5 (adolescence) level of developmental maturity.

Resistance Training Principles for Young Athletes

Principle 1: Children should be encouraged to participate in regular exercise that involves repetitive movements against an opposing force. It is important to note that children can develop strength through a variety of activities, including (a) participation in sports, (b) weight training, (c) manual resistance exercises, and (d) simply playing.

Principle 2: Power lifting, or lifting in a competitive setting to determine the maximum amount of weight an individual can lift is not recommended for children.

Principle 3: The primary focus of resistance training should, at least initially, be (a) focused at developing proper technique, (b) learning the exercises, and (c) developing an interest for resistance training.

Principle 4: Before any resistance is utilized, proper technique should be demonstrated for each exercise. The next step is to gradually apply resistance or weight until the child can lift the weight for the repetition range (i.e., 8 to 12).

Principle 5: Children should perform 8 to 12 repetitions in upper-body exercises, and 15 to 20 in lower-body exercises. Once children are able to perform an exercise for a predetermined maximum number of repetitions per set, then the resistance or maximum number of repetitions should be increased.

Principle 6: One to 3 sets of each exercise should be performed, utilizing approximately 8 to 10 different exercises. In the early stages of training, one set of each exercise should be performed until the child has demonstrated proper form and is acclimated to resistance training.

Principle 7: Children should be encouraged to rest for 1 to 2 min between exercises.

Principle 8: Two to three exercise sessions per week is recommended, followed by at least one day of rest between workouts.

Principle 9: As children develop strength, the training stimulus will need to be adjusted. To maintain maximal stimulus, the resistance and/or number of repetitions must be increased.

Principle 10: Training programs should be designed with specific goals and objectives in mind. The exercises chosen should reflect the desired outcome. For the majority of children, specificity of training is not as important as it will be in later years. Children should participate in a variety of activities to develop a wide range of skills.

Principle 11: A brief warm-up period should precede the exercise session and a brief cool-down should follow the exercise session. Warm-up exercises increase the temperature of muscle and improve its elasticity, both of which improve the muscle's ability to perform work, as well as reduce the risk of muscle and/or joint injury. Cool-down activities lower muscle temperature and metabolic rate.

during resistance training, the following suggestions are recommended:

- Medical clearance/physical needs must be obtained.
- Children should be properly supervised at all times.
- Children should not be allowed to exercise unless the weight training facility is safe for them.
- Children should never perform single maximal lifts or sudden explosive movements, or try to compete with other children.
- Children should be taught to breathe properly during exercise movements.

- Children should never be allowed to use any equipment that is broken or damaged, or which doesn't fit them properly.
- Children should rest for approximately 1 to 2 min between each exercise, more if necessary. In addition, children should have scheduled rest days between each training day.
- Children should be encouraged to drink plenty of fluids before, during, and after exercising.
- Children need to be told that they need to communicate with their coach, parent, or teacher when they feel tired, or when they have been injured.

FOCUS BOX 17.4

Exercise Recommendations for Children

1. Although children are generally quite active, children generally choose to participate in activities that consist of short-burst, high-energy exercise. Children should be encouraged to participate in sustained activities that use large muscle groups.
2. The type, intensity, and duration of exercise activities need to be based on the maturity of the child, medical status, and previous experiences with exercise.
3. Regardless of age, the exercise intensity should start out low and progress gradually.
4. Because of the difficulty in monitoring children's heart rates, the modified Borg Scale offers a more practical method of monitoring exercise intensity in children.
5. Children are involved in a variety of activities throughout the day. Because of this, a specific time should be dedicated to sustained aerobic activities.
6. The duration of the exercise session will vary depending on the age of the children, their previous exercise experience, and the intensity of the exercise session.
7. Because it is often quite difficult to get children to respond to sustained periods of exercise, the session periods need to be creatively designed.

Sample Exercise Recommendation

Mode   Children should be encouraged to participate in sustained activities that use large muscle groups (i.e., swimming, jogging, aerobic dance). Other activities, such as recreational, sport, and fun activities that develop other components of fitness (speed, power, flexibility, muscular endurance, agility, and coordination) should be incorporated into a fitness program.

Intensity   Exercise intensity should start out low and progress gradually. There are currently no universal recommendations available for the use of children's training heart rate during exercise. The Borg Scale of perceived exertion offers a more practical method of monitoring exercise intensity with children.

Frequency   Two to three days of endurance training will allow adequate time to participate in other activities, and yet be sufficient enough to cause a training effect.

Duration   Because children will be involved in a variety of activities during and after school, a specific amount of time should be dedicated to endurance training. Endurance exercise activities should be gradually increased to 30 to 40 min per session. With younger children, it will be necessary to start out with less time initially.

WEBSITE BOX

Chapter 17: Growth, Development, and Exercise

The newest information regarding exercise physiology can be viewed at the following sites.[*]

mdnet.de/asthma/
   Information-packed site with links to all topics on asthma, including a module to help calculate reference lung function values for children.

aap.org/
   Homepage of the American Academy of Pediatrics.

pedi.resp-pulmonary-com/
   Informative and educational site on pediatric issues, especially pulmonary care and lung function testing.

genetic.org/hgf/
   Homepage of the Human Growth Foundation that provides information on human growth-related disorders.

[*]Unless indicated, all URLs preceded by http://www.

Note: These URLs were valid at the time of publication, but could have changed or been deleted from Internet access since that time.

SUMMARY

- There is currently a movement among youth fitness experts to use **criterion-referenced fitness standards** that are based on established fitness and health relationships. Criterion-referenced standards for children have been developed by the Institute for Aerobic Research. On the basis of criterion-referenced fitness standards, U.S. children appear to be reasonably fit, but have below-average upper-body strength.

- The only secular trends in youth fitness that have been analyzed with a high degree of accuracy is skinfold data. There appears to have been a systematic increase in skinfold thickness among 6- to 9-year-old boys and girls from the 1960s and 1970s to the 1980s. Gortmaker and colleagues estimated that obesity had increased from 17.6% in the 6 to 11 age group between 1963 and 1965 to 27.1% between 1976 and 1980. The cause of the increase in body fat over the years has been related to decreased habitual physical activity and increased television viewing.

- Exercise capacity and maximal oxygen uptake (VO_{2max}) increase throughout childhood. The increase in endurance capacity is due to enhanced oxygen transport and enhanced metabolic capacities. In addition, as running economy improves, children are able to run at a lower percentage of VO_{2max}. When American children are compared to children from other countries (Europe, Great Britain, Australia, Canada), foreign children appear to have better cardiovascular endurance. The reason for the discrepancy is not clear.

- Serum cholesterol levels and obesity rates are high in American children. As many as 40% of children ages 5 to 8 show at least one heart disease risk factor (high cholesterol, physical inactivity, obesity, or high blood pressure).

- Children do not grow at a uniform rate throughout the course of their development. There is a rapid increase in height, followed (particularly in boys) by a rapid increase in body mass over the period of **puberty** (the **pubertal growth spurt**). Further, there are substantial interindividual differences in biological age at any given calendar age, with corresponding variations in the timing and magnitude of the pubertal growth spurt. These factors have implications for the fitness professional in terms of appropriate procedures for the standardization of fitness testing and programming. It can be argued that a child's level of **maturation** is more important than age when used to categorize youth sports and athletics.

- There is a rapid rate of growth during the adolescent years, referred to as the **peak height velocity (PHV).** PHV usually occurs 2 years earlier for girls than boys. Girls tend to be slightly bigger and heavier than boys from 2 years to 10 years of age. Strength and body proportions of boys and girls are essentially equal until the beginning of the adolescent period. During puberty, hormonal changes begin

to cause significant variation between the sexes. Increased testosterone release in males causes an increase in lean body mass, whereas in females an increase in estrogen causes an increase in body fat deposition, breast development, and a widening of the hips.

- When aerobic power is expressed per kilogram of body mass, scores commonly decrease over much of childhood, with the rate of loss accelerating at puberty; this has led to the inference that because of insufficient or inadequate school programs of physical education, aerobic fitness deteriorates once a child sits behind a classroom desk. However, there is no fundamental biological reason why maximal oxygen intake should develop as a constant linear function of a child's body mass. When a height^2 comparison is made, aerobic power remains relatively stable throughout childhood.

- As children mature, maximal oxygen uptake levels increase. Until maturity is reached, a relative rather than an absolute expression should be used to compare peak aerobic power in children. Values for VO_{2max} increase at about the same rate in both sexes until age 12. After which, boys continue to increase their maximal oxygen uptake until the age of 18, whereas girls show little improvement after age 14. Numerous researchers have demonstrated improvements in VO_{2max} following endurance training, with changes ranging from 5 to 18%, depending on the mode of training, the intensity of the exercise, and the length of study.

- Young children have a distinctly lower anaerobic capacity when compared to adolescents and adults. Some of the reasons for these differences may be related to (1) low levels of male hormones, (2) a lower glycolytic capacity, (3) lower lactate production during exercise, (4) a decreased capacity to buffer acidosis during exercise, (5) lower rates of glycogenolysis during exercise, and (6) a lower lactate threshold. As children mature, the ability to increase anaerobic capacity improves.

- Adequate strength is considered an important part of health-related fitness and optimal physiological function for both children and adults. It is also recognized as an important contribution to improved motor performance, self-image, and athletic performance for both children and adults. Weltman studied the safety and effectiveness of resistance training in 26 prepubescent children. Weltman and his colleagues found no evidence of damage to the epiphysis, bone, or muscle following a 14-week supervised strength-training program. Dr. Weltman concluded that "supervised strength training using hydraulic strength-training equipment is safe and effective in prepubertal boys."

- Numerous health-related benefits following resistance training by children have been reported in the literature.

SUMMARY

In addition to improvements in muscular strength, other fitness and performance-related effects of resistance training include (1) increased flexibility, (2) favorable improvements in body composition, (3) reduction in serum lipids, (4) reductions in blood pressures, and (5) improvements in cardiorespiratory function. With further research, additional benefits may be realized.

■ Children are not as efficient in dissipating heat as adults because of (1) a lower sweat rate at rest and at exercise,

(2) greater energy expenditure during exercise, and (3) a lower cardiac output at any given metabolic level. Children can acclimatize to hot conditions, but the process takes considerably more time (repeated exposure) than with adults. Special precautions should always be taken when children are exercising in extreme environmental conditions because the risk of thermal injury is much greater in children than in adults.

STUDY QUESTIONS

1. What do we know about the fitness and health status of today's children compared to previous years/decades?

2. What is a criterion-referenced fitness standard?

3. Is coronary heart disease a childhood or adult disease? Explain.

4. Identify and explain the different phases of growth and indicate how they differ between boys and girls.

5. Should sports and athletics be categorized by maturation or age? Explain.

6. What is a better expression of VO_2 for children, mL/kg body weight or mL/height^2? Explain.

7. A coach comes up to you and asks, "Are children as trainable as adults?" In several paragraphs give your response with specific documentation.

8. Speculate on why children have a lower anaerobic capacity than adults.

9. List five benefits of resistance training in children and adolescents.

10. Is resistance training too dangerous for children to perform, both pre- and postpubescent? Explain.

11. Discuss some concerns regarding children exercising in hot or humid environments.

APPLICATIONS

1. Identify research supporting the need for early coronary artery disease prevention in children.

2. Describe a school- and home-based prevention program for children.

3. What are the roles of pediatricians in cardiovascular disease prevention in children? What are the roles of parents?

REFERENCES

1. Amateur Athletic Union. *Physical fitness program.* AAU House, Indianapolis, IN, 1981.

2. American Academy of Pediatrics. Strength training, weight and power lifting, and body building by children and adolescents. *Pediatrics* 86(5):801–803, 1990.

3. American Alliance for Health, Physical Education and Recreation. *AAHPER youth fitness test manual.* Washington, DC, 1965.

4. American Alliance for Health, Physical Education and Recreation. *Physical best: A physical fitness education and assessment program.* Author, Reston, VA, 1988.

5. American College of Sports Medicine. Position stand for the recommended quantity and quality of exercise for developing and maintaining cardiorespiratory and muscular fitness in healthy adults. *Med. Sci. Sports Exerc.* 10:vii–x, 1978.

6. American College of Sports Medicine. Opinion statement on physical fitness in children and youth. *Med. Sci. Sports Exerc.* 20:422–423, 1988.

7. American College of Sports Medicine. Position stand for the recommended quantity and quality of exercise for developing and maintaining cardiorespiratory and muscular fitness in healthy adults. *Med. Sci. Sports Exerc.* 22(10):265–274, 1990.

8. American Orthopaedic Society for Sports Medicine. *Proceedings of the Conference on Strength Training and the Prepubescent,* B. Cahill (ed.). Chicago, 1988.

9. Araki, T., Y. Toda, K. Matsushita, and A. Tsujino. Age differences in sweating during muscular exercise. *Jap. J. Phys. Fit. Sports Med.* 28:239–248, 1979.

10. Atha, J. Strengthening muscle. *Exerc. Sport Sci. Rev.* 91:1–73, 1981.

11. Bar-Or, O. *Pediatric sports medicine for the practitioner: From physiological principles to clinical applications.* Springer-Verlag, New York, Preface, 1983.

12. Bar-Or, O. Trainability of the prepubescent child. *Phys. Sportsmed.* 5:65–82, 1989.

13. Blimkie, C. J., P. Roche, and O. Bar-Or. The anaerobic-to-aerobic power ratio in adolescent boys and girls. In J. Rutenfranz, R. Mocellin, and F. Klimt (eds.), *Children and exercise XII.* Human Kinetics, Champaign, IL, 1986, pp. 3–9.

14. Blimkie, C. J. R., J. Ramsay, D. Sale, D. MacDougall, K. Smith, and S. Garner. Effects of 10 weeks of resistance training on strength development in prepubertal boys. In S. Oseid and K. H, Carlsen (eds.), *International Series on Sport Sciences: Children and exercise XIII.* Human Kinetics, Champaign, IL, 1989, pp. 183–197.

15. Cahill, B. R., and E. H. Griffith. Effect of preseason conditioning on the incidence and severity of high school football knee injuries. *Am. J. Sports Med.* (6)4:180–184, 1978.

16. Caine, D. J. Growth plate injury and bone growth: An update. *Pediatr. Exerc. Sci.* 2:209–229, 1990.

17. Canada Fitness Survey. *Fitness and lifestyles in Canada.* Government of Canada, Fitness and Amateur Sport, Ottawa, Ont.

18. Cureton, K. J., and G. L. Warren. Criterion-referenced standards for youth health-related fitness tests: A tutorial. *Res. Quar. Exerc. Sport* 61:7–19, 1990.

19. Docherty, D., H. A. Wenger, and M. L. Collis. The effects of resistance training on aerobic and anaerobic power in young boys. *Med. Sci. Sports Exerc.* (19):389–392, 1987.

20. Enos, W. F., R. H. Holmes, and J. Beyer. Coronary artery disease among United States soldiers killed in action in Korea. *JAMA* 152:1090–1093, 1953.

21. Gilliam, T. B., V. L. Katch, W. G. Thorland, and A. W. Weltman. Prevalence of coronary heart disease risk factors in active children, 7 to 12 years of age. *Med. Sci. Sports Exerc.* 9(1):21–25, 1977.

22. Gortmaker, S. L., W. H. Dietz, A. M. Sobol, and C.A. Wehler. Increasing pediatric obesity in the United States. *Am. J. Dis. Child.* 141: 535–540, 1987.

23. Grodjinovsky, A., O. Inbar, R. Dotan, and O. Bar-Or. Training effect on the anaerobic performance of children as measured by the Wingate anaerobic test. In K. Berg, and B. Eriksson (eds.), *Children and Exercise International Series on Sports Science.* University Park Press, Baltimore, 1980, 10:139–145.

24. Gumps, V. L., D. Segal, J. B. Halligan, and G. Lower. Bilateral distal radius and ulnar fracture in weightlifting. *Am. J. Sports Med.* 10:375–379, 1982.

25. Hagberg, J. M., A. A. Ehsani, B. Golding, A. Hernandez, D. R. Sinacore, and J. O. Holoszy. Effect of weight training on blood pressure and hemodynamics in hypertensive adolescents. *J. Pediatr.* 104(1):47–151, 1984.

26. Henjia, W. F., A. Rosenberg, D. J. Buturusis, and A. Krieger. Prevention of sports injuries in high school students through strength training. *NSCA J.* 4(1):28–31, 1982.

27. Inbar, O. *Acclimatization to dry and hot environments in young children 8–10 years old.* Doctoral dissertation, Columbia University, New York, 1978.

28. Institute for Aerobic Research. FITNESSGRAM. Dallas, 1987.

29. Kannel, W. B., and T. R. Dawber. Atherosclerosis as a pediatric problem. *J. Pediatr.* 80:544–554, 1972.

30. Khoury, P., J. A. Morrison, K. Kelly, M. Mellies, R. Horvitz, and C. J. Glueck. Clustering and interrelationships of coronary heart disease risk factors in schoolchildren, ages 6 to 19. *Am. J. Epidemiol.* 112(4):524–538, 1980.

31. Lauer, R. M., W. E. Connor, P. E. Leaverton, M. A. Reiter, and W. R. Clarke. Coronary heart disease risk factors in school children: The Muscatine study. *J. Pediatr.* 86(5):697–706, 1975.

32. Lohman, T. G. Advances in body composition assessment. Human Kinetics, Champaign, IL, 1992.

33. Macek, M. Aerobic and anaerobic energy output in children. In J. Rutenfranz, R. Mocellin, and F. Klimt (eds.), *Children and exercise XII,* Human Kinetics, Champaign, Il, 1986, pp. 3–9.

34. Malina, R. M., and C. Brouchard. *Growth, maturation, and physical activity.* Human Kinetics, Champaign, IL: 1991.

35. Mellies, M. J., P. M. Laskarzewski, T. Tracy, and C. J. Glueck. Tracking of high- and low-density-liproprotein cholesterol from childhood to young adulthood in a single large kindred with familial hypercholesterolemia. *Metabolism* 34:747–753, 1985.

36. McMillan, G. C. Development of arteriosclerosis. *Am. J. Cardiol.* 31:542–546, 1973.

37. McNamara, J. J., M. A. Molot, J. F. Stremple, and R. T. Cutting. Coronary artery disease in combat casualties in Vietnam. *JAMA* 216:1185–1187.

38. Meredith, M.D. *FITNESSGRAM user's manual.* Institute for Aerobics Research, Dallas, 1987.

39. Micheli, L. J. Strength training in the young athlete. In E. W. Brown, and C. F. Crystal (eds.), *Competitive sports for children and youth: An overview of research and issues.* Human Kinetics, Champaign, IL, 1988, pp. 99–106.

40. National Strength and Conditioning Association. Position paper on pre-pubescent strength training. *Nat. Strength Condition. Assoc. J.* 7:27–29, 1985.

41. Newman, W. P., et al. Relation of serum lipoprotein levels and systolic blood pressure to early atherosclerosis. *N. Eng. J. Med.* 314: 138–144, 1986.

42. Nielsen, B., K. Nielsen, M. Brhendt Hansen and A. Asmussen. Training of function muscular strength in girls 7–19 years old. In K. Berg and B.K. Erikson (eds.), *Children and exercise.* University Park Press, Baltimore, 1980, 9:69–78.

43. Pate, R. R., and J. G. Ross. Factors associated with health related fitness. *J. Phys. Educ. Rec. Dance* 58(9):93–95, 1987.

44. Pate, R. R., J. G. Ross, T. A. Baumgartner, and R. E. Sparks. The modified pull-up test. *J. Phys. Educ. Rec. Dance* November/December:72, 1987.

45. Pate, R. R. and R. J. Shephard. Characteristics of physical fitness in youth. In C. V. Gisolfi, and D. R. Lamb (eds.),

REFERENCES

Perspectives in exercise science and sports medicine. Benchmark Press, Carmel, IN, 1989, pp. 1–46.

46. Pate, R. R., and D. S. Ward. Endurance exercise trainability in children and youth. In W. A. Grana, J. A. Lombarade, B. J. Sharkey, and J. A. Stone (eds.), *Advances in sports medicine and fitness.* Year Book, Chicago, 1990, pp. 37–55.

47. Pate, R. R., M. L. Burgess, J. A. Woods, J. G. Ross, and T. Baumgartner. Validity of field tests of upper-body muscular strength. *Res. Quar. Exerc. Sport* 64(1):18, 1993.

48. Payne, G. V., and J. R. Morrow. Exercise and VO₂max in children: A meta-analysis. *Res. Quar. Exerc. Sport* 64(3):305–313, 1993.

49. Queary, J. L., and L. L. Laubach. The effects of muscular strength/endurance training. *Technique* 12:9–11, 1992.

50. Reiff, G. G., W. R. Dixon, D. Jacoby, X. G. Ye, C. G. Spain, and P. A. Hunsicker. President's Council on Physical Fitness and Sports, *National school population fitness survey.* Research Project 282–84–0086, University of Michigan, Ann Arbor, 1985.

51. Risser, W. L., J. M. H. Risser, and D. Preston. Weight-training injuries in adolescents. *Am. J. Dis. Child.* 144(9):1015–1017, 1990.

52. Robinson, T. N., et al. Does television viewing increase obesity and reduce physical activity? Cross-sectional and longitudinal analysis among adolescent girls. *Pediatrics* 91(2):273–279, 1993.

53. Ross, J. G., and G. G. Gilbert. The National Children and Youth Fitness Survey: A summary of the findings. *J. Phys. Educ. Rec. Dance* 56(1):45–50, 1985.

54. Ross, J. G. and R. R. Pate. The National Children and Youth Fitness Survey II: A summary of the findings. *J. Phys. Educ. Rec. Dance* 58(9):51–56, 1987.

55. Ross, J. G., R. R. Pate, T. G. Lohman, and G. M. Christenson. Changes in the body composition of children: Summary of findings from the National Children and Youth Fitness Study II. *J. Phys. Educ. Rec. Dance* November/December: 77, 1987.

56. Rotstein, A, R. Dotan, and O. Bar-Or. Effect of training on anaerobic threshold, maximal aerobic power and anaerobic performance of preadolescent boys. *Int. J. Sports Med.* 7:281–286, 1986.

57. Rowland, T. W. Aerobic responses to endurance training in prepubescent children: A critical analysis. *Med. Sci. Sports Exerc.* 17:493–497, 1985.

58. Ryan, J. R, and G. G. Salciccioli. Fracture of the distal radial epiphysis in adolescent weight lifters. *Am. J. Sports Med.* 4:26–27, 1976.

59. Siegel, J. Fitness in prepubescent children: Implications for exercise training. *Natl. Strength Condition Assoc. J.* 10(3), 43–48, 1988.

60. Siegel, J. A., D. N. Camaione, and T. G. Manfredi. The effects of upper body resistance training on prepubescent children. *Pediatr. Exerc. Sci.* 1:145–154, 1989.

61. Sinclari, D. *Human growth after birth,* 4th ed. Oxford University Press, New York, 1985, p. 14.

62. Vrijens, J. Muscle strength development in the pre- and post-pubescent age. *Med. Sport* 11:157–161, 1978.

63. Wells, C. L. The effects of physical activity on cardiorespiratory fitness in children. In G. A. Stull, and H. M. Eckert (eds.), *American Academy of Physical Education papers.* Human Kinetics, Champaign, IL, 1986, pp. 114–126.

64. Weltman, A., et al. The effects of hydraulic resistance strength training in pre-pubescent males. *Med. Sci. Sports Exerc.* (18):629–638, 1986.

65. Wilkins, K. E. The uniqueness of the young athlete: Musculoskeletal injuries. *Am. J. Sports Med.* 8:377–382, 1980.

66. Wilmore, J. H., and J. J. McNamara. Prevalence of coronary disease risk factors in boys, 8 to 12 years of age. *J. Pediatr.* 84:527–533, 1974.

67. Woynarowska, B., D. Mukherjee, A. F. Roche, and R. M. Siervogel. Blood pressure changes during adolescence and subsequent adult blood pressure levels. *Hypertension* 7:695–701, 1985.

RECOMMENDED READINGS

Rowland, T. *Developmental exercise physiology.* Human Kinetics, Champaign, IL, 1996.

Roberts, S. O., and B. Weider. *Strength and weight training for young athletes.* Contemporary Books, Chicago, 1993.

Exercise and Aging

hrough exercise, proper care, and regular check-ups, people are now living longer and more productive lives. Individuals who are worried about the gradual decline in their health and physical capabilities typically associated with the aging process need to become more active! Reports have indicated that athletically and nutritionally fit individuals can be as many as 10 to 20 biological years younger than their true chronological age. Anti-aging gimmicks are prevalent in the U.S. Unfortunately there is no fountain of youth or magic anti-aging pill. However, exercise appears to be the closest thing to an antiaging pill known. Current exercise guidelines encourage older individuals to participate in exercise that strengthens and improves not only the cardiovascular system, but also the musculoskeletal system. Today individuals in their 70s, 80s, and even 90s perform weekly strength training exercises to increase bone density and muscle strength. In fact, some studies have seen an increase of 200 to 300 percent in muscle function in this population! Exercise is an important endeavor throughout the life span. The enormous increase in the older segments of our population have given rise to tremendous opportunities for further research in this area and employment opportunities for fitness professionals.

OBJECTIVES

After studying this chapter, you should be able to:

- Explain how normal aging affects physiological systems.
- List specific recommendations for exercise testing and training for aging individuals.
- Explain the difference between chronological and biological aging, and the effect exercise has on both.
- Describe important health promotion strategies for elderly people.
- Describe appropriate exercise guidelines for individuals with arthritis and osteoporosis.

KEY TERMS

natural life span
life expectancy
healthy life
quality of life

longevity
aging
chronological age
biological age

osteoporosis
osteoarthritis
rheumatoid arthritis

Defining Aging

*A*ging is not merely the passage of time, but rather the manifestation of biological events that occur over a span of time. There is no perfect definition of aging. Aging should not be viewed as a sickness, but as a natural process. Everything on this planet ages to some degree with time, not just human beings. The human life span is the maximum possible length of life that a member of the human species can reach under optimal conditions. As premature death has been reduced in this century, an increasing proportion of the population has lived through the **natural life span,** which is suggested to be around the age of 85.

Life Expectancy in the United States

How long should people live? This is a question that has been asked for centuries and will continue to generate interest and debate. **Life expectancy** is the average, statistically predicted, length of life for an individual. Today, the life expectancy for the majority of men in developed countries is about 71 years, and about 78 years for women. In the near future, it has been estimated that as many as 50% of all deaths will occur after the age of 80. Modern medicine and health promotion activities have helped increase the life span of people.

One of the most serious problems facing all Americans is how to continue to provide quality health care to an ever-increasing elderly population. It has been estimated that health care costs for institutionalized elderly alone for 1990 was $75 billion (22). One possible way to reduce these costs is to keep the aging population as healthy as possible. Another important measure is length of **healthy life.** Although people aged 65 and older have 16.4 years of life remaining on average, they have only about 12 years of healthy life remaining (12). Thus health promotion activities should not be excluded from this population.

Another measure is the **quality of life.** This includes an individual's ability to perform activities of daily living (ADLs), such as walking, bathing, dressing, and eating. The ability to perform ADLs decreases with age. It is clear however, that individuals can lead long, quality lives, but they need to do all of the things adults need to do to stay healthy (exercise, eat right, not smoke, etc).

Increasing Life Expectancy

Longevity is defined in the *Random House Dictionary* as "a long duration of life." How long an individual lives depends on a variety of factors, some include heredity, environmental factors, availability of good medical and health services, and individual responsibility for health maintenance. To date, a fountain of youth has not been discovered. Perhaps the only fountain of youth we can rely on at the present time is the research supporting the health-related benefits of proper nutrition, moderate use of alcohol, use of seat belts, not drinking and driving, and regular exercise.

Aging is unfortunately associated with disease and disability. Most humans today ultimately die from cancer and heart disease. Even though certain physiological changes are inevitable with aging, it appears that the rate of decline from the effects of aging *can* be reduced. Because the majority of people over the age of 65 die from heart disease, cancer, and stroke, preventive strategies initiated even later in adult life may help improve the "quality" of elderly people. It is becoming increasingly clear that regular, "lifelong" physical activity is an important component of preventive health strategies.

Understanding Aging

Aging is a normal biological process. All multicellular organisms undergo changes with time. Aging has been defined as a progressive loss of physiological capacities that eventually culminates in death. Most physiological functions decline with age, but to different extents. The causes of human aging still remain relatively unclear. It appears that aging results from both internal and external forces. In some organs such as the brain, cells die and are not replaced. In other tissues, the cell function changes; for example, cross-linkages develop between adjacent collagen fibrils, decreasing elasticity and facilitating mechanical injury of the affected tissue. Blood vessels become progressively affected by atherosclerosis and arteriosclerosis, thereby decreasing oxygen supply to all body organs. Regardless of the many different causes of aging, death occurs from an infection or environmental stress that cannot be tolerated by an older individual. Aging may simply be due to the wearing out of nonreplaceable body components, such as teeth and kidney function. Finally, it appears that there is really nothing that can be done to prevent aging, and that the rate and effects of aging vary among individuals.

Altering the Aging Process

Have you ever noticed how some people tend to look much older than their age, and others tend to look much younger than their age? In order to better understand this phenomenon, it is important to look at two different ways to categorize age. **Chronological age** can be divided into young, middle, and old age. Birthdays typically chronicle one's age. **Biological age** is assessed by variables such as maximal oxygen uptake, muscle strength, or flexibility. Thus, whereas someone may be 65 years of age, he or she may have a biological age of 45 based on his or her fitness and health status. The im-

FIGURE 18.1

FIGURE 18.1

Decreases in the function of several important physiological functions with increasing age.

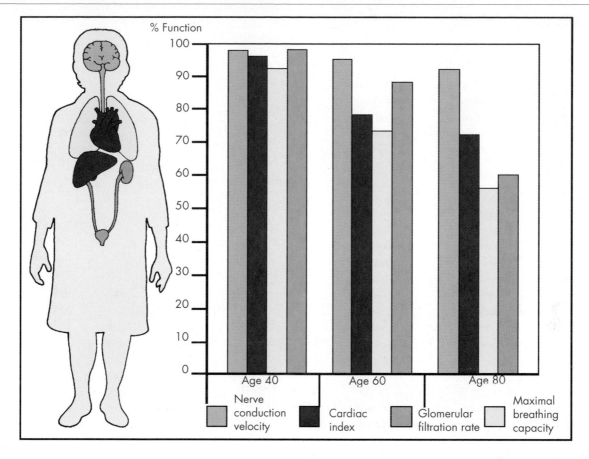

portance of regular exercise and health promotion cannot be emphasized enough when looking at the association of chronological versus biological age. Biological age may be altered by maintaining a regular physical fitness program.

Normal Physiological Changes with Aging and the Effects of Exercise

Figure 18.1 describes some of the changes that occur in all organ systems with age. Table 18.1 lists some of the effects of exercise and aging on selected body systems. To what extent these changes are affected by exercise is not completely understood.

Cardiovascular Changes with Age

It is difficult to separate the effects of aging alone on the cardiovascular system. Deconditioning and disease also play a significant role in changes in the cardiovascular system over time. Both structural and functional changes occur to the cardiovascular system with increasing age. Both functional

natural life span the estimated biological life span an individual should expect to achieve, which is suggested to be around the age of 85

life expectancy the average, statistically predicted, length of life for an individual; the life expectancy for the majority of men in developed countries is about 71 years, and about 78 years for women

healthy life the amount of healthy life an individual has left before death; people aged 65 and older have 16.4 years of life remaining on average, including about 12 years of healthy life remaining

quality of life an individual's ability to perform daily activities (ADLs) such as walking, bathing, dressing, and eating

longevity a long duration of life; how long an individual lives depends on a variety of factors including heredity, environmental factors, availability of good medical and health services, and individual responsibility for health maintenance

aging a progressive loss of physiological capacities that eventually culminates in death.

chronological age can be divided into young, middle, and old age; birthdays typically chronicle one's age

biological age assessed by variables such as maximal oxygen uptake, muscle strength, or flexibility

TABLE 18.1

Effects of exercise and aging on select body systems

BODY SYSTEM	EXERCISE	AGING
Circulatory		
Cardiovascular		
Maximal oxygen consumption	Increase	Decrease
Maximal heart rate	Increase	Decrease
Cardiac output	Increase	Decrease
Blood pressure	Same or decrease	Increase
Vascular resistance	Decrease	Increase
Blood Components		
Serum lipids		
Total cholesterol	?*	Increase
Triglycerides	Decrease	Increase
LDL cholesterol	?	Increase?
HDL cholesterol	Increase	Decrease?
Immune system	Increase	Decrease
Musculoskeletal		
Muscles		
Strength	Increase	Decrease
Endurance	Increase	Unchanged
Flexibility	Increase	Decrease
Bony structures		
Bone mineral content	Increase	Decrease
Body composition		
Lean body mass	Increase	Decrease
Adipose tissue	Decrease	Increase
Regulatory Systems		
Metabolic		
Basal Metabolic Rate	Increase	Decrease
Heat gain	Increase	Decrease
Heat loss	Increase	Decrease
Nervous		
Sleep	Increase?	Decrease
Anxiety/depression	Decrease?	Increase?
Cognitive functioning	Increase	Decrease

*? = Inconclusive or inadequate evidence.

TABLE 18.2

Changes in cardiovascular function with increasing physiological age

Structural Changes	
Left ventricular size	Increases
Contraction and relaxation times	Increases
Left ventricular function	Decreases
Cardiac valve function	Decreases
Electrical conduction system function	Slows
Elasticity of the arteries	Decreases
Blood vessels	Increase and dilate
Artery walls	Thickens
Resting Functional Changes	
Resting heart rate	No change
Blood pressure	Increases
Myocardial compliance	Decreases
Systolic function	Decreases
Diastolic function	Decreases
Stroke volume	Decreases
Cardiac output	Decreases
Oxygen consumption	Decreases
A-aO$_2$ difference	Increases
Effects of Cardiac Changes During Exercise	
VO$_{2max}$	Decreases
a-vO$_2$ difference	Narrowed
Peak HR	Lower
Ejection fraction	Less increase
End-diastolic volume	Decreases

and structural changes result in relatively minor changes in cardiovascular function at rest, but significant differences in circulatory responses to exercise. Table 18.2 lists some of the physiological age changes in cardiovascular function and structure.

Maximal Oxygen Uptake

With normal aging, maximal oxygen uptake (VO$_{2max}$) declines approximately 8 to 10% per decade after age 30 (18) (fig. 18.2). To determine the effect of exercise on loss of maximal oxygen uptake and aging, researchers followed a group of men (aged 44 to 79) who exercised on a regular ba-

sis for a period of 25 years (7). During this time the subjects reported the amount of exercise they did monthly and had their maximal oxygen uptake tested on a regular basis. At the end of the study, it was found that the total group's cardiovascular function was one-half the average loss in maximal oxygen consumption 0.24 mL/min/kg body weight per year compared to 0.45 mL/min/kg body weight per year. These individuals had 60% greater maximal oxygen capacity compared to predicted values for similar ages.

The decline in maximal oxygen uptake has been associated with a decrease in maximal heart rate and stroke volume (thus a decrease in maximal cardiac output), with only a slight decrease in a-vO$_2$ difference. Figure 18.3 shows the relation between aging changes in the cardiorespiratory system and reduced exercise capacity. It is clear however, that aerobic capacity can be improved at any age. One study involved a group of 30 elderly women (mean age 73.6 years) who walked 5 days per week for 30 to 40 min per session at 60% of their heart rate reserve and demonstrated a 12.6% increase in maximal oxygen uptake, compared to a matched control group (26). A 6-month walking program (heart rate < 120 bpm) increased VO$_{2max}$ by an average of 12%, whereas high-intensity training (75% of heart rate reserve) improved VO$_{2max}$ by 18% in 63-year-olds (20). Reduction in aerobic capacity during aging can be altered by exercise training.

FIGURE 18.2

Declining cardiovascular functions are the main contributors to decreases in exercise performance in the elderly.

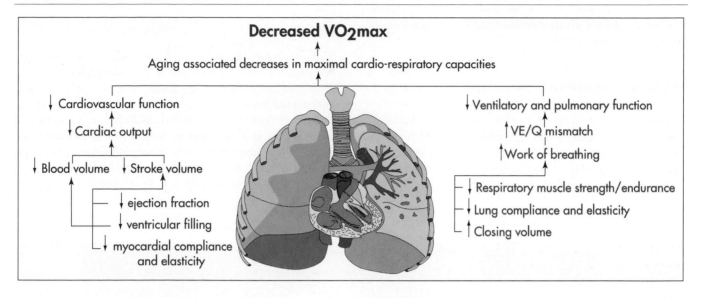

Decreased VO₂max

Aging associated decreases in maximal cardio-respiratory capacities

↓ Cardiovascular function

↓ Cardiac output

↓ Blood volume   ↓ Stroke volume

↓ ejection fraction

↓ ventricular filling

↓ myocardial compliance and elasticity

↓ Ventilatory and pulmonary function

↑ VE/Q mismatch

↑ Work of breathing

↓ Respiratory muscle strength/endurance

↓ Lung compliance and elasticity

↑ Closing volume

FIGURE 18.3

Representations of the relative amount of bone mineral in different populations. The 0% reference line is based on the peak bone mineral content of an adolescent male.

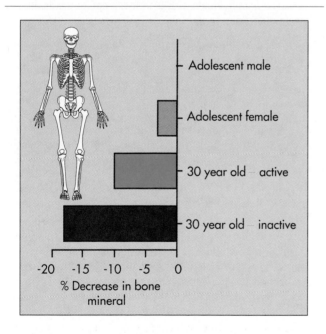

Adolescent male

Adolescent female

30 year old — active

30 year old — inactive

-20   -15   -10   -5   0
% Decrease in bone mineral

TABLE 18.3

Structural and functional changes to the pulmonary system with age

Structural Changes	
Alveolar elastic recoil	Decreases
Respiratory muscle strength	Decreases
Alveolar surface area	Decreases
Pulmonary blood volume	Decreases
Residual lung volume	Increases
Functional Changes	
Maximal ventilation (VE)	Decreases
Ventilatory equivalent (VE/VO₂)	Increases
Expiratory flow rate	Decreases
Forced expiratory volume (1 s)	Decreases
Maximal voluntary ventilation	Decreases
Vital capacity	Decreases
Residual lung volume	Increases
Alveoli and alveolar ducts	Increase in size

Pulmonary Changes with Age

Aging also causes significant changes in the structure and function of the pulmonary system. Individuals can be limited in their ability to participate in moderate to strenuous physical activity because of limitations in their pulmonary system, cardiovascular system, or a combination. Table 18.3 lists some of the structural and functional changes to the pulmonary system with age.

The changes in lung function obviously make it harder for older individuals to move air in and out of the lungs. During exercise, ventilation differs between young and old individuals. At low workloads older persons tend to increase ventilation by increasing tidal volume, rather than breathing frequency. In older individuals, the increase in tidal volume may serve as a compensatory mechanism. High lung volumes decrease the resistance to inspiratory flow and improve elastic recoil. The increased elastic recoil improves expiratory flow. With aging, the ventilatory requirements during activities increases. A greater ventilation is needed for a given workload and for a given level of oxygen consumption (23).

Musculoskeletal System

Of perhaps greater concern to older individuals than age-related changes in cardiovascular and pulmonary function, are the age-related changes that occur to the musculoskeletal system. The loss of bone and muscle strength often lead to serious and life-threatening injuries. Many of the age-related changes that occur in the musculoskeletal system are the result of physical inactivity.

Bones

With age, bones become more fragile. Serious and often debilitating fractures are common in the elderly. By the age of 90 as many as 32% of women and 17% of men will have sustained a hip fracture, and between 12 and 20% of this group will die of related complications. With age, the loss of calcium results in a decrease in bone mass. Bone mass decreases by approximately 10% from peak bone mass to age 65, and by 20% by age 80. In women the loss is higher, amounting to approximately 20% by 65 and 30% by age 80.

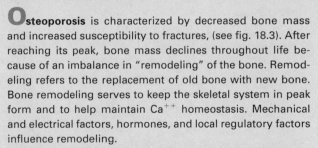

FOCUS BOX 18.1

Osteoporosis

Osteoporosis is characterized by decreased bone mass and increased susceptibility to fractures, (see fig. 18.3). After reaching its peak, bone mass declines throughout life because of an imbalance in "remodeling" of the bone. Remodeling refers to the replacement of old bone with new bone. Bone remodeling serves to keep the skeletal system in peak form and to help maintain Ca^{++} homeostasis. Mechanical and electrical factors, hormones, and local regulatory factors influence remodeling.

Osteoporosis is a major public health problem. The treatment for osteoporosis tries to prevent or retard bone mineral loss. In recent years, scientists have identified several measures that may help reduce the toll of osteoporosis. Estrogen replacement is the only one of these measures in which there is well-documented evidence of its effectiveness in the prevention of fractures from osteoporosis. Although complete proof is lacking that the other measures—such as increased calcium intake—prevent bone loss leading to fractures, many believe that current data are sufficient to suggest that these measures be adopted. New guidelines (August 1997) from the Food and Nutrition Board of the National Academy of Science suggest that calcium needs differ depending on age. In general, adults ages 19 to 50 should get at least 1000 mg a day to maximize "peak bone mass," according to the guidelines. Weight-bearing exercises—walking, jogging, weight training—are thought best for strengthening bones. But at least one study has shown that swimming—a non-weight-bearing exercise—also helped a group of women build bone mass. Exercise also builds muscle strength and agility, which can reduce the risk of falls and fractures. It's important, however, for anyone who has already suffered a fracture to begin a rehabilitation and exercise program in consultation with a physician.

Exercise Guidelines
The greater the physical stress and compression on a bone, the greater the rate of bone deposition (this is why weight-bearing exercise is recommended). Because most individuals who suffer from osteoporosis are elderly, the reader is directed to the exercise guidelines and recommendations for the elderly listed later in this chapter. Additionally, resistance training is an important component in the prevention of osteoporosis. For individuals with diagnosed osteoporosis, the following guidelines apply:

   No jumping, high-impact jogging, running, jarring
   No spinal flexion, crunches, rowing machines
   No trampolines, step aerobics
   No wood gym floors that may get slippery from
    sweat drops
   No abduction/adduction—legs against resistance
    (machines especially)
   No movement of leg sideways or across body
   No pulling on neck when hands are behind head

Case Study
History
Alice is a 58-year-old accountant. She has recently been diagnosed with early onset osteoporosis. She does not currently exercise. She has modified her diet and is taking calcium supplements and estrogen replacement therapy. She was a former smoker, having quit 1 year ago. As the vice president of her company she has very little time to exercise.

Goals
Prevent her disorder from progressing, make her bones stronger, and increase her functional capacity.

Exercise Recommendations
Walking, swimming, or cycling. Intensity, duration, and frequency based on fitness assessment or treadmill test. Comprehensive resistance training and flexibility program also highly recommended. Tailor the workout to accommodate her schedule so that she will stick with the program.

Men tend to lose bone mass by about 1% per year after the age of 50, whereas women begin to lose bone mass in their early 30s with a 2 to 3% decline per year after menopause. Researchers have found that older women (50 to 73 years of age) who exercised for 1 h twice weekly for 8 months increased their bone mineral content by 3.5%, whereas the sedentary controls of similar age lost 2.7% during the same period (8a). Regular physical activity and resistance training appear to have beneficial effects on the rate of age-related bone loss (21) (see focus box 18.1).

Skeletal Muscle

Muscle mass declines with age, resulting in decreased muscle strength and endurance. Muscular strength begins to decline around age 40 with an accelerated decline after age 60. For each decade after the age of 25, 3 to 5% of muscle mass is lost. Muscle force and grip strength decrease significantly with age. After age 74, 28% of men and 66% of women may not be able to lift objects weighing more than 4.5 kg (5). The loss of muscle strength in elderly people can significantly affect the quality and length of life. Simple chores such as taking out the trash or making the bed can be terribly taxing in elderly individuals. The loss of muscle mass has been attributed to changes in lifestyle and the decreased use of the neuromuscular system.

Can Elderly People Gain Strength?

The answer is yes! Significant strength gains are possible in the elderly. The result from a 1988 study performed at Tufts University found that in a group of 60- to 72-year-old untrained men, participating in 12 weeks of strength training (8 repetitions/set, 3 sets/day, 3 days/week at 80% of their 1 RM), there was a 107% increase in knee extensor strength and a 227% increase in knee flexor strength following 12 weeks of training (5). This study demonstrated that strength gains do occur in older men, and these gains are associated with significant muscle hypertrophy and muscle protein turnover. A low-intensity exercise program in 60- to 71-year-old men and women has been shown to significantly improve strength, balance, and flexibility (2). Fiatarone and Evans found that 100 frail men and women in their 80s and 90s, all of whom had at least one chronic illness, improved their weight lifting capacity by 118 percent in a 10-week strength training program (28). In addition to improved strength, their walking speed increased by 12% and their ability to climb stairs by 28%. The researchers of this study state, "Muscle-training can prevent loss of independence and prevent people from becoming chair- or bed-bound."

Flexibility

With normal aging, connective tissue becomes stiffer, and joints become less mobile. Loss of flexibility with age may also be the result of underlying degenerative disease processes such as arthritis. Flexibility does decrease with age; however, there is no evidence that the biological processes associated with aging are responsible for this loss. Loss of flexibility is more likely the result of diminishing physical activity. Flexibility can be improved at any age through exercises that promote the elasticity of the soft tissues. Researchers have recently demonstrated that flexibility can be significantly improved in 57- to 85-year-old women following an exercise program that included static stretching and range-of-motion exercises (17).

What Is Arthritis?

Although there are different forms of arthritis, the most common forms are rheumatoid and osteoarthritis. **Osteoarthritis**, also referred to as *degenerative joint disease*, is a degenerative process caused by the wearing away of cartilage, leaving two surfaces of bone in contact with each other. Osteoarthritis is very common in older individuals, affecting 85% of all people in the United States over the age of 70. **Rheumatoid arthritis** is caused by an inflammation of the membrane surrounding joints. It is often associated with pain and swelling in one or more joints. Rheumatoid arthritis affects about 3% of all women and 1% of all men in the United States. See table 18.4 and focus box 18.2.

TABLE 18.4	
Classification of functional capacity for arthritis	
Class 1:	Complete ability to carry on all usual duties without handicaps
Class 2:	Adequate ability for normal activities despite handicap, discomfort, or limited motion at one or more joints
Class 3:	Ability limited to little or none of the duties of usual occupational or to self-care
Class 4:	Incapacitated, largely or wholly; bedridden or confined to a wheelchair; little or no self-care

osteoporosis characterized by decreased bone mass and increased susceptibility to fractures; primarily caused by decreased bone mass, which increases the susceptibility to fractures

osteoarthritis also referred to as degenerative joint disease; a degenerative process caused by the wearing away of cartilage leaving two surfaces of bone in contact with each other

rheumatoid arthritis caused by an inflammation of the membrane surrounding joints; often associated with pain and swelling in one or more joints

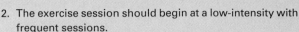

FOCUS BOX 18.2

Arthritis

Exercise is recommended for clients with arthritis to help preserve muscle strength and joint mobility, to improve functional capabilities, to relieve pain and stiffness, to prevent further deformities, to improve overall physical conditioning, to reestablish neuromuscular coordination, and to mobilize stiff or contracted joints. Fitness programs should be carefully designed in conjunction with a physician or physical therapist. The exercise prescription needs to be developed on the basis of the functional status of the individual. For example, someone in functional class I should be able to perform most activities that a typical healthy person can. For those in functional class II, initially non-weight-bearing activities are recommended, such as cycling, warm-water exercise, and eventually walking. Individuals in functional class 3 should benefit from a cycling or warm-water aquatic program. Exercise should be avoided during an acute arthritic flare.

Arthritic individuals often report fatigue and some discomfort as common complaints following exercise. Exercise programs need to balance rest, immobilization of affected joints, and exercise to reduce the severity of the inflammatory joint disease.

The American College of Rheumatology (www.rheumatology.org) offers the following advice on exercise and arthritis.

Research shows that many people with arthritis can safely participate in appropriate, regular exercise programs and achieve better aerobic fitness. Low impact exercises, such as swimming and water aerobics, may be particularly well-tolerated by people with arthritis. Improved strength, endurance and flexibility, and better ability to walk or perform daily tasks are all benefits of exercise. A comprehensive exercise program for a person with arthritis includes flexibility, strengthening and aerobic activities. The content and progression of the program depends upon individual needs and capabilities. Persons with long-standing or severe disease or multiple joint involvement should undertake exercise in collaboration with the health care team. The most successful exercise programs begin with the knowledge and support of people like rheumatologists who are experienced with both arthritis and exercise. Your local Arthritis Foundation is an additional source of information on local exercise programs for arthritis patients.

Exercise Guidelines

1. Individuals with arthritis should be encouraged to participate in activities where quick or excessive movement can be avoided, such as low-impact exercise, stationary cycling, rowing, and water exercise classes.

2. The exercise session should begin at a low-intensity with frequent sessions.

3. Exercise intensity and duration should be reduced during periods of inflammation or pain.

4. Arthritic individuals may need an extended warm-up and cool-down period.

5. The exercise session should be modified in terms of intensity and duration according to how well the client responds to the exercise, changes in medication, and the disease and pain levels.

6. Try to tailor the ROM movements to focus on the arthritic joints.

7. Have the individual take a day or two of rest if he or she continues to complain about pain during or following an exercise session. Use a 2-h pain rule to adjust exercise levels.

8. Arthritic individuals are encouraged to participate in different forms of aerobic exercise such as swimming, cycling, and walking.

9. Proper body alignment during exercise is important.

10. Poor posture plus decreased joint mobility and strength disrupt the performance of efficient, controlled, and integrated movement. Misaligned body positions and awkward movement affect walking gait, increase energy expenditure, and increase fatigue.

11. Pain is quite normal in people with arthritis. Individuals should be instructed to work just up to the point of pain, but not past it. Simple movements for healthy people can be quite painful for individuals with arthritis.

12. Use isometric strengthening exercises. These strengthen the joint structures and surrounding muscles while placing the least amount of stress on the joint itself.

13. It is essential to put all joints through a range of motion at least once a day to maintain mobility.

14. Arthritic individuals need to report any changes in their medications, medical plan, or response to exercise.

15. Individuals with rheumatoid arthritis should not exercise during periods of inflammation.

16. Proper body mechanics should always be taught and reinforced.

17. Regular rest periods should be stressed during exercise sessions.

18. If severe pain persists following exercise, have the client consult with the physician.

19. Remember that arthritic clients may be more limited by joint pain than by cardiovascular function.

Body Composition

Lean body weight declines and body fat increases with age (fig. 18.4). The changes in body composition resulting from age are primarily due to a decrease in the basal metabolic rate and physical activity habits of the elderly. On average, there is a 10% reduction in basal metabolic rate between early adulthood to retirement age, and a further 10% decrease after that (11). The reduction in basal metabolic rate with age is probably the main factor related to the de-

FIGURE 18.4

Changes in total body protein with increasing age in men and women.

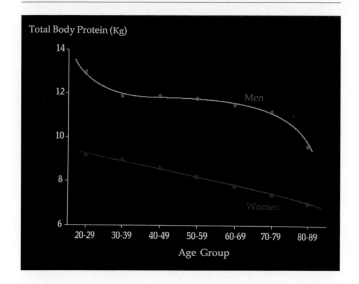

jects, the decreased thermal regulatory capacity in the heat is probably the result of a less efficient sweating mechanism. Older persons generally have less body water and a reduced thirst mechanism, together increasing their risk for dehydration during exercise (3). Older individuals should be encouraged to gradually acclimatize to different environmental conditions, because the acclimatization process may take longer.

Exercise Testing Considerations for the Elderly

Before starting an exercise program, elderly individuals should first see their physicians. Although many of the principles of prescribing exercise to the elderly are the same for any group, special care should be given when setting up a fitness program for older participants. A preexercise evaluation may involve a complete medical history, physical, and treadmill test. The results of the treadmill test can be used to develop the exercise prescription.

Exercise Prescription Considerations for the Elderly

Although the principles of exercise design for the elderly are similar for any group, special care should be given when setting up a fitness program for older participants. Focus box 18.3 lists important considerations when setting up an exercise prescription for elderly clients. For most elderly patients, low-impact exercise is advisable. Exercise programs should be tailored to combine endurance, muscle strength, and joint mobilization in the exercise sessions. Older individuals should be encouraged to become more physically active in all of their daily activities (use the stairs, walk to the store, etc.). Older individuals should be encouraged to bend, move, and stretch in order to keep joints flexible.

According to the American College of Sports Medicine, the goals for exercise in the elderly should include:

. . . maintenance of functional capacity for independent living, reduction in the risk of cardiovascular disease, retardation of the progression of chronic diseases, promotion of psychological well-being, and provision of opportunities for social interaction.

Intensity

The intensity of the exercise program should start out low, perhaps as low as 30 to 40% of VO_{2max}. Because low-intensity exercise is associated with lower risk of injury and initial cardiorespiratory and thermoregulatory stress, it should be encouraged in the elderly population. Elderly individuals should know how to monitor their intensity levels (i.e.,

cline in lean body mass. It has been estimated that muscle mass loss can be as high as 10 to 12% with advancing age (1). The dramatic changes in body composition with age are also due to changes in overall body weight. A loss of 9 kg of muscle mass combined with an increase in 3.4 kg of body fat has been demonstrated in men in their eighth decade compared to men in their fifth decade (24). By age 75, the typical composition is 8% bone, 15% muscle, and 40% adipose tissue (19).

It has been demonstrated that regular physical activity reverses the adverse changes in body composition typically experienced by most elderly individuals. Exercise has been shown to preserve lean body mass, decrease fat stores, and stimulate protein synthesis (9). Lean body mass has been shown to be maintained until age 65 in middle-aged and older athletes (7). In one research study looking at the influence of age and endurance training on metabolic rate, researchers found a higher resting metabolic rate (6%), normalized per kilogram of fat-free weight, in endurance-trained older men compared to untrained men (16). Other researchers have found similar results.

Thermoregulation

Older individuals appear to have a less efficient thermal control system. Both heat gain and heat loss are not as effective in older individuals. There are higher mortality and morbidity rates for heat-related illness in the elderly, compared to younger populations (4). Older subjects tend to have higher rectal temperatures and heart rates when exercising in the heat compared to younger subjects (25). In sedentary sub-

FOCUS BOX 18.3

Exercise Guidelines for Seniors

■ The pace of all movement should be slow to moderate. For choreographed routines, steps should be simple and repeated often. Fast transitions from one type of movement to another should be avoided to prevent postural hypotension and subsequent dizziness, falling, or fainting.

■ Several modes and positions of exercise should be used. Some positions include standing, sitting, standing with a chair for balance, and floor exercise using a mat. Before initiating floor exercise, feedback should be solicited from the group on whether the exercise is desirable. Some adults feel awkward or embarrassed if they have difficulty getting up from the floor in front of their peers. Instruction in how to get up from the floor may be necessary.

■ A variety of equipment should be used to achieve program objectives and sustain motivation. Examples include wands or dowels, surgical tubing, and towels or rubber strips for flexibility and range of motion; Frisbees and low walking beams for balance and coordination; and 1-lb. weights for strength.

■ The pressor reflex should be avoided by keeping the overhead position of the arms to a minimum.

■ Special precautions should be taken for all participants who take medications. These include cardiovascular drugs, such as beta-blockers, calcium-channel blockers, and diuretics, which affect exercise tolerance. Hypoten-

sion may develop if a participant exercises soon after taking nitroglycerin. The dose, type, and time of administration of insulin may need to be changed to prevent hypoglycemia. Medical approval and ongoing medical consultation for persons taking prescription drugs are recommended.

■ The exertion level of all participants should be continually monitored. Heart rate monitoring using the radial or carotid pulse should be taught. Permission to rest and get a drink of water should be given throughout the exercise class. Participants should be told frequently to progress at their own rate.

■ In addition to the instructor, one additional staff member should always be present to observe participants' physical reactions and to assist with any major or minor emergency.

■ The use of layered clothing should be suggested to prevent overheating or cooling. Older adults are less tolerant of the heat and cold.

■ A microphone should be used when conducting a program in a large area if the acoustics are poor. Lower tones can be more readily heard by the older adult.

■ For charts that will be viewed from a distance, such colors as yellow, orange, and red are seen more clearly.

■ The instructor should be certified in CPR and a well-defined and routinely practiced procedure for emergencies should exist.

breathing rate, heart rate or RPE). Elderly subjects may need a longer period of adjustment before exercising at higher-intensity levels. Abrupt changes in exercise intensity are not recommended. Elderly people are more prone to exercise-related injuries, and they tend to need more time to recover compared to younger participants.

Duration

The duration of an exercise program should start out with short (10 to 15 min periods) and gradually progress from there. In addition to the duration of the exercise program itself, elderly people need additional warm-up and cool-down time, perhaps as much as 10 min or more. As the intensity of the exercise sessions increase gradually over time, the duration of each exercise session can increase.

Frequency

In many cases, such as with persons who have arthritis or peripheral vascular disease, frequency of exercise training may be daily. Because many individuals can exercise only

for short periods at a time because of structural and functional limitations, exercise training sessions will have to be shorter and less intense, and thus more frequent. As functional capacity improves, the duration and intensity of exercise training session can be increased, and the frequency reduced.

Type

A comprehensive fitness program, including cardiorespiratory, flexibility, and strength training is recommended. However, the type of exercise may need to be modified, depending on preexisting medical and/or health conditions. For example, for elderly individuals with degenerative joint disease, non-weight-bearing activities such as stationary cycling, water exercises, and chair exercises should be recommended. Individuals with orthostatic hypotension will benefit from sustained moderate activities with short rest intervals. Emphasis should be placed on movements that minimize changing body positions. The type of exercise needs to reflect the type and number of limitations they possess. Activities that involve a high degree of competition are discouraged initially.

Progression

The majority of elderly exercisers need to progress SLOWLY! Changes in an exercise program need to be based on how well the individual is responding to the current regime, the medical and health limitations of the individual, and individual goals. Exercise programs should be reviewed on a regular basis to ensure they are meeting the needs of the participant.

Special Precautions in Exercising for Elderly Clients

Particular care should be given when prescribing weight lifting exercises for those with high blood pressure, heart dis-ease, or arthritis. Incorporate an extended warm-up and cool-down period, approximately 10 to 15 min. The elderly often have a more difficult time when exercising in extreme environmental conditions. Some elderly individuals with arthritis or poor joint mobility may have to participate in non-weight-bearing activities, such as cycling, swimming, and chair and floor exercises.

WEBSITE BOX

Chapter 18: Exercise and Aging

The newest information regarding exercise physiology can be viewed at the following sites.*

arfa.org/index.htm
  Excellent site providing comprehensive information on many topics within exercise physiology.

agingresearch.org/
  Information-packed site on research on human aging, with an emphasis on how to live longer and healthier lives.

agingresearch.org/john_glenn/index.asp
  Superb education modules on aging and exposure to microgravity.

mediconsult.com/
  Information source for any medical condition, including asthma.

afar.org/pub.html
  Free publications about aging provided by the American Federation for Aging Research.

agenet.com/
  Internet information and referral network on anything and everything to do with aging.

mediconsult.com/
  Information source for any medical condition, including age-related diseases and degeneration.

worldhealth.net/
  Homepage of the American Academy of Anti-Aging Medicine.

---

*Unless indicated, all URLs preceded by http://www.

Note: These URLs were valid at the time of publication, but could have changed or been deleted from Internet access since that time.

SUMMARY

■ As premature death has been reduced in this century, an increasing proportion of the population has lived through the **natural life span,** which is suggested to be around the age of 85.

■ Today, the **life expectancy** for the majority of men in developed countries is about 71 years, and about 78 years for women.

■ One of the most serious problems facing all Americans is how to continue to provide quality health care to an ever-increasing elderly population. Although people aged 65 and older have 16.4 years of life remaining on average, they have about 12 years of **healthy life** remaining.

■ **Quality of life** includes an individual's ability to perform daily activities (ADLs) such as walking, bathing, dressing, and eating.

■ An individual's **longevity** depends on a variety of factors including heredity, environmental factors, availability of good medical and health services, and individual responsibility for health maintenance.

■ Although there are many advanced theories, **aging** may simply be due to the wearing out of nonreplaceable body components, such as teeth and kidney function.

■ Whereas someone might have a **chronological age** of 65, he or she may have a **biological age** of 45, based on his or her fitness and health status.

SUMMARY

- Functional changes to the cardiovascular system include a decrease in maximal heart rate; an increase in blood pressure, vascular resistance, and myocardial oxygen consumption requirements; and a decreased stroke volume and cardiac output.

- With normal aging, maximal oxygen uptake (VO_{2max}) declines approximately 8 to 10% per decade after age 30. It appears that aerobic capacity can be improved at any age.

- Changes in the pulmonary conduction system (excluding pathological changes) are minimal, and generally do not affect functional performance of the lung. One of the most dramatic affects of aging is the progressive loss of elastic recoil, which leads to a progressive increase in residual lung volume.

- Functional changes in the pulmonary system include a decrease in maximal ventilation (VE) and a substantial increase in ventilatory equivalent (VE/VO_2) in older individuals. With aging, the ventilatory requirements during activities increase. A greater ventilation is needed for a given workload and for a given level of oxygen consumption.

- With age, the loss of calcium results in a decrease in bone mass. **Osteoporosis,** or a gradual loss or thinning of bone with aging, is a major concern to the elderly. Men tend to lose bone mass by about 1% per year after the age of 50, whereas women begin to lose bone mass in their early 30s with a 2 to 3% decline per year after menopause.

- Muscle mass declines with age, resulting in decreased muscular strength and endurance. For each decade after the age of 25, 3 to 5% of muscle mass is lost.

- With normal aging, connective tissue becomes stiffer, and joints become less mobile. Physical training has been associated with a decrease in flexibility. Flexibility can be improved at any age.

- Exercise is recommended for clients with arthritis to help preserve muscle strength and joint mobility, to improve functional capabilities, to relieve pain and stiffness, to prevent further deformities, to improve overall physical conditioning, to reestablish neuromuscular coordination, and to mobilize stiff or contracted joints. **Osteoarthritis,** also referred to as *degenerative joint disease,* is a degenerative process caused by the wearing away of cartilage, leaving two surfaces of bone in contact with each other. Osteoarthritis is very common in older individuals over the age of 70. **Rheumatoid arthritis** is caused by an inflammation of the membrane surrounding joints. It is often associated with pain and swelling in one or more joints.

- Lean body weight declines and body fat increases with age.

- Older individuals appear to have a less efficient thermal control system. Both heat gain and heat loss are not as effective in older individuals. Trained elderly subjects tend not to display such large discrepancies in thermal regulation versus their sedentary counterparts.

- Before starting an exercise program, elderly individuals should first see their physicians. Although many of the principles of prescribing exercise to the elderly are the same for any group, special care should be given when setting up a fitness program for older participants.

STUDY QUESTIONS

1. Define the terms life expectancy, natural life span, healthy life, quality of life, longevity, and aging.

2. What is the difference between chronological age and biological age, and how does exercise and health promotion strategies alter them?

3. List at least two normal aging effects on the various physiological systems (cardiovascular, pulmonary, metabolic, etc.) and discuss how exercise possibly effects these normal changes.

4. List two specific recommendations to consider before, during, and following exercise testing of an elderly client.

5. What are the general exercise guidelines for intensity, duration, mode, frequency, and rate of progression for elderly clients?

6. Does exercise training prevent arthritis and osteoporosis? If so, how?

7. Does exercise training help in the treatment of arthritis and osteoporosis? If so, how?

APPLICATIONS

1. Sit down one day in a populated area like a shopping mall, and note how many elderly people you see. What percentage of the people were elderly, say over age 65? Are you surprised at the number of elderly people you see?

2. Visit one of your local health clubs or a senior center and observe an exercise class. Is the instructor following the guidelines and recommendations listed in this book? What, if any, changes would you make in the design of the class?

3. Go to a university or medical school library and get several recent issues of medical journals that focus on elderly people, such as *Geriatrics* or the *Journal of Aging and Physical Activity,* and read some of the articles. Make a list of some of the different topics covered.

4. Sit down and talk with someone you know who is elderly, perhaps a grandparent, and talk to them about the physical changes that they have noticed over time. Do they exercise? What problems, if any, do they have with exercise?

5. Practice setting up an exercise prescription for an elderly client with arthritis or osteoporosis. Have your instructor review it.

REFERENCES

1. Borkan, G. A., D. E. Hults, A. F. Gerzof, A. H. Robbins, and C. K. Silbert. Age changes in body composition revealed by computer tomography. *J. Gerontol.* 38: 673–677, 1983.

2. Brown, M., and J. O. Holloszy. Effects of a low intensity exercise program on selected physical performance characteristics of 60- to 71-year-olds. *Aging* 3(2):129–139, 1991.

3. Eisenman, P. A. Hot weather, exercise, old age, and the kidneys. *Geriatrics* 41:108–114, 1986.

4. Ellis, F. P. Mortality from heat illness and heat-aggravated illness in the United States. *Environ. Res.* 5:1, 1972.

4a. *N. Eng. J. Med.* June 23, 1994.

5. Frontera, W. R., C. N. Meredith, K. P. O'Reilly, H. G. Knuttgen, and W. J. Evans. Strength conditioning in older men: Skeletal muscle hypertrophy and improved function. *J. Appl. Physiol.* 64:1038–1044, 1988.

6. Institute of Medicine. *The second fifty years: Promoting health and preventing disability.* National Academy Press, Washington DC, 1992.

7. Kasch, F.W., et al.: Effect of exercise on cardiovascular aging. *Age and Aging* 22:5–10. 1993.

8. Kavanagh T., and R. J. Shephard. The effects of continued training on the aging process. *Ann. N.Y. Acad. Sci.* 301: 656–670, 1977.

8a. Krolner, B., B. Toft, S. P. Nielsin, and E. Tondevold. Physical exercise as prophylaxis against voluntary vertebral bone loss: A controlled study. *Clin. Sci.* 64:541–646, 1983.

9. McMurray, R. C., V. Ben-Ezra, W. A. Forsythe, and A. T. Smith. Responses of endurance-trained subjects to caloric deficits induced by diet and exercise. *Med. Sci. Sports Exerc.* 17:574–579, 1985.

10. Nakamura, E., T. Moritani, and A. Kanetake. Biological age versus physical fitness age. *Eur. J. Appl. Physiol.* 58:778–785, 1989.

11. National Academy of Sciences, Committee on Dietary Allowances, Food and Nutrition Board. *Recommended dietary allowances.* National Academy of Sciences, Washington, DC, 1980.

12. National Center for Health Statistics. *Health, United States, 1989 and prevention profile.* DHHS Pub. No. (PHS) 90-1232. U.S. Department of Health and Human Services, Hyattsville, MD, 1990.

13. Paffenbarger, R. S., R. T. Hyde, A.L. Wing, and C. C. Hsieh. Physical activity, all-cause mortality and longevity of college alumni. *N. Eng. J. Med.* 314:605–613, 1986.

14. Pandolf, K. B., B. S. Cadarette, M. N. Sawaka, A. J. Young, R. P. Francesconi, and R. R. Gonzales. Thermoregulatory responses of middle-aged and young men during dry-heat acclimation. *J. Appl. Physiol.* 65:65–71, 1988.

15. Pekkanen, J., B. Marti, A. Nissinen, J. Tuomilehto, S. Punsar, and M. J. Karvonen. Reduction of premature mortality by high physical activity: A 20-year follow-up of middle-aged Finnish men. *Lancet* 1:1473–1477, 1987.

16. Poehlman, E. T., T. L. McAuliffe, D. R. Van Houten, and E. Danforth. Influence of age and endurance training on metabolic rate and hormones in healthy men. *Am. J. Physiol.* 59:E66–E72, 1991.

17. Rikli, R. E., and D. J. Edwards. Effects of a three-year exercise program on motor function and cognitive speed in older women. *Res. Quart. Exerc. Sport* 62(1):61–67, 1991.

18. Rogers, M. A., J. M. Hagberg, W. H. Martin, A. A. Ehsani, and J. O. Holloszy. Decline in VO_{2max} with aging in master athletes and sedentary men. *J. Appl. Physiol.* 68:2195–2199, 1990.

19. Rudman, D. Growth hormone, body composition, and aging. *J. Geriatric Soc.* 33:800–807, 1985.

20. Seals, D. R., J. M. Hagberg, B. F. Hurley, A. A. Ehsani, and J. O. Holloszy. Endurance training in older men and women I: Cardiovascular responses to exercise. *J. Appl. Physiol.* 57:1024–1029, 1984.

21. Smith, E. L. Exercise for prevention of osteoporosis: a review. *Phy. Sports Med.* 10(3):72–83, 1982.

22. Spirduso, W. W. *Physical activity and aging: Introduction.* In American Academy of Physical Education Papers: Physical Activity and Aging. Human Kinetics, Champaign, IL, 1989, pp. 1–5.

23. Turlbeck, W. M., and G. E. Anges. Growth and aging of the normal lung. *Chest* 67:35–75, 1975.

24. Tzankoff, S. P., and A. H. Norris. Effect of muscle mass decrease on age-related BMR changes. *J. Appl. Physiol.* 43:1001–1006, 1977.

25. Wagner, J. A., S. Robinson, S. P. Tzankoff, and R. P. Marino. Heat tolerance and acclimatization to work in the heat in relation to age. *J. Appl. Physiol.* 33:616–622, 1972.

REFERENCES

26. Warren, B. J., et al. Cardiorespiratory responses to exercise training in septuagenarian women. *Int. J. Sports Med.* 14(2): 60–65, 1993.

27. U.S. Dept. of Health and Human Services. *Healthy people 2000: national health promotion and disease prevention objectives.* U.S. Government Printing Office, Washington, DC, 1991.

28. Flatarone, M. A., et al. Exercise training and nutritional supplementation for physical frailty in very elderly people. *N. Eng. J. Med.* 1994 Jun 23: 330(25):1769–75.

RECOMMENDED READINGS

Spirduso, W. W. *Physical dimensions of aging.* Human Kinetics, Champaign, IL, 1995.

Journal of Aging and Physical Activity. Human Kinetics, Champaign, IL.

The American College of Sports Medicine. *Exercise management for persons with chronic diseases and disabilities.* Human Kinetics, Champaign, IL, 1997.

Hayflick, L. *How and why we age.* Ballantine Books, New York, 1994.

CHAPTER 19

Exercise in Differing Environments

he number of individuals that are becoming exposed to the physiological demands of both exercise and environmental extremes is increasing every year. There is no better example of this fact than the slopes of the world's highest mountains, where mountaineers are beginning to overcrowd traditional camp locations as they await the few bouts of pleasant weather suited to an assault on a mountain summit. The interaction between exercise and the physiological responses to altered environments is also manifest in our exploration of outer space via the U.S. space shuttles or Russia's MIR space station. For the remainder of us who only dream of such exposures, the need to escape the confines and comfort of residential life can still expose us to temperature changes, moderate altitude, and perhaps altered gravitational forces during air flight or a ride on the modern rollercoasters that seem to defy gravity. The performance of exercise in many environmental extremes complicates how the body can adapt to the changes it is exposed to. The purpose of this chapter is to identify how certain environmental changes alter human physiology, and to summarize the main alterations to physiology when exercising during exposure to altered environmental conditions.

OBJECTIVES

After studying this chapter, you should be able to:

- Explain why increasing altitude is associated with increasing hypoxia.
- Apply fundamental knowledge of pulmonary and cardiovascular physiology to explain the decrease in VO_{2max} with increasing altitude.
- List the changes in physiology during exercise that occur from both acute and chronic altitude exposure.
- Explain why many of the chronic adaptations to prolonged altitude exposure can be detrimental to both intense and prolonged submaximal exercise.
- Identify the dangers involved in exposure to hyperbaric conditions.
- Describe the physiological complications of increasing exercise intensities during scuba diving.
- Explain the importance of adequate hydration during exercise, especially in a hot or humid environment.
- Identify the risks to life and the pathophysiology related to those risks when exercising in a hot or humid environment.
- List the beneficial adaptations resulting from heat acclimation.
- Explain the events that lead to heat illness and heat exhaustion.
- Identify the risks to life and the pathophysiology related to those risks when exercising in a cold or windy environment.
- Explain how chronic exposure to microgravity is detrimental to specific physiological functions.
- List conditions and related occupations that are at risk from exposure to increased gravitational forces.

KEY TERMS

partial pressure	altitude training	rehydration
hypoxia	hyperbaria	wet bulb globe
hypobaric hypoxia	the bends	index (WBGI)
normobaric	dehydration	hypothermia
hypoxia	hyperthermia	microgravity
acute mountain	heat exhaustion	orthostatic
sickness (AMS)	heatstroke	tolerance
acclimatization	voluntary	
acclimation	dehydration	
lactate paradox	water intoxication	

Section I: Exercise When Exposed to Altered Pressure

a. Exercise at Increased Altitude

Altitude, Pressure, and Oxygen Availability

As a person moves from sea level to increasing height above sea level (altitude) there is a decrease in pressure that is slightly exponential in nature (fig. 19.1). The decrease in pressure occurs because at sea level there is a greater air mass above the earth which forces air molecules closer together, hence generating increased pressure. With higher altitude, the air mass decreases and the gas molecules in air are more "free" to separate and move at random. As a result, the air pressure is less, and for a given volume of air there are fewer molecules of each gas. It is important to realize that *the relative amount of the different gas molecules in air does not change with changes in altitude.* It is because of this fact that the barometric pressure of a given altitude and the fraction of a known gas in air can be used to quantify how much of the air is composed of one gas or another. A gas quantity in air is not expressed as a concentration, but as a **partial pressure.** For example, the partial pressure of oxygen in dry air at sea level (PO_2) is:

$$\textbf{19.1} \qquad (PO_2) = 760 \text{ mmHg} \times 0.2093$$

$$= 159 \text{ mmHg}$$

In adjusting for the water vapor in the lung, the calculation for the inspired partial pressure of oxygen (P_IO_2) is:

$$\textbf{19.2} \qquad P_IO_2 = (760 - 47) \times 0.2093$$

$$= 149 \text{ mmHg}$$

FIGURE 19.1

The decrease in barometric pressure with an increase in altitude above sea level. The pressure for a given altitude may vary by ±10 mmHg because of extremes in climatic conditions. The curve is not linear, and can be estimated by the formula, $P_B = 760 \, [e^{-(m/7924)}]$. However, between the altitudes of sea level and 3000 m the change in pressure with increasing altitude is close to linear, and can be approximated by an 8 mm Hg decrease in atmospheric pressure every 100 m.

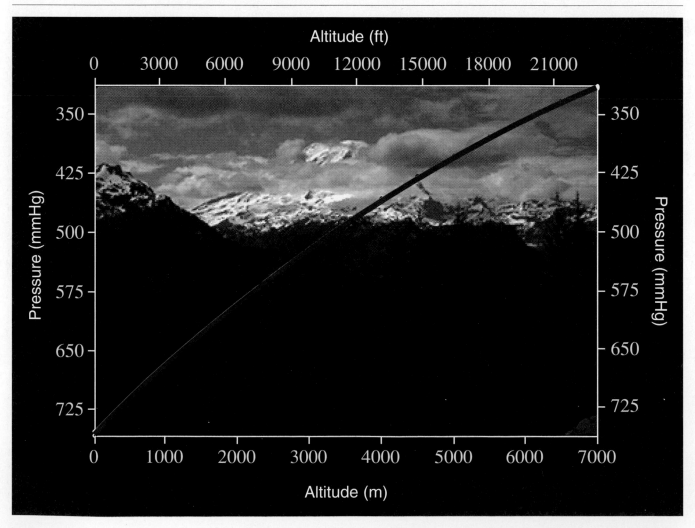

The PO$_2$ in dry air at Pikes Peak, Colorado [4000 m (14,300 ft) or 430 mmHg] is:

19.3

$$PO_2 = 430 \times 0.2093$$

$$= 90 \text{ mmHg}$$

The P$_I$O$_2$ at Pikes Peak is:

19.4

$$P_IO_2 = (430 - 47) \times 0.2093$$

$$= 80 \text{ mmHg}$$

The majority of physiological research on the influences of altitude on human physiology has been focused on the relationship between altitude and the reduction in oxygen content of the air (**hypoxia**). The hypoxia in turn lowers the amount of oxygen bound to hemoglobin in blood, with a resultant reduction in the oxygen content of blood (fig. 19.2). However, there is also evidence that the reduction in barometric pressure might also have independent physiological consequences (77). Unfortunately, we know very little about how a reduced pressure by itself alters human physiology.

The relationships between air pressure, temperature, and volume are presented in appendix D.

partial pressure the pressure of a given gas in a multiple gas mixture

hypoxia (hi-pox'-see-ah) decreased oxygen content of air

FIGURE 19.2

Data showing the conversions from altitude (m and ft) for the conditions of barometric pressure (P$_B$), the inspired partial pressure of oxygen (P$_I$O$_2$), the alveolar partial pressure of oxygen (P$_A$O$_2$), and hemoglobin saturation (SaO$_2$).

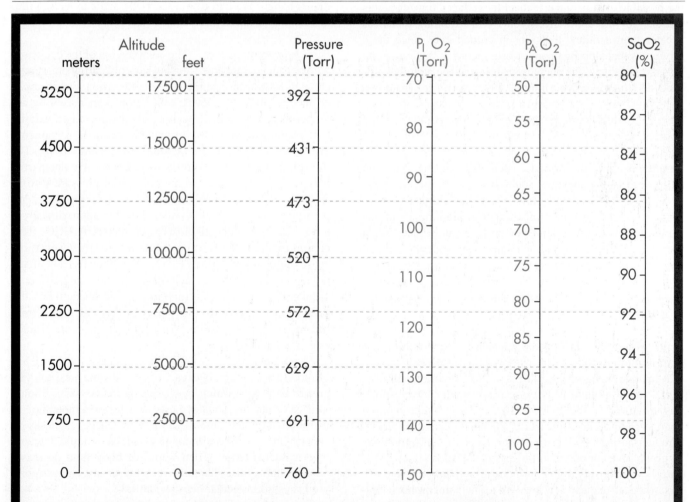

1 Torr = 1 mmHg ; 1 m = 3.28 ft ; P$_B$ = 760[e $^{-(m/7924)}$] ; P$_I$ O$_2$ = (P$_B$- 47) x 0.2093 ; P$_A$ O$_2$ ~ (P$_B$ - 47) x 0.146
SaO$_2$ approximated from %O$_2$ Hb dissociation curve

Why Is There an Interest in Exercise at Increased Altitude?

The interest that humans have had with exposure to high altitude has a long history. Houston (60) noted that historical evidence of high-altitude exploration dates to before Christ, and written reports of the headache accompanying acute mountain sickness have a similar long history. Furthermore, at approximately A.D. 400, Chinese pilgrims documented in writing, we believe for the first time, symptoms of fluid accumulation in the tissues of the lung (pulmonary edema). Ironically, Charles Houston was the physician to "first" report this condition; a difference of over 1500 years!

It was not until the 1968 Mexico City summer olympic games that the impact of altitude on exercise performance was to receive considerable media attention and, therefore, be catapulted into public awareness. During preparation of the Mexico City Olympics, concerns existed for possible beneficial effects of the lower pressure and air resistance at the altitude of 2300 m (P_B = 569 mmHg) (fig. 19.2) for events involving speed and power (e.g., jumping, throwing, and sprinting). Conversely, there was obvious concern for the possible detrimental effects of the reduced oxygen at this altitude for the endurance events (e.g., running distances greater than a mile). It has been argued ever since these Olympics that Bob Beaman's world record in the long jump was attributable to the decreased air resistance at higher altitude, and that the relatively impaired performance (based on winning times) for running distances in excess of a mile were attributable to hypoxia. The 2300-m altitude with an approximate hemoglobin-oxygen saturation at rest of 96% (98% at sea level) clearly had a negative impact on endurance exercise performance. Scientists and the public at large were asking questions such as: Why is endurance exercise impaired at moderate altitude? At what altitude does endurance exercise become impaired? Can training at altitude improve endurance exercise performance at altitude? What are the acute physiological responses to moderate altitude exposure? What are the adaptations that occur because of prolonged altitude exposure? The answers to these and other questions will be provided in the following sections of the chapter.

Acute Adaptations to Altitude Exposure

Research on human altitude exposure consists of several different models that include being on location at actual altitude, experiencing artificial altitude in a hypobaric chamber, or breathing gas mixtures of below-normal oxygen content without changing atmospheric pressure. When the hypoxia occurs by a reduction in barometric pressure, it is termed **hypobaric hypoxia** and applies to on-location and altitude chamber studies. Conversely, hypoxia induced by breathing hypoxic gas when at or near sea level is termed **normobaric hypoxia.**

When first exposed to increased altitude, certain physiological functions of the body change from normal during rest, as well as during exercise. The magnitude of these responses vary depending on the level of activity performed at altitude and on the magnitude of the altitude. Unfortunately, adequate research has not been completed to profile how many of the body's physiological and biochemical functions during rest and exercise change with small increments in altitude above sea level. Altitudes at which most published research has been conducted have been 4300 m (Pikes Peak) and simulated altitudes used in studies on a laboratory-based simulation of an ascent to the peak of Mt. Everest (Operation Everest II) (> 5500 m). For example, of the 27 studies completed to quantify the reduction in VO_{2max} during acute exposure to hypoxia, less than 25% were conducted between sea level and 2500 m. This fact is unfortunate because most people who live and exercise at altitude do so at altitudes of less than 2500 m.

Changes at Rest   When exposed to increasing altitude and the associated reductions in blood oxygen transport capacities, there are immediate changes in ventilation, cardiac function, and blood flow redistribution that function to oppose the hypoxic exposure (fig. 19.3). Nevertheless, some of these changes are harmful to the body and can lead to life-threatening sickness (focus box 19.1).

Cardiopulmonary function   The combination of the decreased barometric pressure and decreased arterial partial pressure of oxygen (P_aO_2) cause an increase in ventilation. For example, at 4300 m above sea level, ventilation is increased by approximately 30% (78, 124). Because this increased ventilation occurs without a proportionate increase in oxygen consumption (VO_2), it is called hyperventilation. The hypoxia-induced hyperventilation reduces alveolar partial pressure of CO_2 (P_ACO_2), arterial partial pressure of CO_2 (P_aCO_2), and blood bicarbonate (HCO_3^-), prompting a temporary respiratory alkalosis that lasts for approximately 2 days. The respiratory alkalosis is corrected by HCO_3^- excretion by the kidneys (*renal compensation*). However, because of the lowered blood HCO_3^- the blood has a dramatic reduction in buffering capacity. Despite these negative consequences of the hyperventilation, there is a benefit because of a raised P_AO_2 and P_aO_2 above values calculated from barometric pressures, thereby making the absolute altitude effectively much lower.

Exposure to low altitudes will increase fluid loss via evaporative cooling because of the lower pressure and greater ease with which water changes state from a liquid to a gas state (e.g., water boils at a lower temperature at increasing altitude!) and *renal diuresis*. These responses increase with increased altitude, and can cause rapid development of dehydration. Such a loss of body fluid decreases blood volume, raises hematocrit and viscosity, and can compromise cardiovascular hemodynamics.

The hypoxia of moderate to extreme altitude is known to stimulate the release of erythropoietin (EPO) from special PO_2 sensitive cells within the kidneys (117). Although the degree of hypoxia needed for increased erythropoietin

FIGURE 19.3

During exposure to altitudes between 3 and 4300 m, research has documented near-immediate changes in cardiovascular, respiratory, and metabolic parameters at rest and during submaximal and maximal exercise. Changes are expressed as a percent of prealtitude exposure. Positive values represent an increase; negative values represent a decrease. During chronic exposure to altitudes between 3 and 4300 m, many physiological variables change relative to the values during acute exposure.

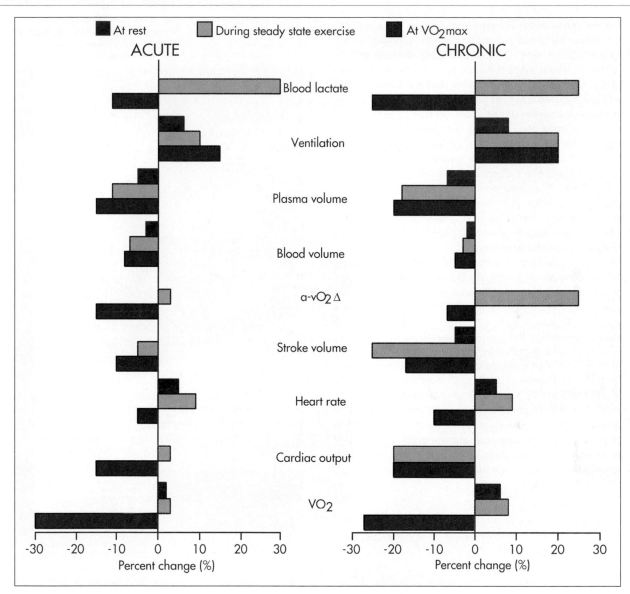

production and release is not known, it is known that a hypoxia sufficient to lower hemoglobin saturation to below 85% required 120 min of exposure before a detectable increase in EPO (1, 35, 68). During continuous and more prolonged altitude exposure at 4300 m (Pikes Peak), peak EPO concentrations occurred after 2 days, and then decreased to near-preexposure levels by day 7 (1). Unfortunately, no research has been completed that has evaluated the 24-h pulsatility of EPO in response to normoxia and hypoxia. This is unfortunate, for as with most pulsatile hormones, the most significant hypoxia-induced increase in EPO and biological response may occur during the sleep cycle.

Another hematological response during hypoxia is an increased production of 2,3-bisphosphoglycerate (2,3-BPG) by erythrocytes (72). Increases in whole blood 2,3-BPG concentrations lower the oxy-hemoglobin (Hb-O_2) dissociation curve, thus increasing oxygen release at the tissues.

hypobaric hypoxia decreased oxygen availability because of decreased barometric pressure

normobaric hypoxia decreased oxygen availability at normal barometric pressure because of a lowered oxygen fraction of inspired air

FOCUS BOX 19.1

The Pathophysiology of Acute Mountain Sickness

Exposure to moderate to extreme altitudes can result in symptoms of headache, lethargy, and nausea. The condition characterized by these symptoms when exposed to increased altitude is termed **acute mountain sickness (AMS)**. The susceptibility to AMS is known to vary among individuals, and is believed to be the result of multiple acute adaptations to the hypoxia and hypobaria of altitude.

AMS is more severe during more extreme hypoxia. Apart from hypoxia itself, the two most important additional contributors to AMS are an *inadequate hyperventilation* and an *inadequate diuresis,* which cause a relative, fluid retention. Exercise is believed to exacerbate the development of AMS (128) (fig. 19.4). The symptoms of AMS are alleviated with supplemental oxygen, pharmacological stimulants to acid-base balance and ventilation (e.g., acetazolamide) (37, 50, 125, 131), or relocation to lower altitudes. The latter strategy is the most successful treatment!

Despite the assumption that endurance conditioning might delay the development of AMS, or reduce the severity of symptoms, there is no experimental evidence to support this. In fact, endurance-trained individuals often have a greater rate of ascent and perform more intense exercise during ascent, which in turn often causes an earlier onset and more severe symptoms of AMS.

AMS should not be regarded as a clinically minor disorder. If not treated appropriately, AMS may develop into the more life-threatening conditions of *pulmonary edema* or *cerebral edema*. Pulmonary edema results from sustained increases in pulmonary blood pressure, causing an increase in water flux from the pulmonary vasculature (52). The etiology of cerebral edema is less clear, but is believed to be a result of prolonged increases in cerebral blood flow.

FIGURE 19.4

Hikers ascending from a base camp of 4200 m in the northwestern Himalayas of Ladakkh, India. At this location, the elevation was approximately 5000 m above sea level.

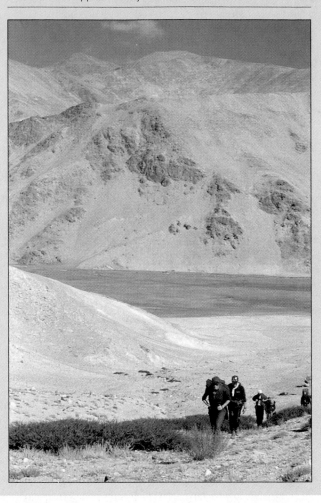

During exposure to moderate to extreme altitudes, the reduced concentration of oxygen in arterial blood (C_aO_2) lowers the effective diffusion gradient for oxygen at the tissues, and despite increases in 2,3-BPG there is a decreased a-v$O_2\Delta$. To maintain a given VO_2, heart rate increases. During exposure to high altitudes, cardiac stroke volume decreases in response to an increased peripheral vascular resistance and increased circulating catecholamines, which in turn further increases resting heart rate (139) (fig. 19.3). On the basis of the principles of the Fick equation, the relatively large increase in heart rate during hypoxia causes resting cardiac output to increase at altitude even though stroke volume decreases (fig. 19.3).

Changes During Submaximal and Incremental Exercise

The consequences of exercise at altitude not only depend on the altitude, but also on the type and intensity of exercise. Research has measured changes in VO_{2max} and various indices of exercise performance at different altitudes. Because of the impact of altitude on blood oxygen content and the known effects of these changes on cardiorespiratory endurance, research has predominantly investigated the effects of altitude on endurance exercise. However, comment will also be made to how acid-base responses to acute altitude exposure may also influence intense exercise performance.

Submaximal exercise   Cardiorespiratory function. For a given submaximal exercise intensity at moderate to severe altitude, there is a larger ventilation response than when compared to sea level (see fig. 19.3). This change is in response to the greater stimulation to ventilation at increased altitude, which is beneficial in raising P_AO_2 and arterial saturation of hemoglobin (SaO_2).

During exposure to hypoxia equivalent to 4300 m above sea level, a given absolute submaximal exercise intensity approximating 50% VO_{2max} at sea level increased steady-state VO_2, cardiac output, and heart rate, and decreased stroke volume compared to sea level values. The increase in VO_2 (worse economy) during exercise at moderate to high altitude is because of the increased work of breathing in combination with additional circulating catecholamines. Cardiac output increases during submaximal exercise at moderate to extreme altitude because of a lowered a-v$O_2\Delta$ secondary to the low SaO_2 (126, 139), as is expected from the Fick equation.

Despite the relative hypoxia, muscle blood flow in working muscle during exercise at altitude is not greater than at sea level for given exercise intensities (9, 54, 139). This response has been explained by the increased hematocrit during both acute (from a decreased plasma volume) and chronic exposure (from polycythemia), which appears to normalize oxygen provision for a given blood flow volume.

Incremental exercise to VO₂max

Cardiopulmonary function. During moderate to severe altitude exposure, the exercise intensity attained during incremental exercise to exhaustion decreases and, as will be explained in subsequent sections, VO2max decreases. Nevertheless, for a given VO2, ventilation is greater at altitude (103, 104, 142).

Relative to VO_2, maximal cardiac output, stroke volume, and muscle blood flow are not depressed at altitude as compared to sea level (102), indicating that cardiovascular function is well maintained during moderate to severe altitude exposure. Consequently, any decrease in VO_{2max} must be related to a combination of a reduced oxygen content of the blood and an impairment in oxygen extraction by the working muscles (136, 138). The lowered maximal cardiac output and stroke volume at altitude may simply reflect the lower exercise intensity at VO_{2max}.

VO₂max. Decreases in VO_{2max} are similar for simulated hypobaric hypoxia, acute exposure to high-altitude locations, and breathing hypoxic gas (4, 20, 107, 109). Data from field studies, altitude chambers, and exercise laboratories at different altitudes using inspired air of lowered oxygen content have been used to derive a relationship between altitude and VO_{2max}. Such a compilation has revealed that VO_{2max} decreases at altitudes as low as 700 m above sea level at a rate of approximately 9.2% every additional 1000-m increase in altitude (fig. 19.5). This fact, along with evidence of a clear relationship between VO_{2max} and blood oxygen content (40), has been interpreted as support for the overwhelming influence of the severity of hypoxia on VO_{2max} decrement.

Despite the simplicity of a single relationship between the altitude (hypoxia) and VO_{2max} decrement for all individuals, research shows that such a description is incorrect (44, 45, 71, 107, 120, 138, 141). Depending on certain features of an individual, the decrement in VO_{2max} during acute exposure to hypoxia may be more or less than previously described (107). For example, highly endurance-trained athletes have been shown to have a reduction in sea level VO_{2max} at 580 m above sea level (44, 45). Furthermore, it has been known for many years that the more cardiorespiratory endurance-trained an individual is (higher sea level VO_{2max}), the greater the decrement in VO_{2max} during hypoxia (71, 107, 120, 141). Robergs and colleagues (107) recently investigated the variables associated with the decrement in VO_{2max} during hypoxia and found that for a given sea level VO_{2max}, individuals with a smaller lean body mass, larger lactate threshold, less hypoxemia, and who were male, had a smaller decrement. Clearly, multiple factors, and not just the oxygen content of the blood, combine to influence a person's tolerance of hypoxia during exercise.

Energy metabolism. Research has shown that exposure to moderate and high altitudes does not increase the degradation of muscle glycogen during exercise to exhaustion, and muscle lactate concentrations at VO_{2max} are not higher compared to sea level (46, 47). In fact, maximal muscle lactate concentrations are actually lower at moderate and high altitudes. These data indicate that the muscle's capacity for glycolysis or the stimulation of glycolysis is decreased at altitude (103). The factor(s) responsible for this change is unknown.

There is a surprisingly small amount of research that has assessed changes in the lactate threshold during hypoxia (57, 69, 129). Each of these studies have shown no significant change in the LT expressed as % VO_{2max} for sea level and moderate to extreme hypoxia. However, as the number of subjects in these studies was relatively small (5 to 12), these results can be questioned. Conversely, there are consistent findings of an increased blood lactate response to submaximal exercise during acute hypoxic exposure (69, 104). Consequently, both the decrease in VO_{2max} and the increase in submaximal lactate accumulation and associated acidosis during moderate to severe hypoxia may independently decrease tolerance to prolonged exercise.

Because the LT changes in concert with reductions in VO_{2max} at altitude, it is no surprise that exercise times to exhaustion for a given exercise intensity decreases at moderate to extreme altitudes. For example, Faulkner and associates (38, 39) reported that running time trials of 1 to 3 mi were approximately 2 to 13% slower at 2300 m than at sea level.

Chronic Adaptations to Altitude Exposure

Acclimatization and Acclimation Because repeated exposure to many environmental conditions can induce chronic

acute mountain sickness the illness that accompanies acute altitude exposure, typically expressed by symptoms of headache and lethargy

FIGURE 19.5

The relative decrease in VO_{2max} during acute exposure to increased altitude. When data from research to 1998 are combined, VO_{2max} expressed as a percent of sea level appears to decrease linearly after approximately 700 m above sea level. At these altitudes, the decrement in VO_{2max} approximates 9.2% every additional 1000 m additional increase in altitude (~3% every 1000 ft above 2300 ft). However, data of VO_{2max} decrement at altitudes between sea level and 1500 m reveal a more curvilinear response, with considerable variability. The background image is of the Indus River and the Himalayan mountains of the Leh Valley in northern India.

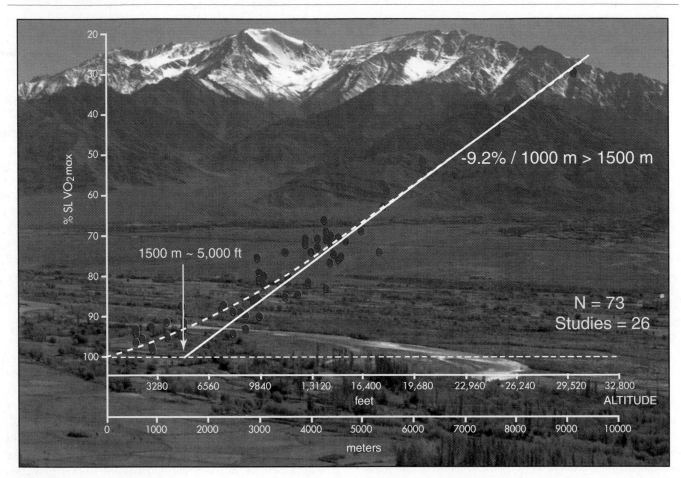

Changes at Rest

Cardiopulmonary function   Ventilation continues to increase during the first 2 weeks of exposure to an increased altitude, regardless of severity (73, 116) (see fig. 19.3). This continued increase in ventilation is retained at altitude even when breathing hyperoxic gas mixtures, and is also retained for several days after a return to sea level (116).

Chronic exposure to increased altitude is known to cause an increase in erythropoiesis because of the previously described acute increase in circulating erythropoietin. The time duration for the stimulation of erythropoiesis and the appearance of mature erythrocytes is 7 days (117). Thus, at least 1 week is required for the polycythemia of altitude exposure to become meaningful.

The polycythemia of altitude exposure in combination with altitude-induced reductions in plasma volume can increase hematocrit from approximately 46% at sea level to over 54% after 15 days of exposure at 4300 m (58, 139) (see

adaptations of the body that are beneficial (e.g., mild altitude, hot or humid conditions) as well as harmful (e.g., extreme altitude, microgravity, air pollution), research is being performed to evaluate whether exercise training can increase the adaptability of the body to altered environments, and therefore decrease the stress of these exposures. When individuals are chronically exposed to an altered environment, adaptations occur as part of a process known as **acclimatization.** Depending on the extreme nature of the environmental change and the biological response, this process may take several days to months. The time required for acclimatization is problematic, and intermittent exposure to artificial environmental conditions has been shown to stimulate similar adaptations to acclimatization. The adaptations resulting from these artificial exposures occur as part of a process known as **acclimation.** The details from research on acclimatization and acclimation to specific environmental changes will be presented in the sections on chronic adaptations that follow.

fig. 19.3). Compared to acute altitude exposure, the chronic increase in hematocrit and the increased saturation of hemoglobin can increase C_aO_2 by 30 mL/L. These changes in blood composition occur without a change in total blood volume because the increased red blood cell mass is offset by the reduced plasma volume (139).

Muscle morphology and metabolic capacities   The hypoxia of moderate to severe altitude exposure raises the question of whether chronic exposure to hypoxia induces adaptations in skeletal muscle that improve oxygen diffusive or utilization capacities. Such changes would include increases in capillary density, smaller muscle fiber areas, increased myoglobin stores, and increased mitochondrial density.

Early research on muscle adaptation to high altitude revealed increased stores of myoglobin and increased muscle enzyme activities (106). These findings were interpreted to indicate an improvement in skeletal muscle morphology and aerobic metabolism after altitude acclimatization. Unfortunately, more recent research has questioned the occurrence of beneficial muscle adaptation to high altitude. Green and colleagues (46–48) reported a decrease in muscle fiber area and an increased muscle capillary density after chronic exposure to high altitude (> 4800 m). However, these changes occurred with no increases in enzyme activity from the glycogenolytic, glycolytic, β-oxidation, or TCA cycle pathways. In fact, after exposure to the extreme altitude of 7260 m, muscle enzymatic activities actually decreased (47).

After 21 days of acclimatization to 4300 m, individuals increased their dependence on blood glucose at rest (13). However, despite an increased reliance on carbohydrate catabolism, resting muscle glycogen stores are not decreased (46, 47). Because the muscle glycogen data were obtained from research that required subjects to be mostly sedentary during acclimatization, it remains unclear how daily physical activity at increased altitude may influence muscle glycogen synthesis, especially when inadequate food intake is typical during moderate to severe altitude exposure (17).

Body composition   Prolonged exposure to moderate to extreme altitudes is associated with a loss in lean body mass and total body weight (17). This response has been explained in part by a reduced caloric intake, an increased basal metabolic rate, dehydration, and decreased gastrointestinal function (poor nutrient absorption) (17). Body weight during 21 days of exposure at 4300 m can be better preserved when caloric intake is increased to account for the increase in basal metabolic rate (17). Such an increase in calories amounted to approximately 340 Kcal/day. Clearly, *food and fluid intake should be increased when one is exposed to increased altitude.*

Changes During Submaximal and Incremental Exercise

Cardiopulmonary function   For a given VO_2, ventilation is increased further after acclimatization to increased altitude (58, 143). For example, after 15 days at 4300 m maximal ventilation increased to 205 L/min compared to 186 L/min during acute exposure (58). On the basis of previous explanations, an increased ventilation relative to VO_2 increases $P_{A}O_2$.

Despite the improvements in blood oxygen transport from the sustained hyperventilation of chronic altitude exposure, there is evidence that muscle blood flow and cardiac output decrease during submaximal exercise at 4300 m because of an increased sympathetic stimulation and reduced leg blood flow during exercise (9, 139) (see fig. 19.3). The data indicate that *the body may preserve a given oxygen transport to contracting muscle* for a given VO_2 (9).

During exercise to exhaustion, maximal cardiac output decreases further during chronic altitude exposure (9, 31, 102, 109, 139). Nevertheless, as will be described below, VO_{2max} values at moderate and high altitude increase after acclimatization.

VO_{2max}   The early research on Saltin and associates (109) and Horstman and colleagues (58) indicated that after as little as 14 days of exposure to an altitude of 4300 m, VO_{2max} increases. The reported increases are not large and approximate 10%, which is small compared to the reductions in VO_{2max} that normally exceed 20% for altitudes greater than 3000 m (fig. 19.5). Because acute moderate to severe altitude exposure can reduce maximal cardiac output, maximal limb blood flow, and C_aO_2, the fact that acclimatization to altitude does not cause large changes in VO_{2max} is not surprising. In fact, the increase in VO_{2max} after moderate to high-altitude acclimatization is remarkable given the previously described decreases in pulmonary and cardiovascular function at VO_{2max}. The increase in VO_{2max} must therefore be due to the improvements in hematology and muscle metabolic capacities that accompany prolonged moderate to high-altitude exposure.

Energy metabolism   Compared to acute altitude exposure, acclimatization to moderate to extreme altitude decreases muscle glycogen degradation for a given submaximal intensity (13–15, 48), and increases the utilization of blood glucose (14, 15).

Ironically, despite the hypoxia and increased reliance on carbohydrate during moderate to intense exercise at altitude after acclimatization, there is a decreased circulating blood lactate compared to exercise during acute exposure (10, 15, 80) (fig. 19.3). This was initially an unexpected finding, and has been termed the **lactate paradox** (10, 15, 80, 104). Research has indicated that the lowered maximal blood lactate response can be explained by an increased lactate uptake by

---

acclimatization (a'kly-ma-ty-za'shun) the process of chronic adaptation to a given environmental stress

acclimation (a'kli-ma'shun) the process of chronic adaptation to an artificially imposed environmental stress

lactate paradox the decreased maximal lactate production by contracting skeletal muscle after chronic altitude exposure

active and inactive skeletal muscle, the heart, kidney, and liver (15), and a reduced ability of the central nervous system to support exercise at high intensities (67).

Short-Term Intense Exercise Performance

The question of whether acute altitude exposure alters the capacity for short-term intense exercise has not received widespread research interest. However, because of the decreases in blood bicarbonate concentrations during acute and chronic altitude exposure, one could speculate that muscle metabolism during intense exercise could be impaired.

Di Prampero and associates (34) studied the effects of simulated altitude on the ability to generate maximal power during 10 s of cycling. Mechanical power output over time was no different for exercise at sea level, during normobaric hypoxia with an inspired partial pressure of oxygen (P_IO_2) equivalent to 3000 m, and during hypobaric hypoxia at 4500 (fig. 19.6). Thus, for very short-duration intense efforts, the muscles' abilities to regenerate ATP at high rates are not impaired during acute exposure to moderate to high altitude.

For more prolonged intense exercise, where there is an increased contribution from glycolysis and lactate production, acclimatization of sea level caucasian subjects to 5350 m not only decreased maximal blood lactate accumulation, but also increased the blood acidosis experienced at given blood lactate values (19, 20) (fig. 19.6). Such a reduced buffer capacity of the blood is directly related to the decreased blood bicarbonate concentration during acute and chronic altitude exposure.

Does Living at Altitude Improve Exercise Tolerance at Altitude?

A useful research design in altitude physiology has been to compare the physiology at moderate- or high-altitude exposure of altitude natives and sea level residents. Maresh and associates (78) exposed moderate-altitude natives (1830 to 2200 m) and sea level residents (both groups citizens of the United States) who were of similar cardiorespiratory fitness to a simulated altitude of 4270 m. Altitude natives reported fewer symptoms of acute mountain sickness, experienced half the decrement in VO_{2max} and maximal blood lactate accumulation, and had larger maximal ventilation compared to sea level residents during maximal exercise testing at altitude. The lactate threshold did not differ between the groups at altitude. The results indicated that individuals who have lived at moderate altitude all their lives responded better to acute altitude exposure than did sea level residents. As no measures of hematology, pulmonary function, or muscle metabolic capacities were completed, the reasons for these differences were not addressed.

Interestingly, similar evidence of improved acute adaptation to increased altitude exists for residents of altitudes as low as 1600 m (Denver, Colorado). Reeves and colleagues (103) indicated that when exposed to 4300 m, residents of Denver have a lower resting P_ACO_2 and a higher HbO_2 saturation, and achieved stable P_ACO_2 and SaO_2 values earlier

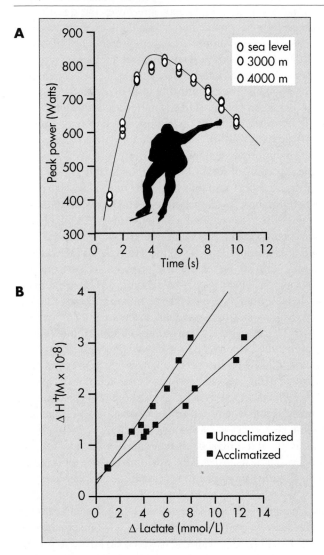

FIGURE 19.6

(a) The maximal power output during 10 s of "all-out" effort during cycle ergometry performed at sea level and at 3000 m above sea level. Adapted from Green et al. (47). (b) During more prolonged intense exercise, individuals that have acclimatized to an altitude of 5350 m have a lower maximal blood lactate concentration yet a lower blood buffering capacity as indicated by a greater decrease in blood pH relative to an increase in blood lactate. Adapted from Di Prampero et al. (34).

than sea level residents. Clearly, *living at altitudes that are low to moderate provides improved tolerance and responsiveness to increased altitude exposure.*

Living and Training at Altitude to Improve Exercise Performance

Ever since the Mexico City Olympic games, the potential for enhanced performance from high-**altitude training** has been a topic of widespread debate. Interest in this topic had originally focused on two topics: (1) whether altitude training can improve sea level performance and (2) whether altitude training can improve performance at altitude. More recently, the concept of living (or at least sleeping) at altitude and training at sea level has received research interest (*sleep high and train low*).

Altitude Training and Altitude Performance   Prior to and following the Mexico City games, researchers demonstrated that training at high altitude was essential for improved endurance performance at altitude. For example, acclimatization to moderate altitudes was associated with 5 to 10% improvements in VO_{2max} compared to acute exposure (38, 39, 100).

During this time (1970s) the obvious question to ask was why exercise performance in endurance events at altitude could be improved with prolonged altitude exposure. Findings of increased hematocrit and hemoglobin concentrations of blood after prolonged altitude exposure provided indirect evidence (now known to be incorrect) of improved blood oxygen transport capacities, and the notion that altitude training may be beneficial for even sea level exercise performance was reinforced.

Altitude Training and Sea Level Performance   Scientific studies of changes in VO_{2max} and exercise performance at sea level after altitude acclimatization have produced results that both confirm (32, 38, 39) and negate (16, 51) the benefit of altitude training. For example, exposure of athletes to altitudes between 2300 and 3300 m above sea level for 2 weeks resulted in an increased VO_{2max} on return to sea level and improved performance in the 1500-m and 1-mi races (32, 38, 39). Conversely, studies where athletes were exposed to 4000 m and 3100 m for 20 to 63 days revealed slower running times at sea level and reduced or unchanged VO_{2max} values (2, 16, 51).

On the basis of the previous explanations of acute and chronic adaptations to altitude, there is clear evidence that *if living at altitude were to provide any potential benefit, it would be for residing at low to moderate altitude*. Living at high altitudes is accompanied by reduced pulmonary function and capacities, reduced cardiovascular capacities, losses in muscle enzyme capacities, and decreases in lean body mass. These are all detrimental occurrences for the optimal development of cardiorespiratory endurance. In addition, to reap the benefits from improved training quality at lower altitudes, yet retain the chronic mild hypoxic stimulus of living at moderate altitudes, it has been recommended that *athletes should live at moderate altitudes, yet train at lower altitudes* (73, 74, 130), a concept referred to as "sleep high, train low."

A global statement concerning the scientific evaluation of exercise training at altitude would be that *there is no consistent scientific evidence to support training at altitude to improve sea level performance*. Conversely, training at altitude to improve altitude performance provides a definite advantage for cardiorespiratory endurance. The influence of altitude training for more intense exercise performance has not adequately been addressed by research. Despite these statements, Olympic class and professional athletes from around the world travel to moderate altitudes to complete altitude training to improve sea level performance. Athletes also willingly expose themselves to normobaric hypoxia during sleep by breathing hypoxic gas mixtures. In doing so, world records and personal best times are achieved, which reinforces the perceived benefits of altitude exposure to endurance performance. Clearly, there may be positive aspects of altitude training that science has yet to detect. For this reason, scientific interest in altitude training and athletic performance continues.

b. Exercise During Hyperbaria

Exposure of the body to increased pressure, or **hyperbaria,** can be accomplished with submersion under water or when placed within a hyperbaric chamber. When one is submerged under seawater, the pressure increases 1 atmosphere (atm) (760 mmHg) every 10 m. In freshwater, the pressure increase is not as great because of the different water density, and approximates 1 atm every 10.4 m of depth (84). Exposure to hyperbaria occurs for individuals who work beneath the surface of the ocean or beneath the ground in deep mines, or who conduct experimental clinical or applied research in hyperbaric chambers. Obviously, the development of the self-contained underwater breathing apparatus (scuba) in the 1943, and its widespread recreational use allowed large numbers of individuals to become exposed to the inherent risks of hyperbaric exposure. The physical, physiological, and medical concerns of exposure to hyperbaria, especially when applied to scuba, which involves exercise, are therefore worthy of inclusion in a text that focuses on the physiology of exercise.

When the body is submerged in water to the level of the neck, acute cardiovascular adaptations occur in response to the increased compressive forces that are exerted on the skin, resulting in decreased cutaneous blood flow, increased central blood volume, increased venous return, and a lowered heart rate. In addition, during face immersion in water an additional neurological reflex is excited (diving reflex) that also lowers heart rate. Consequently, it can be argued that immersion of the body in water improves cardiovascular function. However, this statement may be premature, because immersion for as little as 15 min up to 3 h followed by on-land incremental exercise decreases VO_{2max} (65). One theory suggests that prolonged water immersion decreases plasma volume because of an increased urine volume, and this may be detrimental to exercise performance when one returns to dry land (65).

When exercise is performed in water versus on land, results indicate that because of the increased resistance provided by the water, VO_2 is higher for a given amount of

---

altitude training exercise training in hypoxic environments

hyperbaria (hi-per-bar'i-ah) increased barometric pressure

physical power output, yet, for a given VO$_2$, heart rate is lower when one is under water.

The need to remain under water for extended periods of time requires the use of a scuba, or modifications of the scuba, to provide a continual supply of oxygen and removal of carbon dioxide. During these conditions, knowledge of the gas laws is vital to understanding how the pulmonary and cardiovascular systems respond to hyperbaria. For example, Boyle's law concerns the inverse relationship between pressure and volume for a constant gas temperature, Charles's law concerns the direct proportionality between gas volume and temperature, and Dalton's law concerns how the total pressure of a gas volume represents the sum of the individual pressures of each gas. Boyle's and Dalton's laws are very important to hyperbaric exposures. For example, when submerged under water, the increasing pressure decreases gas volume in all body cavities (Boyle's law). In addition, the increasing pressure increases the total gas pressures in the lung in proportion to their fraction in the air (Charles's law). Thus lung volumes decrease during descent but alveolar gas partial pressures increase during descent.

Breath-Holding During Submersion

During breath-holding (fig. 19.7), P$_A$CO$_2$ increases and P$_A$O$_2$ decreases, as would be expected from the body's continual production of CO$_2$ and consumption of O$_2$. As the most potent ventilatory stimulant is an increasing P$_A$CO$_2$, breath-holding is accompanied by an increasing chemical drive to ventilate. It is this drive that is sensed by the brain and causes what is normally an intolerable need to breathe. Although hyperventilating immediately prior to breath-hold can lower P$_A$CO$_2$ and therefore prolong the time that P$_A$CO$_2$ increases to stimulate ventilation, this maneuver is dangerous because P$_A$O$_2$ continues to decline and can cause a reduced oxygen supply to the brain and unconsciousness. This is a life-threatening occurrence when one is submerged in water, and especially when one performs breath-hold diving where P$_A$O$_2$ can decrease dramatically on ascent (see fig. 19.7)!

In descending to greater depths during breath-hold, the increasing compressive forces decrease lung volumes and pressures in other body cavities. Thus body cavity pressures need to be equalized to the increasing pressure of the environment to prevent the rupture of vessels during excessive constriction (termed "squeeze"). Usually, this is most noticeable for the inner ear and eustachian tube.

During diving to increased pressures, decreases in lung volumes can be tolerated to the point where lung volume equals residual volume. Thereafter, continued increases in pressure are exerted on what is now a closed lung volume, which in turn risks the eventual rupture of the alveoli. Thus the depth limit for breath-hold diving is dependent on the residual volume relative to total lung capacity. Generally, individuals have a lung capacity to residual volume of 4:1 to 5:1 (84), which can be calculated from the known increase in pressure at increased depths and Boyle's law to limit the depth of breath-hold dives to between 30 and 40 m.

FIGURE 19.7

During breath-holding the P$_A$O$_2$ decreases and the P$_A$CO$_2$ increases, as would be expected from metabolism. During breath-holding when diving to increased depths, the increasing water pressure actually increases PO$_2$ despite continued metabolic activity of the body. However, on return to the surface, the decreasing pressure can rapidly decrease P$_A$O$_2$ to dangerous levels, increasing the risk for syncope. Adapted from Young and Young (142).

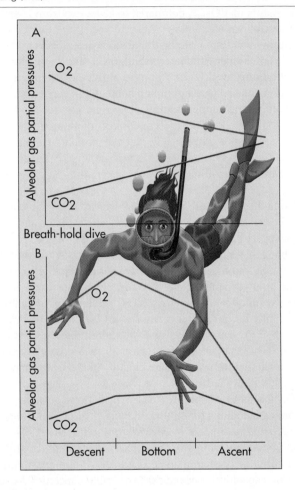

Scuba Diving

The use of the scuba when submerged under water partially decreases the risk for squeeze in body cavities that are "open" to the respiratory passages and stabilizes alveolar gas partial pressures by providing a continual supply of oxygen and allowing removal of carbon dioxide. However, depending on the depth and duration of the dive, added problems arise that can impair exercise performance.

In breathing self-contained air through a regulator that equilibrates air pressure to that of the environment, the increasing depth increases the pressure of the air inhaled. This phenomenon increases the density of the gas, which in turn increases the work of breathing. This change causes divers to hypoventilate, which in turn can cause altered acid-base balance, headache, and impaired cognitive function. Thus at depths causing pressures to exceed 6 atm, air mixtures are altered by including helium and reducing nitrogen, which lowers the density of the gas, decreases the work of breathing, and normalizes ventilation.

Another reason to lower the nitrogen content of the scuba compressed gas is to decrease the health risks of excessive nitrogen retention by the body. Such risks include neurological impairment (i.e., raptures of the deep), as well as increased risk for decompression sickness (**the bends**). Decompression sickness occurs when nitrogen dissolved in body fluids and tissues is forced to escape as bubbles of gas rather than dissolved gas. This occurs because of a too rapid decrease in pressure (too fast an ascent) that causes nitrogen from tissues that have a slow rate of desaturation to oversaturate and therefore force nitrogen to form gas bubbles. Although the general cause of decompression sickness is a too rapid ascent, a rapid ascent is more severe if the dive duration was long (allows more time for nitrogen to saturate tissues), or the dive depth was great (decreases the time required for tissue saturation). Because some tissues (e.g., fat) desaturate slowly, the longer and deeper the dive, the more time that is required for the safe desaturation of nitrogen from tissues. For these reasons, dive tables have been developed that recommend durations needed at certain depths during ascent after specific diving depths and times.

Another issue of concern for scuba divers who dive to depths in excess of 2 atm for periods of time in excess of 5 h is the development of oxygen toxicity (84). These conditions do not apply to recreational divers, whose equipment does not accommodate long dive times.

Section II: Exercise and Thermal Stress

a. Exercise in Hot or Humid Environments

Continuous or intermittent exercise performed for prolonged periods of time is associated with increased sweat rates and a reduction in body water or **dehydration.** When exercise is performed in hot or humid environments, the potential for dehydration is increased. In addition, the heat generation from exercise in combination with the heat stress from the environment can also increase the risk of excessive body heat storage (**hyperthermia**), resulting in cardiovascular complications, central nervous system and motor function impairment, and in extreme circumstances even death.

It is important to understand how and why the body functions deteriorate during exercise-induced dehydration and hyperthermia, how these deteriorations influence exercise performance, how to best prevent them or reduce their severity, and how to best recover from them. These issues form the basic structure of the following sections.

Acute Adaptations During Exercise

Changes in Body Temperatures   The change in core temperature during exercise is influenced by the metabolic rate (ex-

ercise intensity), the environmental temperature, and an individual's effectiveness for increasing evaporative heat loss (76, 89, 92, 113) (fig. 19.8). For a range of environmental heat stress conditions, the change in core temperature is not influenced by the environment but mostly by the metabolic heat load of the exercise. However, as exercise intensity increases, core temperature rises abruptly (76). In addition, the actual core temperature response for an individual is influenced by that individual's cardiorespiratory fitness, and therefore the degree of acclimatization to heat exposure (113).

Exercise-Induced Evaporative Heat Loss and Dehydration
During prolonged submaximal exercise in a hot or humid environment, a person's sweat rate can increase to between 2 and 3 L/h. Depending on gender and body size, the total blood volume may be 5 L, the plasma volume may be 2.75 L, and the total body water may be 35 L (fig. 19.9). Obviously, compared to the total body water the blood cannot lose a large volume of water during exercise. Figure 19.10 illustrates the sources of fluid lost during exercise-induced dehydration. Initially, the largest volume of water is lost from interstitial fluid. As dehydration increases, there is an increasing contribution from intracellular fluid. Although the relative loss (to total loss) of fluid from the plasma remains constant during dehydration, more severe dehydration represents a larger volume of fluid loss, and therefore a larger volume reduction in each compartment. Because plasma volume represents the smallest fluid compartment, a given volume change in plasma is a large fluid loss relative to the small absolute plasma volume. A 4% decrease in body weight for a person weighing 70 kg approximates a 7-kg fluid loss. A 10% volume of this loss equals 700 mL, or 25% of the plasma volume. As will be discussed, fluid losses from plasma of this magnitude have detrimental cardiovascular repercussions.

Despite the large fluid volume losses during exercise at high sweat rates, the electrolyte losses are not physiologically significant (26, 28–30), as was presented in chapter 11.

The decreasing fluid volumes of the body also have detrimental effects on sweating and therefore evaporative cooling. As the body becomes dehydrated, sweat rates actually decrease, and body core temperature increases. In fact, when dehydration becomes severe the sweat response can dramatically decrease and increase risk for heat injury (see focus box 19.2). Such a decreased sweat response occurs from a combination of the diminished function of the sweat gland and an increased plasma osmolality (retards fluid leaving the blood), rather than from an altered central nervous system regulation of sweat gland function (132).

---

the bends decompression sickness following too rapid an ascent from water submersion

dehydration decreased body water content

hyperthermia (hy'per-ther-my'ah) a body core temperature above 37°C

FIGURE 19.8

During exercise, heat loss to the surroundings can occur by radiation, convection, conduction, and evaporative cooling.

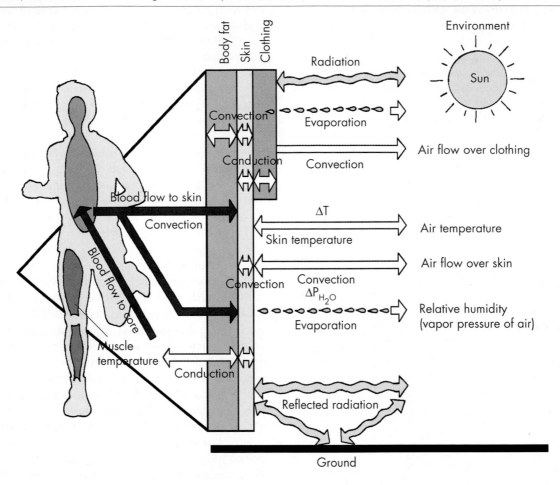

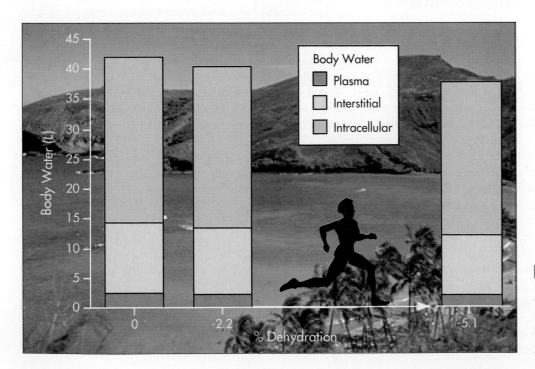

FIGURE 19.9

Body water is distributed within the vascular system (plasma and lymph), fluid spaces between cells (interstitium), and cells (intracellular).

FIGURE 19.10

During exercise-induced dehydration, body water is lost from intracellular, interstitial, and vascular fluid compartments, with greater losses from interstitial and intracellular water. As dehydration increases, a larger portion of water loss comes from cells. However, because of the small volume of plasma and the multiple roles of plasma for optimal cardiovascular function and thermoregulation, even small losses of plasma can have major negative consequences to exercise.

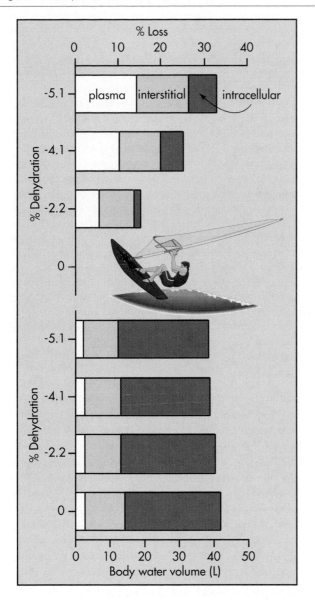

Given the decreasing fluid volume in each of the body's fluid compartments and the increasing core temperature, how do these losses influence cardiovascular function, muscle metabolism, and exercise performance?

Changes in Cardiovascular Function   Increasing dehydration causes a continued increase in core temperature, increases in heart rate because of reductions in venous return and stroke volume, decreases in cardiac output, and increases in a-vO$_2\Delta$ (126). Nadel and colleagues (87) have re-

ported a strong association between stroke volume and the % decrease in plasma volume (reflecting dehydration).

The decreased central cardiovascular function during dehydration is accompanied by alterations in peripheral blood flow to the skin and to the contracting skeletal muscles. For example, an important cardiovascular response to exercise in neutral and hot environments is to increase cutaneous blood flow, thereby improving heat loss from the body. With increasing dehydration, neural reflexes respond to a decreasing blood volume and systemic blood pressure and induce an increasing splanchnic and cutaneous vasoconstriction, which increases the central blood volume at the expense of a decreased capacity for heat transport to the skin (135). Consequently, if exercise is continued, skin temperatures may decrease because of evaporative, convective, and radiative cooling despite an increasing core temperature and increasing average body temperature.

Changes in Muscle Metabolism   As dehydration and core temperatures increase during exercise in a hot environment, the increased heat load, altered redistribution of the cardiac output, and increased catecholamine release have the potential to alter muscle metabolism. Fink and associates (41) demonstrated that during cycling in a hot or cold environment, greater muscle glycogen degradation occurred in the hot environment, as well as greater blood lactate accumulation.

The authors hypothesized that the altered muscle metabolism was because of a reduced muscle blood flow and accompanied hypoxia. More recent research has shown that muscle blood flow does not decrease during exercise in the heat (89, 110), and that muscle glycogen does not decrease more during exercise in a hot environment compared to neutral thermal conditions (89, 144). The increased blood lactate accumulation has been a consistent research finding and may relate to an increased fast-twitch motor unit recruitment in combination with decreased blood lactate removal (113).

Dehydration Can Compromise Exercise Performance   Cardiovascular indications of dehydration occur with as little as 1% dehydration; however, more severe dehydration to 3% is required before detriments in VO$_{2max}$ are detected (114, 115). This statement was based on a review of research that measured VO$_{2max}$ in neutral and hot environments; however, the decrements in VO$_{2max}$ reported by different studies have been extremely variable. The reason for the variability in research results is probably due to differences in environmental heat stress between studies (112, 113). The added fatigue during exercise in the heat when dehydrated is related to the decreased maximal cardiac output and a central nervous system impairment because of the increased core temperature (115).

Submaximal exercise performance is also impaired in a hot environment. Exhaustion occurs at a reduced exercise time and at a lower core temperature when one is dehydrated during exercise in a hot environment compared to neutral

F O C U S   B O X   1 9 . 2

Heat Illness, Heat Exhaustion, and Heatstroke

The increasing hyperthermia that accompanies exercise, regardless of the state of dehydration, can lead to a series of system and cellular changes that increase risk for exhaustion, organ failure (especially the kidney and liver), and death (61–63). Although hyperthermia can occur without severe dehydration, dehydration exacerbates the condition.

When one is dehydrated and hyperthermic, cardiovascular function is compromised because of a decreased plasma and total blood volume, and in combination with the increased core temperature, these produce symptoms of central nervous system disturbances such as *lethargy, dizziness*, and *lack of coordination*. This symptomology marks the condition that is commonly referred to as **heat exhaustion**. Although there is hyperthermia, the hyperthermia is not usually extreme during heat exhaustion, with the compromised cardiovascular system being the main cause of symptomology (64).

If dehydration and body heat storage continue beyond heat exhaustion, as is often the case during competitive exercise, the increasing hyperthermia (> 39.5°C) causes symptoms to develop into *disorientation, confusion, psychoses*, and eventually *coma*, along with elevated serum enzymes (118). These symptoms mark the phase of the heat illness spectrum termed **heatstroke** (fig. 19.11).

Individuals vary in their tolerance of a hot environment; however, research has not been able to provide an accurate prediction of susceptibility to heat illness other than being sedentary, overweight, dehydrated, and unacclimatized to the heat. The completion of a heat tolerance test (exercise in a controlled temperature and humidity environment) is the most accurate method to evaluate a predisposition to heat injury. However, such procedures are not cost-effective when evaluating large numbers of individuals for heat tolerance. Research has shown that an individual previously exposed to heatstroke is more susceptible to another bout of heat illness (36, 61), and this observation has been explained by residual or permanent damage to the hypothalamus.

The symptoms of heat illness are believed to be multifaceted, and in the severe symptoms of heatstroke, are explained by cellular changes that are due to high core temperatures between 40 and 44°C (61). The rising core temperature increases the rates of metabolic reactions, increases ion fluxes across membranes, and decreases the efficiency of mitochondrial respiration. Accompanied changes are an increase in lactate production and acidosis, decreased excitability and contractility of skeletal and cardiac muscle, and increased leakage from skeletal muscle of K^+, Ca^{++}, and the enzymes creatine kinase and lactate dehydrogenase (61–63, 118). During severe cases of heatstroke, cell leakage and damage is so severe that large proteins circulate in the blood and eventually cause damage to the liver and kidneys. During these conditions, muscle cells swell and become necrotic, and this symptom of severe heat injury is termed *rhabdomyolisis*.

---

thermal stress (114, 115). These responses are understandable, given the previously described acute cardiovascular adaptations during prolonged exercise in the heat.

Improving Exercise Tolerance During Exposure to Hot or Humid Environments

Given the devastating results of dehydration to exercise tolerance in both neutral and hot environments, fluid ingestion during exercise is vital to decrease the rate of exercise-induced dehydration and its physiological consequences. Numerous research studies have shown the benefit of fluid ingestion during exercise in a hot environment. In addition, the body can acclimatize to hot or humid environments, or be acclimated in order to tolerate exercise in a hot or humid environment.

Fluid Intake   Numerous studies have shown the benefits of fluid ingestion during exercise in hot environments (8, 26, 29, 33, 49, 81, 82, 83, 91, 94, 99, 105, 108, 114). In fact, this topic was researched as early as 1944 using military personnel (99) and the study is considered a classic reference in the importance of hydration during exercise. Basically, ingesting fluid retards the development of dehydration (i.e., it is not totally prevented), dampens the increase in heart rate (8,

24, 29), improves venous return and cardiac output (95), retains an increased cutaneous blood flow (94), dampens the increase in core temperatures (8, 33), and delays the onset of fatigue.

As with the topics of fluid, electrolyte, and carbohydrate intake during exercise (chapter 11), similar questions have been raised regarding the best type of fluid to ingest during exercise in a hot environment. On the basis of the work of Gisolfi and Duchman (43), the ability of carbohydrate-electrolyte solutions to increase intestinal water absorption should indicate the superiority of carbohydrate-electrolyte drinks above water alone during exercise in the heat. Despite this evidence, research has shown a similar benefit from carbohydrate drinks and water (18, 33, 81, 82, 94, 108), and electrolyte drinks and water (8), to generate changes in sweating, core temperatures, and cardiovascular responses to exercise in the heat. However, carbohydrate intake during exercise did increase blood glucose concentrations and caused improved exercise performance (33, 81, 82) as would be expected from the findings presented in chapter 11.

A possible explanation for the similar physiological benefits of the ingestion of water and carbohydrate solutions during exercise in the heat is an impairment of either gastric emptying or intestinal absorption of carbohydrate solutions

FIGURE 19.11

Exercise in a hot or humid environment can increase the risk of heat illness. Initially, the symptoms of heat illness are represented by general sensations of fatigue resulting from a compromised cardiovascular system. If exercise or another heat stress is continued, the sweat response can decrease, resulting in increased rate of heat storage and the development of heatstroke.

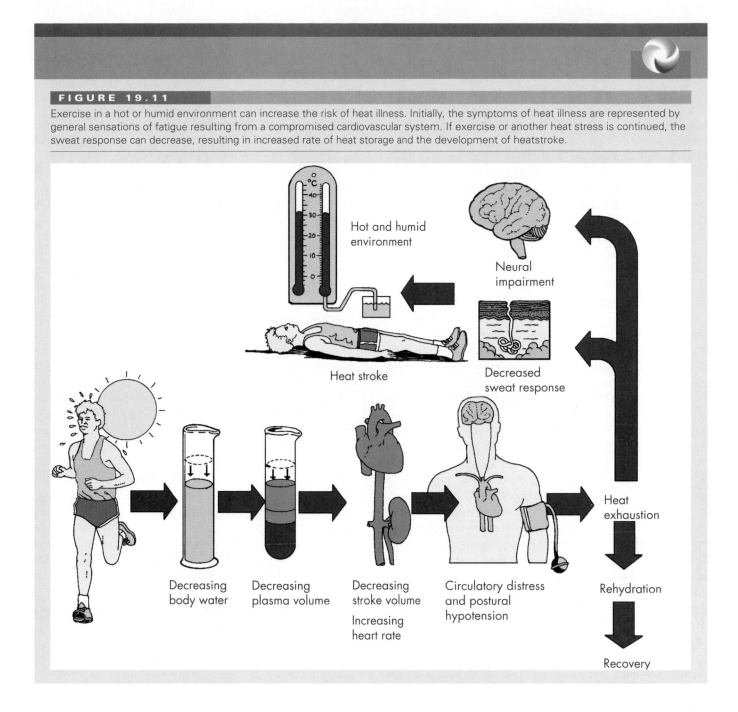

Hot and humid environment

Neural impairment

Heat stroke

Decreased sweat response

Decreasing body water

Decreasing plasma volume

Decreasing stroke volume

Increasing heart rate

Circulatory distress and postural hypotension

Heat exhaustion

Rehydration

Recovery

during heat stress, which in turn would minimize hydration effect differences compared to water alone. Ryan and colleagues (108) measured the gastric emptying of water and drinks with different carbohydrate concentrations during 3 h of cycling at 60% VO_{2max} in the heat. The results revealed that all drinks emptied at similar rates over the total duration of exercise. However, using a more sensitive gastric-emptying technique (double-sampling to provide gastric-emptying rates in 10-min intervals), Rehrer and associates (105) reported that during exercise in the heat when dehydrated there is increased gastric distress causing a reduced gastric emptying of a 7% carbohydrate solution compared to when normally hydrated. There was no comparison made to plain

water. Clearly, the known benefit of ingesting carbohydrate solutions to improve fluid delivery to the body has not been verified during dehydration.

An important research finding of studies evaluating fluid intake during exercise in hot environments is that *ad libitum*

heat exhaustion decreased exercise tolerance that is due to a combination of dehydration, a reduced plasma volume and cardiovascular compromise, and hyperthermia

heatstroke the progression from heat exhaustion when body core temperature increases to values that impair central nervous system and damages peripheral tissues

fluid intake is less effective than forced drinking to replace fluid lost through sweating (49, 99). This developing dehydration despite the availability of fluid has been termed **voluntary dehydration.** However, there have also been cases where individuals have ingested too much water, causing **water intoxication** and the development of *hyponatremia* (decreased serum sodium to < 130 mEq/L) (49, 56).

Heat Acclimation and Acclimatization   The reproducibility of the cardiovascular compromise during prolonged exercise in the heat has enabled researchers to use these responses to evaluate individual tolerances to exercise in hot environments, as well as adaptations to exercise in a hot environment that occur after acclimatization or acclimation. Standard heat tolerance tests (HTTs) have been developed to provide a reference protocol from which to compare physiological responses to exercise in the heat under different conditions. For example, Houmard and colleagues (59) reported that HTTs have generally involved low-intensity exercise (< 40 to 50% VO_{2max}) in a hot and dry environment (~ 40°C and 30% relative humidity) for between 60 to 100 min. Individuals with a greater increase in core temperature and heart rate are less tolerant of exercise in a hot environment.

The utility of HTTs has also been demonstrated when determining acclimatization or acclimation to exercise in a hot environment (6). Typically, subjects demonstrate improved heat tolerance after endurance training in a hot environment for 60 to 100 min for 4 to 10 days (59). In addition, evidence indicates that even endurance-trained athletes who live in cool or temperate climates have experienced partial heat acclimation. However, even when these individuals are artificially heat acclimated, further improvements are detected (5, 42, 95). The more intense the exercise training, and therefore the more extreme the heat load, the greater is the apparent benefit to heat acclimation. Consequently, highly endurance-trained individuals have near maximal heat acclimation regardless of their environmental climatic conditions (5, 95). However, research by Avellini and associates (7) revealed that endurance training will improve heat acclimation only if there is training-induced hyperthermia. Swimmers who trained and improved VO_{2max} by training in cold water did not have improved heat acclimation compared to athletes trained in warm water, or on land. For individuals who train in a hot environment, exercise training does not need to be intense because the added heat stress seems to be adequate to maximally stimulate the adaptive mechanisms of heat acclimation (59). Thus *a person's VO_{2max} is a poor reflection of heat acclimation*, because cardiorespiratory endurance is not the causal factor that stimulates heat acclimation.

Chronic Adaptations

The adaptations associated with heat acclimation are similar to those of standard endurance training that stress thermoregulation and consist of an increased plasma volume, early onset of sweating during exercise (85, 86), an increased submaximal exercise stroke volume (7), more dilute sweat electrolyte composition (28, 29), and decreased muscle glycogen degradation (30) (table 19.1). As previously explained, these adaptations have implications to thermoregulation, cardiovascular function, and muscle metabolism during prolonged exercise.

Rehydration from Dehydration   Given that maximal sweat rates exceed the maximal ability of the body to absorb water (see chapter 11), prolonged exercise or exercise in a hot or humid environment will always lead to some degree of dehydration. Ideally, this dehydration should be small if preventive strategies are adhered to, such as frequent ingestion of fluids.

The condition of dehydration is accompanied by increased serum concentrations of the hormones ADH and aldosterone (chapter 9). The hormones increase fluid conservation by decreasing urine volumes and ADH along with angiotensin II, and raise peripheral vascular resistance to maintain systemic blood pressures. A fluid loss from the body amounting to 4% body weight, or 3 L for a euhydrated 75-kg adult, must be replaced as rapidly as possible for optimal **rehydration.** Early research on the topic of rehydration revealed that this process was not simple, as rehydration was incomplete after 4 h of recovery even when ingested volumes during rehydration equaled the volume of water lost during dehydration (24). Furthermore, rehydration was most effective when a carbohydrate electrolyte solution was used compared to distilled water (24).

More recent research has combined neuroendocrine physiology, renal physiology, cardiovascular physiology, and muscle metabolism to determine the optimal procedure for rehydration from exercise-induced dehydration (43). Nose and colleagues (93) reported that sodium replacement with water increased fluid replacement during rehydration compared to water alone. Similarly, the addition of carbohy-

---

TABLE 19.1

Chronic adaptations to exercise and exercise in a hot environment that improve acclimation to exercise in the heat

ACCLIMATION ADAPTATION	PHYSIOLOGICAL BENEFIT
↑ Plasma volume	↑ Blood volume
	↑ Venous return
	↑ Cardiac output
	↓ Submaximal heart rate
	More sustained sweat response
	↑ Capacity for evaporative cooling
Earlier onset of sweating	Improved evaporative cooling
↓ Osmolality of sweat	Electrolyte conservation (mainly sodium)
↓ Muscle glycogen degradation	↓ Likelihood for muscle fatigue during prolonged exercise

drate to solutions for purposes of rehydration also increases drink osmolality and, on the basis of the research on Costill and Sparks (24), should also improve fluid replacement. However, more recent research using carbonated and non-carbonated solutions indicated that neither carbonation or carbohydrate improved rehydration compared to water (70). Additional research is required to determine how best to re-hydrate the body during recovery from exercise. An optimal drink would be one that retains a high percentage of the ini-tial volume within the body, and especially within the vascu-lar space, without being removed by the kidney and lost as urine.

Evaluating Environmental Conditions for Risks of Heat Injury

When combining the risks of exercise in a hot environment to the development of dehydration and the occurrence of heat illness, prevention of dehydration and hyperthermia is of primary importance. The American College of Sports Medicine (3) devised a scoring system derived from weighted temperatures that reflect the environmental ther-mal conditions of dry heat, radiative heat, and the potential for evaporative cooling.

This index of risk to thermal injury is based on the fol-lowing temperatures:

Dry bulb temperature: measure of air temperature
Black bulb temperature: measure of the potential for ra-diative heat gain
Wet bulb temperature: measure of the potential for evap-orative cooling

The index developed by ACSM places the greatest im-portance on the wet bulb temperature, because of the over-whelming influence of evaporative cooling on body heat gain, with the next-highest importance placed on radiative heat gain, and then air temperature. The adjusted tempera-ture is termed the wet bulb globe temperature (WBGT).

19.5 $WBGT = (0.7 \times Tw) + (0.2 \times Tb) + (0.1 \times Td)$

where Tw = wet bulb temperature, Tb = black bulb temper-ature, and Td = dry bulb temperature.

Because the WBGT is not really a temperature, expres-sion of the rating as a temperature can lead to confusion. Rather, *the WBGT is an index of the risk to heat illness for a given environmental condition*, and therefore should really be termed the **wet bulb globe index (WBGI)**. Table 19.2 lists the range of WBGI values that are associated with dif-ferent risks for heat injury.

b. Exercise in Cold Environments

The thought of being exposed to cold temperatures conjures images and feelings of discomfort. Typically, we dress our-selves to decrease sensations of cold when exposed to a cold environment. We even do this prior to exercising and, there-

TABLE 19.2

The relative risks for heat injury at different ranges of the WBGI (Wet Bulb Globe Index)

WBGI	RECOMMENDATIONS
23–28	**High risk for heat injury: red flag** Make runners aware that heat injury is possible, especially for those with a history of susceptibility to heat illness.
18–23	**Moderate risk for heat injury: amber flag** Make runners aware that the risk for heat injury will increase during the race.
< 18	**Low risk for heat injury: green flag** Make runners aware that although risk is low, there is still a possibility for heat injury to occur.
< 10	**Possible risk for hypothermia: white flag** Make individuals aware that conditions may cause excessive heat loss from the body, especially for individuals who will have slow race times and when conditions are wet and windy.

Source: Adapted from American College of Sports Medicine (3).

fore, the actual exposure to cold is minimized and the poten-tial impact of exercise in the cold is reduced. Furthermore, because dressing the body for insulation during exercise ac-tually minimizes the potential for heat loss from evaporative cooling, radiation, and convection, exercise in cold environ-ments can actually lead to exercise-induced hyperthermia, exercise-induced dehydration, and therefore the symptoms that accompany heatstroke. These events can occur even when environmental temperatures are below freezing!

Acute Adaptations to Cold Exposure

When not prepared for exposure to cold, skin and core tem-peratures decrease, which in turn stimulate peripheral temper-ature receptors and the central receptors of the hypothalamus. The neural response to cold involves the stimulation of shiv-ering, which induces involuntary skeletal muscle twitches that can increase basal metabolic rate and, therefore, heat produc-tion severalfold (97). The peripheral response to cold involves vasoconstriction of the cutaneous and skeletal muscle circula-tions, which of course decreases blood flow and therefore heat transfer from the core to the periphery. This latter response es-sentially increases the insulative properties of the dermal and

voluntary dehydration the progressive development of dehy-dration despite the availability of fluid to drink *ad libitum*

water intoxication excess drinking of fluid (typically plain wa-ter) that lowers the concentration of serum sodium, increas-ing the risk for developing hyponatremia

rehydration the process of returning fluids to the body

wet bulb globe index (WBGI) used to rate the relative risk of heat injury associated with given environmental conditions

skeletal muscle layers of the body. However, because vasco-constriction does not occur in the cerebral circulation, there is a large potential for heat loss from the head which can amount to 25% of the total heat loss from the body (97). The rate of heat loss increases when one is submerged in cold water because water has up to four times the thermal conductivity of air at the same temperature. Further increases in heat loss occur in water when there is water movement over the body because of the increased contribution of convective heat loss.

Heat loss from an individual will be less if there is more subcutaneous body fat. This relationship is more accurate in water than in air (123). Similarly, the critical water and air temperature below which the body increases basal metabolic rate is lower in individuals with more subcutaneous fat (123, 134).

Exercise During Cold Exposure

If submaximal exercise is performed and heat production is inadequate to match heat loss from the body, the increased VO_2 resulting from shivering increases submaximal VO_2 (97). However, as previously explained, typically when humans exercise in the cold, the increased clothing prevents excessive heat loss, and there is a net body heat gain. Unfortunately, the extent of body heat gain, sweating, and dehydration has not been extensively researched under the more realistic conditions of exercise in the cold when overdressed! However, as indicated in figure 19.12, it is known that the amount of clothing required to maintain thermal balance decreases with an increase in exercise intensity. Thus individuals should dress in layers during exercise in the cold, and once they are warm they should be able to remove layers causing a decrease in clothing insulation that matches the required insulative needs for the exercise condition (97).

During conditions that lower the body core temperature during water immersion, incremental exercise swimming performed to exhaustion results in a lower VO_{2max} (85, 86). Performance is also decreased during intense dynamic exercise when muscle is cooled. Bergh and Ekblom (11) reported a decrease in maximal strength and power output after muscle cooling, with explanations of this phenomenon based on increased tissue viscosity, decreased speed of ATP breakdown, regeneration, and contraction cycling, and perhaps impaired electrochemical function.

Can Humans Adapt to Chronic Cold Exposure?

Unlike human adaptations to chronic exposure to altitude or heat, there is minimal adaptation to chronic cold exposure. Research on this topic has compared responses from individuals from different cultures and geographic locations, as well as individuals from warm environments forced to live in cold environments for an extended period of time.

Some of the earliest research on cold acclimatization was performed on the Australian aborigines (55). Although the central Australian aborigines at the time of these studies

---

FIGURE 19.12

During exercise in a cold environment, there is a need to increase the insulative properties of the clothing. However, the insulation required in clothing decreases as exercise intensity increases. Adapted from Sharkey (119).

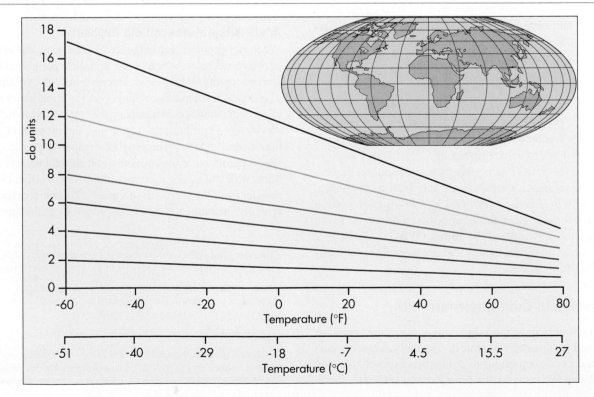

lived outdoors in a desert environment where day temperatures could exceed 40°C, night time temperatures would drop below freezing. Despite these temperature fluctuations, the aborigine people wore no clothing and slept on the ground with minimal structural protection from the elements. During exposure to cold, shivering did not occur and the basal metabolic rate in the aborigines did not increase. Rather, the aborigines had an increased vasoconstriction of the cutaneous and skeletal muscle circulations, and experienced larger decreases in temperatures of the skin and core than European subjects exposed to the same conditions (53). These responses, although initially appearing to be maladaptations that were due to the larger decrease in core temperature, conserved energy and, from this perspective, may have been an important adaptation for survival.

A total body response to cold exposure similar to that of the Australian aborigines occurs in the Korean pearl divers. In these women, core temperatures decrease to approximately 35°C during repeat dives, yet these women have a lower shivering threshold temperature than European subjects. It seems that shivering is really a poor response to total body cold exposure because it increases blood flow to the more active skeletal muscle, and actually increases the rate of heat loss. Shivering is therefore counterproductive when the total body is exposed to the cold, especially cold-water exposure which as previously explained has a greater thermal conductance than air (144).

The arctic Eskimo has been an obvious race of interest in research on adaptation to cold. However, data indicate that there are no unusual total body responses evident in the Eskimo compared to Europeans (144). However, the Eskimo, like other races and Europeans who routinely expose body parts to cold-water immersion, demonstrate a decreased vasoconstriction and warmer finger temperatures during exposure of the bare hand to cold (144). In addition, there is less of an increase in systemic blood pressure during hand immersion in cold water (cold-pressor test). These responses do not occur when other body parts are exposed to cold-water immersion. Thus this evidence indicates a potential adaptation to cold exposure in the body part routinely exposed to cold.

Windchill

Air movement over the surface of the body increases heat loss. This fact is expressed by the windchill index, which adjusts air temperatures to lower values based on wind velocity (table 19.3). For example, when exposed to an air temperature of 10°C and a wind velocity of 32 km/h, the adjusted windchill temperature approximates 0°C (freezing).

The windchill issue is important to consider, especially after exercise in a cold environment. For example, just as it was important to take off layered clothing during exercise, the need to add layered clothing after exercise is vital. After exercise, the moistened clothing and skin can cause a rapid

---

TABLE 19.3

Air temperatures and air temperatures adjusted for windchill caused by increased wind velocity

		AIR TEMPERATURE											
°C		10	4	-1	-7	-12	-18	-23	-29	-34	-40	-45	-51
(°F)		(50)	(40)	(30)	(20)	(10)	(0)	(-10)	(-20)	(-30)	(-40)	(-50)	(-60)
WIND SPEED													
KMH	MPH	WINDCHILL ADJUSTED TEMPERATURE											
0	0	10 (50)	4 (40)	-1 (30)	-7 (20)	-12 (10)	-18 (0)	-23 (-10)	-29 (-20)	-34 (-30)	-40 (-40)	-45 (-50)	-51 (-60)
8.0	5	9 (48)	3 (37)	-3 (27)	-9 (16)	-14 (6)	-21 (-5)	-26 (-15)	-32 (-26)	-38 (-36)	-44 (-47)	-49 (-57)	-56 (-68)
16.1	10	4 (40)	-2 (28)	-9 (16)	-16 (4)	-23 (-9)	-29 (-21)	-36 (-33)	-43 (-46)	-50 (-58)	-57 (-70)	-64 (-83)	-71 (-95)
9.3	15	2 (36)	-6 (22)	-13 (9)	-21 (-5)	-28 (-18)	-38 (-36)	-43 (-45)	-50 (-58)	-58 (-72)	-65 (-85)	-73 (-99)	-80 (-112)
32.2	20	0 (32)	-8 (18)	-16 (4)	-23 (-10)	-32 (-25)	-39 (-39)	-47 (-53)	-55 (-67)	-63 (-81)	-71 (-96)	-79 (-110)	-87 (-124)
40.2	25	-1 (30)	-9 (16)	-18 (0)	-26 (-15)	-34 (-29)	-42 (-44)	-51 (-59)	-59 (-74)	-67 (-88)	-76 (-104)	-83 (-118)	-92 (-133)
48.3	30	-2 (28)	-11 (13)	-19 (-2)	-28 (-18)	-36 (-33)	-44 (-48)	-53 (-63)	-62 (-79)	-70 (-94)	-78 (-109)	-87 (-125)	-96 (-140)
56.4	35	-3 (27)	-12 (11)	-20 (-4)	-29 (-20)	-37 (-35)	-45 (-49)	-55 (-67)	-63 (-82)	-72 (-98)	-81 (-113)	-89 (-129)	-98 (-145)
64.4	40	-3 (26)	-12 (10)	-21 (-6)	-29 (-21)	-38 (-37)	-47 (-53)	-56 (-69)	-65 (-85)	-73 (-100)	-82 (-116)	-91 (-132)	-100 (-148)

Little risk (for properly clothed person)   Increasing risk (cover up fully)   Greatest risk (exercise indoors)

heat loss, which would be increased in windy conditions. The development of postexercise hypothermia is a definite risk, and can be prevented by replacing wet clothes with dry clothes of even greater insulative properties.

Hypothermia and Frostbite

Decreases in core temperature, or **hypothermia,** are potentially life-threatening. As previously explained, body core temperatures can decline during exposure to cold water, and cold air, with increased risk as wind velocity increases. Symptoms of developing hypothermia are weakness, fatigue, decreased shivering, incoherency, and loss of communication skills. These initial symptoms should signal to other individuals the need to remove the person from the cold and start to reheat the person as soon as possible. Once unconsciousness occurs, the next symptom of hypothermia, the chances for successful treatment in the field decrease dramatically. Obviously, the risk of hypothermia on land increases during moist and windy conditions. The risk for hypothermia when submerged in water increases exponentially with decreases in water temperature (134).

On the basis of table 19.3, the risk for frostbite increases when skin is exposed to extremely cold temperatures. Appropriate clothing needs to be worn to protect the areas most prone to frostbite: the fingers, toes, ears, and nose.

Section III: Human Function and Performance During Gravitational Challenge

a. Microgravity

Human exercise performed in outer space is a modern example of exercise in an extreme environment. The earth has a gravitational force (*g*) that can be used as a standard force of 1*g*. Astronauts are exposed to gravitational forces less than 1*g*. For example, the moon has a gravitational force equal to 0.17*g*, whereas a spacecraft and the objects within it (e.g., the space shuttle of NASA, focus box 19.3) are exposed to zero gravity (0*g*) when outside a planetary orbit.

Ever since the first human space exploration, when astronauts returned to earth unable to walk after leaving the spacecraft, it was evident that prolonged exposure to **microgravity** was detrimental to human function. It was obvious that science had to determine what functions of the body were compromised in microgravity, and why. These were difficult challenges because it is very expensive to generate microgravity conditions on earth and therefore conduct research in microgravity. However, researchers have devised methods that are used to mimic the stresses placed on the body during microgravity. The most common method is *head down bed rest* for prolonged periods of time. The results of research using these methods have supplemented knowledge obtained from actual spaceflight research.

Physiological Effects of Exposure to Microgravity

The condition of microgravity unloads the work done by the body's muscles that maintain posture against the force of gravity. Similarly, microgravity environments unload the stress of weight bearing on bones and decrease the demands placed on the cardiovascular system during periods of muscle activity. For example, the lower the resistance that is applied to muscle during contraction, the lower the metabolic load, and thus the need for physiological adjustments to supply nutrients and remove waste products is reduced. Exposure to microgravity for extended periods of time risks atrophy of muscle and bone, decreases function of skeletal muscle (biochemical capacities and contractile function), compromises cardiovascular function, and alters body composition (88).

The muscle atrophy accompanying exposure to microgravity closely resembles the atrophy from disuse or immobilization (12, 133). Muscle strength and muscle fiber areas decrease, causing a reduced ability to perform work. Not surprisingly, declining muscle function also occurs with enhanced bone mineral loss in bones that are weight bearing. Such mineral losses approximate 4% and are similar again to studies of bed rest (140).

Extensive changes occur in cardiovascular function during exposure to microgravity. The decreased gravitational force decreases resistance to blood flow from the lower limbs and periphery to the heart, which decreases venous volume, increases arterial volume, increases systemic blood pressures, and stimulates the right atrium to release atrial natriuretic peptides that inhibit ADH release (see chapter 13). These factors combine to result in a renal diuresis, and decreasing plasma and blood volume.

During the prolonged spaceflights of *Salyut 1* (23 days), *Salyut 4* (63 days), and *Salyut 6* (140 days) missions, resting stroke volumes and heart rates did not change from preflight values during the complete exposures. However, when exercising, heart rates increased after 41 days and stroke volumes decreased after 62 days of exposure, yet these changes were only small at 10% and 12%, respectively (22, 23). Clearly, the renal diuresis accompanying microgravity does not pose drastic limitations to rest or exercise conditions when remaining in microgravity, even for extended periods of time. Interestingly, astronauts of the *Skylab 4* mission who exercised daily did not show any decreases in cardiovascular function during exercise throughout their 84-day exposure to zero gravity (111). This difference may indicate the beneficial role of exercise in microgravity for preserving cardiovascular function.

The detriment of the chronic adaptations of the body to microgravity is not seen until return to earth and therefore

---

hypothermia (hy′po-ther-mi′ah) a decreased body temperature below 37°C

microgravity (my-kro-grav′i-ti): conditions of decreased gravitational force

FOCUS BOX 19.3

John Glenn's Return to Space: Investigating the Connections Among Aging, Human Physiology, and Microgravity

On October 29 1998, the National Aeronautics and Space Administration (NASA) launched the space shuttle *Discovery* into orbit (fig. 19.13) for a 9-day mission. Although this was a routine mission, and functioned to perform now-routine satellite retrieval and basic science operations, it was one of the most publicized and interest-generating missions in the history of the space shuttle program. The unique quality of this mission was the inclusion of John Glenn, born on July 18, 1921 (fig. 19.14), among the crew.

On February 20, 1962, John Glenn was the first U.S. astronaut to orbit the earth (fig. 19.15). John completed three orbits of the earth during a 5-h flight, and was awarded the Space Congressional Medal of Honor for this feat. John Glenn was never offered another opportunity to return to space during his additional 3 years of service with the military and he retired from the Marine Corps in 1965. Since that time, he served four consecutive terms as a state senator from Ohio.

Why did John Glenn return to space? This answer is based on the similarity between the chronic adaptations to microgravity and the aging process, and the increasing age of our populations. For example, the average age of citizens in most Western societies is increasing dramatically. Within the United States in 1963 there were 17 million people over the age of 65 years. In 1998 there were twice that amount, and the number of Americans 85 years and older is projected to increase from 3.3 million in 1998 to 18.9 million by the year 2050 (88). It is not a surprise to find that as we age there are certain degenerative processes that decrease the effectiveness of how we function in our daily activities, and also during exercise.

One of the key scientific findings of human space exploration is that microgravity seems to induce a degeneration of many body systems similar to the aging process. The scientific interest in John Glenn's return to space at the age of 77 years is his relatively older age, how his age will influence his loss in function of many body systems, and the rate at which these functions will return to/approach normal. Of course, it is difficult to extrapolate scientific findings when using just one subject, especially when the subject is extremely different from the average 77-year-old male. Not surprisingly, this scientific flaw has been a major criticism of the promotion of the *Discovery's* research on aging. Nevertheless, a single subject is better than none, and John Glenn's willingness to provide his body to better direct and stimulate further research on aging is a testament to his commitment to the space program.

FIGURE 19.13

The space shuttle *Endeavour* being prepared for launching at the Kennedy Space Center, Cape Canaveral, Florida.

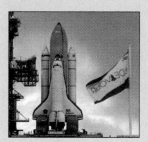

FIGURE 19.14

John Glenn (1998).

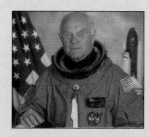

FIGURE 19.15

John Glenn (circa 1962).

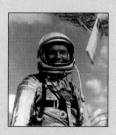

FIGURE 19.16

A photograph of a pilot in a g suit, designed to compress the lower limbs and abdomen to improve venous return to the heart during severe flight maneuvers.

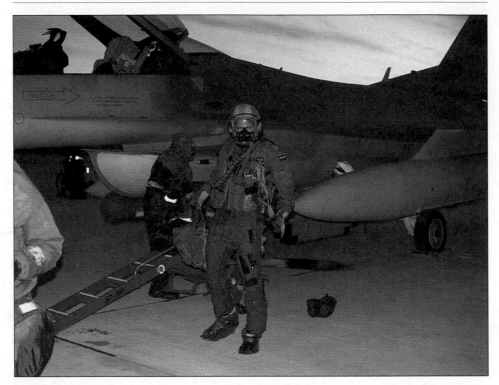

breathing that intermittently increases systemic blood pressures and intrathoracic pressure, which in turn improves the pumping of blood back to the right atrium.

Interestingly, research has shown that aerobic fitness does not improve a person's tolerance of a challenged venous return to the heart (**orthostatic tolerance**) (21, 121, 122). In fact, endurance training decreases orthostatic tolerance (127), whereas resistance training may actually improve orthostatic tolerance (121). The reasons for these findings have been explained by a reduced capacity for reflex vasoconstriction when endurance-trained. Possible causes of this difference are a resetting of the baroreceptors because of an increased total blood volume, an increased venous capacitance, or a depressed sympathetic nervous system and neuroendocrine response to cardiovascular challenge (127).

the return to gravity. Astronauts have "detrained" their tolerance and regulation of venous return to the heart against gravity, and episodes of syncope are common during the initial days after their return to earth. The muscle atrophy and reduced strength confounds their functional abilities, and because of the difficulty in measuring short-term changes in bone mineral density, it remains unclear how exposure to microgravity will influence bone mineral homeostasis in the decades following exposure to microgravity.

b. Increased Gravitational Forces

Exposing the lower body to negative pressures (LBNP) mimics conditions that many fighter pilots become exposed to during aerial maneuvers that increase the gravitational forces (positive g's) on the body. Because the pilots are seated, rapid turning of a plane can effectively increase the gravitational forces that retard blood flow to the heart and brain. If venous return is too compromised, pilots can experience syncope and therefore risk their lives and those of their copilots. This risk is so real that fighter pilots are rated on their g tolerance; the higher the g tolerance, the more extreme the maneuvers that can be performed prior to syncope and, therefore, the more effective the pilot should be in air combat.

To decrease the risk of syncope, pilots wear a special suit (a g suit) with bladders that inflate around the legs and waist, effectively assisting in the pumping of blood back to the heart (fig. 19.16). Pilots also perform a modified form of

Section IV: Exercise and Air Pollution

Research and observation combine to indicate the potential for air pollution to adversely affect exercise performance (98). This fact is important given the increasing urbanization and potential for air pollution in the major cities of most developed and developing countries. The potential negative effects of air pollution depend on the type of pollutant, its particulate size, water solubility, effects on pulmonary function, and concentration relative to dose response characteristics. Examples of common air pollutants are listed in table 19.4.

Of the known air pollutants, carbon monoxide is the most abundant, and because it has 200 times the affinity for hemoglobin than oxygen, it has high potential for detriment to health and exercise performance. However, despite this fact, CO inhalation resulting in up to 20% COHb does not impair submaximal exercise performance. Conversely, CO inhalation causing 4% COHb has been shown to decrease VO_{2max}. The detrimental effects of carbon monoxide inhalation are greater when exposed to increased altitudes (96), as would be expected based on the previous material presented in this chapter.

The inhalation of air containing ozone at concentrations greater than the NAAQS recommendations (table 19.4) has not been shown to impair submaximal exercise performance, yet it will induce increased discomfort and decreased lung function

(96). During exercise performed to VO_{2max}, there is evidence for a detriment when breathing air with ozone as high as 0.75 ppm (96); however, this was an extremely high ozone concentration and therefore lacks application to exercise outdoors.

Sulfur dioxide is released into the atmosphere during the combustion of fossil fuels. Sulfur dioxide is highly water soluble and can be converted to sulfuric acid. Together, the sulfur oxides and their derivatives exert their negative functions by irritating the lung, and thereby decreasing ventila-tory flow rates (96). Nitrogen dioxide is also produced from the combustion of fossil fuels and when handling fertilizers. The effects of nitrogen dioxide on exercise performance have not been extensively researched.

orthostatic tolerance the ability to withstand gravitational force in opposing blood flow back to the heart

TABLE 19.4

Examples of air pollutants that can impair exercise performance

POLLUTANT	UPPER HEALTHY LIMIT*	DETRIMENT
Carbon monoxide (CO)	9 ppm	Greater affinity for hemoglobin than oxygen
Carbon dioxide (CO_2)		Hyperventilation, acid-base disturbance, headache
Ozone (O_3)	0.12 ppm	Decreased lung function, headache
Sulphuric acid (H_2CO_4)		Irritates upper respiratory tract
Sulfur oxide (SO_2)	0.14 ppm	↑ Exercise-induced bronchospasm
Nitrogen dioxide (NO_2)		Lung irritant
Suspended particles	150 μg/m³	Aggravation of asthma and obstructive lung diseases

*Determined by the National Average Air Quality Standards of the United States of America.

Sources: Adapted from Pandolf (96) and Pierson et al. (98).

WEBSITE BOX

Chapter 19: Exercise in Differing Environments

The newest information regarding exercise physiology can be viewed at the following sites.*

NASA.org/
  Homepage of NASA.

http://microgravity.msfc.nasa.gov/
  Research program concerned with how microgravity influences the human body.

http://zeta.lerc.nasa.gov/sedhome.htm
  Another research program concerned with how microgravity influences the human body.

Princeton.edu/~oa/altitude.html
  Princeton University's information on high-altitude physiology and illnesses.

http://hyperion.advanced.org/15215/Foe/Dehydration/index.html
  All you ever needed to know about dehydration.

http://quickcare.org/gast/dehydrate.html
  Even more on dehydration.

mteverest.com/
  Organized list of all the links you could ever find that pertain to Mt. Everest.

millcom.com/~kbayne/denali.html
  All the information you need to plan and mount an assault on Denali (Mt. McKinley).

lnch.com/~diper/ak.html
  More information about Mt. McKinley, including excellent maps.

marketnet.com/mktnet/wound/hbo2.html
  Interesting site that explains the medical use of hyperbaric oxygen therapy (HBOT) for improving wound healing, treating carbon monoxide poisoning, and treating the bends.

curtin.edu.au/curtin/dept/physio/pt/edres/exphys/e552_96/
  Index of brief reviews of exercise physiology by students from Curtin University, Australia. Topics include nutrition, ergogenic aids, environmental physiology, training, and clinical applications.

agingresearch.org/john_glenn/index.asp
  Superb education modules on aging and exposure to microgravity.

uhms.org/
  Homepage of the Undersea and Hyperbaric Medical Society.

arfa.org/index.htm
  Excellent site providing comprehensive information on many topics within exercise physiology.

hyperbaricmedicine.org/
  Homepage of the American College of Hyperbaric Medicine.

*Unless indicated, all URLs preceded by http://www.

Note: These URLs were valid at the time of publication, but could have changed or been deleted from Internet access since that time.

- When a person is exposed to increasing altitude there is an exponential decrease in air pressure which decreases the amount (**partial pressure**) of oxygen in a given volume of air. The term used for conditions of a reduced oxygen content is **hypoxia.**

- When the hypoxia occurs because of a reduction in barometric pressure, it is termed **hypobaric hypoxia,** and therefore applies to on-location and altitude chamber studies. Conversely, hypoxia induced by breathing hypoxic gas when at or near sea level is termed **normobaric hypoxia.**

- The combination of the decreased barometric pressure and decreased P_aO_2 causes an increase in ventilation. The hypoxia-induced hyperventilation reduces P_ACO_2, P_aCO_2 and blood HCO_3^-, inducing a temporary respiratory alkalosis that lasts for approximately 2 days. The respiratory alkalosis is corrected by HCO_3^- excretion by the kidneys (*renal compensation*). There is a benefit to hyperventilation because of a raised P_AO_2 and P_aO_2 above values calculated from barometric pressures, thereby making the absolute altitude effectively much lower.

- Exposure to higher altitude will increase fluid loss via evaporative cooling because of the lower pressure and greater ease with which water changes from a liquid to a gas state (e.g., water boils at a lower temperature at increasing altitude!).

- Exposure to moderate to extreme altitudes can result in symptoms of headache, lethargy, and nausea. The condition characterized by these symptoms when exposed to increased altitude is termed **acute mountain sickness (AMS).** Apart from hypoxia itself, the two most important additional contributors to AMS are an *inadequate hyperventilation* and an *inadequate diuresis,* which causes a relative fluid retention.

- Depending on certain features of an individual, the decrement in VO_{2max} during acute exposure to hypoxia is very individualistic. For a given sea level VO_{2max}, individuals with a smaller lean body mass, larger lactate threshold, and less hypoxemia may have a smaller decrement.

- When individuals are chronically exposed to an altered environment, adaptations occur as part of a process known as **acclimatization.** The adaptations resulting from these artificial exposures occur as part of a process known as **acclimation.**

- Research has shown that exposure to moderate and high altitudes does not increase the degradation of muscle glycogen during exercise to exhaustion, and muscle lactate concentrations are not higher compared to sea level. In fact, maximal muscle lactate concentrations are actually lower at moderate and high altitudes, a condition that has been termed the **lactate paradox.**

- Ventilation continues to increase during the first 2 weeks of exposure to an increased altitude, regardless of severity. Chronic exposure to increased altitude is known to cause an increase in erythropoiesis because of the previously described acute increase in circulating erythropoietin. The time duration for the stimulation of erythropoiesis and the appearance of mature erythrocytes is 7 days (131)—a process termed polycythemia.

- Prolonged exposure to moderate to extreme altitudes is associated with a loss in lean body mass and total body weight. This response has been explained in part by a reduced caloric intake, an increased basal metabolic rate, dehydration, and decreased gastrointestinal function (poor nutrient absorption). Clearly, *food and fluid intake should be increased when one is exposed to increased altitude.*

- For very short-duration intense efforts (< 10 s), the muscles' abilities to regenerate ATP at high rates are not impaired during acute exposure to moderate to high altitude. For more prolonged intense exercise, where there is an increased contribution from glycolysis and lactate production, maximal blood lactate accumulation is decreased and there is a greater blood acidosis for given blood lactate values.

- There has been interest in whether individuals who complete **altitude training** perform better at sea level or at altitude. Individuals who have lived at low to moderate altitude all their lives respond better to acute altitude exposure than do sea level residents, as indicated by a smaller decrement in sea level VO_{2max}. There is clear evidence that *if living at altitude was to provide any potential benefit, it would be for residing at low to moderate altitude.* In addition, to reap the benefits from improved training quality at lower altitudes, yet retain the chronic mild hypoxic stimulus of living at moderate altitudes, it has been recommended that *athletes should live at moderate altitudes, yet train at lower altitudes,* a concept referred to as "sleep high, train low."

- Exposure of the body to increased pressure, or **hyperbaria,** can be accomplished when submerged under water, or when placed within a hyperbaric chamber. When submerged under seawater, the pressure increases 1 atmosphere (atm) (760 mmHg) every 10 m. In freshwater, the pressure increase is not as great because of the different water density, and approximates 1 atm every 10.4 m of depth (84). Risk for a too-rapid ascent during submersion can lead to decompression sickness commonly referred to as **the bends.**

- Body submersion can result in a decreased cutaneous blood flow, increased central blood volume, increased venous return, and lowered heart rate. It is theorized that prolonged water immersion decreases plasma volume because of an increased urine volume, and this may be detrimental to exercise performance when returning to dry land.

■ Continuous or intermittent exercise performed for prolonged periods of time is associated with increased sweat rates, and a reduction in body water or **dehydration.** The heat generation from exercise in combination with the heat stress from the environment can also increase the risk of excessive body heat storage (**hyperthermia**).

■ During prolonged submaximal exercise in a hot or humid environment, a person's sweat rate can increase to between 2 and 3 L/h. Initially, the largest volume of water is lost from interstitial fluid. As dehydration increases, there is an increasing contribution from intracellular fluid. Despite the large fluid volume losses during exercise at high sweat rates, the electrolyte losses are not physiologically significant.

■ When one is dehydrated and hyperthermic, cardiovascular function is compromised because of a decreased plasma and total blood volume and, in combination with the increased core temperature, these produce symptoms of central nervous system disturbances such as *lethargy*, *dizziness*, and *lack of coordination*. This symptomology marks the condition that is commonly referred to as **heat exhaustion.** If dehydration and body heat storage continues beyond heat exhaustion, symptoms can develop into *disorientation*, *confusion*, *psychoses*, and eventually *coma*, along with elevated serum enzymes. These latter symptoms mark the phase of the heat illness spectrum termed **heatstroke.**

■ Cardiovascular indications of dehydration occur with as little as 1% dehydration; however, more severe dehydration to 3% is required before detriments in VO_{2max} are detected. Submaximal exercise performance is also impaired in a hot environment. Exhaustion occurs at a reduced exercise time and at a lower core temperature when one is dehydrated during exercise in a hot environment compared to neutral thermal stress.

■ An important research finding of studies evaluating fluid intake during exercise in hot environments is that *ad libitum* fluid intake is less effective than forced drinking to replace fluid lost through sweating. This developing dehydration despite the availability of fluid has been termed **voluntary dehydration.** However, there have also been cases where individuals have ingested too much water, causing **water intoxication** and the development of *hyponatremia* (decreased serum sodium to < 130 mEq/L).

■ Typically, subjects demonstrate improved heat tolerance after endurance training in a hot environment for 60 to 100 min for 4 to 10 days. The more intense the exercise training, and therefore the more extreme the heat load, the greater is the apparent benefit to heat acclimation. The heat load is the most important factor that will cause heat acclimation. Consequently, *a person's VO_{2max} is a poor reflection of heat acclimation*, because cardiorespiratory endurance is not the most important causal factor.

■ The adaptations associated with heat acclimation are similar to those of standard endurance training that stress thermoregulation and consist of an increased plasma volume, early onset of sweating during exercise, an increased submaximal exercise stroke volume, more dilute sweat electrolyte composition, and decreased muscle glycogen degradation.

■ A fluid loss from the body amounting to 4% body weight, or 3 L for a euhydrated 75-kg adult, must be replaced as rapidly as possible for optimal **rehydration.** An optimal rehydration drink would be one that retains a high percentage of the initial volume within the body, and especially within the vascular space, without being removed by the kidney and lost as urine.

■ The American College of Sports Medicine (3) devised a scoring system derived from weighted temperatures that reflect the environmental thermal conditions of dry heat, radiative heat, and the potential for evaporative cooling. This index of risk to thermal injury is based on the following temperatures: *dry bulb temperature*: measure of air temperature; *black bulb temperature*: measure of the potential for radiative heat gain; and *wet bulb temperature*: measure of the potential for evaporative cooling. The adjusted temperature is termed the **wet bulb globe index (WBGI).**

$$WBGI = (0.7 \times Tw) + (0.2 \times Tb) + (0.1 \times Td)$$

where Tw = wet bulb temperature, Tb = black bulb temperature, and Td = dry bulb temperature.

■ The amount of clothing required to maintain thermal balance decreases with an increase in exercise intensity. Thus, individuals should dress in layers during exercise in the cold, and once they are warm they should be able to remove layers causing a decrease in clothing insulation that matches the required insulative needs for the exercise condition.

■ Air movement over the surface of the body increases heat loss. This fact is expressed by the windchill index, which adjusts air temperatures to lower values based on wind velocity. For example, when exposed to an air temperature of 10°C and a wind velocity of 32 km/h, the adjusted windchill temperature approximates 0° C (freezing).

■ Decreases in core temperature, or **hypothermia,** are potentially life-threatening. Symptoms of developing hypothermia are weakness, fatigue, decreased shivering, incoherency, and loss of communication skills. These initial symptoms should signal to other individuals the

SUMMARY

need to remove the person from the cold and start to re-heat the person as soon as possible.

■ The earth has a gravitational force (g) that can be used as a standard force of $1g$. Astronauts are exposed to gravitational forces less than $1g$. For example, the moon has a gravitational force equal to $0.17g$, whereas a spacecraft and the objects within it are exposed to zero gravity ($0g$) when outside a planetary orbit.

■ Ever since the first human space exploration, when astronauts returned to earth unable to walk after leaving the spacecraft, it was evident that prolonged exposure to **microgravity** was detrimental to human function. For example, exposure to microgravity for extended periods of time risks atrophy of muscle and bone, decreases function of skeletal muscle (biochemical capacities and contractile function), compromises cardiovascular function, and alters body composition.

■ To decrease the risk of syncope, fighter pilots wear a special suit (a g suit) with bladders that inflate around the legs and waist, effectively assisting in the pumping of blood back to the heart. Pilots also perform a modified form of breathing that intermittently increases systemic blood pressures and intrathoracic pressure, which in turn improves the pumping of blood back to the right atrium. Interestingly, research has shown that aerobic fitness does not improve a person's tolerance of a challenged venous return to the heart (**orthostatic tolerance**).

■ Research and observation combine to indicate the potential for air pollution to adversely affect exercise performance. Examples of common air pollutants are carbon monoxide (CO), carbon dioxide (CO_2), ozone (O_3), sulphuric acid (H_2CO_4), sulfur oxide (SO_2), nitrogen dioxide (NO_2), and suspended particles.

STUDY QUESTIONS

1. Explain the terms hypobaria, hypoxia, hypobaric hypoxia, normobaric hypoxia.

2. How does an increase in altitude influence air pressure, the oxygen content of the air, and the oxygen content of arterial blood?

3. Whether VO_{2max} increases after chronic altitude exposure remains a controversial topic. What chronic adaptations to high-altitude exposure would support an increase in VO_2max, and what chronic adaptations would oppose an increase in VO_{2max}?

4. Explain the "lactate paradox."

5. Is short-term intense exercise impaired at moderate to high altitudes? If so, what types and durations of exercise are not affected/impaired, and why?

6. Explain the concept of *sleep high and train low*, as applied to increasing the benefits of altitude exposure on sea level performance.

7. Explain the dangers of breath-holding during underwater exercise.

8. Using each of Boyle's and Charles's laws, explain the dangers of scuba diving.

9. What is dehydration, and why is it such a concern during exercise in warm to hot environments?

10. What are the differences between *acclimatization* and *acclimation?*

11. Explain the importance of cutaneous vasodilation to improved evaporative heat loss.

12. Explain the WBGI.

13. Why is the issue of exercise in a cold environment of limited relevance to most individuals?

14. Is the shivering response to cold exposure an appropriate mechanism for retaining body heat, regardless of whether on land or in water? Explain.

15. Is there evidence of human adaptation to cold environments? Explain.

16. Why is exposure to microgravity detrimental to human physiology on return to gravity? What interventions have been attempted to decrease the effects? Have they been successful?

17. What has research revealed about the effects of carbon monoxide and ozone on exercise performance?

APPLICATIONS

1. How would you determine if an athlete was likely to experience considerable detriment in VO_{2max} during a race at altitude (7500 ft)?

2. Is acclimation to heat stress a practice that all individuals who are anticipating future exposure to hot or humid environments should complete? Explain.

3. What are the human physiological challenges to the success of the proposed space station project of NASA?

REFERENCES

1. Abbrecht, P. H., and J. K. Littell. Plasma erythropoietin in men and mice during acclimatization to different altitudes. *J. Appl. Physiol.* 32(1):54–58, 1972.

2. Adams, W. C., G. W. Mack, G. W. Langhans, and E. R. Nadel. Effects of equivalent sea-level and altitude training on VO_{2max} and running performance. *J. Appl. Physiol.* 39:262, 1975.

3. American College of Sports Medicine. Position stand on the prevention of thermal injuries during distance running. *Med. Sci. Sports Exerc.* 16(5): ix–xiv, 1985.

4. Anderson, H. T., E. B. Smeland, J. O. Owe, and K. Myhre. Analyses of maximum cardiopulmonary performance during exposure to acute hypoxia at simulated altitude-sea level to 5000 meters (760–404 mmHg). *Aviat. Space Environ. Med.* 56:1192–1197, 1985.

5. Armstrong, L. E., and K. B. Pandolf. Physical training, cardiorespiratory physical fitness and exercise-heat tolerance. In K. B. Pandolf, M. N. Sawka, and R. R. Gonzalez (eds.), *Human physiology and environmental medicine at terrestrial extremes.* Cooper Publishing Group, Carmel, 1986, pp. 199–226.

6. Armstrong, L. E., R. W. Hubbard, J. P. DeLuca, and E. L. Christensen. Heat acclimatization during summer running in the United States. *Med. Sci. Sports Exerc.* 19(2):131–136, 1987.

7. Avellini, B. A., Y. Shapiro, S. M. Fortney, C. B. Wenger, and K. B. Pandolf. Effects on heat tolerance of physical training in water and on land. *J. Appl. Physiol.* 53(5):1291–1298, 1982.

8. Barr, S. I., D. L. Costill, and W. J. Fink. Fluid replacement during prolonged exercise: Effects of water, saline, or no fluid. *Med. Sci. Sports Exerc.* 23(7):811–817, 1991.

9. Bender, P. R., et al. Oxygen transport to exercising leg in chronic hypoxia. *J. Appl. Physiol.* 65(6):2592–2597, 1988.

10. Bender, P. R., et al. Decreased exercise muscle lactate release after high-altitude acclimatization. *J. Appl. Physiol.* 67(2):1456–1462, 1989.

11. Bergh, U., and B. Ekblom. Influence of muscle temperature on maximal muscle strength and power output in human skeletal muscle. *Acta Physiol. Scand.* 107:33–37, 1979.

12. Booth, F. W. Effects of limb immobilization on skeletal muscle. *J. Appl. Physiol.* 52(5):1113–1118, 1982.

13. Brooks, G. A., et al. Increased dependence on blood glucose after acclimatization to 4300 m. *J. Appl. Physiol.* 70(2):919–927, 1991.

14. Brooks, G. A., et al. Decreased reliance on lactate during exercise after acclimatization to 4300 m. *J. Appl. Physiol.* 71:333–341, 1991.

15. Brooks, G. A., et al. Muscle accounts for glucose disposal but not blood lactate appearance during exercise after acclimatization to 4300 m. *J. Appl. Physiol.* 72(6):2435–2445, 1992.

16. Buskirk, E. R., J. Kollias, R. F. Akers, E. K. Prolop, and E. P. Reategui. Maximal performance at altitude and on return from altitude in conditioned runners. *J. Appl. Physiol.* 23:259–266, 1967.

17. Butterfield, G. E., J. Gates, S. Fleming, G. A. Brooks, J. R. Sutton, and J. T. Reeves. Increased energy intake minimizes weight loss in men at high altitude. *J. Appl. Physiol.* 72(5):1741–1748, 1992.

18. Carter, J. E., and C. V. Gisolfi. Fluid replacement during and after exercise in the heat. *Med. Sci. Sports Exerc.* 21(5):532–539, 1989.

19. Cerretelli, P., A. Veicsteinas, and C. Marconi. Anaerobic metabolism at high altitude: The lactacid mechanism. In W. Brendel and R.A. Zink (eds.), *High-altitude physiology and medicine.* Springer-Verlag, New York, 1982, pp. 94–102.

20. Cerretelli, P. O_2 breathing at altitude: Effects on maximal performance. In W. Brendel and R. A. Zink (eds.), *High-altitude physiology and medicine.* Springer-Verlag, New York, 1982, pp. 9–15.

21. Convertino, V. A., T. M. Sather, D. J. Goldwater, and W. R. Alford. Aerobic fitness does not contribute to prediction of orthostatic tolerance. *Med. Sci. Sports Exerc.* 18(5):551–556, 1986.

22. Convertino, V. A. Potential benefits of maximal exercise just prior to return from weightlessness. *Aviat. Space Environ. Med.* 58:568–572, 1987.

23. Convertino, V. A. Physiological adaptations to weightless: Effects of exercise and work performance. *Exerc. Sport Sci. Rev.* 18:119–166, 1990.

24. Costill, D. L., and K. E. Sparks. Rapid fluid replacement following thermal dehydration. *J. Appl. Physiol.* 34(3):299–303, 1973.

25. Costill, D. L., and W. J. Fink. Plasma volume changes following exercise and thermal dehydration. *J. Appl. Physiol.* 37(4):521–525, 1974.

26. Costill, D. L. R. Cote, T. Miller, and S. Wynder. Water and electrolyte replacement during repeated days of work in the heat. *Aviat. Space Environ. Med.* 46(6):795–800, 1975.

REFERENCES

27. Costill, D. L., R. Cote, and W. J. Fink. Muscle water and electrolytes following varied levels of dehydration in man. *J. Appl. Physiol.* 40(1):6–11, 1976.

28. Costill, D. L. Sweating: Its composition and effects on body fluids. *An. New York Acad. Sci.* 301:160–174, 1977.

29. Costill, D. L. Water and electrolyte requirements during exercise. *Clin. Sports Med.* 3(3):639–648, 1984.

30. Costill, D. L. Muscle metabolism and electrolyte balance during heat acclimation. *Acta Physiol. Scand.* 128(Suppl. 556):111–118, 1986.

31. Cymerman, A., et al. Operation Everest II: Maximal oxygen uptake at extreme altitude. *J. Appl. Physiol.* 66:2446–2453, 1989.

32. Daniels, J., and N. Oldridge. The effects of alternate exposure to altitude and sea level on world-class middle distance runners. *Med. Sci. Sports Exerc.* 2(3):107–112, 1970.

33. Davis, J. M., D. R. Lamb, R. R. Pate, C. A. Slentz, W. A. Burgess, and W. P. Bartoli. Carbohydrate-electrolyte drinks: Effects on endurance cycling in the heat. *Am. J. Clin. Nutr.* 48:1023–1030, 1988.

34. Di Prampero, P. E., P. Mognoni, and A. Veicsteinas. The effects of hypoxia on maximal anaerobic alactic power in man. In W. Brendel and R.A. Zink (eds.), *High-altitude physiology and medicine.* Springer-Verlag, New York, 1982, pp. 88–93.

35. Eckardt, K., U. Boutellier, A. Kurtz, M. Shopen, E. A. Koller, and C. Bauer. Rate of erythropoietin formation in humans in response to acute hypobaric hypoxia. *J. Appl. Physiol.* 66(4):1785–1788, 1989.

36. Epstein, Y. Heat intolerance: Predisposing factor or residual injury? *Med. Sci. Sports Exerc.* 22(1):29–35, 1990.

37. Evans, W. O., S. M. Robinson, D. H. Horstman, R. E. Jackson, and R. B. Weiskopf. Amelioration of the symptoms of acute mountain sickness by staging and acetazolamide. *Aviat. Space Environ. Med.* 47(5):512–516, 1976.

38. Faulkner, J. A. Effects of training at moderate altitude on physical performance capacity. *J. Appl. Physiol.* 23:85, 1967.

39. Faulkner, J. A., J. Kollias, C. B. Favour, E. R. Buskirk, and B. Balke. Maximal aerobic capacity and running performance at altitude. *J. Appl. Physiol.* 24:685–691, 1968.

40. Ferretti, G., C. Moia, J.-M. Thomet, and B. Kayser. The decrease of maximal oxygen consumption during hypoxia in man: A mirror image of the oxygen equilibrium curve. *J. Physiol.* 498(1):231–237, 1997.

41. Fink, W. J., D. L. Costill, and P. J. Van Handel. Leg muscle metabolism during exercise in the heat and cold. *Eur. J. Appl. Physiol.* 34:183–190, 1975.

42. Gisolfi, C. V., and J. S. Cohen. Relationships among training, heat acclimation, and heat tolerance in men and women: The controversy revisited. *Med. Sci. Sports Med.* 11(1):56–59, 1979.

43. Gisolfi, C. V., and S. M. Duchman. Guidelines for optimal replacement beverages for different athletic events. *Med. Sci. Sports Exerc.* 24(6):679–687, 1992.

44. Gore, C. J., et al. Reduced performance of male and female athletes at 580 m altitude. *Eur. J. Appl. Physiol.* 75:136–143, 1997.

45. Gore, C. J., et al. Increased arterial desaturation in trained cyclists during maximal exercise at 580 m altitude. *J. Appl. Physiol.* 80(6):2204–2210, 1996.

46. Green, H. J., J. R. Sutton, P. M. Young, A. Cymerman, and C. S. Houston. Operation Everest II: Muscle energetics during maximal exhaustive exercise. *J. Appl. Physiol.* 66:142–150, 1989.

47. Green, H. J., J. R. Sutton, A. Cymerman, P. M. Young, and C. S. Houston. Operation Everest II: Adaptations in human skeletal muscle. *J. Appl. Physiol.* 66:2454–2461, 1989.

48. Green, H. J., J. R. Sutton, E. E. Wolfel, J. T. Reeves, G. E. Butterfield, and G. A. Brooks. Altitude acclimatization and energy metabolic adaptations in skeletal muscle during exercise. *J. Appl. Physiol.* 73(6):2701–2708, 1992.

49. Greenleaf, J. E. Problem: Thirst, drinking behavior, and involuntary dehydration. *Med. Sci. Sports Exerc.* 24(6):645–656, 1992.

50. Grissom, C. K., R. C. Roach, F. H. Sarnquist, and P. H. Hackett. Acetazolamide in the treatment of acute mountain sickness: Clinical efficacy and effect on gas exchange. *An. Intern. Med.* 116:461–465, 1992.

51. Grover, R. F., J. V. Weil, and J. T. Reeves. Cardiovascular adaptations to exercise at high altitude. *Exerc. Sport Sci. Rev.* 14:269–302, 1986.

52. Groves, B. M., et al. Operation Everest II: Elevated high-altitude pulmonary resistance unresponsive to oxygen. *J. Appl. Physiol.* 63(2):521–530, 1987.

53. Hammel, H. T., R. W. Elsner, D. H. LeMessurier, H. T. Anderson, and F. A. Milan. Thermal and metabolic responses of the Australian aborigine exposed to moderate cold in summer. *J. Appl. Physiol.* 14:605–615, 1959.

54. Hartley, L. H., J. A. Vogel, and M. Landowne. Central, femoral, and brachial circulation during exercise in hypoxia. *J. Appl. Physiol.* 34(1):87–90, 1973.

55. Hicks, C. S. Terrestrial animals in cold: Exploratory studies of primitive man. In D. B. Dill, E. F. Adolph, and C. G. Wilber (eds.), *Handbook of physiology, Sect. 4: Adaptation to the environment.* American Physiological Society, Washington D.C., 1964, pp. 405–412.

56. Hiller, W. D. B. Dehydration and hyponatremia during triathlons. *Med. Sci. Sports Exerc.* 21(5):S219–S221, 1989.

57. Hogan, M. C., R. H. Cox, and H. G. Welch. Lactate accumulation during incremental exercise with varied inspired oxygen fractions. *J. Appl. Physiol.* 55:1134–1140, 1983.

58. Horstman, D. H., R. Weiskopf, and R. E. Jackson. Work capacity during 3-week sojourn at 4300 m: Effects of relative polycythemia. *J. Appl. Physiol.* 49:311–318, 1980.

59. Houmard, J. A., D. L. Costill, J. A. Davis, J. B. Mitchell, D. D. Pascoe, and R. A. Robergs. The influence of exercise intensity on heat acclimation in trained subjects. *Med. Sci. Sports Exerc.* 22(5):615–620, 1990.

60. Houston, C. S. High adventure: The romance between medicine and mountaineering. *Exerc. Sport Sci. Rev.* 22:1–22, 1994.

61. Hubbard, R. W., and L. E. Armstrong. The heat illnesses: Biochemical, ultrastructural and fluid-electrolyte considera-

tions. In K. B. Pandolf, M. N. Sawka, and R. R. Gonzalez (eds.), *Human physiology and environmental medicine at terrestrial extremes.* Cooper Publishing Group, Carmel, 1986, pp. 305–360.

62. Hubbard, R. W. Heatstroke pathophysiology: The energy depletion model. *Med. Sci. Sports Exerc.* 22(1):19–28, 1990.

63. Hubbard, R. W. An introduction: The role of exercise in the etiology of exertional heatstroke. *Med. Sci. Sports Exerc.* 22(1):2–5, 1990.

64. Hughes, R. L., M. Clode, R. H. T. Edwards, T. L. Goodwin, and N. L. Jones. Effects of inspired O_2 on cardiopulmonary and metabolic responses to exercise in man. *J. Appl. Physiol.* 24:366, 1968.

65. Kame, V. D., and D. R. Pendergast. Effects of short-term and prolonged immersion on the cardiovascular responses to exercise. *Aviat. Space Environ. Med.* 66:20–25, 1995.

66. Karvonen, J., and J., Saarela. The effect of sprint training performed in a hypoxic environment on specific performance capacity. *J. Sports Med.* 26:219–224, 1986.

67. Kayser, B., M. Narici, T. Binzoni, B. Grassi, and P. Cerretelli. Fatigue and exhaustion in chronic hypobaria: Influence of exercising muscle mass. *J. Appl. Physiol.* 76(2):634–640, 1994.

68. Knaupp, W., S. Khilnani, J. Sherwood, S. Scharf, and H. Steinberg. Erythropoietin response to acute normobaric hypoxia in humans. *J. Appl. Physiol.* 73(3):837–840, 1992.

69. Koistinen, P., T. Takala, V. Martikkala, and J. Leppaluoto. Aerobic fitness influences the response of maximal oxygen uptake and lactate threshold in acute hypobaric hypoxia. *Int. J. Sports Med.* 26(2):78–81, 1995.

70. Lambert, C. P., et al. Fluid replacement after dehydration: Influence of beverage carbonation and carbohydrate content. *Int. J. Sports Med.* 13(4):285–292, 1992.

71. Lawler, J., S. Powers, and D. Thompson. Linear relationship between VO_{2max} and VO_{2max} decrement during exposure to acute hypoxia. *J. Appl. Physiol.* 64(4):1486–1492, 1988.

72. Lenfant, C. P. Effect of chronic hypoxic hypoxia on the O_2-Hb dissociation curve and respiratory gas transport in man. *Resp. Physiol.* 7:7, 1969.

73. Levine, B. D., et al. The effect of normoxic and hypobaric hypoxic endurance training on the hypoxic ventilatory response. *Med. Sci. Sports Exerc.* 24(7):769–775, 1992.

74. Levine, B. D., and J. Stray-Gunderson. A practical approach to altitude training: Where to live and train for optimal performance enhancement. *Int. J. Sports Med.* 13:S209–S212, 1992.

75. Libert, J. P., V. Candas, J. C. Sagot, J. P. Meyer, J. J. Vogt, and T. Ogawa. Contribution of skin thermal sensitivities of large body areas to sweating response. *Jap. J. Physiol.* 34:75–88, 1984.

76. Lind, A. R. A physiological criterion for setting thermal environmental limits for everday work. *J. Appl. Physiol.* 16:51–56, 1963.

77. Loepkky, J., M. V. Icenogle, P. Scotto, R. A. Robergs, H. Hinghofer-Szalkay, and R. C. Roach. Ventilation during simulated altitude, normobaric hypoxia and normoxic hypobaria. *Resp. Physiol.* 107:231–239, 1997.

78. Maresh, C. M., B. J. Noble, K. L. Robertson, and W. E. Sime. Maximal exercise during hypobaric hypoxia (447 Torr) in moderate-altitude natives. *Med. Sci. Sports Exerc.* 15:360–365, 1983.

79. Martin, D., and J. O'Kroy. Effects of acute hypoxia on the VO_{2max} of trained and untrained subjects. *J. Sports Sci.* 11:37–42, 1993.

80. Mazzeo, R. S., et al. β-Adrenergic blockade does not prevent the lactate response to exercise after acclimatization to high altitude. *J. Appl. Physiol.* 76(2):610–615, 1994.

81. Millard-Stafford, M., P. B. Sparling, L. B. Rosskopf, B. T. Hinson, and L. J. Dicarlo. Carbohydrate-electrolyte replacement during a simulated triathlon in the heat. *Med. Sci. Sports Exerc.* 22(5):621–628, 1990.

82. Millard-Stafford, M., P. B. Sparling, L. B. Rosskopf, and L. J. Dicarlo. Carbohydrate-electrolyte replacement improves distance running performance in the heat. *Med. Sci. Sports Exerc.* 24(8):934–940, 1992.

83. Montain, S. J., and E. F. Coyle. Fluid ingestion during exercise increases skin blood flow independent of increases in blood volume. *J. Appl. Physiol.* 73(3):903–910, 1992.

84. Muza, S. R. Hyperbaric physiology and human performance. In K. B. Pandolf, M. N. Sawka, and R. R. Gonzalez (eds.), *Human physiology and environmental medicine at terrestrial extremes.* Cooper Publishing Group, Carmel, 1986, pp. 565–590.

85. Nadel, E. R., K. B. Pandolf, M. F. Roberts, and J. A. J. Stolwijk. Mechanism of thermal activation to exercise and heat. *J. Appl. Physiol.* 37(4):515–520, 1974.

86. Nadel, E. R., E. Holmer, U. Bergh, P. O. Åstrand, and J. A. J. Stolwijk. Energy exchanges of swimming man. *J. Appl. Physiol.* 36:465–471, 1974.

87. Nadel, E. R., S. F. Fortney, and C. B. Wenger. Circulatory and thermal regulations during exercise. *Fed. Proc.* 39:1491–1497, 1980.

88. NASA. NASA Facts: Parallel Processes? The study of human adaptation to space helps us understand aging. http://shuttle.nasa.gov/future/sts95/aging.html.

89. Nielsen, B., and M. Nielsen. Body temperature during work at different environmental temperatures. *Acta Physiol. Scand.* 56:120–129, 1962.

90. Nielsen, B., G. Savard, E. A. Richter, M. Hargreaves, and B. Saltin. Muscle blood flow and muscle metabolism during exercise and heat stress. *J. Appl. Physiol.* 69(3):1040–1046, 1990.

91. Noakes, T. D. Fluid replacement during exercise. *Exerc. Sport Sci. Rev.* 21:297–330, 1993.

92. Noakes, T. D., et al. Metabolic rate, not percent dehydration, predicts rectal temperature in marathon runners. *Med. Sci. Sports Exerc.* 23(4):443–449, 1991.

93. Nose, H., G. W. Mack, X. Shi, and E. R. Nadel. Role of osmolality and plasma volume during rehydration in humans. *J. Appl. Physiol.* 65:325–331, 1988.

94. Owen, M. D., K. C. Kregel, P. T. Wall, and C. V. Gisolfi. Effects of ingesting carbohydrate beverages during exercise in the heat. *Med. Sci. Sports Exerc.* 18(5):568–575, 1986.

REFERENCES

95. Pandolf, K. B. Effects of physical training and cardiorespiratory fitness on exercise-heat tolerance: Recent observations. *Med. Sci. Sports Exerc.* 11:60–65, 1979.

96. Pandolf, K. B. Air quality and human performance. In K. B. Pandolf, M. N. Sawka, and R. R. Gonzalez (eds.), *Human physiology and environmental medicine at terrestrial extremes*. Cooper Publishing Group, Carmel, 1986, pp. 591–630.

97. Pate, R. R. Special considerations for exercise in cold weather. *Gatorade Sports Science Exchange* 10(1):1–5, 1988.

98. Pierson, W. E., D. S. Covert, J. Q. Koenig, T. Namekata, and Y. S. Kim. Implications of air pollution effects on athletic performance. *Med. Sci. Sports Exerc.* 18(3):322–327, 1986.

99. Pitts, G. C., R. E. Johnson, and F. C. Consolazio. Work in the heat as affected by intake of water, salt and glucose. *Am. J. Physiol.* 142:253–259, 1944.

100. Pugh, L. G. C. E., M. B. Gill, and S. Lahirim. Muscular exercise at great altitudes. *J. Appl. Physiol.* 19:431–440, 1964.

101. Ramanathan, N. L. A new weighting system for mean surface temperature of the human body. *J. Appl. Physiol.* 19(5):531–533, 1964.

102. Reeves, J. T., et al. Operation Everest II: Preservation of cardiac function at extreme altitude. *J. Appl. Physiol.* 63:531–539, 1987.

103. Reeves, J. T., et al. Adaptations to hypoxia: Lessons from Operation Everest II. In W. Simmons (ed.), *Man in extreme environments*. Mosby-Year Book, St. Louis, 1991, pp. 334–361.

104. Reeves, J. T., et al. Oxygen transport during exercise at altitude and the lactate paradox: Lessons from Operation Everest II and Pikes Peak. *Exerc. Sport Sci. Rev.* 20:275–296, 1992.

105. Rehrer, N. J., E. J. Beckers, F. Brouns, F. Ten Hoor, and W. H. M. Saris. Effects of dehydration on gastric emptying and gastrointestinal distress while running. *Med. Sci. Sports Exerc.* 22(6):790–795, 1990.

106. Reynafarje, C. Myoglobin content and enzymatic activity of muscle and altitude adaptation. *J. Appl. Physiol.* 17:301–305, 1962.

107. Roberts, R. A., R. Quintana, D. Parker, and C. Frankel. Multiple variables determine the decrement in VO_{2max} during acute hypobaric hypoxia. *Med. Sci. Sports Exerc.* 30(6):869–879, 1998.

108. Ryan, A. J., T. L. Bleiler, J. E. Carter, and C. V. Gisolfi. Gastric emptying during prolonged cycling exercise in the heat. *Med. Sci. Sports Exerc.* 21(1):51–58, 1989.

109. Saltin, B., R. F. Grover, C. G. Blomqvist, L. H. Harley, and R. L. Johnson, Jr. Maximal oxygen uptake and cardiac output after 2 weeks at 4300 m. *J. Appl. Physiol.* 45:400–409, 1968.

110. Savard, G. K., B. Nielsen, I. Laszcynska, B. E. Larsen, and B. Saltin. Muscle blood flow is not reduced in humans during moderate exercise and heat stress. *J. Appl. Physiol.* 64:649–657, 1988.

111. Sawin, C. F., J. A. Rummel, and E. L. Michel. Instrumented personal exercise during long-duration space flights. *Aviat. Space Environ. Med.* 46:394–400, 1975.

112. Sawka, M. N., and C. B. Wenger. Physiological responses to acute exercise-heat stress. In K. B. Pandolf, M. N. Sawka, and R. R. Gonzalez (eds.), *Human physiology and environmental medicine at terrestrial extremes*. Cooper Publishing Group, Carmel, 1986, pp. 97–152.

113. Sawka, M. N. Body fluid responses and hypohydration during exercise-heat stress. In K. B. Pandolf, M. N. Sawka, and R. R. Gonzalez (eds.), *Human physiology and environmental medicine at terrestrial extremes*. Cooper Publishing Group, Carmel, 1986, pp. 227–265.

114. Sawka, M. N., A. J. Young, W. A. Latzka, P. D. Neuffer, M. D. Quigley, and K. B. Pandolf. Human tolerance to heat strain during exercise: Influence of hydration. *J. Appl. Physiol.* 73(1):368–375, 1992.

115. Sawka, M. N. Physiological consequences of hypohydration: Exercise performance and thermoregulation. *Med. Sci. Sports Exerc.* 24(6):657–670, 1992.

116. Schoene, R. B., R. C. Roach, P. H. Hackett, J. R. Sutton, A. Cymerman, and C. S. Houston. Operation Everest II: Ventilatory adaptation during gradual decompression to extreme altitude. *Med. Sci. Sports Exerc.* 22(6):804–810, 1990.

117. Schooley, J. C., and L. J. Mahlmann. Hypoxia and the initiation of erythropoietin production. *Blood Cells* 1:429–448, 1975.

118. Shapiro, Y., and D. S. Seidman. Filed and clinical observations of exertional heat stroke patients. *Med. Sci. Sports Exerc.* 22(1):6–14, 1990.

119. Sharkey, B. *Physiology of fitness*. 2nd ed. Human Kinetics, Champaign, IL, 1984.

120. Shephard, R. J., E. Bouhlel, H. Vandewalle, and H. Monod. Peak oxygen intake and hypoxia: Influence of physical fitness. *Int. J. Sports Med.* 9:279–283, 1988.

121. Smith, M. L., and P. B. Raven. Cardiovascular responses to lower body negative pressure in endurance and static exercise-trained men. *Med. Sci. Sports Exerc.* 18(5):545–550, 1986.

122. Smith, M. L., D. L. Hudson, and P. B. Raven. Effects of muscle tension on the cardiovascular responses to lower body negative pressure in man. *Med. Sci. Sports Exerc.* 19(5):436–442, 1987.

123. Smith, R. M., and J. M. Hanna. Skinfolds and resting heat loss in cold air and water: temperature equivalence. *J. Appl. Physiology* 39(1):93–102, 1975.

124. Squires, R. W., and E. R. Buskirk. Aerobic capacity during acute exposure to simulated altitude, 914–2286 meters. *Med. Sci. Sports Exerc.* 14:36–40, 1982.

125. Stager, J. M., A. Tucker, L. Cordain, B. J. Engebretsen, W. F. Brechue, and C. C. Matulich. Normoxic and acute hypoxic exercise tolerance in man following acetazolamide. *Med. Sci. Sports Exerc.* 22(2):178–184, 1990.

126. Stenberg, J. Hemodynamic response to work at simulated altitude, 4000 m. *J. Appl. Physiol.* 21:1589, 1966.

127. Stevens, G. H. J., B. H. Foresman, X. Shi, S. A. Stern, and P. B. Raven. Reduction in LBNP tolerance following prolonged endurance exercise training. *Med. Sci. Sports Exerc.* 24(11):1235–1244, 1992.

128. Sutton, J. R., and G. Coates. Pathophysiology of high-altitude illnesses. *Exerc. Sport Sci. Rev.* 111:210–231, 1983.

129. Sutton, J. R., et al. Operation Everest II: Oxygen transport during exercise at extreme simulated altitude. *J. Appl. Physiol.* 64(4):1309–1321, 1988.

130. Sutton, J. R. Exercise training at high altitude: Does it improve endurance performance at sea level? *Gatorade Sports Science Exchange* 6(4):1–4, 1993.

131. Swenson, E. R., and J. M. B. Highes. Effects of acute and chronic acetozolamide on resting ventilation and ventilatory responses in men. *J. Appl. Physiol.* 74(1):230–237, 1993.

132. Thaysen, J. H., and I. L. Schwartz. Fatigue of the sweat glands. *Clin. Sci.* 11:1719–1725, 1955.

133. Thornton, W. E., and J. A. Rummel. Muscular deconditioning and its prevention in space flight. In R. S. Johnson and S. F. Dietlen (eds.), *Biomedical results from Skylab* (NASA SP-377). National Aeronautics and Space Administration, Washington DC, 1977, pp. 191–197.

134. Toner, M. M., and W. D. McArdle. Physiological adjustments of man to the cold. In K. B. Pandolf, M. N. Sawka, and R. R. Gonzalez (eds.), *Human physiology and environmental medicine at terrestrial extremes*. Cooper Publishing Group, Carmel, 1986, pp. 361–400.

135. Tripathi, A., G. W. Mack, and E. R. Nadel. Cutaneous vascular reflexes during exercise in the heat. *Med. Sci. Sports Exerc.* 22(6):796–803, 1990.

136. Wagner, P. D., G. E. Gale, R. E. Moon, J. R. Torre-Bueno, B. W. Stolp, and H. A. Saltzman. Pulmonary gas exchange in humans exercising at sea level and simulated altitude. *J. Appl. Physiol.* 61(1):260–270, 1986.

137. Wagner, P. D. Muscle O_2 transport and O_2 dependent control of metabolism. *Med. Sci. Sports Exerc.* 27(1):47–53, 1995.

138. Wagner, P. D. A theoretical analysis of factors determining VO_{2max} at sea level and altitude. *Resp. Physiol.* 106:329–343, 1996.

139. Wolfel, E. E., et al. Oxygen transport during steady-state submaximal exercise in chronic hypoxia. *J. Appl. Physiol.* 70(3):1129–1136, 1991.

140. Wronski, T. J., and E. R. Morey. Alterations in calcium homeostasis and bone during actual and simulated space flight. *Med. Sci. Sports Exerc.* 15(5):410–414, 1983.

141. Young, A. J., A. Cymerman, and R. L. Burse. The influence of cardiorespiratory fitness on the decrement in maximal aerobic power at high altitude. *Eur. J. Appl. Physiol.* 54:12–15, 1985.

142. Young, A. J., and P. M. Young. Human acclimatization to high terrestrial altitude. In K. B. Pandolf, M. N. Sawka, and R. R. Gonzalez (eds.), *Human physiology and environmental medicine at terrestrial extremes*. Cooper Publishing Group, Carmel, 1986, pp. 497–544.

143. Young, A. J., and P. M. Young. Human acclimatization to high terrestrial altitude. In K. B. Pandolf, M. N. Sawka, and R. R. Gonzalez (eds.), *Human performance physiology and environmental medicine at terrestrial extremes*. Benchmark Press, Indianapolis, 1988, pp. 497–543.

144. Young, A. J. Energy substrate utilization during exercise in extreme environments. *Exerc. Sport Sci. Rev.* 18:65–117, 1990.

RECOMMENDED READINGS

Adams, W. C., G. W. Mack, G. W. Langhans, and E. R. Nadel. Effects of equivalent sea-level and altitude training on VO_{2max} and running performance. *J. Appl. Physiol.* 39:262, 1975.

American College of Sports Medicine. Position stand on the prevention of thermal injuries during distance running. *Med. Sci. Sports Exerc.* 16(5): ix–xiv, 1985.

Anderson, H. T., E. B. Smeland, J. O. Owe, and K. Myhre. Analyses of maximum cardiopulmonary performance during exposure acute hypoxia at simulated altitude-sea level to 5000 meters (760–404 mmHg). *Aviat. Space Environ. Med.* 56:1192–1197, 1985.

Armstrong, L. E., R. W. Hubbard, J. P. DeLuca, and E. L. Christensen. Heat acclimatization during summer running in the United States. *Med. Sci. Sports Exerc.* 19(2):131–136, 1987.

Bender, P. R., et al. Oxygen transport to exercising leg in chronic hypoxia. *J. Appl. Physiol.* 65(6):2592–2597, 1988.

Bender, P. R., et al. Decreased exercise muscle lactate release after high-altitude acclimatization. *J. Appl. Physiol.* 67(2):1456–1462, 1989.

Brooks, G. A., et al. Decreased reliance on lactate during exercise after acclimatization to 4300 m. *J. Appl. Physiol.* 71:333–341, 1991.

Buskirk, E. R., J. Kollias, R. F. Akers, E. K. Prolop, and E. P. Reategui. Maximal performance at altitude and on return from altitude in conditioned runners. *J. Appl. Physiol.* 23:259–266, 1967.

Cerretelli, P., A. Veicsteinas, and C. Marconi. Anaerobic metabolism at high altitude: The lactacid mechanism. In W. Brendel, and R. A. Zink. (eds.), *High-altitude physiology and medicine*. Springer-Verlag, New York, 1982, pp. 94–102.

Convertino, V. A. Potential benefits of maximal exercise just prior to return from weightlessness. *Aviat. Space Environ. Med.* 58:568–572, 1987.

Convertino, V. A., T. M. Sather, D. J. Goldwater, and W. R. Alford. Aerobic fitness does not contribute to prediction of orthostatic tolerance. *Med. Sci. Sports Exerc.* 18(5):551–556, 1986.

Cymerman, A., et al. Operation Everest II: Maximal oxygen uptake at extreme altitude. *J. Appl. Physiol.* 66:2446–2453, 1989.

Faulkner, J. A. Effects of training at moderate altitude on physical performance capacity. *J. Appl. Physiol.* 23:85, 1967.

Faulkner, J. A., J. Kollias, C. B. Favour, E. R. Buskirk, and B. Balke. Maximal aerobic capacity and running performance at altitude. *J. Appl. Physiol.* 24:685–691, 1968.

RECOMMENDED READINGS

Ferretti, G., C. Moia, J.-M. Thomet, and B. Kayser. The decrease of maximal oxygen consumption during hypoxia in man: A mirror image of the oxygen equilibrium curve. *J. Physiol.* 498(1):231–237, 1997.

Gisolfi, C. V., and J. S. Cohen. Relationships among training, heat acclimation, and heat tolerance in men and women: The controversy revisited. *Med. Sci. Sports Med.* 11(1):56–59, 1979.

Gore, C. J., et al. Reduced performance of male and female athletes at 580 m altitude. *Eur. J. Appl. Physiol.* 75:136–143, 1997.

Greenleaf, J. E. Problem: Thirst, drinking behavior, and involuntary dehydration. *Med. Sci. Sports Exerc.* 24(6):645–656, 1992.

Horstman, D. H., R. Weiskopf, and R. E. Jackson. Work capacity during 3-week sojourn at 4300 m: Effects of relative polycythemia. *J. Appl. Physiol.* 49:311–318, 1980.

Lawler, J., S. Powers, and D. Thompson. Linear relationship between VO_{2max} and VO_{2max} decrement during exposure to acute hypoxia. *J. Appl. Physiol.* 64(4):1486–1492, 1988.

Levine, B. D., and J. Stray-Gunderson. A practical approach to altitude training: Where to live and train for optimal performance enhancement. *Int. J. Sports Med.* 13:S209–S212, 1992.

Montain, S. J., and E. F Coyle. Fluid ingestion during exercise increases skin blood flow independent of increases in blood volume. *J. Appl. Physiol.* 73(3):903–910, 1992.

Nadel, E. R., S. F. Fortney, and C. B. Wenger. Circulatory and thermal regulations during exercise. *Fed. Proc.* 39:1491–1497, 1980.

Noakes, T. D., et al. Metabolic rate, not percent dehydration, predicts rectal temperature in marathon runners. *Med. Sci. Sports Exerc.* 23(4):443–449, 1991.

Owen, M. D., K. C. Kregel, P. T. Wall, and C. V. Gisolfi. Effects of ingesting carbohydrate beverages during exercise in the heat. *Med. Sci. Sports Exerc.* 18(5):568–575, 1986.

Pitts, G. C., R. E. Johnson, and F. C. Consolazio. Work in the heat as affected by intake of water, salt and glucose. *Am. J. Physiol.* 142:253–259, 1944.

Pugh, L. G. C. E., M. B. Gill, and S. Lahirim. Muscular exercise at great altitudes. *J. Appl. Physiol.* 19:431–440, 1964.

Robergs, R. A., R. Quintana, D. Parker, and C. Frankel. Multiple variables determine the decrement in VO_{2max} during acute hypobaric hypoxia. *Med. Sci. Sports Exerc.* 30(8):869–879, 1998.

Sawka, M. M. Physiological consequences of hypohydration: Exercise performance and thermoregulation. *Med. Sci. Sports Exerc.* 24(6):657–670, 1992.

Sutton, J. R., et al. Operation Everest II: Oxygen transport during exercise at extreme simulated altitude. *J. Appl. Physiol.* 64(4):1309–1321, 1988.

Wolfel, E. E., et al. Oxygen transport during steady-state submaximal exercise in chronic hypoxia. *J. Appl. Physiol.* 70(3):1129–1136, 1991.

CHAPTER 20

Gender and Exercise Performance

oday, more than ever before, the issue of gender equality/inequality in athletics and sports is a topic of considerable debate and scientific inquiry. Historically, social thought assumed that the "more delicate" female body would be unable to tolerate running long distances such as in the Olympic marathon. However, an accumulating body of research indicates otherwise and, since 1984, women have been competing in the marathon. Similar gender transitions in athletic competition have occurred in the Hawaii Ironman, and cases where female adolescents want gender equality in sports participation during high school and university competition are becoming more common in the United States. The increased acceptance of female participation in sports and athletics has been supported by changes in societal expectations of women, as well as by scientific research of how women respond to exercise. Most of this research reveals that women can have physiological responses to exercise that differ from men, which in most circumstances offers no detriment to health and well-being, and in some instances may be advantageous. In addition, the special functions of women that relate to reproductive function and pregnancy have been important areas of research that have identified the benefits and dangers of excessive exercise. The purpose of this chapter is to summarize the structural and functional differences between men and women, identify how these variations influence different types of exercise, and introduce research findings on topics important to the gender-specific effects of exercise on the human body.

OBJECTIVES

After studying this chapter, you should be able to:

- Identify the main differences in structure and function between males and females.
- Explain how specific gender differences in structure or function influence exercise performance.
- Explain the importance of lean body mass to specific functional differences between genders.
- List the role of estradiol for the female and explain the importance of the menstrual cycle to the health of the female.
- Explain the benefits and risks to the mother and fetus when exercising during pregnancy.

KEY TERMS

menstrual cycle
follicular phase
ovulatory phase
luteal phase

17β-estradiol
progesterone
athletic
  amenorrhea

female athlete triad
testosterone

A General Comparison of Male and Female Structure and Function

igure 20.1 illustrates the external appearance of the postpubescent male and female, and lists the data of measurements pertinent to exercise performance. These pictures and data represent average representations of males and females and, because of this, ranges for certain parameters are listed. Also, there are females whose comparisons with males will differ in ways other than those indicated in figure 20.1, and vice versa. However, for males and females of similar training and relative fitness, the relative differences between genders are valid.

The data of figure 20.1 present several main areas of functional differences between males and females. Body composition is known to influence prolonged exercise (endurance) as well as short-term intense exercise performance. Body composition may also influence thermoregulatory capacities, which can also be affected by the difference in sweat gland density between males and females. The distinct capacities of the cardiovascular system of the male and female have the potential to amount to differences in oxygen transport capabilities. The hormonal variations between males and females cause differences in substrate use during exercise and in the control of ventilation at rest, during exercise, and when exposed to high altitude. Finally, these parameters combine to present different overall concerns for males and females participating in strenuous exercise training. The organization of this chapter is based on these general areas of structure and function.

Gender Differences in Cardiorespiratory Endurance

Cardiorespiratory endurance concerns the function of the heart, lungs, vasculature, and skeletal muscle to exchange gases in the lungs, transport gases and metabolites in blood, and exchange gases and metabolites between the blood and

---

FIGURE 20.1

An illustration and data of the differences between males and females. These differences can be grouped on the basis of structural and functional criteria. Compared to the male, the female generally has a higher percentage of body fat, and this fat is distributed especially around the hips and thighs, whereas the male's fat is distributed around the waist and stomach. Males have a larger lean body mass, even when expressed relative to total body weight, and are taller than the average female. The male has a narrower pelvic region than the female. The female has fewer sweat glands than the male, a smaller heart, lower percentages of slow-twitch motor units, a smaller blood volume, and a lower hemoglobin concentration and hematocrit. Females have ovaries that produce estrogen and progesterone, whereas males have testes that produce testosterone. These hormones exert different metabolic and regulatory functions on the body, especially during exercise.

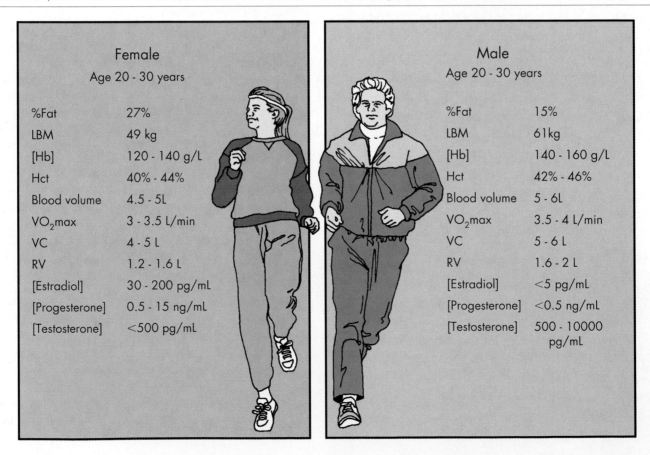

	Female Age 20 - 30 years			**Male** Age 20 - 30 years
%Fat	27%		%Fat	15%
LBM	49 kg		LBM	61kg
[Hb]	120 - 140 g/L		[Hb]	140 - 160 g/L
Hct	40% - 44%		Hct	42% - 46%
Blood volume	4.5 - 5L		Blood volume	5 - 6L
VO$_2$max	3 - 3.5 L/min		VO$_2$max	3.5 - 4 L/min
VC	4 - 5 L		VC	5 - 6 L
RV	1.2 - 1.6 L		RV	1.6 - 2 L
[Estradiol]	30 - 200 pg/mL		[Estradiol]	<5 pg/mL
[Progesterone]	0.5 - 15 ng/mL		[Progesterone]	<0.5 ng/mL
[Testosterone]	<500 pg/mL		[Testosterone]	500 - 10000 pg/mL

skeletal muscle. As explained in chapters 6 and 7, the greater the capacity of the body to perform these functions, the greater is the body's cardiorespiratory endurance. These capacities involve central cardiovascular and pulmonary function, peripheral vascular function, and skeletal muscle fiber type and metabolic capacities.

Cardiovascular and Pulmonary Function

There is evidence of gender differences in pulmonary function. Females have a smaller lung volume and pulmonary capillary volume than the male, causing lower maximal pulmonary ventilation (38, 39). However, as will be explained below, it is unclear whether these differences are simply a reflection of a smaller body mass.

Research on exercise-induced hypoxemia has been biased by predominantly male subject selection (19, 32). Whether this condition occurs more or less in females than males is unclear; however, Robergs and colleagues (33) revealed that both moderately to well-trained men and women experience a similar degree of exercise-induced hypoxemia at sea level and at altitudes up to 2500 m. Nevertheless, McClaren and associates (25) reported that, compared to males, females tend to have a greater hypoxemia during incremental exercise to VO_{2max} because of mechanical constraints caused by relatively small lung volumes and maximal expiratory flow rates. Clearly, more research must be done on the ventilatory limitations to exercise between genders, especially at higher altitude.

Cardiovascular capacities are known to differ between males and females. Generally, females have a smaller heart, with lower filling volumes, and maximal stroke volumes, and cardiac outputs (28, 31). When combined with a lower blood hemoglobin concentration, hematocrit, and total blood volume, the female is at a definite disadvantage for transporting oxygen to skeletal muscles during exercise. The cardiovascular differences between the genders are best expressed by the relationship between cardiac output and oxygen consumption during exercise. For a given VO_2, females have a larger cardiac output than males because of a lower a-$vO_2\Delta$ secondary to the reduced oxygen delivery (15).

The fact that females have a lower cardiovascular capacity than males does not mean that females have a reduced ability to adapt to endurance training. Pellicia and colleagues (31) reported that females also adapt to endurance training by improving the pumping effectiveness of the heart, as indicated by increased end-diastolic dimensions. These increases are similar to the adaptability of the male, and indicate that gender differences in cardiovascular structure and function are due to genetic and related hormonal differences during the phases of growth, development, and sexual maturity. In fact, *when cardiovascular parameters are expressed relative to body surface area or lean body mass, gender differences are less pronounced* (31).

Skeletal Muscle Structure and Function

Limited data exist that compare the fiber type proportions of males and females. The data that do exist pertain to elite ath-

letes and, because of genetic bias and athletic selection, it is unclear how valid these data reflect true gender difference issues. For example, it has been reported that females tend to have a lower slow-twitch fiber type proportion in the gastrocnemius muscle (8, 9).

Maximal Oxygen Consumption

The measure of VO_{2max} is known to be very different in equally trained males and females. Given the previously detailed roles of both muscular endurance and central cardiovascular function in determining VO_{2max} (chapters 6 and 7), this is not surprising.

Maximal oxygen consumption (VO_{2max}) is higher in comparably trained males than females, with the difference being dependent on the expression of VO_2 (fig. 20.2) (8, 9, 12, 15, 26, 39, 40). For example, Tarnopolsky and associates (40) compared females and males on training, age, and distance events, and females had a 21% lower VO_{2max} (4.38 vs. 3.42 L/min for males and females, respectively). However, when VO_2 was expressed relative to lean body mass the ability to consume oxygen was similar (74.9 vs. 74.7 mL/kg LBM/min for males and females, respectively). Nevertheless, when accounting for all the research on this topic, and adjusting for fat-free mass and training status, the gender difference in VO_{2max} is reduced on average to approximately a 15% larger value for the male (15, 39). This suggests that although lean body mass is important in explaining gender differences in VO_{2max}, other factors are also influential.

Submaximal Oxygen Consumption

Numerous researchers have reported contradictory findings concerning steady state oxygen consumption for a given submaximal running velocity (1, 14, 37). However, in the most extensive study of elite male and female long-distance runners, Daniels and Daniels (12) documented a significantly lower VO_2 at a given running velocity for males compared to females, resulting in a 6 to 7% advantage for males. Thus, for a given running velocity, elite male runners are consuming 6 to 7% less oxygen while remaining at steady state. When combined with a higher VO_{2max}, and therefore a potentially higher relative intensity at the lactate threshold, males can remain at steady state while running at a faster speed. In using the averaged data from Daniels and Daniels (12) and assuming a lactate threshold of 85% VO_{2max}, the maximal steady-state running speed for the male and female athletes were 288.7 and 333.8 m/min. Over the length of the 10,000-m race, this difference amounts to a time difference of 4 min 42 s, or a 13% performance advantage for the male.

Gender Differences in Endocrine Function and Metabolism During Exercise

Figure 20.3 illustrates and compares the changes in basal body temperature and circulating anterior pituitary and gonadal hormone concentrations in the female relative to the

FIGURE 20.2

The differences in VO_{2max} between males and females when expressed in absolute or relative terms.

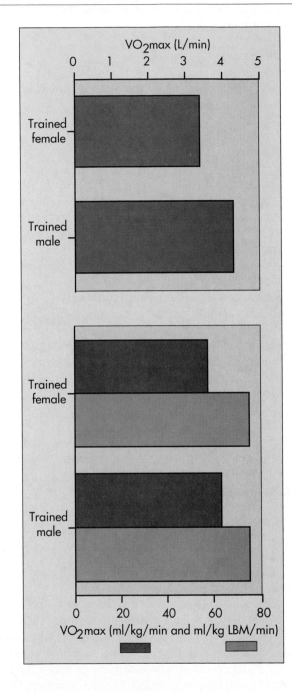

latory phase, which results in the release of the ovum and may last 3 days; and the luteal phase, which extends from ovulation to the onset of menstrual bleeding. The luteal phase is generally more consistent in duration, lasting approximately 13 days. However, as will be discussed in subsequent sections, the duration of the luteal phase is known to decrease in certain female athletes and can be relatively more variable in length than the follicular phase (22, 23).

The distinct phases of the menstrual cycle are important because there are differences in hormone concentrations during these phases that are influential in regulating fuel mobilization during exercise. During the early to midfollicular phase, the female has low concentrations of estrogen (specifically 17β-estradiol, or simply estradiol) and progesterone. Estradiol inhibits glucose uptake by tissues and indirectly favors lipid catabolism. Progesterone is a known stimulant to ventilation, and has some effect in decreasing the metabolic actions of estradiol. Consequently, *during the early follicular phase the female is endocrinologically most like the male*.

During the ovulatory and luteal phases, the increased estradiol and progesterone concentrations have the potential to alter substrate use and ventilation at rest and during exercise. Compared to males, when exercising at a given percent of VO_{2max}, females catabolize more fat than males (35, 40), and rely less on muscle glycogen (40). For example, during 15.5 km of running at 65% VO_{2max}, females use 25% less muscle glycogen than the equally trained males, and 30% less urea nitrogen excretion (less protein catabolism) (40) (fig. 20.4). Although the topic of catabolism of endogenous lipids within skeletal muscle is unclear, data indicate that females may be able to utilize more of their intramuscular store of triacylglycerols than the male for a given relative submaximal exercise intensity (5, 40). These differences are reduced for highly trained females, possibly because of their

menstrual cycle. Males have negligible concentrations of estrogen and progesterone. Conversely males have higher concentrations of testosterone (fig. 20.1). These comparisons highlight the large endocrinological differences between males and females, and also indicate the dramatic variation in endocrine function during the menstrual cycle of the female.

There are three phases within the menstrual cycle: the **follicular phase,** which begins with the onset of menstruation and has a variable length of between 9 to 23 days; the **ovu-**

menstrual cycle the monthly variation in gonadal hormones of the female that result in the release of an ovary and the eventual expulsion of the ovary and developing placenta during menstruation

follicular phase the phase of the menstrual cycle beginning with the onset of menstruation and ending at the start of ovulation, usually 9 to 23 days in duration

ovulatory phase the phase of the menstrual cycle involved with ovulation, usually 3 days in duration

luteal phase the phase of the menstrual cycle beginning with the end of ovulation and ending at the start of menstruation, usually 13 days in duration

17β-estradiol the most biologically active estrogen steroid hormone that influences lipid metabolism, bone growth, and the development of female secondary sex characteristics. Estrogens are produced by the ovary of the female and, to a lesser extent, by the adrenal cortex and testes of the male

progesterone (pro-jes'ter-own) a steroid hormone synthesized by the developing follicle of the ovary and released during the luteal phase of the menstrual cycle

FIGURE 20.3

The changing hormonal concentrations during the menstrual cycle.

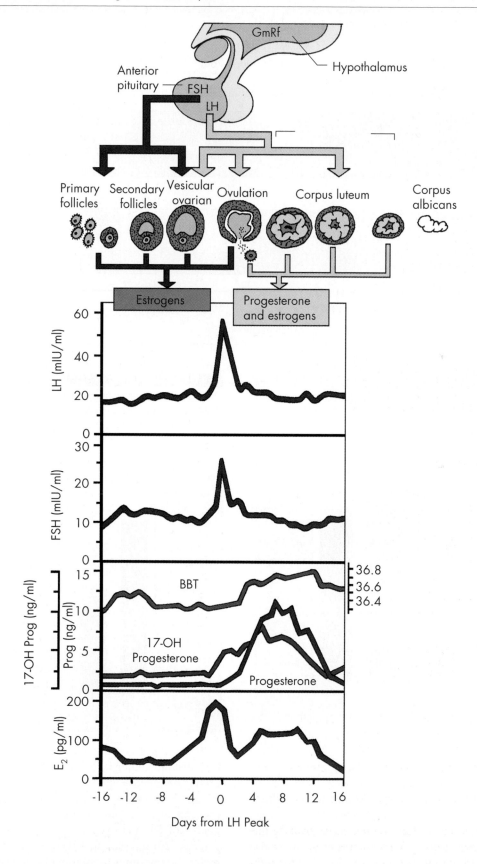

FIGURE 20.4

The decrease in muscle glycogen is less for females than males during equivalent relative exercise intensities. In addition, females are less dependent on amino acid oxidation during prolonged exercise. It is assumed that the difference in energy substrate utilization between males and females resides in the greater use of intramuscular stores of lipid.

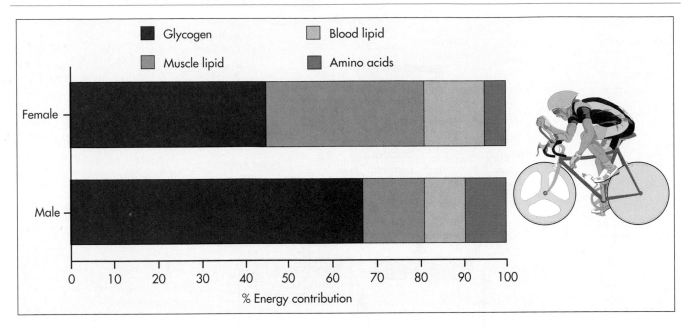

FIGURE 20.5

A comparison of muscular power between males and females, and how gender differences are removed when power is expressed relative to lean body mass.

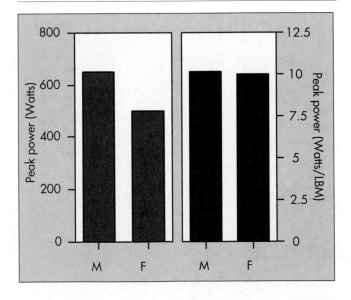

FIGURE 20.6

The increase in muscle strength and hypertrophy for males and females in response to 16 weeks of weight training. Although the absolute changes are greater for the male, there are no gender differences in these changes relative to pretraining values.

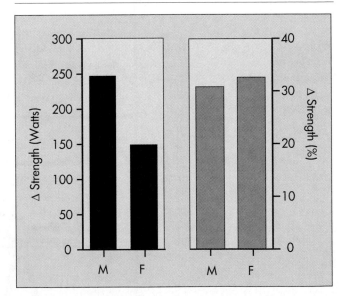

shortened luteal phase and lower circulating estrogen concentrations (35).

Given the endocrinological potential for metabolic differences in females during the different phases of the menstrual cycle, what has research revealed on this topic? During the luteal phase there are increases in circulating free fatty acids, glycerol and blood lipoprotein lipase activity (36). In addi-

tion, insulin binding is lowered during the luteal phase, compromising glucose uptake and eventual carbohydrate catabolism. Unfortunately, studies involving exercise have been less conclusive in identifying metabolic differences among phases of the menstrual cycle (29, 35). Kanaley and colleagues (20) reported that there were no differences in the metabolic responses to 90 min of running at 60% of VO_{2max}

during the follicular or luteal phase of the menstrual cycle. These similarities existed despite large differences in circulating estrogen and progesterone concentrations. These findings may be explained by antagonistic effects of progesterone compared to estrogen, as well as the intrinsic (insulin-independent) increase in skeletal muscle glucose uptake by contracting skeletal muscle. More research should be completed on this topic before a statement can be made in confidence regarding the need to control the phase of the menstrual cycle in order to compare female and male metabolic responses to exercise.

Gender Differences in Muscular Strength and Power

The greater lean body mass in males compared to females is a major determinant of the greater muscular strength of males. However, *differences in strength and power between genders are removed when either measure is expressed relative to lean body mass* (fig. 20.5). This fact stresses the importance of muscle mass on intense exercise performance, regardless of gender.

Although it has been widely accepted that females respond less to strength training than males, research does not support this claim. Cureton and associates (10) demonstrated that males and females who participated in a 16-week weight training program experienced equal muscle hypertrophy, and equal muscular strength improvement when expressed relative to pretraining values (fig. 20.6).

Research in animal models has indicated that estrogens provide a protective effect against muscle damage during exercise (41). Such damage has been associated with an antioxidant role of estrogen, thereby stabilizing membrane proteins. Unfortunately, past research of muscle damage during exercise has not provided gender comparisons. Clearly, this is an important area of future research.

Gender Differences in Exercise at Extreme Environments

Males and females not only exercise under normal environmental conditions, but also when exposed to climatic extremes (high temperature and humidity vs. cold temperatures) or high altitude. Exercise under these conditions demands additional physiological adaptations that research has shown to differ between genders.

Thermoregulation

It has generally been accepted that women sweat less than men, and that this difference is due to a lower sweat output from each sweat gland. However, research has not shown any difference in the change in sweat rate, core temperature, and cardiovascular responses between genders during exercise in a hot environment (6, 27). This is especially true when sweat rate is expressed relative to core temperature (18).

There is some evidence to indicate that sweat electrolyte content (Na^+ and Cl^-) is less in the female; however, it re-

mains unclear whether these differences are due to a different aldosterone response, a real although not experimentally verified greater sweat rate in the male, or some effect of estrogen on the rate of electrolyte reabsorption by the sweat gland (27).

With regard to gender differences in acclimatization to dry heat, research does indicate that females may adapt better than the similarly trained and fit male (18). After 11 days of 120 min of exercise in dry heat (43°C), females ($n = 4$) had less of an increase in core temperature and could exercise for longer than the males ($n = 6$). However, when males and females perform exercise of equal absolute intensity in a hot environment, females have higher rectal temperatures and heart rates compared to men (37). Thus, when referring to *relative exercise intensities,* females tolerate and adapt to heat stress better than males. When referring to *absolute intensities,* and therefore an *absolute heat load,* males tolerate heat stress better than females.

Adaptation to High Altitude

Progesterone is a potent stimulant to ventilation, and it is well known that females have a greater hypoxic stimulus to ventilation than men because of higher circulating progesterone concentrations (38). Such an increased sensitivity to ventilation during hypoxia should provide the female with greater potential to increase P_AO_2 and improve acute adaptation to high altitude. Conversely, because females are known to retain water during the menstrual cycle, and their tendency to become slightly edematous is recognized as an increased risk for developing acute mountain sickness and the life-threatening conditions of pulmonary and cerebral edema, it remains to be shown whether females are more susceptible to AMS during specific phases of the menstrual cycle (16).

Given these physiological differences between genders, do females adapt differently than males at high altitude? Unfortunately we do not know the answer to this question. The most thorough investigation of females at high altitude was completed in 1966 (17). This study, actually a series of studies located at Pikes Peak, Colorado (4300 m above sea level), revealed that females have a higher ventilation than males during altitude exposure, and that iron supplementation was necessary to induce a polycythemic response in females during prolonged exposure to high altitude.

Limited research has been completed comparing males and females in measurements of VO_{2max} and blood hemoglobin saturation (SaO_2) during exercise at altitude (2, 30, 33). Roberas and associates (33) completed the most thorough study on this topic and revealed that females have less of a decrement in VO_{2max} than males with increasing altitude above sea level (fig. 20.7). There was no indication that females had greater ventilation than males, or maintained a higher SaO_2. Gender differences in fitness and body size (males greater than females) explained most of the gender difference in the change in VO_{2max}; however, additional factors unrelated to pulmonary function must also be involved.

FIGURE 20.7

Females have less of a decrement in VO_{2max} for given increases in altitude than males. However, as explained in the text, these differences are more due to body size and sea level fitness differences than to gender alone.

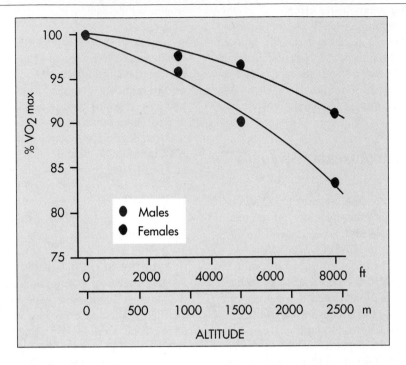

Special Concerns for Females Who Exercise

Women who exercise have an increased likelihood of improved health and decreased risk for developing degenerative diseases (heart disease, osteoporosis, etc.). However, because of the relative delicacy of the neuroendocrinological regulation of the female hypothalamic-pituitary-ovarian axis, chronic exercise can lead to menstrual cycle irregularities. In addition, the pregnant female and her fetus have special needs that exercise may impose upon. These and other special needs of the female athlete will be explained in the following sections.

Athletic Amenorrhea and Bone Mineral Status

A subgroup of women who exercise have been reported to have a shortened luteal phase of the menstrual cycle (22, 23). The degree of luteal phase shortening has been shown to correspond to the intensity of training (duration and frequency of training), with more intense training exacerbating the decrease in the length of the luteal phase. Comment was given to these responses in chapter 9.

For females who train too hard, increasing the likelihood of a negative energy balance (13, 29), there is a risk that the luteal phase will continue to shorten and that they will eventually experience a cessation of the menstrual cycle, a condition called **athletic amenorrhea.** The endocrinological events that are be-

lieved to inhibit the regulation of the menstrual cycle at the level of the hypothalamic-pituitary axis were explained in chapter 9, and are discussed in focus box 20.1.

The cessation of the menstrual cycle has ramifications for the female other than a natural means of birth control. The absence of a surge in FSH (follicle-stimulating hormone) and LH (luteinizing hormone) prevents development of the ovarian follicle, from which estradiol and progesterone are produced. The inability of the female to produce ovarian estradiol chronically lowers circulating estradiol concentrations, which increases the rate of bone resorption from the skeleton, thereby increasing the risk of *premature osteoporosis* (11). Furthermore, evidence also exists that connects females with menstrual irregularities to a higher incidence of musculoskeletal injury (24). The multifaceted causes and related health implications of athletic amenorrhea have been detailed in the American College of Sports Medicine (29) position on the "female athletic triad" (focus box 20.1).

The amenorrheic female has a few alternatives that decrease the deleterious effects of this condition. First, she can reduce her training, which has been shown to reestablish the menstrual cycle. The female can also retain her training and seek medical advice about a suitable estradiol supplement. Estrogen patch treatment is effective in increasing serum 17β-estradiol (35). Despite this fact, females are generally prescribed an oral birth control pill. Because of the length of time required to detect changes in bone mineral density, conclusive data are not available on the effectiveness of birth control pill or patch use in retarding the development of osteoporosis.

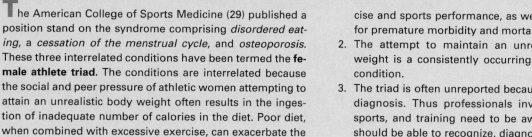

FOCUS BOX 20.1

The Female Athlete Triad

The American College of Sports Medicine (29) published a position stand on the syndrome comprising *disordered eating*, a *cessation of the menstrual cycle*, and *osteoporosis*. These three interrelated conditions have been termed the **female athlete triad.** The conditions are interrelated because the social and peer pressure of athletic women attempting to attain an unrealistic body weight often results in the ingestion of inadequate number of calories in the diet. Poor diet, when combined with excessive exercise, can exacerbate the endocrine response to the exercise and dietary stress, causing a cessation of the menstrual cycle (amenorrhea) (13). The amenorrhea causes a reduction in circulating estrogen, producing an increase in bone mineral loss, which when sustained over long periods of time contributes to the development of osteoporosis.

De Cree (13) commented that the female athlete triad is not necessarily typical of all athletic women who experience exercise-related menstrual irregularities (ERMI). For example, some women experience ERMI simply from excessive exercise without caloric restriction, or a decrease in body fat or total weight. Thus, the proposed mechanism for the ERMI and amenorrhea of the female athlete triad is a disturbance of the hypothalamic-gonadotropin-releasing hormone axis. This disturbance is believed to be secondary to chronic increases in circulating catecholamine, cortisol, and opioid hormones.

The ACSM position on the female athlete triad contains nine key features, which are summarized below:

1. The female athlete triad is a serious syndrome that can affect elite athletes, as well as nonelite physically active girls and women. The triad can result in declining exercise and sports performance, as well as increase the risk for premature morbidity and mortality.

2. The attempt to maintain an unrealistically low body weight is a consistently occurring characteristic of this condition.

3. The triad is often unreported because of denial and poor diagnosis. Thus professionals involved with exercise, sports, and training need to be aware of the triad, and should be able to recognize, diagnose, and provide treatment recommendations.

4. Screening for the triad should involve the following: menstrual change, disordered eating, weight change, cardiac arrhythmias, depression, or skeletal stress fractures. Because of the specific nature of these symptoms, collaboration with health care professionals (dietitians, clinicians) is recommended.

5. Professionals involved with exercise, sports, and training should promote and provide exercise training and support functions that do not exacerbate any one of the components of the triad.

6. Parents should not pressure their daughters to lose weight. Thus, in addition to the client/athlete, parents and/or additional family members are also a target audience for education and prevention of the triad.

7. Sport-governing bodies should accept the responsibility of recognizing and preventing the triad in their female athletes.

8. Physically active girls and women should be educated about the triad and appropriate ways to ensure proper nutrition and training practices.

9. Further research on the prevalence, causes, prevention, and treatment of the symptoms of the triad is needed.

Exercise During Pregnancy

The health benefits of exercise and the increasing participation by women in exercise have raised the concern of the role of exercise for the mother and fetus during pregnancy. Initial inquiry into this topic concerned the effects of exercise on uterine and fetal blood flow, core and fetal temperature fluctuations, carbohydrate metabolism, and protection from the physical shock accompanying certain movements (e.g., running) (fig. 20.8).

One method to assess fetal responses during exercise performed by the mother is to record changes in fetal heart rate. Initial research performed on sheep has documented increases in fetal heart rate; however, it is unclear whether similar responses in humans are due to ischemic hypoxia or simply a result of increased catecholamine levels. The difficulty of performing research on pregnancy and exercise using human subjects has resulted in similar vague findings for temperature changes and glucose metabolism (2, 6, 42).

Despite the often publicized dangers of exercise during pregnancy, there is evidence of benefits (table 20.1). Exercise by the pregnant female may develop increased capacities for supporting the fetus, such as improved cardiovascular function and carbohydrate metabolism. Although there have been statements by the medical community concerning the possibility that exercise training may decrease the duration of labor and, therefore, possibly the risks associated with childbirth, no experimental evidence exists to support this (6, 21).

Based on a metanalysis of the effects of exercise during pregnancy on the mother and fetus, no evidence exists to indicate that exercise performed 3 times per week for up to a 45-min duration at a heart rate of 144 b/min is harmful (21).

athletic amenorrhea the absence of a menstrual cycle induced by endocrinological responses from exercise training that inhibit the release of follicle-stimulating hormones from the anterior pituitary gland

FIGURE 20.8

A summary of the potential risks to the fetus from a pregnant woman who exercises, as well as the potential benefits obtained when a pregnant women exercises throughout her term.

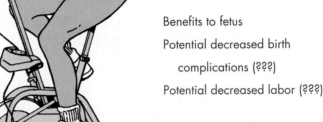

Exercise during pregnancy

Risks to mother

Hypoglycemia

Hyperthermia

Musculoskeletal injury

Benefits to mother

Improved insulin sensitivity

Improved body fat control

Psychosocial interactions

Potential decreased birth
    complications (???)

Potential decreased labor (???)

Risks to fetus

Hypoglycemia

Hyperthermia

Decreased placental
    blood flow

Physical shock

Benefits to fetus

Potential decreased birth
    complications (???)

Potential decreased labor (???)

TABLE 20.1

Physiological changes resulting from pregnancy and potential benefits of exercise during pregnancy

CHANGES DURING PREGNANCY	POTENTIAL BENEFITS OF EXERCISE
↑ Body weight	Improved posture
↑ Heart size	↓ Weight gain
Altered center of gravity	Back pain
↑ Plasma volume (45%)	↓ Anxiety and depression
Physiological anemia	↓ Risk for gestational diabetes
↑ Heart rate, stroke volume, cardiac output	Improved digestion and intestinal motility
↓ Peripheral vascular resistance	↓ "Postpartum belly"
↓ Venous compliance	

Source: Adapted from American College of Sports Medicine (2), Bonen et al. (4), and Clapp et al. (7).

The American College of Gynecology recommends a similar frequency and intensity of exercise, but with a duration of not more than 15 min (1, 21). It is assumed that women who have symptoms of infection, cardiovascular disease, or other illnesses may not be suitable for the aforementioned recommendations. In addition, exercise performed for longer durations, at higher intensities, at altitude or during increased thermal stress (hot or humid conditions) may be unsafe. Because of the decrease in the potential for trauma, non-weight-bearing exercises such as cycling, swimming, or other water-based exercises are recommended for the pregnant female. However, because of the risk of hyperthermia when exercising in a swimming pool with warm water, pregnant females should exercise in cool water (< 85°F).

Given the importance of exercise intensity and duration to the specific benefits and dangers to the mother and fetus, it is important to recognize that what may be good for the mother may be detrimental to the fetus (fig. 20.8). The risk may be in the impairment of fetal well-being, and this needs to be of primary concern. Future research needs to more clearly identify exercise intensities and conditions associated with unacceptable risk to fetal well-being.

Special Concerns for Males Who Exercise

Detrimental effects from excessive exercise also exist for male reproductive function. Overtraining can result in significant reductions in serum **testosterone,** presumably because of a hindered hypothalamic-pituitary-gonadal axis, similar to the endocrine negative inhibition of athletic amenorrhea in the female (32). The chronic reductions in testosterone are associated with decreased sperm counts, but not to

levels conducive to reduced fertility (32). Nevertheless, De Souza and colleagues (14) revealed that the magnitude of reduction in sperm count was highly correlated to training mileage in runners; the greater the training mileage the lower the sperm count.

> **female athlete triad** the syndrome comprising disordered eating, a cessation of the menstrual cycle, and increased risk for osteoporosis
>
> **testosterone (tes-tos'ter-own)** a steroid hormone synthesized by the testes, which induces development of male secondary sex characteristics and increased muscle mass

---

WEBSITE BOX

Chapter 20: Gender and Exercise Performance

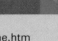

The newest information regarding exercise physiology can be viewed at the following sites.*

arfa.org/index.htm
  Excellent site providing comprehensive information on many topics within exercise physiology.
io.com/~brenda/cycles/index.html
  A Web-based application to help track a woman's monthly menstrual cycle and time of ovulation.
Aomc.org/HOD2/general/general-PREMENST.html
  Explanation of PMS and related links.
bcdg.org/
  Informative site providing diverse information on breast cancer.
http://ww2.cancer.org/bcn/index.html
  Breast cancer network of the American Cancer Society.
mediconsult.com/
  Information source for any medical condition, including menopause, osteoporosis, testicular cancer, etc.

mayohealth.org.mayo/9712/htm/raloxifene.htm
  Information on estrogen replacement therapy.
acor.org/diseases/TC/
  Testicular Cancer Research Center.
pregnancycalendar.com/
  Information on pregnancy, including a calendar service for estimating due date.
musculardevelopment.com/oct/andro1.html
  Excellent overview of testosterone and adrostenedione, including the biochemical pathway of steroid synthesis.

---

*Unless indicated, all URLs preceded by http://www.

Note: These URLs were valid at the time of publication, but could have changed or been deleted from Internet access since that time.

SUMMARY

- Females have a smaller lung volume and pulmonary capillary volume than males, causing lower maximal pulmonary ventilation. Generally, females have a smaller heart, with lower filling volumes, maximal stroke volumes, and cardiac outputs. When combined with a lower blood hemoglobin concentration, hematocrit, and total blood volume, the female is at a definite disadvantage for transporting oxygen to skeletal muscles during exercise. However, *when cardiovascular parameters are expressed relative to body surface area or lean body mass, gender differences are less pronounced.*

- Maximal oxygen consumption (VO_{2max}) is higher in comparably trained males than females. However, when VO_{2max} is expressed relative to lean body mass, the abil-

ity of males and females to consume oxygen is less discrepant, with males retaining a 15% larger value. For a given running velocity, elite male runners consume 6 to 7% less oxygen while remaining at steady state.

- Females experience changes in basal body temperature and circulating anterior pituitary and gonadal hormone concentrations during the **menstrual cycle.** There are three phases within the menstrual cycle: the **follicular phase,** which begins with the onset of menstruation and has a variable length of between 9 to 23 days; the **ovulatory phase,** which results in the release of the ovum and may last 3 days; and the **luteal phase,** which extends from ovulation to the onset of menstrual bleeding.

SUMMARY

- During the early to midfollicular phase, the female has low concentrations of estrogen (specifically **17β-estradiol,** or simply estradiol) and **progesterone.** Estradiol inhibits glucose uptake by tissues, and indirectly favors lipid catabolism. Progesterone is a known stimulant to ventilation, and has some effect in decreasing the metabolic actions of estradiol. Consequently, *during the early follicular phase the female is endocrinologically most like the male.*

- Compared to males when exercising at a given percent of VO_{2max}, females catabolize more fat than the male and rely less on muscle glycogen. Data indicate that females may be able to utilize more of their intramuscular store of triacylglycerols than the male for a given relative submaximal exercise intensity. These differences are reduced for highly trained females.

- The greater lean body mass in males compared to females is a major determinant of the greater muscular strength of males. However, *differences in strength and power between genders are removed when either measure is expressed relative to lean body mass.* This fact stresses the importance of muscle mass on intense exercise performance, regardless of gender.

- It has generally been accepted that women sweat less than men, and that this difference is due to a lower sweat output from each sweat gland. However, research has not shown any difference in the change in sweat rate, core temperature, and cardiovascular responses between genders during exercise in a hot environment.

- Progesterone is a potent stimulant to ventilation, and it is well known that females have a greater hypoxic stimulus to ventilation than men because of higher circulating progesterone concentrations. Such an increased sensitivity to ventilation during hypoxia should provide the female with greater potential to increase P_AO_2 and improve acute adaptation to high altitude. Conversely, because females are known to retain water during the menstrual cycle, their tendency to become slightly edematous is recognized as an increased risk for developing acute mountain sickness and the life-threatening conditions of pulmonary and cerebral edema.

- Females have less of a decrement in VO_{2max} than males with increasing altitude above sea level. This gender difference is not related to pulmonary function.

- A subgroup of women who exercise has been reported to have a shortened luteal phase of the menstrual cycle. The degree of luteal phase shortening has been shown to correspond to the intensity of training (duration and frequency of training), with more intense training exacerbating the decrease in the length of the luteal phase. For females who train too hard, there is the likelihood that the luteal phase will continue to shorten and that they will eventually lose their menstrual cycle, a condition called **athletic amenorrhea.** In addition, amenorrhea is often associated with unrealistic attempts to lose body weight, poor diet, excessive/inappropriate exercise training goals, and an increased risk of developing osteoporosis. These interrelated symptoms comprise a syndrome that has been termed the **female athlete triad.**

- Exercise by the pregnant female may develop increased capacities for supporting the fetus, such as improved cardiovascular function and carbohydrate metabolism. Although there have been statements by the medical community concerning the possibility that exercise training may decrease the duration of labor and, therefore, possibly the risks associated with childbirth, no experimental evidence exists to support this. Because of the decrease in the potential for trauma, non-weight-bearing exercises such as cycling, swimming, or other water-based exercises are recommended for the pregnant female.

- Detrimental effects from excessive exercise also exist for male reproductive function. Overtraining can result in significant reductions in serum **testosterone,** presumably because of a hindered hypothalamic-pituitary-gonadal axis, similar to the endocrine negative inhibition of athletic amenorrhea in the female. The chronic reductions in testosterone are associated with decreased sperm counts, with the magnitude of reduction in sperm count being positively related to training mileage.

STUDY QUESTIONS

1. What are the differences in body composition between males and females? Explain how these differences might influence exercise performance.

2. Why do females have lower cardiovascular and oxygen transport capacities than males?

3. Why do normally menstruating females catabolize more lipid at a given submaximal exercise intensity compared to males?

4. What are the phases of the menstrual cycle, how long are they, and how do they differ endocrinologically?

5. If you were conducting a study comparing male and female metabolic responses to exercise, at what phase of the menstrual cycle should the females be in, and why?

APPLICATIONS

1. List the health benefits to the female from participating in a strength and/or endurance exercise training program.

2. Based on the material presented in this chapter, should females have different standards than men for entry into certain vocations that involve life-threatening conditions (e.g., military, fire department, police force)?

3. What are the connections between athletic amenorrhea, osteoporosis, and low circulating estradiol concentrations?

4. What are some concerns about the pregnant female who wants to exercise, and what are the current recommendations for pregnant females who exercise?

REFERENCES

1. American College of Gynecologists. *Exercise during pregnancy and the postpartum period.* ACOG Technical Bulletin No. 189, Feb. 1994.

2. American College of Sports Medicine. *ACSM's guidelines for exercise testing and prescription.* Williams & Wilkins, Baltimore, 1996.

3. Bhambani, Y., and M. Singh. Metabolic and cinematographic analysis of walking and running in men and women. *Med. Sci. Sports Exerc.* 17:131–137, 1985.

4. Bonen, A., P. Campagna, L. Gilchrist, D. C. Young, and P. Beresford. Substrate and endocrine responses during exercise at selected stages of pregnancy. *J. Appl. Physiol.* 73(1): 134–142, 1992.

5. Bunt, J. C. Metabolic actions of estradiol: Significance for acute and chronic exercise responses. *Med. Sci. Sports Exerc.* 22(3):286–290, 1990.

6. Clapp, J. F., III, M. Wesley, and R. H. Sleamaker. Thermoregulatory and metabolic responses to jogging prior to and during pregnancy. *Med. Sci. Sports Exerc.* 19(2):124–130, 1987.

7. Clapp, J. F., III, R. Rokey, J. L. Treadway, M. W. Carpenter, R. M. Artal, and C. Warrnes. Exercise in pregnancy. *Med. Sci. Sports Exerc.* 24(6):S294–S300, 1992.

8. Costill, D. L., W. J. Fink, and M. L. Pollock. Muscle fiber composition and enzyme activities of elite distance runners. *Med. Sci. Sports Exerc.* 8:96–100, 1976.

9. Costill, D. L., W. J. Fink, M. Flynn, and J. Kirwan. Muscle fiber composition and enzyme activities in elite female distance runners. *Int. J. Sports Med.* 8:103–106, 1987.

10. Cureton, K. J., M. A. Collins, D.W. Hill, and F. M. Mcelhanon, Jr. Muscle hypertrophy in men and women. *Med. Sci. Sports Med.* 20(4):338–344, 1988.

11. Dalsky, G. P. Effect of exercise on bone: Permissive influence of estrogen and calcium. *Med. Sci. Sports Exerc.* 22(3):281–285, 1990.

12. Daniels, J., and N. Daniels. Running economy of elite male and elite female runners. *Med. Sci. Sports Exerc.* 24(4):483–489, 1992.

13. De Cree, C. Sex steroid metabolism and menstrual irregularities in the exercising female: A review. *Sports Med.* 25(6):369–406, 1998.

14. De Souza, M. J., J. C. Arce, L. S. Pescatello, H. S. Scherzer, and A. A. Luciano. Gonadal hormones and semen quality in male runners. A volume threshold effect of endurance training. *Int. J. Sports Med.* 15(7):383–391, 1994.

15. Froberg, K., and P. K. Pedersen. Sex differences in endurance capacity and metabolic response to prolonged, heavy exercise. *Eur. J. Appl. Physiol.* 52:446–450, 1984.

16. Hackett, P. H., R. D. Rennie, S. E. Hofmeidter, R. F. Grover, and J. T. Reeves. Fluid retention and relative hypoventilation in acute mountain sickness. *Respiration* 43:321–329, 1982.

17. Hannon, J. P., J. L. Shields, and C. W. Harris. High altitude acclimatization in women. In R. E. Goddard (ed.), *The effects of altitude on physical performance.* Chicago Athletic Institute, 1966, 37–44.

18. Horstman, D. H., and E. Christensen. Acclimatization to dry heat: Active men vs. active women. *J. Appl. Physiol.* 52(4):825–831, 1982.

19. Johnson, B. D., K. W. Saupe, and J. A. Dempsey. Mechanical constraints on exercise hyperpnea in endurance trained athletes. *J. Appl. Physiol.* 73(3):874–886, 1992.

20. Kanaley, J. A., R. A. Boileau, J. A. Bahr, J. E. Misner, and R. A. Nelson. Substrate oxidation and GH responses to exercise are independent of menstrual phase and status. *Med. Sci. Sports Exerc.* 24(8):873–880, 1992.

21. Lokey, E. A., Z.V. Tran, C. L. Wells, B. C. Myers, and A. C. Tran. Effects of physical exercise on pregnancy outcomes: A meta-analytic review. *Med. Sci. Sports Exerc.* 23(11):1234–1239, 1991.

22. Loucks, A. B. Effects of exercise training on the menstrual cycle: Existence and mechanisms. *Med. Sci. Sports Exerc.* 22(3):275–280, 1990.

23. Loucks, A. B., et al. The reproductive system and exercise in women. *Med. Sci. Sports Exerc.* 24(6):S288–S293, 1992.

24. Lloyd, T., et al. Women athletes with menstrual irregularity have increased musculoskeletal injuries. *Med. Sci. Sports Exerc.* 18(4):374–379, 1986.

25. McClaren, S. R., C. A. Harns, D. F. Pegelow, and J. A. Dempsey. Smaller lungs in women affect exercise hyperpnea. *J. Appl. Physiol.* 84(6):1872–1881, 1998.

26. Maughan, R., and L. Leiper. Aerobic capacity and fractional utilization of aerobic capacity in elite and nonelite male and female marathon runners. *Eur. J. Appl. Physiol.* 52:80–87, 1983.

27. Meyer, F., O. Bar-Or, D. MacDougall, and G. J. F. Heigenhauser. Sweat electrolyte loss during exercise in the heat: Effects of gender and maturation. *Med. Sci. Sports Exerc.* 24(7):776–781, 1992.

REFERENCES

28. Mitchell, J. H., et al. Acute response and chronic adaptation to exercise in women. *Med. Sci. Sports Exerc.* 24(6): S258–S265, 1992.

29. Otis, C. L., B. Drinkwater, M. Johnson, A. Loucks, and J. Wilmore. American College of Sports Medicine position stand: The female athlete triad. *Med. Sci. Sports Exerc.* 29(5):i –ix, 1997.

30. Paterson, D. J., H. Pinnington, A. R. Pearce, and A. L. Morton. Maximal exercise cardiorespiratory responses of men and women during acute exposure to hypoxia. *Aviat. Space Environ. Med.* 58:243–247, 1987.

31. Pellicia, A., B. J. Maron, A. Spataro, M. A. Proschan, and P. Spirito. The upper limit of physiologic cardiac hypertrophy in highly trained elite athletes. *N. Eng. J. Med.* 324(5):295–301, 1991.

32. Powers, S. K., D. Martin, and S. Dodd. Exercise-induced hypoxemia in elite endurance athletes: Incidence, causes and impact on VO_{2max}. *Sports Med.* 16(1):14–22, 1993.

33. Robergs, R. A, R. Quintana, D. L. Parker, and C. C. Frankel. Multiple variables explain the variability in the decrement in VO_{2max} during acute hypobaric hypoxia. *Med. Sci. Sports Exerc.* 30(6):869–879, 1998.

34. Roberts, A. C., R. D. McClure, R. I. Weiner, and G. A. Brooks. Overtraining effects male reproductive status. *Fert. Steril.* 60(4):686–692, 1993.

35. Ruby, B. C., and R. A. Robergs. Gender differences in substrate utilization during exercise. *Sports Med.* 17(6):393–410, 1994.

36. Ronkainen, H. R. A., A. J. Pakarinen, and A. J. I. Kauppila. Adrenocortical function of female endurance runners and joggers. *Med. Sci. Sports Exerc.* 18(4):385–389, 1986.

37. Shapiro, Y., K. B. Pandolf, B. A. Avellini, N. A. Pimental, and R. F. Goldman. Physiological responses of men and women to humid and dry heat. *J. Appl. Physiol.* 40:786–796, 1980.

38. Shoene, R. B., H. T. Robertson, D. J. Peirson, and A. P. Peterson. Respiratory drives and exercise in menstrual cycles of athletic and nonathletic women. *J. Appl. Physiol.* 50:1300–1305, 1981.

39. Sparling, P. B. A meta-analysis of studies comparing maximal oxygen uptake in men and women. *Res. Quart. Exerc. Sport.* 51(3):542–552, 1980.

40. Tarnopolsky, L. J., J. D. MacDougall, S. A. Atkinson, M. A. Tarnopolsky, and J. R. Sutton. Gender difference in substrate for endurance exercise. *J. Appl. Physiol.* 68(1):302–308, 1990.

41. Tiidus, P. M. Can estrogens diminish exercise-induced muscle damage? *Can. J. Appl. Physiol.* 20(1):26–38, 1995.

42. Wolfe, L. A., I. K. M. Brenner, and M. F. Mottola. Maternal exercise, fetal well being, and pregnancy outcome. *Exerc. Sport Sci. Rev.* 22:145–151, 1994.

RECOMMENDED READINGS

American College of Gynecologists. *Exercise during pregnancy and the postpartum period.* ACOG Technical Bulletin No.189, Feb. 1994.

American College of Sports Medicine. *ACSM's guidelines for exercise testing and prescription.* Williams & Wilkins, Baltimore, 1996.

Bunt, J. C. Metabolic actions of estradiol: Significance for acute and chronic exercise responses. *Med. Sci. Sports Exerc.* 22(3):286–290, 1990.

Clapp, J. F., III, M. Wesley, and R. H. Sleamaker. Thermoregulatory and metabolic responses to jogging prior to and during pregnancy. *Med. Sci. Sports Exerc.* 19(2):124–130, 1987.

Dalsky, G. P. Effect of exercise on bone: Permissive influence of estrogen and calcium. *Med. Sci. Sports Exerc.* 22(3): 281–285, 1990.

Daniels, J., and N. Daniels. Running economy of elite male and elite female runners. *Med. Sci. Sports Exerc.* 24(4):483–489, 1992.

De Souza, M. J., J. C. Arce, L. S. Pescatello, H. S. Scherzer, and A. A. Luciano. Gonadal hormones and semen quality in male runners. A volume threshold effect of endurance training. *Int. J. Sports Med.* 15(7):383–391, 1994.

Froberg, K., and P. K. Pedersen. Sex differences in endurance capacity and metabolic response to prolonged, heavy exercise. *Eur. J Appl. Physiol.* 52:446–450, 1984.

Loucks, A. B., et al. The reproductive system and exercise in women. *Med. Sci. Sports Exerc.* 24(6):S288–S293, 1992.

Lloyd, T., et al. Women athletes with menstrual irregularity have increased musculoskeletal injuries. *Med. Sci. Sports Exerc.* 18(4):374–379, 1986.

Mitchell, J. H., et al. Acute response and chronic adaptation to exercise in women. *Med. Sci. Sports Exerc.* 24(6):S258–S265, 1992.

Ruby, B. C., and R. A. Robergs. Gender differences in substrate utilization during exercise. *Sports Med.* 17(6):393–410, 1994.

Tarnopolsky, I. J., J. D. MacDougall, S. A. Atkinson, M. A. Tarnopolsky, and J. R. Sutton. Gender difference in substrate for endurance exercise. *J. Appl. Physiol.* 68:302–308, 1990.

Wolfe, L. A., I. K. M. Brenner, and M. F. Mottola. Maternal exercise, fetal well being, and pregnancy outcome. *Exerc. Sport Sci. Rev.* 22:145–151, 1994.

CHAPTER 21

Exercise, Weight Control, Health, and Disease

he connections between regular exercise/physical activity and health were not always as obvious as they are today. In fact, as recently as the early 1980s medical and public attitudes toward exercise were quite different. To run 5 mi, swim 1 mi in the ocean, or cycle 50 mi along the coast, and to do these several times each week were viewed to be characteristics of abnormal behavior. After all, the objectives of "modern society" were to make life easier to live, not more laborious. Physicians were not demanding that their patients exercise more to combat hypertension, excess body fat, or heart disease, and their was no media support to promote exercise and an active lifestyle. However, thanks to the continued research efforts of physical educators and exercise physiologists, and certain "more enlightened" physicians, the connections between an active lifestyle and overall health became more recognized. During the two decades from 1980 to the present, the evidence that exercise can not only prevent disease, but also reverse many disease processes has accumulated to such a degree that now almost all medical organizations have published statements on how important exercise is in the prevention and treatment of their diseases of interest. The purpose of this chapter is to present a brief review of the research that has supported the importance of exercise in weight control, the prevention and treatment of certain diseases, and health maintenance.

OBJECTIVES

After studying this chapter, you should be able to:

- Identify the causes of obesity.
- Describe the health implications of obesity and overweight.
- Explain the role of exercise in treating and preventing weight loss and weight maintenance.
- List specific recommendations for exercise training for obese individuals.
- Explain the role of exercise in the treatment and prevention of selected chronic diseases.
- Identify some important health promotion and disease prevention strategies.

KEY TERMS

mortality	myocardial	risk factors
epidemiology	infarction	hypertension
overweight	claudication	arteriosclerosis
BMI	pulmonary edema	angina
obesity	atherosclerosis	stroke

A Short History of Exercise and Health

*T*he relatively recent recognition of the beneficial nature of exercise to health and well-being can be initially viewed as evidence of the inability of past research to provide connection(s) between exercise and health. However, this conclusion is far from the truth. As early as the 1880s evidence existed concerning the protective effect that regular physical activity provided against premature death from heart disease and stroke (1). Furthermore, the discipline of exercise physiology was already being developed on the basis of the emphasis on how exercise influences the incidence and development of symptoms of heart disease (2).

The first half of the twentieth century was largely influenced by both world wars, and therefore exercise physiology was focused on military training. However, after World War II there was a reemphasis on the influence of exercise on heart disease. A major study on the association between exercise and cardiovascular disease was conducted in England during the 1950s (3). The incidence and severity of cardiovascular disease in London bus conductors and bus drivers was compared. Because London buses have two levels, conductors have to walk throughout the bus and up and down stairs repeatedly every day. Conversely, bus drivers remain seated throughout the workday.

Not surprisingly, results indicated that the conductors were more physically fit than the drivers, and had a lower incidence of coronary heart disease (CHD) with reduced death (**mortality**) and early mortality from CHD. Similar results were found from the same researchers in their study of the leisure-time exercise habits of civil servants (4). The authors concluded:

Physical activity of work provides protection against ischemic heart disease. Men in physically active jobs have less ischemic heart disease during middle age, what disease they have is less severe, and they tend to develop it later than similar men in physically inactive jobs.

Similar research and findings were also obtained in the United States, with additional evidence for not just the benefits of exercise, but for different quantities of exercise. Paffenbarger and colleagues studied the work-based physical activity patterns and the health records of San Francisco longshoremen (fig. 21.1) (5). The anti-CHD benefits of physical activity were greatest in men who expended more than 8500 kcal/week. The same researchers then compared leisure-time versus work-related physical activity and risk for CHD in 16,936 alumni of Harvard University between 1962 and 1972 (fig. 21.2). Once again the beneficial effects of physical activity were seen with an increase in energy expenditure, especially for individuals who expended more than 2000 kcal/week.

FIGURE 21.1

Death rates from coronary heart disease per 10,000 man-years of work for 3,686 San Francisco longshoremen, 1951 to 1972, by work activity and age at death.

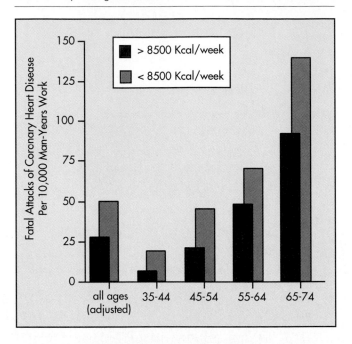

FIGURE 21.2

Incidence rates of coronary heart disease (nonfatal and fatal) per 10,000 man-years of observation among 16,936 Harvard Alumni, 1962 to 1972.

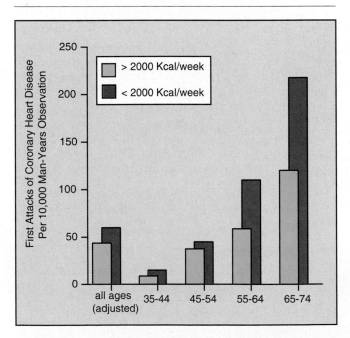

Since the classic studies of Morris and Paffenbarger, there have been hundreds of additional studies that have identified exercise and physical activity as associated with a reduced incidence and severity of CHD. However, it must be highlighted that these studies have just provided evi-

TABLE 21.1

A summary of the disease processes and illnesses combated by regular exercise and physical activity

CHRONIC DISEASE	IMPACT OF EXERCISE/ PHYSICAL ACTIVITY
CHD	Prevention, rehabilitation, diagnosis
Hypertension	Prevention, rehabilitation
Obesity	Prevention, rehabilitation
Stroke	Prevention, rehabilitation
Peripheral vascular disease	Prevention, rehabilitation, diagnosis
Cancers	
Colon	Prevention, rehabilitation
Breast	Prevention, rehabilitation
Prostate	Prevention, rehabilitation
Lung	Prevention, rehabilitation
Diabetes	
Non-insulin- dependent	Prevention, rehabilitation
Osteoporosis	Prevention, rehabilitation
Lower back pain	Prevention, rehabilitation
Chronic obstructive pulmonary disease	Prevention, rehabilitation, diagnosis
Asthma	Prevention, rehabilitation, diagnosis

dence of an association. Such research is called cross-sectional research, and when applied to the study of health it is termed **epidemiology.** No details of why a proposed association exists can be drawn from epidemiology research and, because of the nature of the research, the interpretation of cause and effect between exercise and prevention of CHD is not automatic. These limitations exist because the research relies on study of large numbers of subjects and grouping subjects based on variables of interest, rather than controlling the level of exercise and physical activity. Such control cannot be done on human subjects because it would be unethical to restrain people from being active for years and even decades, have them eat poor diets, force them to smoke cigarettes, make them gain or lose excessive amounts of body fat, insist that they develop diabetes, and so forth!

How then do researchers know that physical activity actually protects against CHD? Could it be some other variable that differs among groups? Well, there is always the possibility, but epidemiologists can use statistics that can essentially control for other variables. For example, Morris and Paffenbarger adjusted their data based on scores for other variables that could influence the development of CHD. Thus the connection between increased physical activity and reduced CHD was not made because subjects who were exercising more had a better diet, better genetics, were not diabetic, or did not smoke. In addition, the findings from studies like those of Morris and Paffenbarger can be used to develop more controlled animal re-

search, where manipulating the daily physical activity, diet, and emotional stress over a lifetime is realistic and "relatively" less ethically questionable. Finding similar results from animal research adds credibility to the less-controlled human epidemiological findings.

Exercise and Health

A good place to start is with the definition of health. The World Health Organization defines health as:

A state of complete physical, mental, and social well-being and not merely the absence of disease or infirmity.
　　　　　　　　—World Health Organization, 1947

The WHO's definition of health takes into account not only the condition of your body, but also your mental and social well-being. Today, many consider the term wellness as a better measure of overall health and well-being. Wellness is defined as:

An approach to personal health that emphasizes individual responsibility for well-being through the practice of health-promoting behaviors.

The wellness model includes emotional, social, intellectual, spiritual, and physical dimensions. Each component of the wellness model is important to the maintenance of good health and well-being. Participating in wellness activities will enhance your quality of life and overall potential.

Clearly, the development and maintenance of health involves processes that are additional to the presence or absence of disease. However, research has mainly focused on how exercise influences disease processes because these processes can be quantified using valid measurement tools. Conversely, it is harder to validly quantify the quality of life of a person who is not ill with a recognized disease or illness. This is unfortunate, because for many people the benefits of exercise are not quantifiable and relate to improving a person's demeanor, enjoyment, social relationships, family interactions, and so forth.

Table 21.1 summarizes the disease processes that regular exercise and physical activity are known to have a positive impact on. Obviously, exercise is important in combating coronary heart disease. However, research shows us that exercise also benefits diseases and illnesses such as obesity,

mortality the epidimological and vital statistics term for death

epidemiology (epp' a-dee' me-ology) the study of the nature, cause, control, and determinants of the frequency and distribution of disease, disabilities, and death in human populations

FOCUS BOX 21.1

Some Health Facts on Physical Inactivity: A Summary of the Surgeon General's Report

A New View of Physical Activity

People who are usually inactive can improve their health and well-being by becoming even moderately active on a regular basis.

Physical activity need not be strenuous to achieve health benefits.

Greater health benefits can be achieved by increasing the amount (duration, frequency, or intensity) of physical activity.

Some Facts About Physical Inactivity

Sedentary lifestyles double the risk of heart disease.

In terms of heart disease risk, physical inactivity is equivalent to smoking a pack of cigarettes per day.

More people are at risk for developing heart disease because of physical inactivity, than are all people for smoking, high blood pressure, and high cholesterol (combined).

Physical inactivity reduces your life span.

Physical inactivity is associated with a higher incidence of chronic diseases such as diabetes, arthritis, osteoporosis, and obesity.

Physical activity declines dramatically with age and during adolescent years.

Fitness Trends over the Years

In high school, enrollment in daily physical education classes dropped from 42% in 1991 to 25% in 1995.

Only 19% of all high school students are physically active for 20 min or more in physical education classes every day during the school week.

In 1995 the CDC conducted the first national survey to simultaneously examine six areas of health behavior by college students. The consensus of the study was that 21% were overweight.

Only 4 out of 10 said they had participated in vigorous physical activity for at least 20 min on 3 or more of the 7 days prior to the survey.

Only 22% of adults engage in leisure-time activities at or above the level recommended for health benefits in the U.S. Public Health Service's health and disease prevention goals and objectives for the nation.

The Benefits of Regular Physical Activity

Reduces the risk of dying prematurely.

Reduces the risk of dying from heart disease.

Reduces the risk of developing diabetes.

Reduces the risk of developing high blood pressure.

Helps lower blood pressure in people who have high blood pressure.

Reduces the risk of developing colon and other forms of cancer.

Reduces depression and anxiety.

Helps control weight.

Helps build and maintain healthy bones, muscles, and joints.

Helps older adults become stronger and better able to move without falling.

Promotes psychological well-being.

---

stroke, specific (but not all) cancers, non-insulin-dependent diabetes, osteoporosis, and obstructive pulmonary diseases.

Is Physical Inactivity Really Such a Serious Problem in the United States?

In 1996 the U.S. Department of Health and Human Services, the Centers for Disease Control and Prevention (CDC), and the President's Council on Physical Fitness and Sports teamed up with the surgeon general and released the first surgeon general's report on physical activity and health (see focus box 21.1). This document reported that more than 60% of adults do not achieve the recommended amount of regular physical activity needed to improve and *maintain* one's health. In fact, 25% of all adults are not active at all. The number of Americans who do not participate in regular exercise has been called an epidemic. Many health and fitness experts consider physical inactivity one of the top public health burdens in the

United States. Individuals that choose to, or are forced to, lead a physically inactive life, dramatically increase their risk for a variety of chronic diseases and reduce their life spans.

Defining Physical Fitness

The simplest definition for health-related physical fitness is *the ability of the body's systems (heart, lungs, blood vessels, and muscles) to function efficiently to resist disease and to be able to participate in a variety of activities without undue fatigue.* An individual who is physically fit has sufficient stamina to pursue most, if not all, of the activities they want to participate in over the course of the day, week, month, and year. Such activities include work, family activities, leisure activities (including exercise), and other recreational activities. The five components of health-related physical fitness are *muscular strength, muscular endurance, cardiorespiratory endurance, flexibility, and body composition.* A comprehensive fitness program should have activities that develop and maintain each of the five components.

How Much Exercise Is Enough?

The American College of Sports Medicine, in conjunction with the Centers for Disease Control and Prevention and the President's Council on Physical Fitness and Sports, recently issued a new recommendation on increased physical activity for Americans. The recommendation states: "Every American adult should accumulate 30 minutes or more of moderate-intensity physical activity over the course of most days of the week. Because most Americans do not presently meet the standard described above, almost all should strive to increase their participation in moderate and/or vigorous physical activity." The ACSM/CDC position statement on exercise is perhaps the most powerful single event to have occurred in the last decade in the field of sports medicine and exercise physiology. The consensus statement means that a little bit of daily physical activity results in health-related benefits. Examples of activities that can contribute to the 30 min total are walking up stairs (instead of taking the elevator), gardening, raking leaves, walking at lunch. In addition, more typical forms of exercise are also encouraged, such as running, swimming, cycling, working out at a health club, and playing tennis. Individuals should strive to participate in activities that improve and maintain the key components of health-related fitness. Figure 21.3 presents a convenient way to consider the quantity and quality of exercise needed to maintain good health and well-being.

Exercise, Diet, and Weight Control

Obesity is perhaps the most prevalent chronic health problem in the United States today. As many as 33% of the population is overweight (above their desired weight). Most Americans seem obsessed with their weight. If you ask most Americans whether or not they are satisfied with their weight, more than likely most will say No! At any given time, 20% of the U.S. population is taking part in some form of weight-loss program (6). Americans spend over $30 billion annually on various weight-loss methods, most of which fail. Excess body weight is associated with numerous health-related problems, including increased risk for coronary artery disease, diabetes, and hyperlipidemia. However, the primary reason most people are not happy with their weight is based on appearance.

An obsession with obesity can also be unhealthy. The majority (95%) of dieters are unsuccessful at keeping the weight off after dieting. Repeated weight loss and weight gain, referred to as the "yo-yo effect," can lead to long-term detrimental alterations in metabolism. In addition, an obsession with weight and weight loss can lead to practices of self-imposed starvation (anorexia nervosa) or binge eating followed by emaciation caused by purging (bulimia), which are both serious medical problems. The importance of maintaining a healthy body weight and eating nutritiously is important, but not an easy task for anyone.

Excess Weight

Excess weight is a serious medical, health, and social issue. Since the evolution of industrialized societies, the incidence of obesity has risen dramatically. There is no longer a need to hunt or pick one's food, we just drive by a window or go to a "super" market. The ease of obtaining food, combined with the fact that most people today work in sedentary professions, has led to an epidemic of obesity in the United States, and other nations as well. Today it takes a conscious effort to increase one's physical activity level and choose foods that are healthy. Even most well-educated people do not believe they have the time or knowledge to eat healthy and get enough exercise.

Two terms are often used to classify excess weight: overweight and obesity. The National Center for Health Statistics has defined someone as being **overweight** if she or he has a BMI of 27.8 or more for men and 27.3 or more for women (7). A normal BMI has been classified as 20.0 for men and 25.0 for women. These classifications of overweight are based on **BMI** measurements corresponding to approximately 20% or more above the 1983 Metropolitan Life Insurance Company tables. Newer guidelines suggest a BMI of 20 to 25 for most middle-aged adults (8). BMIs in this range have the lowest risk for disease and premature death (see focus box 21.2).

Obesity literally means "excess fat." **Obesity** refers to excess body fat versus body weight. An ideal body fat percentage for good health is between 10 to 15% for young men and between 20 to 25% for young women. Body fat percentages greater than 20% for men or 30% for women are considered an indication of obesity.

Thus *overweight* and *obesity* should not be used interchangeably. The dissociation between being overweight and obese was demonstrated as far back as the 1940s when researchers studied a group of professional football players. When they compared the players' weights to early actuary weight tables, the majority of the players were considered seriously overweight. But when they tested the players' body compositions, the majority of them had body fat percentages under 20%, meaning that they simply did not fit the "normal" standards for the weight charts (9).

Health Implications of Obesity

It is estimated that obesity affects one of every three persons in the United States and is said by some to be this country's number one health problem. Obesity is associated with

---

overweight being above a weight as defined by a particular chart or reference group

BMI weight in kilograms divided by height in meters squared

obesity excess fat

FIGURE 21.3

The Physical Activity Pyramid.

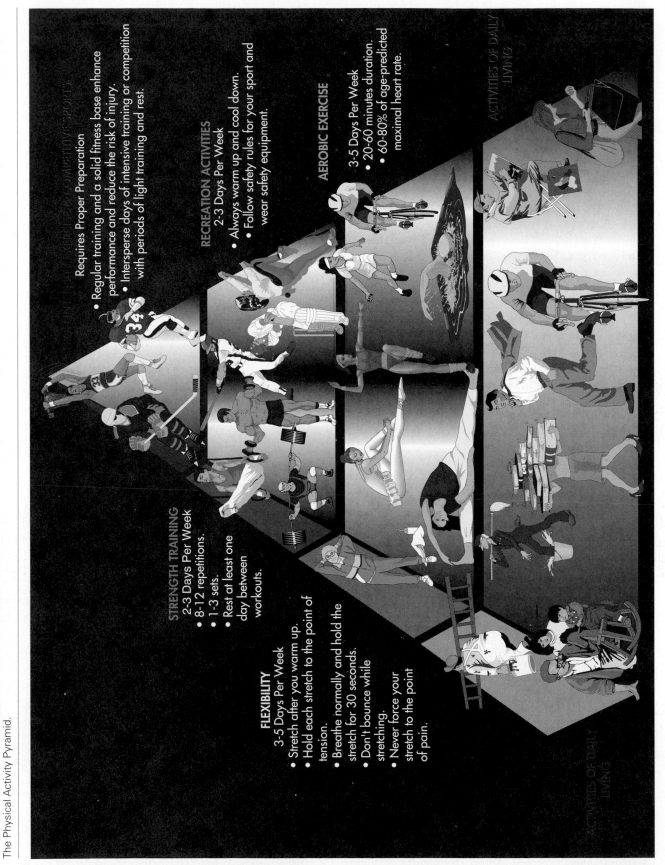

COMPETITIVE SPORTS

Requires Proper Preparation
- Regular training and a solid fitness base enhance performance and reduce the risk of injury.
- Interspese days of intensive training or competition with periods of light training and rest.

RECREATION ACTIVITIES
2-3 Days Per Week
- Always warm up and cool down.
- Follow safety rules for your sport and wear safety equipment.

AEROBIC EXERCISE
3-5 Days Per Week
- 20-60 minutes duration.
- 60-80% of age-predicted maximal heart rate.

STRENGTH TRAINING
2-3 Days Per Week
- 8-12 repetitions.
- 1-3 sets.
- Rest at least one day between workouts.

FLEXIBILITY
3-5 Days Per Week
- Stretch after you warm up.
- Hold each stretch to the point of tension.
- Breathe normally and hold the stretch for 30 seconds.
- Don't bounce while stretching.
- Never force your stretch to the point of pain.

ACTIVITIES OF DAILY LIVING

ACTIVITIES OF DAILY LIVING

ACTIVITIES OF DAILY LIVING

FOCUS BOX 21.2

Finding Your BMI

1. Multiply your weight by 705:
    e.g., 140 lb × 705 = 98,700
2. Divide the answer by your height:
    98,700 / 65 in = 1,518

3. Divide the answer by your height again:
    1,518 / 65 = 23.4
4. Final result = BMI of 23.4

higher risk for diabetes mellitus, hypertriglyceridemia, decreased levels of high-density lipoprotein cholesterol, and increased levels of low-density lipoprotein cholesterol, gallbladder disease, chronic hypoxia, some forms of cancer, sleep apnea, and degenerative joint disease (10).

Obesity is a major contributor to such illnesses as hypertension, hypercholesterolemia, and diabetes (11), and is an independent risk factor for cardiovascular disease (12). Numerous population studies have confirmed that obesity is associated with numerous health and medical problems. NHANES II (National Health and Nutrition Examination Survey) found that the prevalence of hypertension among overweight adults was 2.9 times higher than among nonoverweight adults. Data from the Framingham study found that in men, for every 10% increase in relative weight, blood pressure increased by 6.5 mm Hg, a 15% gain resulting in an 18% increase in systolic blood pressure (13).

It is estimated that approximately ⅓ of all cases of hypertension are due to obesity (14).

Fat Distribution

Obesity is clearly associated with increased medical and health risks. However, exactly where the excess fat is stored is also related to overall mortality and increased risk for cardiovascular disease. In general, women tend to store fat in the lower half of the body around the hip and thigh area (*gynoid obesity*), whereas men tend to store fat on the upper part of the body around the abdominal area (*android obesity*). Android obesity compared to gynoid obesity is associated with greater risk of developing diabetes, hypertension, and heart disease (15).

Weight Loss

Dieting has become a national pastime for Americans. Even though most people know that dieting alone is ineffective in achieving long-term success, dieting is still the method of choice for most overweight individuals. It has been estimated that as many as 40% of adult women and 20% of adult men report they are currently trying to lose weight at any one time (16).

In order to maintain ideal body weight, energy consumed (food consumed daily) needs to equal energy output

(daily physical activity habits). When these are equal, one is said to be in energy balance. In order to gain or lose weight, each side of the equation needs to be adjusted. To lose 1 lb per week requires a 3500 caloric negative balance. Several possible combinations are possible to achieve this goal:

Reduce caloric intake by 500 calories per day.
Reduce caloric intake by 250 calories and increase energy expenditure by 250 calories per day.
Increase caloric expenditure by 500 calories per day.

The safe recommended weight loss per week is 2.2 lb.

The Role of Exercise in Weight Loss and Weight Control

Exercise appears to play a critical role in the loss and maintenance of body weight (17, 18). The metabolic mechanisms by which exercise contributes to weight loss and/or maintenance includes increased energy expenditure, enhanced fat mobilization by increasing adipose tissue activity, a small increase in postexercise resting metabolic rate, possibly an increased thermogenic response to food if exercise is in close proximity to a meal, minimized loss of lean body weight, improved psychological functioning, retardation of the decline in basal metabolic rate with dietary restrictions, and possibly better appetite control (19).

Exercise alone or in combination with a sensible diet produces the best long-term weight loss results. Exercise can contribute up to a 300 to 400 kcal deficit per exercise bout. Keeping food intake constant with an exercise program conducted 3 times per week (at an intensity and duration eliciting 300 to 400 kcal/session) could result in a 16-lb weight loss in 1 year. The benefits of exercise in weight loss and weight control is really quite minimal, but if exercise training is combined with modest caloric restriction, the negative energy balance is even greater. Exercise is important because it helps maintain resting metabolic rate and fat-free mass. Regular exercise may also help control appetite and improve psychological outlook when trying to lose weight.

Exercise, Health, and Disease

Cardiovascular Diseases

Cardiovascular diseases continue to be the leading cause of death in the Western world (American Heart Association, 1998). According to 1994 estimates, 57,490,000 Americans have one or more forms of cardiovascular disease. In 1994 alone, cardiovascular diseases claimed 954,720 lives or 41.8 of all deaths. This year as many as 1,500,000 Americans will have a new or recurrent heart attack, and about ⅓ of them will die. From another perspective, more than two of every five Americans die of cardiovascular disease. The good news is that death rates from cardiovascular disease have been on the decline. From 1984 to 1994, death rates from cardiovascular disease have declined 22.4%. The reduction in death rates from cardiovascular diseases can be linked to lifestyle changes among Americans and advances in medical treatments. Cardiovascular disease is still a major killer. And, fortunately, cardiovascular disease is highly preventable.

Exercise plays an important role in preventing heart disease, as well as in the rehabilitation of individuals with heart disease. The major risk factors for coronary heart disease—hypertension, smoking, high cholesterol—are all positively affected by exercise. Furthermore, physical inactivity is now recognized as a major contributor to the atherosclerotic process.

There are several different types of cardiovascular disease, including coronary artery disease (CAD), peripheral vascular disease (PVD), and congestive heart failure (CHF). CAD can cause impaired heart function, and eventually heart attack (**myocardial infarction**). PVD can cause pain in the peripheral musculature (**claudication**) during even mild physical activity. CHF is characterized by a progressive deterioration of the function of the heart muscle (myocardium), resulting in poor exercise tolerance, and impaired lung function because of a worsening accumulation of fluid in the lungs (**pulmonary edema**).

Coronary heart disease develops over decades, the incidence of which is increased exponentially with the existence of specific traits, illnesses, and other diseases identified in table 21.2. CHD is the most prevalent of the cardiovascular diseases, and accounts for the majority of all deaths (all cause mortality) in developed countries (fig. 21.4). CHD involves the narrowing of one or more arteries of the heart, called coronary arteries. These arteries narrow because of the accumulation of fatty, fibrous, and calcified deposits within the blood vessels. These deposits are referred to as plaque, and the disease process causing plaque development is termed **atherosclerosis.**

The origin of the study of coronary artery disease in the United States began in a small town in Massachusetts. In the late 1940s residents of Framingham began to be screened in an effort to determine common patterns or risk factors of cardiovascular disease (21). Since the start of the Framingham study, hundreds of studies have investigated specific causes of coronary artery disease, which has led to the development of **risk factors** for coronary artery disease. The risk factors that research has shown to be causal to the development of CHD are termed *primary* risk factors. The risk factors that research has shown to contribute to the severity of the primary risk factors and hence the development of CHD are termed *secondary* risk factors. The more risk factors that are present, the greater the risk (exponential increase) for developing CHD, or having CHD.

It is tempting to rate the risk factors on how important they are to the development of CHD. This has proven difficult to do, which is logical because of the multiple factors that can combine to cause CHD. For example, animal research indicates that hypercholesterolemia is pivotal to the severity of atherosclerosis and progression of CHD. The initial applied result of these findings was to immediately raise concerns over controlling dietary cholesterol intake, the prescription of blood cholesterol–lowering medications, and routine blood cholesterol measurement. However, simply addressing what might appear to be a laboratory-determined important risk factor can remove emphasis away from more easily, and less expensively alterable risk factors. The best example of this is physical inactivity. Within the United States, more than two-thirds of the population are classified as being physically inactive. Given this high incidence, and the fact that physical inactivity can worsen many of the other risk factors for CHD, it is becoming more recognized that physical inactivity may be the single most detrimental risk factor for CHD (fig. 21.5). Ironically, physical inactivity is also the cheapest and potentially simplest risk factor to modify.

The generalized results of research on whether different types of exercise training and physical activity alter risk factors are presented in table 21.3. These results are generaliza-

TABLE 21.2			
Risk factors for the development of coronary artery disease			
PRIMARY RISK FACTORS	**MODIFIABLE**	**SECONDARY RISK FACTORS**	**MODIFIABLE**
Physical inactivity	Yes	Age	No
Cigarette smoking	Yes	Gender	No
Hypertension	Yes	Family history	No
Diabetes	Yes	Obesity	Yes
Hypercholesterolemia	Yes	Emotional stress	Yes

FIGURE 21.4

Rates of death from leading causes (1992).

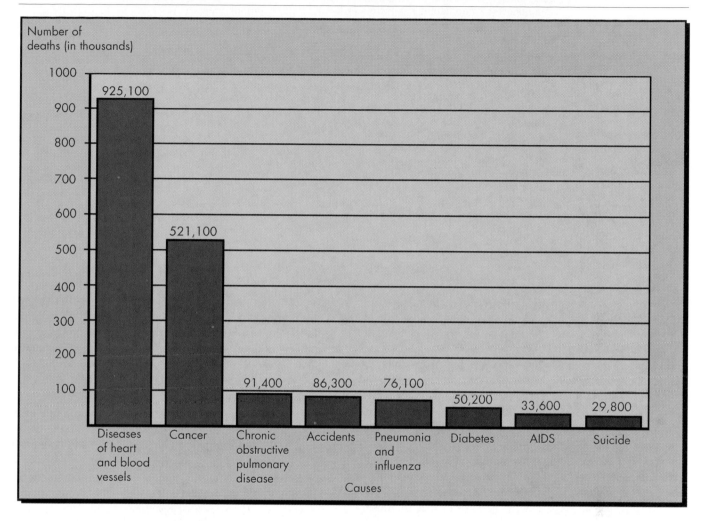

FIGURE 21.5

Population attributable risk by risk factor.

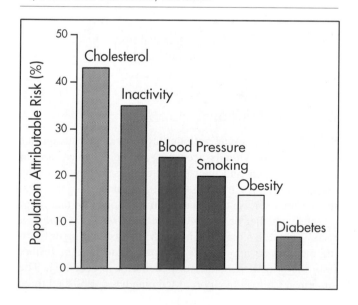

tions because it is difficult to summarize all types of training (intensity, frequency, duration) in one table. Furthermore, as will be explained in subsequent sections, the role of physical activity in altering specific risk factors is not well researched. However, we know that regular physical activity, as distinct from more intense exercise training, has some protection against premature death from CHD (22).

myocardial infarction heart attack

claudication ischemic pain in the lower extremities associated with exercise, which is due to reduced blood flow resulting from atherosclerosis in the femoral arteries

pulmonary edema accumulation of fluid in the lung

atherosclerosis (ather oh' scler row' sis) caused by a narrowing of the coronary arteries which supply the heart muscle with blood and oxygen

risk factors factors associated with increased risk for acquiring a disease or disability

TABLE 21.3

Summary of whether different types of exercise training and physical activity alter specific "modifiable" risk factors for CHD

RISK FACTOR	EXERCISE TRAINING		DAILY PHYSICAL ACTIVITY†
	ENDURANCE*	STRENGTH*	
Physical activity	⇑	⇑	⇑
Cigarette smoking	⇔	⇔	⇔
Hypertension	⇓	⇔	⇔
Diabetes	⇓	⇓	⇔
Hypercholesterolemia	⇓	⇔	⇔
Obesity	⇓	⇓	⇔
Emotional stress	⇓	⇓	⇓

*Assumes at least 3 times/week at intensities sufficient to cause a physiological training stimulus.

†At lest 30 min of accumulated physical activity/day.

Benefits of Exercise in Individuals with Established Coronary Artery Disease

Clearly, regular physical activity reduces the risk of CAD. How effective is exercise at treating CAD? Initially, extended bed rest was recommended for patients recovering from a myocardial infarction. The thinking at that time was that the heart takes approximately 6 weeks to heal after a heart attack, and that any undue stress might compromise that healing process. Although the heart may be healing, the rest of the body is slowly deteriorating. Bed rest results in (1) a decrease in work capacity, (2) a decreased adaptability to changes in position, (3) a decrease in blood volume, (4) a decrease in muscle mass, (5) an increase in risk for thromboembolism, and (6) a decrease in respiratory and pulmonary function (see focus box 21.3).

In the early 1940s, physicians began to experiment with early mobilization after a cardiac event, and the results were favorable. Early mobilization of cardiac patients resulted in fewer complications, faster recovery, and reduction in many of the other related complications of bed rest mentioned above. Today, exercise is a standard therapeutic modality in the treatment of cardiac disease. In almost all cases, individuals recovering from a myocardial infarction, cardiac surgery, or other cardiac procedure, should benefit from a supervised cardiac rehabilitation program and eventually outpatient exercise.

The Clinical Practice Guideline, *Cardiac Rehabilitation*, was developed under the direction of the Agency for Health Care Policy and Research and the National Heart, Lung and Blood Institute of the U.S. Department of Health and Human Services. It provides broad recommendations, on the basis of evaluations of the scientific evidence pertaining to the various components of cardiac rehabilitation. In this landmark document, the following conclusions were made regarding the benefits of exercise training:

The scientific data clearly establish that improvements in objectively measured exercise tolerance result from cardiac rehabilitation exercise training; therefore, appropriately prescribed and conducted exercise training should be a key component of cardiac rehabilitation services for coronary patients with angina, myocardial infarction, CABG and PTCA. The beneficial effect of cardiac rehabilitation exercise training on exercise tolerance is one of the most clearly established favorable outcomes in the panel's view. The most consistent benefit appeared to occur with exercise training at least three times per week for 12 weeks' duration. The duration of aerobic exercise training sessions varied from 20 to 40 minutes, at an intensity approximately 70 to 85% of baseline maximal exercise test heart rate. No statistically significant increase in cardiovascular complications or other serious adverse outcomes were reported in any randomized controlled trials that evaluated the role of exercise training in patients with coronary disease.

—Adapted from Clinical Practice Guideline, *Cardiac Rehabilitation*

Risk Stratification

Several medical organizations have developed categories that stratify individuals according to their medical and/or health conditions and their potential risks for injury during exercise testing or training (23). In essence, risk stratification before exercise testing or training is one tool that helps establish whether or not *the benefits outweigh the potential risks!* There are situations in which exercise testing or training may not be appropriate at a particular time, or further tests may need to be performed before proceeding. The American College of Sports Medicine has established three

FOCUS BOX 21.3

Benefits of Exercise in the Prevention and Treatment of Coronary Artery Disease

Maintain or Increase Myocardial Oxygen Supply

Delay progression of coronary artery disease (possible).

Improve lipoprotein profile (increase HDL-C/LDL-C ratio, decrease triglycerides) (probable).

Improve carbohydrate metabolism (increase insulin sensitivity) (probable).

Decrease platelet aggregation and increase fibrinolysis (probable).

Decrease adiposity (usually).

Increase coronary collateral vascularization (unlikely).

Increase epicardial artery diameter (possible).

Increase coronary blood flow (myocardial perfusion) or distribution (possible).

Decrease Myocardial Work and Oxygen Demand

Decrease heart rate at rest and submaximal exercise (usually).

Decrease systolic and mean systemic arterial pressure during submaximal exercise (usually) and at rest (usually).

Decrease cardiac output during submaximal exercise (probable).

Decrease circulating plasma catecholamine levels at rest (probable) and at submaximal exercise (usually).

Increase Myocardial Function

Increase stroke volume at rest and in submaximal and maximal exercise (likely).

Increase ejection fraction at rest and during exercise (likely).

Increase intrinsic myocardial contractility (possible).

Increase myocardial function resulting from decreased afterload (probable).

Increase myocardial hypertrophy (probable); but this may not reduce CHD risk.

Increase Electrical Stability of Myocardium

Decrease regional ischemia at submaximal exercise (possible).

Decrease catecholamines in myocardium at rest (possible) and at submaximal exercise (probable).

Increase ventricular fibrillation threshold due to reduction of cyclic AMP (possible).

---

categories of risk stratification (*apparently healthy, increased risk and known disease*) (23).

Individuals who fall into the apparently healthy category are at the least risk for problems during exercise. Routine testing for coronary artery disease in asymptomatic low-risk individuals remains controversial because of the limited ability to detect disease in this group. Individuals who are at increased risk have symptoms suggestive of possible cardiopulmonary or metabolic disease (such as chest pain, diabetes, etc.) and/or have two or more major coronary risk factors and thus are at greater risk during exercise. A physician may need to be present when testing high-risk individuals, depending on the medical history of the individual. Individuals with documented evidence of cardiovascular, pulmonary, or metabolic disease are at the greatest risk during exercise. A physician always needs to be present when testing an individual with known disease or is at high risk for heart disease.

Following hospital discharge, some patients who are low risk (no complications in hospital and have good functional capacity) may have home exercise prescribed. These patients would benefit by participating in a moderate exercise program at a fitness facility, in addition to the home exercise regime. Patients who, following hospital discharge, fall into higher-risk categories (complications in the hospital, a large MI, poor functional capacity < 4 METs) should be referred to a supervised cardiac rehabilitation program first. Once they complete the program and decrease their risk factor profile (table 21.2), they can begin exercise with less supervision.

Hypertension

Hypertension, or elevated blood pressure, is one of the most prevalent chronic diseases in the United States. Simply defined, hypertension is a chronically elevated blood pressure greater than 140/90 mmHg. More specifically, a person with hypertension is defined as having a blood pressure reading greater than 140/90 mmHg on two or more separate occasions, or currently taking antihypertensive medications (ACSM). As many as 50 million Americans have chronically elevated blood pressure, or are taking antihypertensive medication (NHANES III: The Fifth Report of the Joint National Committee on Detection, Evaluation, and Treatment of High Blood Pressure). Hypertension is related to the development of heart disease, increased severity of atherosclerosis, stroke, congestive heart failure, left ventricular hypertrophy, aortic aneurysms, and peripheral vascular disease.

The majority of individuals with high blood pressure are not on any therapy to control their blood pressure, and do not even know they have a problem. The cause of 90 to 95% of the cases of high blood pressure are not known, but once detected, can be controlled. Many of the risk factors for hypertension can be controlled. Hypertension is a serious medical

hypertension two or more high blood pressure readings > 140/90 mmHg, descriptive of need to take hypertensive medications

problem if left untreated. Hypertensive individuals have a 3 to 4 times risk of developing coronary artery disease, and up to 7 times the risk of having a stroke. Hypertension can be caused by several disease processes, with diseases of the kidney, inappropriately regulated blood vessels, and deterioration (hardening) of peripheral arteries (**arteriosclerosis**) being the major causes.

The detrimental effects of hypertension are on the heart and brain. The heart must work harder (by generating more pressure) to pump blood around the body. This increases the heart's demand for oxygen, can damage coronary blood vessels, and if atherosclerotic disease is present, will increase the likelihood for insufficient blood flow (ischemia), the onset of **angina,** and the occurrence of a myocardial infarction (MI). Hypertension can also escalate to values (especially during specific types and intensities of exercise) that increase the risk of damage to small blood vessels or cause blood clots to form, and if this occurs in the brain it can cause **stroke.**

Exercise can protect against and be an effective treatment for hypertension by increasing the number of capillaries in skeletal muscle and thereby lowering resistance to blood flow, improving the neural regulation of blood vessels, which will also reduce peripheral resistance, or reducing the work of the heart at rest and during exercise. In fact, a review of 33 studies involving exercise training and its effects on hypertension revealed that endurance training can cause a reduction of approximately 10 mmHg in both systolic and diastolic pressures (24). Similar results are also possible in individuals whose blood pressure is caused by renal disease.

Prolonged low-intensity (aerobic) exercise is therefore recommended as a nonpharmacological method for decreasing hypertension (ACSM).

The available evidence indicates that endurance exercise training by individuals at high risk for developing hypertension will reduce the rise in blood pressure that occurs with time. Thus, it is the position of the American College of Sports Medicine that endurance exercise training is recommended as a nonpharmacological strategy to reduce the incidence of hypertension in susceptible individuals. The exercise recommendations to achieve this effect are generally the same as those prescribed for developing and maintaining cardiovascular fitness in healthy adults. However, exercise training at somewhat lower intensities appears to lower blood pressure as much, or more, than exercise at higher intensities, which may be more important in specific hypertensive populations.

> —Adapted from the American College
> of Sports Medicine Position Stand
> on Physical Activity, Physical
> Fitness, and Hypertension

Resistance training for strength is potentially contraindicated because of the risk of alarmingly high increases in blood pressure during contractions. Use of resistance training with low-resistance settings, assuming correct breathing patterns, may provide benefit, especially for individuals who need to improve their abilities to perform activities of daily living. However, it should also be stated that severe hypertension does not appear to be reversible by exercise alone. In addition to regular aerobic exercise, the Joint National Committee on Detection, Evaluation, and Treatment of High Blood Pressure makes the following recommendations to lower and control blood pressure. (Also see focus box 21.4.)

Lose weight if overweight.
Limit alcohol intake to < 1 oz per day.
Reduce sodium intake to less than 2.3 g per day.
Stop smoking.
Reduce dietary fat, saturated fat, and cholesterol.
Maintain adequate dietary potassium, calcium, and magnesium intake.

Diabetes

Diabetes mellitus is a disease that results in the diminished capacity of the pancreas to secrete insulin in response to a given glucose stimulus, and/or the decreased capacity of cells to respond to insulin and increase glucose uptake. The net result of either condition is the same, that of an increased blood glucose concentration, a decreased ability to use glucose as a fuel, and subsequent alterations in the metabolism of carbohydrate, fat, and protein. The highly elevated blood glucose causes diabetics to be at increased risk for kidney failure, nerve damage, and eye problems and eventual blindness. The reduced ability to use glucose causes large increases in blood triacylglycerols, predisposes individuals to physical inactivity, and thereby increases risk for CHD.

There are four types of diabetes: insulin-dependent (IDDM), non-insulin-dependent (NIDDM), gestational (GDM), and impaired glucose tolerance (IGT). IDDM generally occurs in childhood and involves the destruction of the insulin secreting β cells of the pancreas. Consequently, IDDM requires regular injections of insulin along with a controlled diet to regulate blood glucose.

NIDDM is the most common form of diabetes, affecting 90% of the diabetic population. NIDDM predominantly (75%) occurs in overfat adults, and involves the reduced insulin-stimulated ability of cells to take up glucose from the blood, termed reduced *insulin sensitivity*. The connection between NIDDM and being overfat reveals the main aspects of treatment—diet and exercise to lower blood lipids, decrease body fat, improve cardiovascular function, and increase the ability of skeletal muscle to use glucose without the need of insulin. The key elements of the type of exercise training to be performed by individuals with NIDDM are therefore those specific to combating hypercholesterolemia, obesity, and CHD. The unique benefit of exercise training to individuals with NIDDM is its ability to allow skeletal muscle to take up glucose without the need for insulin. This response is localized to the muscles exercised, associated with

FOCUS BOX 21.4

Exercise Guidelines and Recommendations for Hypertension

1. Avoid holding breath and straining during exercise (Valsalva maneuver).
2. Weight training should be used as a supplement to endurance training, not as the primary exercise.
3. Exercise intensity may need to be monitored by the RPE (rate of perceived exertion) scale because medications can alter the accuracy of the training heart rate during exercise.
4. Individuals with hypertension should be instructed to move slowly when transitioning from the floor to standing because they are more susceptible to orthostatic hypotension if they are taking antihypertensive medication.
5. Both hypertensive and hypotensive responses are possible during and after exercise for individuals with hypertension.

6. Individuals with severe hypertension need to be carefully monitored during exercise initially, and possibly long term.

Exercise Mode

Endurance activities, such as walking, running, cycling, swimming, and so on.

Exercise Intensity

50 to 60% VO_{2max}, gradually increasing to 70 to 85% VO_{2max}.

Exercise Frequency

4 to 5 days/week.

Exercise Duration

20 to 30 min.

---

a given bout of exercise, and can be retained for extended periods of time if sufficient exercise training (duration and frequency) is performed (focus box 21.5).

Hypercholesterolemia

Hypercholesterolemia refers to a condition of above-normal concentrations of cholesterol in the blood. Blood cholesterol can be divided into *total* cholesterol, high-density lipoprotein (*HDL*) cholesterol, and low-density lipoprotein (*LDL*) cholesterol. Normal and abnormal concentrations of the blood cholesterols are provided in table 21.4. The general term used to describe an elevation in one or more of the blood lipids is *hyperlipidemia*.

Cross-sectional research data have indicated that a 1% decrease in total cholesterol is associated with a 2% reduction in risk for CHD. In addition, for each 1 mg/dL increase in HDL there is a 2 and 3% reduction in risk for CHD for men and women, respectively. The total cholesterol link to CHD is based on the availability of cholesterol for deposition in the process of atherosclerosis. Conversely, increased HDL cholesterol decreases CHD risk as the lipoprotein molecule responsible for HDL cholesterol removes excess cholesterol from blood vessels. This cholesterol is then recirculated to the liver where the cholesterol is removed from the blood and catabolized. Research from the Framingham study has shown that elevated blood triacylglycerides are an independent risk for CHD, presumably because of their incorporation into atherosclerotic plaques.

The evidence for the benefit of exercise and physical activity on blood lipid concentrations has been obtained from both cross-sectional and experimental (where exercise is controlled in the same subjects, or two groups of subjects) research. For example, physically active men and women have lower total cholesterol and total to HDL ratios than their sedentary counterparts (25). Similarly, individuals who increase their physical activity through endurance exercise training develop lower total and LDL blood cholesterol, and higher HDL cholesterol concentrations compared to control subjects (26). Research of blood cholesterol changes following resistance training has produced conflicting findings, and at this time no comment can be made for recommending resistance exercise as a means to normalize blood lipid profiles (27).

Peripheral Vascular Disease

Peripheral vascular disease is atherosclerosis that occurs in arteries of the peripheral vasculature. The associated reductions in the inner diameter of the arteries reduces blood flow and, during times of increased metabolic demand such as exercise, can cause leg pain (claudication) and severely compromised exercise tolerance. Endurance exercise training can be a preventive and rehabilitative strategy for peripheral vascular disease because of reductions in blood lipids and improved vascularization and endurance metabolic adaptations of muscle. A supervised exercise program has been shown to improve claudication and overall physical activity levels. Clinical studies have demonstrated improved: (1) treadmill time, (2) oxygen uptake, (3) improved physical functioning, and (4) level of activity.

arteriosclerosis (are tear ee oh' scler row' sis) deterioration (hardening) of peripheral arteries

angina chest pain caused by an imbalance between blood supply and demand to the heart

stroke reduced blood flow to the brain, resulting in permanent brain damage

FOCUS BOX 21.5

Exercise Guidelines for Individuals with Diabetes

Individuals with diabetes mellitus should participate in regular physical activity and preferably perform exercise training as described below.

- Do not inject insulin into the muscle groups to be exercised.
- Check blood glucose regularly.
- Always carry a rapid-acting (simple carbohydrate) food to correct hypoglycemia.
- Consume carbohydrate snacks during exercise. Take extra precautions to care for feet.

Exercise Mode

Endurance activities, such as walking, running, cycling, swimming, and so on.

Exercise Intensity

50 to 60% VO_{2max}, gradually increasing to 70% VO_{2max}.

Exercise Frequency

5 to 7 days/week (IDDM); 4 to 5 days/week (NIDDM).

Exercise Duration

20 to 30 min (IDDM); 40 to 60 min (NIDDM).

IDDM

General Exercise Recommendations for Type 1 Diabetes

Component	Recommendations
Type	Aerobic: walking, jogging, cycling, stair climbing, cross-country skiing, etc.
	Strength (moderate level resistance training): circuit programs using light weights with 10–15 repetitions
Intensity	60–90% maximum heart rate or 50–85% VO_{2max}
Duration	20–60 min plus 5–10 min warm up and cool-down period
Frequency	Daily in order to ensure optimal blood glucose control
Timing	The timing of exercise is particularly important for individuals with IDDM. Both insulin therapy and blood glucose level at the time of exercise need to be considered. Avoid exercise at time of peak insulin action.

NIDDM

General Exercise Recommendations for Type 2 Diabetes

Component	Recommendations
Type	Aerobic: walking, jogging, cycling, stair climbing, cross-country skiing, etc.
	Strength (moderate level resistance training): circuit programs using light weights with 10–15 repetitions
Intensity	60–90% maximum heart rate or 50–85% VO_{2max}
Duration	20–60 min plus 5–10 min warm up and cool-down period
Frequency	3–5 times per week; daily if on insulin therapy

TABLE 21.4

Normal and abnormal concentrations of blood cholesterols and triacylglycerol

BLOOD LIPID	CONCENTRATIONS
Total Cholesterol	
Desirable	< 200 mg/dL (mmol/L)
Borderline high	200–239 mg/dL (mmol/L)
High	> 240 mg/dL (mmol/L)
HDL Cholesterol	
Desirable	> 35 mg/dL (mmol/L)
Low	< 35 mg/dL (mmol/L)
LDL Cholesterol	
Optimal	< 100 mg/dL (mmol/L)
Desirable	< 130 mg/dL (mmol/L)
Borderline high	130–159 mg/dL (mmol/L)
High	> 160 mg/dL (mmol/L)
Triacylglycerols	
Desirable	< 200 mg/dL (mmol/L)
Borderline high	200–239 mg/dL (mmol/L)
High	> 240 mg/dL (mmol/L)

Osteoporosis

One of the most devastating diseases of the skeletal system that can be altered by physical activity is *osteoporosis*. Osteoporosis is characterized by a decrease in the bone mineral density of the skeleton, increasing risk for postural deformities and bone fractures. The incidence of osteoporosis is high, affecting approximately 20 million individuals in the United States, with an estimated medical cost of $3.8 billion/year (28). The development of osteoporosis can begin in childhood, where inadequate diet and physical inactivity can combine to prevent adequate bone mineral deposition. During adulthood, there is a gradual loss of bone mineral, and if insufficient bone mineral was there to begin with, an individual is at a tremendously increased risk for fractures later in life. In women, especially those in their teens and early adulthood, social and elite sporting pressures can cause the development of eating disorders, accompanied by the loss of the menstrual cycle that can further increase risk for osteoporosis. The loss of the menstrual cycle (amenorrhea) prevents the body from synthesizing estrogen, which has a protective effect on bone mineral in the female. The combination of diet, endocrinology, and exercise has been termed the *female athletic triad*. The role of estrogen in this triad also makes the postmenopausal female at increased risk for osteoporosis, and partly explains the importance of estrogen replacement therapy for both young (exercise-induced amenorrhea) and elderly (postmenopausal) women.

Assuming a normal diet and, for women, a functional menstrual cycle, both men and women can decrease the rate of bone mineral loss as they age by exercise training and regular physical activity. Greater bone mineral retention occurs when the exercise is weight-bearing (walking, running, roller blading, etc.) versus weight-supported exercise (cycling, swimming, etc.). The goal of exercise in the prevention and treatment of osteoporosis is to (1) increase bone mass during growth years, (2) maintain bone mass or decrease rate of bone loss in adulthood, and (3) decrease the rate/risk of falls in the elderly.

WEBSITE BOX

Chapter 21: Exercise, Weight Control, Health, and Disease

The newest information regarding exercise physiology can be viewed at the following sites.*

arfa.org/index.htm
> Excellent site providing comprehensive information on many topics within exercise physiology.

http://fitnesslink.com/nutri.htm
> Information-packed site on exercise and the mind and body, nutrition, fitness programs, hot to train, and more.

curtin.edu.au/curtin/dept/physio/pt/edres/exphys/e552_96/
> Index of brief reviews of exercise physiology by students from Curtin University, Australia. Topics include nutrition,

ergogenic aids, environmental physiology, training, and clinical applications.

mediconsult.com/
> Information source for any medical condition, including exercise and hypertension, heart disease, diabetes, etc.

---

*Unless indicated, all URLs preceded by http://www.

Note: These URLs were valid at the time of publication, but could have changed or been deleted from Internet access since that time.

SUMMARY

- The connections between regular exercise/physical activity and health were not always as obvious as they are today. During the two decades from 1980 to the present, the evidence for how exercise can not only prevent disease, but also reverse many disease processes has accumulated to such a degree that now almost all medical organizations have published statements on the importance of exercise in the prevention and treatment of their diseases of interest.

- One of the first studies on the association between exercise and cardiovascular disease was conducted in England during the 1950s. This study found that bus conductors were more physically fit than the drivers, and had a lower incidence of coronary heart disease (CHD), with reduced death (**mortality**) and early mortality from CHD.

- Hundreds of studies have provided evidence of an association between exercise and health. Such research is called cross-sectional research, and when applied to the study of health it is termed **epidemiology.** No details of why a proposed association exists can be drawn from epidemiology research and, because of the nature of the research, the interpretation of cause and effect between exercise and prevention of CHD is not automatic.

- Health can be defined in a variety of ways. The World Health Organization defines health as "A state of complete physical, mental, and social well-being and not merely the absence of disease or infirmity." Today, many consider the term wellness a better measure of overall health and well-being. Wellness is defined as an approach to personal health that emphasizes individual responsibility for well-being through the practice of health-promoting behaviors.

- Physical inactivity has been identified as a serious problem in the United States. It has been estimated that as many as 60% of adults do not achieve the recommended amount of regular physical activity needed to improve and maintain one's health.

- Physical fitness is defined as the ability of the body's systems (heart, lungs, blood vessels, and muscles) to function efficiently, as to resist disease and to be able to participate in a variety of activities without undue fatigue.

- The five components of health-related physical fitness are muscular strength, muscular endurance, cardiorespiratory endurance, flexibility and body composition. A comprehensive fitness program should have activities which develop and maintain each of the five components.

SUMMARY

- The American College of Sports Medicine, in conjunction with the Centers for Disease Control and Prevention (CDC) and the President's Council on Physical Fitness and Sports have issued a position stand for the recommendation on increased physical activity for Americans. It encourages Americans to regular physical activity everyday.

- Obesity is perhaps the most prevalent chronic health problem in the United States today. As many as 33% of the population is overweight (above their desired weight). Excess weight is a serious medical, health and social issue.

- The National Center for Health Statistics has defined someone as being **overweight** if they have a BMI of 27.8 or more for men and 27.3 or more for women. A normal **BMI** has been classified as 20.0 for men and 25.0 for women.

- Obesity literally means "excess fat." **Obesity** refers to excess body fat, versus body weight. An ideal body fat percentage for good health is between 10 to 15% for young men and between 20 to 25% for young women. Body fat percentages greater than 20% for men or 30% for women is considered an indication of obesity.

- In general, women tend to store fat in the lower half of the body around the hip and thigh area (*gynoid obesity*), whereas men tend to store fat on the upper part of the body around the abdominal area (*android obesity*). Android obesity compared to gynoid obesity is associated with greater risk of developing diabetes, hypertension, heart disease (15).

- In order to maintain ideal body weight, energy consumed (food consumed daily) needs to equal energy output (daily physical activity habits). When these are equal, one is said to be in energy balance. The safe recommended weight loss per week is 2.2 lb. Exercise appears to play a critical role in the loss and maintenance of body weight.

- Cardiovascular disease continues to be the leading cause of death in the Western world. More than two of every five Americans die of cardiovascular disease. Exercise plays an important role in preventing heart disease, as well as in the rehabilitation of individuals with heart disease.

- There are several different types of cardiovascular disease, including coronary artery disease (CAD), peripheral vascular disease (PVD), and congestive heart failure (CHF). CAD can cause impaired heart function, and eventually heart attack (**myocardial infarction**). PVD can cause pain in the peripheral musculature (**claudication**) during even mild physical activity. CHF is characterized by a progressive deterioration of the function of the heart muscle (myocardium), resulting in poor exercise toler-

ance, and impaired lung function because of a worsening accumulation of fluid in the lung (**pulmonary edema**).

- The major **risk factors** for coronary heart disease— hypertension, smoking, high cholesterol—are all positively affected by exercise. Furthermore, physical inactivity is now recognized as a major contributor to the atherosclerotic process.

- The Clinical Practice Guideline, *Cardiac Rehabilitation*, was developed under the direction of the Agency for Health Care Policy and Research and the National Heart, Lung and Blood Institute of the U.S. Department of Health and Human Services. It provides broad recommendations, on the basis of the evaluation of the scientific evidence pertaining to the various components of cardiac rehabilitation.

- In essence, risk stratification before exercise testing or training is one tool that helps establish whether or not *the benefits outweigh the potential risks!* The American College of Sports Medicine has established three categories of risk stratification (*apparently healthy, increased risk, and known disease*).

- Hypertension, or elevated blood pressure, is one of the most prevalent chronic diseases in the United States. **Hypertension** is defined as a chronically elevated blood pressure greater than 140/90 mmHg. Hypertension can be caused by several disease processes, with diseases of the kidney, inappropriately regulated blood vessels, and deterioration (hardening) of peripheral arteries (**arteriosclerosis**) being the major causes.

- Detrimental effects of hypertension to the heart include ischemia, the onset of **angina,** and myocardial infarction (MI). Damage to the brain can result in **stroke.**

- Exercise can protect against and be an effective treatment for hypertension by either increasing the number of capillaries in skeletal muscle and thereby lowering resistance to blood flow, improving the neural regulation of blood vessels, which will also reduce peripheral resistance, or reducing the work of the heart at rest and during exercise.

- Diabetes mellitus is a disease that results from the diminished capacity of the pancreas to secrete insulin in response to a given glucose stimulus, and/or the decreased capacity of cells to respond to insulin and increase glucose uptake. NIDDM is the most common form of diabetes, affecting 90% of the diabetic population. The connection between NIDDM and being overfat reveals the main aspects of treatment—diet and exercise to lower blood lipids, decrease body fat, improve cardiovascular function, and increase the ability of skeletal muscle to use glucose without the need of insulin.

- *Hypercholesterolemia* refers to a condition of above-normal concentrations of cholesterol in the blood. Research from the Framingham study has shown that elevated blood triacylglycerides are an independent risk for CHD, presumably because of their incorporation into atherosclerotic plaques. The evidence for the benefit of exercise and physical activity on blood lipid concentrations has been obtained from both cross-sectional and experimental (where exercise is controlled in the same subjects, or two groups of subjects) research.

▪ Peripheral vascular disease is **atherosclerosis** that occurs in arteries of the peripheral vasculature. Clinical studies have demonstrated improved (1) treadmill time, (2) oxygen uptake, (3) improved physical functioning, and (4) level of habitual physical activity.

▪ *Osteoporosis* is characterized by a decrease in the bone mineral density of the skeleton, increasing risk for postural deformities and bone fractures. Greater bone mineral retention occurs when the exercise is weight-bearing (walking, running, roller blading, etc.) versus weight-supported exercise (cycling, swimming, etc.).

STUDY QUESTIONS

1. What are primary and secondary risk factors for exercise?

2. How does exercise reduce the risk for developing certain diseases? Do we know for a fact that exercise is responsible for these reductions?

3. Why is physical inactivity recognized as a primary public health problem in the United States today?

4. What kind of global exercise recommendations are being promoted for all Americans?

APPLICATIONS

1. What obstacles do severely obese individuals face in exercising? How would these obstacles influence their motivation to exercise?

2. What are the health risks of exercise for severely obese individuals?

REFERENCES

1. Berryman, J. W., *Out of Many, One: A history of the American College of Sports Medicine*, Human Kinetics, 1995.

2. Massengale, J. D. and R. A. Swanson. *The history of exercise and Sport Science Human Kinetic*s, 1996.

3. Morris, J. N., et al. Coronary heart disease and physical activity of work. *Lancet* 2:1053–1057, 1111–1210, 1953.

4. Morris, J. N., et al. Vigorous exercise in leisure-time and the incidence of coronary heart disease. *Lancet* 1:333–339, 1973.

5. Paffenbarger, R. S., et al. Characteristics of longshoremen related to fatal coronary heart disease and stroke. *Am. J. Public Health.* 61:1362–1370, 1971.

5a. Paffenbarger, R. S., and A. L. Wing. Chronic disease in former college students: XVI. Physical activity as an index of heart attack risk in college alumni. *Am. J. Epidemiol.* 108:161–175, 1978.

6. Storlie, J., and H. A. Jordan (eds.). *Nutrition and exercise in obesity management. LaCrosse Health and Sports Science Symposium.* SP Medical and Science Books, New York, 1984.

7. Najjar, M. F., and M. Rowland. *Anthropometric reference data and prevalence of overweight, United States, 1976–80 Vital and health statistics.* Series 11, No. 238. DHHS Pub. No. (PHS) 87–1688. Public Health Service, U.S. Government Printing Office, Washington, DC, October 1987.

8. Department of Health and Human Consensus Conference on Obesity, April 1, 1992.

9. Welham, W. C., and A. R. Behnke. The specific gravity of healthy men: Body weight divided by volume and other physical characteristics of exceptional athletes and of naval personnel. *JAMA* 118:498–501, 1942

10. Xavier Pi-Sunyer, F. Medical hazards of obesity. *An. Int. Med.* 119(7):655–660, 1993.

11. National Instiues of Health Consensus Development Conference Statement. *Health implications of obesity.* 1985.

12. Hubert, H. B., et al. Obesity as an independent risk factor for cardiovascular disease: 26-year follow-up of participants in the Framingham Study. *Circulation* 67:968–977, 1983.

13. Kannel, W. B., N. Brand, J. J. Skinner, T. R. Dawber, and P. M. McNamara. The relation of adiposity to blood pressure and development of hypertension. The Framingham Study. *An. Int. Med.* 67:48–59, 1967.

14. MacMahon, S. W., R. B. Blacket, G. J. Macdonald, and W. Hall. Obesity, alcohol consumption and blood pressure in Australian men and women. The National Heart Foundation of Australia Risk Factor Prevalence Study. *J. Hyperten.* 2:85–91, 1984.

REFERENCES

15. Ducimetiere, P., and J. L. Richard. The relationship between subsets of anthropometric upper versus lower body measurements and coronary heart disease risk in middle-aged men. The Paris Prospective Study. *Int. J. Obesity* 13:111–112, 1989.

16. Stephenson, M. G., A. S. Levy, N. L. Sass, and W. E. McGarvey. 1985 NHIS findings: Nutrition knowledge and baseline data for the weight-loss objectives. *Public Health Reports* 102:61–67, 1987.

17. Svendson, O., et al. Effect of an energy restrictive diet, with and without exercise, on lean tissue mass, resting metabolic rate, cardiovascular risk factors, and bone in overweight postmenopasual women. *Am. J. Med.* 95:131, 1993.

18. Kayman, S., W. Bruvold, and J. Stern. Maintenance and relapse after weight loss in women: Behavioral aspects. *Am. J. Clin. Nutr.* 52:800, 1990.

19. Brownell, K. D., and C. M. Grilo. Weight management. In J. L. Durstine, et al. (eds), *American College of Sports Medicine's resource manual for guidelines for exercise testing and prescription,* 2nd ed. Lea & Febiger, Philadelphia, 1993, pp. 455–460.

20. American Heart Association. *1998 Heart and stroke facts statistics.* American Heart Association, Dallas, 1998.

21. Dawber, T. R., G. F. Meadors, and F. E. Moore. Epidemiological approaches to heart disease: The Framingham study. *A. J. Public Health* 41:279–286, 1951.

22. Blair, S. N., H. W. Kohl, R. S. Pafffenbarger, D. G. Clark, K. H. Cooper, and L. W. Gibbons. Physical fitness and all-causes mortality: A prospective study of healthy men and women. *JAMA* 262:2395, 1989.

23. Kenney, W. L. *ACSM's Guidelines for exercise testing and prescription,* 5th ed. Williams & Wilkins, Philadelphia, 1995.

24. Hagberg, J. M. Exercise, fitness, and hypertenstion. In, C. Bouchard, R. J. Shepard, T. Stephens, J. R. Sutton, and B. D. McPherson (eds.), *Exercise, fitness and health: A consensus of current knowledge.* Human Kinetics, Champaign, IL, pp. 455–466, 1991.

25. Despres, J. P. and A. Marette. Relation of components of insulin resistance syndrome to coronary disease risk. *Curr Opin, Lipidol.* 5(4):274–289, 1994.

26. Hardman, A. E. Physical activity, obesity and blood lipids. *Int. J. Obes. Metab. Disord.* 23(Suppl.3):S64–71, 1999.

27. McCartney, N. The role of resistance training in patients with cardiac disease. *J. Cardiovasc. Risk* 3(2):160–166, 1996.

28. Christiansen, C. Consensus Development Conference on Osteoporosis. *Am. J. Med.* 95:5A, 1993.

RECOMMENDED READINGS

Stefanick, M. L. Exercise and weight control. In J. Holloszy (ed.), *Exercise and sport sciences reviews: Vol. 21.* Williams & Wilkins, Philadelphia, 1993, pp. 363–398.

American College of Sports Medicine. *Exercise management for persons with chronic diseases and disabilities.* Human Kinetics, Champaign, IL, 1997.

Haskell, W. L., et al. Effects of intensive risk factor reduction on coronary atherosclerosis and clinical events in men and women with coronary artery disease. *Circulation* 89:975–990, 1994.

Kenney, W. L. *ACSM's guidelines for exercise testing and prescription,* 5th ed. Williams & Wilkins, Philadelphia, 1995.

Lilly, L. S., *Pathophysiology of heart disease,* 2nd ed. Williams & Wilkins, Philadelphia, 1998.

Watson, R. R., and M. Eisinger (eds.). *Exercise and disease.* CRC Press, Boca Raton, FL, 1992.

Professional Issues in Career Opportunities

This appendix is not written to "sugar coat" the discipline and profession of exercise physiology. We write the following material with honesty, integrity, and a conviction that as exercise physiologists we are an important component of the increasing societal need to be more physically active. After all, most of the research on exercise and health has been completed by exercise physiologists within university programs that offer physical education or exercise science degrees. However, as will be revealed in the sections to follow, exercise physiology and exercise physiologists have a long way to go before attaining the academic and professional respect they deserve.

We encourage you to read this appendix with the thought that efforts are underway to make a profession in exercise physiology a reality in the near future. If you are motivated by the need to know more about how the body responds to exercise stress, and have an insatiable desire to eventually be in command of this body of knowledge, then we urge you to follow your dreams. It is people like you, who desire to be an exercise physiologist, that will help make the progress of professionalization evolve more rapidly and correctly.

Historical Development

Exercise physiology has a long history that can be dated back to the nineteenth century. The knowledge that exercise is beneficial for health and well-being was documented at a similar time. The historical development of the exercise sciences, especially exercise physiology, has been well reviewed and presented in textbook form, as was discussed in chapter 1. *Any student of exercise physiology who wishes to become an exercise physiologist should read about the historical development of exercise physiology.*

Since 1950, the discipline of exercise physiology was developed within curricula of physical education programs in countries such as the United States, Sweden, Australia, Great Britain, and Canada. The early connection between exercise physiology and sports/athletics can be seen in the content of many of the exercise physiology textbooks from this era. However, several innovative cardiologists and prominent physical educators came together in 1954 with the common recognition that exercise had tremendous potential for use in medical fields to aid in the prevention, treatment, diagnosis, and rehabilitation of several diseases (most notably heart disease). These individuals formed the American College of Sports Medicine (ACSM) with the initial mission to act as a forum for individuals from all professions who had an interest in exercise and the human body. This forum would stimulate and support increased knowledge of how exercise influenced the human body.

The development of ACSM was both positive and negative to the professional development of exercise science and exercise physiology in particular. For example, although ACSM gave all exercise scientists a public forum to express their knowledge and research, it resulted in exercise scientists forming the nucleus of ACSM and neglecting the professional needs of their own discipline and students. The strong involvement of exercise physiologists in ACSM was inevitable given the importance of exercise physiology to the mission of understanding the physiological responses of the body to different exercise stresses. What has resulted from this has been the professional development of other disciplines within sports medicine, such as physical therapy, athletic training, nutrition/dietetics, and so forth. These professions are self-governing with academic program accreditation, certification and licensure, medical recognition in the health care industry, and in certain circumstances insurance coverage for their functions in clinical practice. In the meantime, exercise physiologists have remained unfocused, until recently, on what they need as professionals and how they should act to support the academic programs in exercise physiology and all the graduates of exercise science programs who call themselves exercise physiologists.

As ACSM grew in size and importance during the 1970s and 1980s, and the profession of exercise physiology remained stagnant, the discipline of exercise physiology expanded tremendously. Many university programs recognized the growth of the sciences devoted to a better understanding of sports and athletic performance, and departments and even colleges were developed that specifically focused on the sciences of human movement. Many programs and departments still have names that reflect human movement, kinesiology, sports sciences, human bioenergetics, exercise technology, and exercise science. However, the application of exercise physiology to sports and athletics was not the only purpose of exercise physiology classes. With the growing recognition of the importance of exercise and physical activity to optimal health and well-being during the 1980s, the study of exercise was becoming equally recognized for understanding how exercise and physical activity combated ill health and several disease processes. Exercise physiology therefore became a course not only for physical educators, athletic trainers, and coaches, but also for health professionals who could benefit patients by prescribing regular physical activity. The students of exercise physiology therefore also included students of medicine, physical therapy, nursing, and health promotion, to name just a few.

This transition in students exposed to exercise physiology has been superficially flattering to the discipline, but devastating to the profession of exercise physiology. Without any professional body to protect the discipline and graduates of exercise physiology/science programs, other more developed professions have started to grasp onto the knowledge base of exercise physiology and nurture the incorporation of exercise physiology into their professional duties. The result of this has been the existence of a work environment where Ph.D.-trained exercise physiologists lecture to physical therapy, nursing, medical, and nutrition students. Exercise physiologists are then told by representatives of these fields that their members are the individuals who should act and function as exercise physiologists in the clinical setting.

Despite the development of this professional scenario, recent trends in the professionalization of exercise physiology are underway to correct these errors. Depending on the country in which you live (see appendix B for Internet-based organizations), there may be no organization for any exercise science discipline or organizations may be young and developing. Ironically, it seems that compared to the other major countries that have advanced university degrees in the exercise sciences, the United States is the most disorganized country when it comes to the professional needs of exercise science undergraduate and graduate majors. The end result is that no matter where you live in the world, there is no international consensus on what is exercise science or what is exercise physiology. There is no international effort in progress that will standardize educational requirements for an exercise science degree. However, in Canada (Canadian Society of Exercise Physiologists—CSEP) and the United States (American Society of Exercise Physiologists—ASEP) there are organizations that have recently been formed to standardize educational requirements of exercise physiologists and promote the employment of exercise physiologists.

The result of this chaos in the professional status of exercise science and exercise physiology is that there is limited professional effort to promote employment and employment conditions for graduates of exercise science and exercise physiology programs. When a student is focused on exercise physiology, this is a major concern. The medical disciplines (cardiology, pulmonology, endocrinology, orthopedics, etc.) have their own professional organizations, and the allied health professions also provide professional support to their members (e.g., nutrition/dietetics, physical therapy, nursing). Most of this support occurs in the political arena, where employment conditions are nurtured through lobbying for state funding and insurance coverage. Ironically, even though an undergraduate-trained exercise physiologist is better trained to conduct exercise tests and prescribe exercise training to healthy and diseased individuals, they may be less likely to do so in the future. This is because dieticians, nurses, and physical therapists are currently arguing that they are the most suited to conduct such tests because they are currently recognized clinically, and exercise physiologists are not.

This current educational and professional environment makes a graduate from exercise science or exercise physiology wonder what his or her degree is worth today, and tomorrow! Well, if current trends continue in the future, an exercise science degree may only enable you to be employed in the fitness industry, or to market yourself privately as an exercise specialist. However, problems still exist because your exercise physiology degree is not recognized professionally, and there is no professional organization protecting and publicizing the quality of your qualifications; therefore what is to stop any person from calling himself or herself an exercise physiologist? The result would be competition for your future employment from people who may not have invested the time and money to develop academic and skill competencies. The end result is still fewer job opportunities.

Despite the gray overtones of the previous paragraphs, efforts are underway to change the future of exercise physiology, at least in the United States. These changes may spread to other countries. As of March 1997, the foundation of the American Society of Exercise Physiologists (ASEP) has resulted in work on the development of standards for academic programs, as well as standards for academic and skill competencies of exercise physiologists. By the year 2000, university professors of academic programs in exercise science will be able to have their programs accredited as ASEP certified programs. In addition, graduates (undergraduate, M.S., Ph.D.) of these and programs yet to be accredited will have the choice to become certified as exercise physiologists with ASEP.

Internet Homepages Pertinent to Exercise Physiology

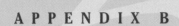

The increasing popularity of disseminating and retrieving information via the World Wide Web (www) of the Internet has revolutionized the social as well as pure sciences. Searching for documents and topical information on the Internet has been described as "surfing." When "surfing the Net," many sites can be found that pertain to exercise physiology and related topics, hence this appendix. The purpose of this appendix is to provide a list of Internet addresses with summaries of what the site can provide the student of exercise physiology, as well as the exercise physiology professional. However, to begin with, a brief introduction to the Internet is provided for the student who has yet to become aware of this method of information dissemination and retrieval.

Because this appendix provides information about the Internet, we have provided information for this and other sections solely from information obtained from the resources on the Internet listed in the references. Many of these resources are also listed in table B.1.

What Is the Internet?

History

The Internet began more than 30 years ago as a vast international network of computers used by scientists and technical researchers. The initial computer language that operated the Internet was complex, and prevented the wide-scale use of the Internet by individuals who did not have the educational training, time, and resources to send and receive information. However, in 1990 two physics researchers at the European Particle Physics Laboratory (CERN), Tim Berners-Lee and Robert Cailliau, developed a computer language and format that could interface the Internet to any computer, anywhere in the world (5).

The next major development of the Internet came after the formulation of computer software that enabled individuals to easily send or retrieve information from the Internet. From 1993 to 1994, the number of sites on the www increased from 130 to 2738 (1–5). Today the number of sites is estimated at 2,215,195 (fig. B.1) (1). Businesses, laboratories, schools, universities, government divisions and services, and private citizens are a few examples of all who can have heir own separate sites (called a web page or homepage) to express whatever information they want. New Internet-based services have been developed (software, web page design, Internet-based sales and registration, etc.) and future applications of the Internet are evolving rapidly every day. Interestingly, the growth of the number of computers that can access the Internet (hosts) is increasing more rapidly than the number of websites (fig. B.1). Comparison of the increases in hosts versus websites indicates that at present there is a greater demand for access to the World Wide Web than for its use to present information.

Structure and Components

Given the enormous potential of the Internet, it is important that one understands how it is structured to work prior to using it.

TABLE B.1		
Resources on the Internet that provide information on what the Internet is and how to use it best		
NAME	**ADDRESS**	**DESCRIPTION**
All about the Internet	http://info.isoc.org/internet	Site of the Internet Society, providing explanations of the Internet and data of the past, present, and forecast future use of the Internet.
An overview of the World Wide Web	http://shell.rmi.net/~kgr/internet	Provides written explanations, presented as separate documents, of specific aspects of using the Internet.
The Internet index	openmarket.com/intindex/	Provides statistics of all aspects of Internet function and use.
Understanding and using the Internet	pbs.org/uti/	A thorough written and pictorial presentation of all features that pertain to the Internet. Excellent!

*Unless the address begins with "http," first type "http://www." followed by the listed address.

FIGURE B.1

Comparison of the growth among websites and computer hosts. Interestingly, the number of computers that can access the Internet has increased more rapidly than the number of websites.

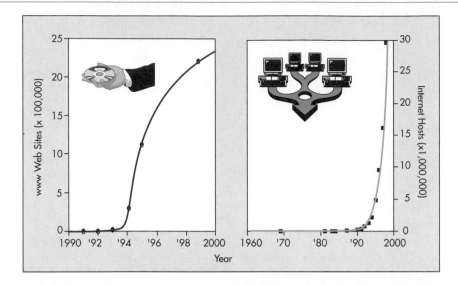

TABLE B.2

Glossary of terms and definitions about the Internet, listed alphabetically

TERM	DEFINITION
ASCII	"American standard code for information exchange," a worldwide standard for the 128 code numbers (consisting of 7 digit binary, 0000000 through 1111111) used by computers to represent all the upper- and lowercase Latin letters, numbers, punctuation, etc.
Bandwidth	How much computer information, usually measured in bits/s, that can be sent through a computer connection. A full page of English text approximates 15,000 bits.
Baud	The number of bits/s that can be sent or received. Usually pertains to an external device such as a modem or printer.
Bit	The smallest unit of computerized data, represented by a single digit binary number (0 or 1).
Bps	Bits/s.
Browser	A type of *client* program located on a computer that is used to look at Internet resources.
Byte	A set of bits that represents a single character.
Client	A software program that is used to contact and retrieve information from a *server* program on another computer. A web browser is a type of client program.
Cyberspace	Currently used to describe the range of information available through computer *networks*.
E-mail	"Electronic mail" that is sent, usually in text, from one person to another.
Ethernet	A common method of networking computers into a local area *network* (LAN).
FTP	"File transfer protocol," a common method of moving files between two *Internet* sites. FTP differs from *E-mail* in that the format of the original document remains intact, and complex documents such as figures can be transferred.
GIF	"Graphic interchange format," a common format for transferring image files between servers or other software.
Gopher	A *client-* and *server*-type program that has been largely surpassed by the *hypertext* of the *World Wide Web*.
Hit	A single request from a web *browser* for a single item.
Homepage	The *web page* that is first retrieved by a *browser*. The homepage is like a combined cover and contents page of a book because it directs the user to other pages of information connected to the *homepage*.
Host	Any computer or *network* that is a site for services available to other computers on the *network*.
HTML	"Hypertext markup language," the coding language used to create *hypertext* documents for use on the *World Wide Web*. HTML files are designed to be viewed using a *World Wide Web client* program such as Netscape or Mosaic.
HTTP	"Hypertext transport protocol," the protocol for moving hypertext files across the *Internet*.
Hypertext	Any text that contains links (words or phrases) to other documents.
Internet	The vast collection of interconnected computer *networks* that use the *TCP/IP* protocols.
IP Number	"Internet protocol number," a unique number consisting of four parts separated by dots that is given to every computer on the *Internet* (e.g., 165.113.245.2).

The Internet is structured by literally thousands of computers (called hosts) that can be connected to send and receive information. As previously identified, the sites within computers are termed *websites* or *homepages* (table B.2). Web pages are located on host computers that allow access to the Internet, and the specific software programs that can connect a computer to the Internet have been termed *servers*. An Internet server can be located on any computer, assuming basic memory and processing speed requirements. Nevertheless, organizations usually have selected computers that function solely to provide 24 h/day access to the Internet.

The program that is run on a computer to access and display information on a web page is termed a *browser*. There are many types of browsers, with Netscape and Mosaic the more popular examples. Access to the website is provided by the website address. The address is referred to as a "uniform resource locator" or *URL* (table B.2). Examples of URLs can be found in tables B.1, B.3, and B.4.

Basic Functions

Because of the modern marvels of computer programming, the Internet functions like an electronic yellow pages directory. However, unlike having to lookup a business or organization and then make a call during working hours, the Internet enables you to communicate with a target entity at any time, send and retrieve information (text and figures), and even arrange purchases or book reservations. All these functions can be conducted in the privacy of your own home or office.

For the scientist, the Internet is analogous to a book where the references are stated and allow you to access them electronically to observe the original sources. Thus the impact of the Internet on science is still in its infancy. Imagine being able to research the publications for your next term paper right from your own home, with no need to take the time to search the shelves of the library, invest your time and money on photocopying, and then have to organize where you store your articles. The world of scientific information retrieval is

TABLE B.2	
Glossary of terms and definitions about the Internet, listed alphabetically	
TERM	**DEFINITION**
ISP	"Internet service provider," an institution that provides access to the *Internet,* usually for money (e.g., America Online, Earthlink).
Java	A network-oriented programming language that was designed to safely download programs from the *Internet* to your computer.
JPEG	"Joint photographic experts group," the most commonly used image format for exporting photographic images.
Login	The account name used to access a computer system.
Modem	A device that connects a phone line to a computer so that computers can connect to one another to send and retrieve information.
Mosaic	The first *browser* of the *World Wide Web.* The code of Mosaic has been licensed by other, now more popular, browsers such as *Netscape.*
Netscape	A *browser* of the *World Wide Web,* and the name of a company.
Network	Two or more computers connected together.
Node	A single computer connected to a *network.*
Password	A code used to gain access to a locked system.
PPP	"Point to point protocol," allows a computer to use a regular telephone line and a modem to make a *TCP/IP* connection and thus be on the *Internet.*
Server	A computer or software package that provides service to *client* software running on other computers. A single computer could be running several different types of *server* software, which is the reason why a *server* is not necessarily just a computer.
TCP/IP	"Transmission control protocol/Internet protocol," a collection of protocols that defines the *Internet.* To be on the *Internet* a computer must have TCP/IP software.
Telnet	The command and program used to *login* from one *Internet* site to another.
Terminal	A device that enables you to send commands to a computer in another location.
UNIX	The most common operating system for servers on the *Internet.* UNIX is designed to be multiuser, and has *TC/IP* built in.
URL	"Uniform resource locator," the standard format for addresses of any resource on the *Internet,* such as a *homepage.* The URL is usually given through a *browser* and typically takes the form of http://www.pbs.com/.
	The "com" extension refers to a company. Other extensions are, "org," which refers to an organization, "edu," which refers to an educational institution, and so on. Codes for countries other than the United States also exist in a URL, such as "au" for Australia and "ca" for Canada.

TABLE B.3

Internet homepages that are pertinent to exercise physiology

DISCIPLINE/ PROFESSION	NAME	ADDRESS*	DESCRIPTION
Biomechanics	Ariel's Cybersport Quarterly	sportscience.org/	Monthly electronic magazine presenting the latest on the electronic analysis of sport biomechanics, especially those of elite athletes.
	Biomechanics World Wide	per.ualberta.ca/biomechanics/ bwwframe.htm	Comprehensive site that provides links to the individual homepages of the world concerned with any aspect of biomechanics. In addition, other services are offered which include links to journals, career opportunities, and applications issues such as sport and exercise, motor control, prosthetics.
Exercise physiology	Exercise Physiology Digital Image Archive	abacon.com/dia/exphys/ home.html	12 excellent quality diagrams can be downloaded free into PowerPoint to use as overhead transparencies or slides (PC and Mac format available).
	Exercise Physiology Links	http://wso.williams.edu/ ~sbennett/exer.html	Provides links for topics such as muscle physiology, fitness, and training.
	The Exercise and Physical Fitness Page	gsu.edu/~wwwfit/	Service page of the Department of Kinesiology and Health of Georgia State University. Provides information on main topics in exercise physiology such as how to train specific components of fitness, understanding body composition, how to use exercise to decrease body fat, etc.
	Masters Athlete Physiology & Performance	kis.hia.no/~stephens/index. html	High-content site dedicated to examining and explaining the physiology and training methods of age group sport and endurance athletes. Contains both pure and applied exercise physiology material.
	Copenhagen Muscle Research Center	nmr.imbg.ku.dk:80/cmrc/	Research site examining many issues that concern oxygen transport to and utilization by contracting skeletal muscle.
	Team Oregon	TeamOregon.com/publications/ marathon/	Comprehensive advice and assistance for marathon training.
Exercise and sport science	Sportscience	sportsci.org/	Probably the most developed and professionally complete Internet site for exercise science issues. The services provided by this site are too numerous to mention. You must check this one out!
Kinesiology	Kinesiology World Wide	umich.edu/~divkines/ kinesworld/complete.html	Provides a complete list of links to kinesiology homepages within the United States, Australia, Canada, Europe, and New Zealand.
	Muscles in Action	med.umich.edu/lrc/Hypermuscle/ Hyper.html	A multimedia interactive site devised to assist students in learning the muscles and actions of the human body.
Nutrition	Nutribase	nutribase.com	An interactive on-line nutrient database, as well as assistance in calculating weight loss, caloric requirements, and tips for dieters.
	Arbor Nutrition Guide	arborcom.com/	Extensive site for obtaining almost anything there is to know about nutrition. You can search within the site, or specifically view contents organized within applied, clinical food and food science divisions.

*Unless the address begins with "http," first type "http://www." followed by the listed address.

†Those concerned with published research databases.

TABLE B.3

Internet homepages that are pertinent to exercise physiology

DISCIPLINE/ PROFESSION	NAME	ADDRESS*	DESCRIPTION
Organizations/ institutions	American College of Sports Medicine (ACSM)	acsm.org	Presents information of the functions and services of ACSM.
	American Society of Exercise Physiologists (ASEP)	css.edu/users/tboone2/asep/ toc.htm	Extensive site devoted to the research and professional needs of exercise physiologists. Contains a newsletter, forum, research journal, information on professionalization, and many links.
	Australian Association for Exercise and Sport Sciences (AAESS)	nor.com.au/business/aaess/ home.htm	Caters to the need to identify, develop, and secure prospective career paths in the exercise sciences.
	Canadian Society for Exercise Physiology (CSEP)	csep.ca/	Developed to promote the generation, synthesis, transfer, and application of knowledge and research related to exercise physiology.
	Gatorade Sports Science Institute (GSSI)	gssiweb.com/site.html	Provides on-line free membership and access to information, services, and commercial products. Items include a reference library, expert summaries on specific topics, information for coaches, newsletter, and publications.
	International Federation of Sports Medicine (FIMS)	fims.org/	Unifies the sports medicine organizations of the world into a collective body for the purpose of promoting the study and development of sports medicine throughout the world.
	American Association for Active Lifestyles and Fitness (AAALF)	aahperd.org/aaalf/aaalf.html	Promotes active lifestyles and fitness through support of research, dissemination of information, networking, and professional development of fitness professionals.
	American Association of Cardiovascular and Pulmonary Rehabillitation (AACVPR)	http://128.220.112.180/aacvppr /aacvpr.html	Professional organization that functions to serve the needs of all professionals in cardiovascular and pulmonary rehabilitation. Provides free access to publications, guidelines, material, and images for slides and/or handouts, etc.
	National Association for Girls and Women in Sport (NAGWS)	aahperd.org/nagws/ nagws.html	Focused to increase the recognition and development of women's collegiate sports. Provides membership information, issues pertaining to title IX, and statistics of women in sports.
	American Association of Health Education (AAHE)	aahperd.org/cgi-bin/counter.pl/ aahe/aahe.html	Provides membership information, publications and communications, and professional information.
	American Association for Health, Physical Education, Recreation and Dance (AAHPERD)	aahperd.org/	Promotes quality education programs to improve health and fitness within the United States. Consists of six other associations (also listed in this table), and provides details of organization efforts and programs, and periodicals, newsletters, and publications.
	American Association for Leisure and Recreation (AALR)	aahperd.org/cgi-bin/counter. pl/aalr/aalr.html	Provides membership information, publications and communications, and professional information.
	American Heart Association (AHA)	amhrt.org/	A huge site, consisting of thousands of items for comprehensive information on heart disease, stroke, family health, medical treatments, prevention, etc.

*Unless the address begins with "http," first type "http://www." followed by the listed address.

†Those concerned with published research databases.

Internet homepages that are pertinent to exercise physiology

DISCIPLINE/ PROFESSION	NAME	ADDRESS*	DESCRIPTION
Organizations/ institutions Cont'd	Centers For Disease Control and Prevention (CDC)	cdc.gov/	A huge site informing the public of the U.S. government's stance on many aspects of health. Provides publications, software, products, grant information, data, statistics, etc.
	National Association of Sport and Physical Education (NASPE)	aahperd.org/naspe/ naspe-main.html	Provides membership information and services, publications and communications, and professional information.
	National Dance Association (NDA)	aahperd.org/nda/nda-main. html	Provides membership information and services, publications and communications, and professional information.
	National Sports Medicine Institute of the United Kingdom (NSMI)	nsmi.org.uk/	Provides advice on the training, nutrition, and physiology of triathlon, rowing, tennis, gymnastics, soccer, hockey, and rugby.
Research publications[†]	British Journal of Sports Medicine	bmipg.com/data/jsm.htm	Presents research of sports medicine, including exercise physiology.
	Canadian Journal of Applied Physiology	humankinetics.com/infok/ journals/cjap/intro.htm	Journal of the Canadian Society for Exercise Physiology.
	European Journal of Applied Physiology	http://link.springer.de/link/ service/journals/00421/index. htm	Presents research of many applications of physiology, with a large component on exercise physiology research.
	International Journal of Sports Nutrition	humankinetics.com/infok/ journals/ijsn/intro.htm	Presents research pertinent to sports nutrition.
	Journal of Applied Physiology	uth.tmc.edu/apabstracts/ 1995/jap/toc.html	Journal of the American Physiological Society.
	Journal of Exercise Physiology online	css.edu/users/tboone2/asep/ toc.htm	Journal of the American Society for Exercise Physiology.
	Journal of Physiology	http://physiology.cap.cam.ac. uk/JPhysiol/index.html	From the British equivalent of the American Physiological Society.
	Journal of Sports Sciences	Chapmanhall.com/js/default. html	Multidisciplinary exercise science research journal.
	Medicine and Science in Sports and Exercise	wwilkins.com/MSSE/index. html	Journal of the American College of Sports Medicine.
	Pediatric Exercise Science	humankinetics.com/infok/ journals/pes/intro.htm	Presents research of how exercise affects children.
	Science and Sport	Elselvier.nl:80/inca/ publications/store/5/0/5/8/2/2/	Multidisciplinary exercise science research journal.
	Sports Medicine	Adis.com/frames8.html	Excellent review journal.
	Strength and Conditioning	humankinetics.com/infok/ journals/s&c/intro.htm	Journal of the National Strength and Conditioning Association.

*Unless the address begins with "http," first type "http://www." followed by the listed address.

[†]Those concerned with published research databases.

not yet to the point where literature searching is that easy, but the potential is there for information to be at the fingertips of anybody with a computer and Internet access.

How to Use the Internet

Many of the resources used to write this section are listed in table B.1. For those of you who are not well versed in the terminology or conceptual functioning of the Internet, just as we were prior to writing this appendix, these resources are a great place to start your education of the World Wide Web.

TABLE B.4

Internet sites that provide numerous links to other resources pertinent to exercise physiology

SITE	ADDRESS*
American Society of Exercise Physiology	css.edu/users/tboone2/asep/
Arbor Nutrition Guide	arborcom.com/
Medicine and sports-related links	mspweb.com/
Sportsci	sportsci.com/

*Unless the address shown begins with "http," first type "http://www." followed by the listed address.

As is true for most new knowledge or skills, the best education is that of experiencing the topic firsthand. The websites presented in table B.1 are a good place to start your inquiries into the Internet. From there we suggest that you then venture into the more exercise physiology–specific sites of tables B.3 and B.4. There are no special directions to follow when using the World Wide Web. Get your feet wet and learn as you go. Hopefully, we have provided the raw ingredients in tables B.1 to B.4 to enable you to understand the language and increase the success you have in finding information that you are interested in. Good luck, and happy "surfing."

Internet Addresses Pertinent to the Exercise Sciences

Table B.3 lists the URLs of many Internet websites, organized by topic and accompanied by a simple description. However, many sites simply have far too much material and additional links to do justice to a table presentation. The websites that offer numerous links have been combined in table B.4. In fact, the websites of table B.4 provide links to most of the sites we have detailed in this appendix.

REFERENCES

1. All About the Internet. http://shell.rmi.net/~kgr/internet/.
2. American Society of Exercise Physiologists Links. http://css.edu.users/tboone2/asep/toc.htm.
3. Sportscience Links. http://www.sportsci.org.
4. The Internet Index. http://www.openmarket.com/intindex/.
5. Understanding and Using the Internet. http://www.pbs.org/uti.

Conversion Units

Depending on the country you are in, you may use different units to measure variables such as height, weight, energy, or pressure. For example, in most of Europe, Australia, Canada, and Great Britain, the metric system of measurement is accepted and used in schools and the workplace. Conversely, in the United States there has been a societal reluctance to convert to metric units despite the U.S. Congress Metric Conversion Act of 1975, which endorsed an international system of measurement (table C.1). Such discrepancies in how individuals report data are not conducive to the optimal dissemination of research findings throughout the world. Consequently, the scientific community has had to reach consensus on how to express the units of different measurements. Consequently, in 1977 the World Health Organization recommended the worldwide adoption of the Système International d'Unités (SI units). The main components of the SI system are presented in table C.1.

The recommended rule for the use of SI units is:

1. Symbols should be written without a period(".").
2. Symbols that are not named after persons should be written in small letters (e.g., "m" for meter and "K" for Kelvin).
3. For differing units that have the same name, unique symbols must be used (e.g., time minute [min] vs. angle minute [']).

TABLE C.1

The main measurements and units of the SI

QUANTITY	BASIC UNIT	SYMBOL
Length	meter*	m
Area	square meter	m^2
Volume	cubic meter	m^3
Mass	kilogram	kg
Number	one	1
Time	second	s
Electric current	ampere	A
Electric charge	coulumb	C
Electric potential, difference, electromotive force	volt	V
Thermodynamic temperature	kelvin	K
Capacitance	farad	F
Electric resistance	ohm	Ω
Conductance	siemens	S
Celsius temperature	degree Celsius	°C
Luminous intensity	candela	cd
Amount of substance	mole	mol
Mass concentration (density)	kilogram per liter	kg/L
Substance concentration	mole per liter	mol/L
Molality	mole per kilogram	mol/kg
Osmolality	osmole per kilogram	Osmol/kg
Number concentration	reciprocol liter	L^{-1}
Pressure	pascal	Pa N/m^2
Surface tension	newtons per meter	N/m
Force	newton	N
Energy, work, heat	joule	J
Frequency	hertz	Hz
Enzyme catalytic activity	katal	kat

Conversion factors for the different units of work, power, force, pressure, mass, length, volume, temperature, frequency, and pH are presented in table C.2.

*US spelling

TABLE C.2

Conversion factors for the different units of work, power, force, pressure, mass, length, volume, temperature, frequency, and pH*

WORK	kJ	kcal	ft./lb	kgm
1 kilojoule (kJ)	1.0	0.2388	737	1786.9
1 kilocalorie (kcal)	4.1868	1.0	3086	426.8
1 foot pound (ft.lb)	0.000077	0.000324	1.0	0.1383
1 kilogram-meter (kgm)	0.009797	0.002345	7.23	1.0

POWER	HORSEPOWER	kgm/min^{-1}	ft.lb/min^{-1}	W	kcal/min^{-1}	kJ/min^{1}
1 horsepower	1.0	4,564.0	33,000.0	745.7	10.694	44.743
1 kgm/min^{-1}	0.000219	1.0	7.233	0.16345	0.00234	0.0098068
1 ft.lb/min^{-1}	0.00003	0.1383	1.0	0.0226	0.000324	0.0013562
1 watt (w)	0.001314	6.118	44.236	1.0	0.014335	0.060
1 kcal/min^{-1}	0.0936	426.78	3086.0	69.697	1.0	4.186
1 kJ/min^{-1}	0.02235	101.97	737.30	16.667	0.2389	1.0

FORCE	lb	kg	N
1 pound (lb)	1.0	0.4545	0.04635
1 kilogram (kg)	2.2	1.0	0.10197
1 Newton (N)	19.614	9.807	1.0

PRESSURE	mmHg	kPa	torr	mBar
1 millimeter of mercury (mmHg)	1.0	0.13333	1.0	0.7502
1 kilopascal (kPa)	7.501	1.0	7.501	5.6272
1 torr	1.0	0.1333	1.0	0.7502
1 millibar (mBar)	1.333	0.1777	1.333	1.0

MASS	oz	g	lb	kg
ounce (oz)	1.0	28.35	0.0625	0.028
gram (g)	0.0353	1.0	0.0022	0.001
pound (lb)	16.0	454	1.0	0.454
kilogram (kg)	35.714	1000	2.204	1.0

TABLE C.2S

Conversion factors for the different units of work, power, force, pressure, mass, length, volume, temperature, frequency, and pH*

LENGTH	in	cm	mm	ft	yd	m	mi	km
inch (in)	1.0	2.54	25.4	0.0833	0.0278	0.0254	6.31×10^{-5}	2.546×10^{-5}
centimeter (cm)	0.3937	1.0	10	0.0324	0.0108	0.01	2.48×10^{-5}	1.0×10^{-5}
millimeter (mm)	0.03937	0.1	1.0	0.00328	0.00984	0.001	6.21×10^{-7}	1.0×10^{-6}
feet (ft)	12	30.48	304.8	1.0	0.3333	0.304	1.894×10^{-4}	0.0003055
yard (yd)	36	91.44	914.4	3	1.0	0.912	5.68×10^{-4}	3.53×10^{-4}
meter (m)	254	100	1000	3.2895	1.0936	1.0	6.214×10^{-4}	0.001
mile (mi)	63,360	16.1×10^{4}	16.1×10^{5}	5280	1760	1610	1.0	1.61
kilometer (km)	39,283	100,000	1.0×10^{6}	3273.32	1,093	1,000	0.62112	1.0

VOLUME	fl oz	tsp	tbsp	c	mL	pt	L	qt	gal
fluid ounce (fl oz)	1.0	6	2	0.125	29.575	0.0625	33.8123	0.03125	0.007812
teaspoon (tsp)	0.1667	1.0	0.3333	0.0208	4.97	0.01042	0.005	0.0052	0.0013
tablespoon (tbsp)	0.5	3	1.0	14.8	14.8	0.03125	0.0149	0.0156	0.0039
cup (c)	8	48	16	1.0	236.6	0.5	0.2366	0.25	0.0625
milliliter (mL)	0.0338	0.2012	0.0676	0.00423	1.0	0.0021	0.001	0.00106	2.64×10^{-4}
pint (pt)	16	96	32	2	473.2	1.0	0.473	0.5	0.125
liter (L)	33.6	201.6	67.2	4.2265	1000	2.1	1.0	0.961	0.246
quart (qt)	32	192	64	4	946.4	2	1.057	1.0	0.25
gallon (gal)	128	768	256	16	3785.6	8	4.065	4	1.0

TEMPERATURE	°F	°C	K
Fahrenheit (°F)	1.0	(°F − 32) × 0.5556	—
Celsius (°C)	(°C × 1.8) + 32	1.0	—
Kelvin (K)	273°K = 32°F	273°K = 0°C	1.0

FREQUENCY	Hz	1/min
Hertz (Hz)	1.0	60
1/minute (min)	0.01667	1.0

pH	pH	[H⁺]
pH	1.0	10^{-pH}
[H⁺] (mol/L)	$-(\log_{10})$	1.0

*For the following conversion tables, the conversion factors represent how one unit of the measure listed down the page equals the number of units of the measure listed across the page. For example, 1 Kjoule equals 0.2388 Kcal and 0.0056 kgm.

Sources: Adapted from Lippert, H. and H. P. Lehmann. SI units in medicine: An introduction to the international system of units with conversion tables and normal ranges. Urban & Schwarzenburg, Baltimore, 1978; and Young, D. S. An. Intern. Med. 106: 114–120, 1987.

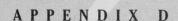

Gas Volumes and Indirect Calorimetry

The measurement of any gas volume necessitates the understanding of how to express the volume relative to the three conditions that influence gas volume: (1) *temperature*, (2) *pressure,* and (3) *water vapor content*. This is especially crucial in exercise physiology because of the importance of measurements of oxygen consumption (VO_2) and carbon dioxide production (VCO_2) during rest and exercise conditions. Furthermore, temperature, pressure, and water vapor content of atmospheric air can change within a day, and can be extremely different depending on terrestrial altitude and climate. Consequently, the expression of gas volumes based on standard conditions is vital for valid comparisons of data collected under different environmental conditions.

The Different Gas Volume Conditions

Gas volumes can be expressed as any one of the conditions of table D.1. Generally, gas volumes are collected under ATPS conditions, and the main conversion of interest is to STPD conditions. However, pulmonary function and lung volume measurements are often expressed relative to BTPS conditions so that gas volumes within the body are quantified.

Conversion Between Gas Volume Conditions

The student of exercise physiology should not have to memorize gas volume conversion equations. The process of converting from one gas condition to another is best accomplished from an understanding of the relationships between gas volume and changes in temperature, pressure, and water vapor. From this understanding will come the ability to generate any conversion equation that is required in laboratory computations.

Temperature

As the temperature of a gas increases, the gas molecules increase in motion, occupying more space and thereby increasing gas volume. This relationship is termed *Charles's law.* To convert a gas volume from one temperature condition to another, the first process is to decipher how the gas volume will

change on the basis of temperature alone (table D.2). Converting from ATPS to STPD will mostly require a decrease in temperature (room temperature gas collection is usually completed in a controlled environment approximating 20°C), which means that the STPD volume will be less than ATPS. This means that a conversion factor less than 1 is required ($273/T_R$). Converting from ATPS to BTPS will mostly require an increase in temperature, which means that the BTPS volume will be greater than ATPS. This means that a conversion factor greater than 1 is required ($310/273$). Determining the temperature conversion factor is as simple as indicated above!

Pressure

As the pressure of a gas increases, the gas molecules are forced to move closer to each other, thereby decreasing gas volume. This relationship is termed *Boyle's law.* When applied to gas volume conversions, the relationship between water vapor and gas volume is also accounted for here. The

TABLE D.1

The different gas volume conditions

CONDITION	TEMPERATURE	PRESSURE	WATER VAPOR
Standard temperature, pressure, dry (STPD)	273 K (0°C)	760 mmHg	0 mmHg
Atmospheric temperature, pressure, saturated (ATPS)	T_A K	P_A	P_{H_2O}
Body temperature, pressure, saturated (BTPS)	310 K (37°C)	P_A	47 mmHg (@37°C)

TABLE D.2

Conversion constants for different gas volumes

CONVERSIONS	TEMPERATURE	PRESSURE
ATPS to STPD	$273/T_A$	$(P_B - P_{H_2O}) / 760$
ATPS to BTPS	$310/T_A$	$(P_B - P_{H_2O \, atm}) / (P_B - P_{H_2O \, body})$
STPD to BTPS	$310/273$	$760 / (P_B - P_{H_2O \, body})$

more water vapor, the less air that remains for the true gases. Consequently, water vapor pressure must be subtracted from the barometric pressure.

The quantification of water vapor pressure is not simple. Typically the relative humidity of the air is measured (for atmospheric air) or known (expired air is always 100% saturated with water vapor) (table D.3). Relative humidity is measured using either a hydrometer or wet and dry bulb temperatures. If a wet and dry bulb temperature approach is used, the relative humidity can be determined from charts, as presented in table D.4. The higher the gas temperature, the more water vapor for a given relative humidity (table D.3). Once the relative humidity is known, a conversion chart is used to convert the relative humidity for a given gas temperature to water vapor pressure.

Data for practicing conversions are provided in the study questions at the end of this appendix.

TABLE D.3

Water vapor pressures (P_{H_2O}) in fully saturated air at different gas temperatures

AMBIENT TEMPERATURE (°C)	WATER VAPOR PRESSURE (mmHg)*
14	12.9
15	13.5
16	14.1
17	14.9
18	15.5
19	16.5
20	17.5
21	18.7
22	19.8
23	21.1
24	22.4
25	23.8
26	25.2
27	26.7
28	28.3
29	30.0
30	31.8
31	33.7
32	35.7
33	37.7
34	39.9
35	42.2
36	44.6
37	47.1
38	49.4
39	52.0
40	54.7

*Water vapor pressure can also be estimated from the formula,
$P_{H_2O} = [13.955 - (0.6584T)] + (0.419T_2)$, where T = temperature °C.

Indirect Calorimetry

As discussed in chapter 4, the computations involved in indirect calorimetry are the "nuts and bolts" of data collection in a typical exercise physiology laboratory. Although most data collection completed today is aided by computer-integrated equipment that does not require the completion of manual calculations, knowledge of the derivation of the equations of indirect calorimetry is recommended to reinforce the basic physiology and math inherent in this process. The equations of indirect calorimetry are presented below.

It is best to start with the fundamental equation for VO_2. Essentially, you are calculating the difference between the oxygen volume inhaled from the oxygen volume exhaled. To do this you need to know both inspired and expired volumes, and inspired and expired gas fractions.

D.1 $$VO_2 = (V_I \times F_IO_2) - (V_E \times F_EO_2)$$

Inspired Ventilation

If you use an indirect calorimetry system where expired ventilation is measured, then the Haldane transformation is used to solve for V_I. This is important because V_I and V_E are not always identical as they change in relation to each other whenever the RER is not 1.0.

The Haldane transformation is based on the fact that gaseous nitrogen is physiologically inert (i.e., it is neither consumed nor produced by the body).

D.2 $$(V_I \times F_IN_2) = (V_E \times F_EN_2)$$

Equation (D.2) is rearranged to eventually get to equation (D.4).

D.3 $$V_I = (V_E \times F_EN_2)/F_IN_2$$

D.4 $$V_I = V_E \times (F_EN_2 /F_IN_2)$$

Equation (D.4) can be further rearranged by assuming that air is solely composed of nitrogen, oxygen, and carbon dioxide (99.9% true!!). Thus, the expired nitrogen (F_EN_2) must be equal to the gas remaining in air once the oxygen and carbon dioxide contents are removed.

D.5 $$V_I = V_E \times [1 - (F_ECO_2 + F_EO_2)]/0.7903$$

If you use a system where inspired volume is measured, and expired volume must be calculated, then the Haldane transformation is rearranged as follows:

D.6 $$(V_I \times F_IN_2) = (V_E \times F_EN_2)$$

D.7 $$V_E = V_I \times (F_IN_2/F_EN_2)$$

D.8 $$V_E = (V_I \times F_IN_2)/F_EN_2$$

D.9 $$V_E = V_I \times 0.7903/[1 - (F_ECO_2 + F_EO_2)]$$

TABLE D.4														
Relative humidity values from temperatures from wet and dry bulb thermometers*														

T_{dry} (°C)	$T_{dry} - T_{wet}$ (°C)														
	1	2	3	4	5	6	7	8	9	10	11	12	13	14	15
	Relative Humidity (RH)														
16	90	81	71	63	54	46	38	30	23	15	8				
17	90	81	72	64	55	47	40	32	25	18	11				
18	91	82	73	65	57	49	41	34	27	20	14	7			
19	91	82	74	65	58	50	43	36	29	22	16	10			
20	91	83	74	66	59	51	44	37	31	24	18	12	6		
21	91	83	75	67	60	53	46	39	32	26	20	14	9		
22	92	83	76	68	61	54	47	40	34	28	22	17	11	6	
23	92	84	76	69	62	55	48	42	36	30	24	19	13	8	
24	92	84	77	69	62	56	49	43	37	31	26	20	15	10	5
25	92	84	77	70	63	57	50	44	39	33	28	22	17	12	8
26	92	85	78	71	64	58	51	46	40	34	29	24	19	14	10
27	92	85	78	71	65	58	52	47	41	36	31	26	21	16	12
28	93	85	78	72	65	59	53	48	42	37	32	27	22	18	13
29	93	86	79	72	66	60	54	49	43	38	33	28	24	19	15
30	93	86	79	73	67	61	55	50	44	39	35	30	25	21	17
31	93	86	80	73	67	61	56	51	45	40	36	31	27	22	18
32	93	86	80	74	68	62	57	51	46	41	37	32	28	24	20
33	93	87	80	74	68	63	57	52	47	42	38	33	29	25	21
34	93	87	81	75	69	63	58	53	48	43	39	35	30	26	23
35	94	87	81	75	69	64	59	54	49	44	40	36	32	28	24
36	94	87	81	75	70	64	59	54	50	45	41	37	33	29	25
37	94	87	82	76	70	65	60	55	51	46	42	38	34	30	26
38	94	88	82	76	71	66	61	56	51	47	43	39	35	31	27
39	94	88	82	77	71	66	61	57	52	48	43	39	36	32	28
40	94	88	82	77	72	67	62	57	53	48	44	40	36	33	29

*From U.S. Weather Bulletin No. 1071.

Example: T_{dry} = 22°C; T_{wet} = 17°C; $T_{dry} - T_{wet}$ = 5°C; RH = 61%

Oxygen Consumption

Once equation (D.5) has been solved, then equation (D.1) can be used to calculate VO_2. This fact is true because, during expired gas indirect calorimetry, you measure or know all the remaining variables (measured = V_E, F_ECO_2, and F_EO_2; known = F_IN_2, F_IO_2).

D.10 $VO_2 = \{V_E \times [1 - (F_ECO_2 + F_EO_2) / 0.7903]$
$\times F_IO_2\} - (V_E \times F_EO_2)$

D.11 $VO_2 = \{V_E \times [1 - (F_ECO_2 + F_EO_2) / 0.7903]$
$\times 0.2093\} - (V_E \times F_EO_2)$

Carbon Dioxide Production

Now that V_I (or V_E) and VO_2 are calculated, the calculation of VCO_2 is relatively simple, and requires only knowledge of F_ICO_2 (0.0003). This fraction is easily remembered as "three zeros and three"! Also, remember that for VCO_2 you are calculating a gas that is produced by the body, not consumed. Thus, you have to *subtract the CO_2 consumed by the body from that produced by the body.*

D.12 $VCO_2 = (V_E \times F_ECO_2) - (V_I \times F_ICO_2)$

Although the product of $V_E \times F_ICO_2$ is usually very small, especially calculation of data acquired during rest conditions, it is important to always account for the volume of inspired CO_2. For example, during maximal exercise conditions with a V_ISTPD = 150 L/min, V_ICO_2 = 45 mL/min, a value large enough to alter VCO_2 and the respiratory exchange ratio!

Respiratory Exchange Ratio

As discussed in chapter 4, the respiratory exchange ratio (RER) is the simple ratio of VCO_2 to VO_2. It is used to gauge the relative intensity of the exercise, and to indirectly determine the carbohydrate and fat oxidation using the nonprotein RER table. It is useful as a gauge of exercise intensity because as the RER approaches 1.0, the exercise intensity is approaching that of the maximal steady state. For example, when the RER increases above 1.0, additional CO_2 is being produced from acid buffering resulting from an increase in ATP regeneration from nonmitochondrial reactions (glycolysis and creatine phosphate). These intensities cannot be tolerated for extended periods of time because of eventual creatine phosphate depletion and the progressive development of more severe acidosis.

D.13 $$RER = VCO_2/VO_2$$

Recommendations

Remember to always convert gas volumes from ATPS to STPD prior to completing your calculations. This is not essential because conversions can always be done for VO_2 and VCO_2. However, this requires added computations and time, and introduces increased risk for error.

Calculating inspired volume separately makes the VO_2 calculation more straightforward. If you have read chapter 4, the VO_2 and VCO_2 calculations are self-explanatory, as is the calculation of the respiratory exchange ratio. It is recommended that you practice these calculations using the data that follow in the study questions.

Study Questions

1. Using the data of table D.5, calculate the gas volumes for the respective gas conditions when collecting air under the respective ATPS conditions.
2. Using data from table D.6, calculate the VO_2, VCO_2, and RER for each condition.

TABLE D.5

Data for calculations of gas volumes under different environmental conditions

VOLUME ATPS (L/min)	T (°C)	P (mmHg)	DRY, WET BULB (°C)	RELATIVE HUMIDITY (%)	STPD (L/min)	BTPS (L/min)
45	21	745		80	?	?
9	18	712	23, 15		?	?
112	28	680		29	?	?
188	22	630	19, 7		?	?

TABLE D.6

Data for calculations of VO_2, VCO_2, and RER for different metabolic conditions*

TIME (min)	V_E STPD (L/min)	F_EO_2	F_ECO_2
0	5.35	0.1658	0.0390
1	17.23	0.1616	0.0389
2	19.5	0.1552	0.0405
3	24.3	0.1470	0.0470
4	27.14	0.1496	0.0484
5	37.5	0.1498	0.0506
6	41.39	0.1564	0.0488
7	49.85	0.1558	0.0497
8	58.37	0.1575	0.0499
9	67.73	0.1625	0.0483
10	75.59	0.1615	0.0506
11	129.24	0.1757	0.0396
12	145.03	0.1784	0.0362
13	170.08	0.1778	0.0362

*These data from a cycle ergometer exercise test to VO_{2max} using a 30 W/min incremental protocol. Subject was a male elite-trained cyclist and weighed 59.2 kg.

Energy Expenditure

The equations for the calculations of VO_2 and VCO_2 from appendix D can be used to also estimate energy expenditure. In fact, the equations of indirect calorimetry were originally derived for this purpose. Remember, we need to calculate energy expenditure from VO_2 and VCO_2 during exercise because we cannot accurately quantify heat production and release from the body during exercise. Values for VO_2 and VCO_2 provide an *indirect method* for calculating energy expenditure, hence the term *indirect calorimetry*.

The basic principle behind using values of VO_2 and VCO_2 for energy-expenditure calculations is the direct relationships between VO_2 and metabolic rate and specific energy yield differences between carbohydrate and fat catabolism. These energy differences between carbohydrate and fat were detailed in chapter 4, and presented in the table of nonprotein RER energy equivalents.

Calculations of energy expenditure cannot be applied to all exercise conditions. For the VO_2 and VCO_2 values to reflect actual energy expenditure, the exercise must be:

1. Performed at steady-state intensities.
2. For at least 3 min to reach steady state.
3. Not accompanied by hyperventilation, which artificially raises VCO_2.
4. Of a duration and nutrition state not associated with large increases in amino acid oxidation (meets steady-state assumptions, is not longer than 60 min, and there is adequate carbohydrate nutrition prior to and during exercise).

If the above criteria are met, then VO_2 and VCO_2 can be used as follows:

E.1   Energy expenditure (kcal/min) = VO_2 (L/min)
$\times$ kcal equivalent (kcal/L)

The kcal equivalent is obtained from the nonprotein RER table of chapter 4. For example, if exercise was performed and the following data were calculated:
VO_2 = 1.5 L/min; VCO_2 = 1.3 L/min; RER = 0.86; kcal/L VO_2 = 4.875 kcal/L.

$$kcal/min = 1.5 \times 4.875 = 7.3125$$

If this exercise was sustained for 60 min then,

$$kcal = 7.3125 \times 60 = 438.75 \; kcal$$

Remember, kcal is not the internationally recognized unit of energy. Data of kcal should be converted to kJ (kilojoules) using the conversion factor of 4.1868.

$$kJ = 438.75 \times 4.1868 = 1836.9585$$

Energy Expenditure During Specific Activities

Many other sources provide energy expenditure for different activities. However, these values are gross approximations and are not very accurate. The most variable component of the energy expenditure equation is the value for oxygen consumption (VO_2). For a given activity and exercise intensity, this value will vary depending on body mass, biomechanical efficiency, and biochemical efficiency. The variability in VO_2 will depend on the exact activity at question. For example, cycling is an exercise mode that would have relatively smaller between-subject variability in VO_2 for a given intensity because body weight is supported and the mechanical actions of cycling are constrained to the design of the bike and are relatively simple. Conversely, the oxygen cost of running at 5 mi/h will vary tremendously between different individuals because of the greater range of potential differences in running style (biomechanical efficiency), and the fact that body weight is not supported and therefore adds to the intensity of the exercise. Many energy expenditure charts account for the role of body mass by expressing energy expenditure values relative to kilograms body mass.

If you need to estimate energy expenditure for a given exercise condition, it is recommended that you use equations that can estimate VO_2 on the basis of other criteria of intensity (speed, incline, etc.). You should then make an intelligent guess at the RER. Remember, the lower the intensity and the longer the duration, RER values will probably be less than 0.85. For more intense exercises that lie closer to the lactate threshold intensity, RER will be between 0.9 and 1.0. You should then use the previous equations to calculate energy expenditure.

Table E.1 provides data for you to calculate energy expenditures and answer the study questions.

TABLE E.1

Energy expenditures for selected exercise conditions

VO$_2$ (L/min)	RER	Duration (min)	kcal
1.85	0.86	90	?
2.65	0.96	35	?
3.4	1.12	4	?
2.0	0.82	2	?
2.50	0.90	45	?

Study Questions

1. Which conditions of table E.1 would you view to provide accurate data of energy expenditure? Why?

2. On the basis of data in chapter 4, if you know that the exercise condition is not ideally suited to calculate energy expenditure, what is more inaccurate, the absolute energy expenditure values you calculate or the energy partitioned to carbohydrate and fat oxidation? Why?

Recommended Dietary Allowances

Food and Nutrition Board, National Academy of Sciences—National Research Council

Recommended dietary allowances,[a] revised 1989 (abridged[*])
(designed for the maintenance of good nutrition of practically all healthy people in the United States)

CATEGORY	AGE (YEARS) OR CONDITION	WEIGHT[b] (kg)	WEIGHT[b] (lb)	HEIGHT[b] (cm)	HEIGHT[b] (in)	PROTEIN (g)	VITAMIN A (µg RE)[c]	VITAMIN E (mg α-TE)[d]	VITAMIN K (µg)	VITAMIN C (mg)	IRON (mg)	ZINC (mg)	IODINE (µg)	SELENIUM (µg)
Infants	0.0–0.5	6	13	60	24	13	375	3	5	30	6	5	40	10
	0.5–1.0	9	20	71	28	14	375	4	10	35	10	5	50	15
Children	1–3	13	29	90	35	16	400	6	15	40	10	10	70	20
	4–6	20	44	112	44	24	500	7	20	45	10	10	90	20
	7–10	28	62	132	52	28	700	7	30	45	10	10	120	30
Males	11–14	45	99	157	62	45	1000	10	45	50	12	15	150	40
	15–18	66	145	176	69	59	1000	10	65	60	12	15	150	50
	19–24	72	160	177	70	58	1000	10	70	60	10	15	150	70
	25–50	79	174	176	70	63	1000	10	80	60	10	15	150	70
	51+	77	170	173	68	63	1000	10	80	60	10	15	150	70
Females	11–14	46	101	157	62	46	800	8	45	50	15	12	150	45
	15–18	55	120	163	64	44	800	8	55	60	15	12	150	50
	19–24	58	128	164	65	46	800	8	60	60	15	12	150	55
	25–50	63	138	163	64	50	800	8	65	60	15	12	150	55
	51+	65	143	160	63	50	800	8	65	60	10	12	150	55
Pregnant						60	800	10	65	70	30	15	175	65
Lactating	1st 6 months					65	1300	12	65	95	15	19	200	75
	2nd 6 months					62	1200	11	65	90	15	16	200	75

[*]NOTE: This table does not include nutrients for which dietary reference intakes have recently been established [see *Dietary Reference Intakes for Calcium, Phosphorus, Magnesium, Vitamin D, and Fluoride* (1997) and *Dietary Reference Intakes for Thiamin, Riboflavin, Niacin, Vitamin B_6, Folate, Vitamin B_{12}, Pantothenic Acid, Biotin, and Choline* (1988)].

[a]The allowances, expressed as average daily intakes over time, are intended to provide for individual variations among most normal persons as they live in the United States under usual environmental stresses. Diets should be based on a variety of common foods in order to provide other nutrients for which human requirements have been less well defined.

[b]Weights and heights of reference adults are actual medians for the U.S. population of the designated age, as reported by NHANES II. The median weights and heights of those under 19 years of age were taken from Hamill et al. (1979) (see pages 16–17). The use of these figures does not imply that the height-to-weight ratios are ideal.

[c]Retinol equivalents. 1 retinol equivalent = 1 µg retinol or 6 µg β-carotene.

[d]α-tocopherol equivalents. 1 mg d-α tocopherol = 1 α-TE.

© Copyright 1998 by the National Academy of Sciences. All rights reserved.

Reprinted with permission from *Recommended Dietary Allowances*, 10th edition. Copyright 1989 by the National Academy of Sciences. Courtesy of the National Academy Press, Washington, D.C.

Food and Nutrition Board, Institute of Medicine—National Academy of Sciences

Dietary reference intakes: recommended levels for individual intake

LIFE-STAGE GROUP	CALCIUM (mg/d)	PHOSPHORUS (mg/d)	MAGNESIUM (mg/d)	D (µg/d)[a,b]	FLUORIDE (mg/d)	THIAMIN (mg/d)	RIBOFLAVIN (mg/d)	NIACIN (mg/d)[c]	B$_6$ (mg/d)	FOLATE (µg/d)[d]	B$_{12}$ (µg/d)	PANTOTHENIC ACID (mg/d)	BIOTIN (µg/d)	CHOLINE[e] (mg/d)
Infants														
0–5 mo	210*	100*	30*	5*	0.01*	0.2*	0.3*	2*	0.1*	65*	0.4*	1.7*	5*	125*
6–11 mo	270*	275*	75*	5*	0.5*	0.3*	0.4*	4*	0.3*	80*	0.5*	1.8*	6*	150*
Children														
1–3 yr	500*	460	80	5*	0.7*	0.5	0.5	6	0.5	150	0.9	2*	8*	200*
4–8 yr	800*	500	130	5*	1*	0.6	0.6	8	0.6	200	1.2	3*	12*	250*
Males														
9–13 yr	1300*	1250	240	5*	2*	0.9	0.9	12	1.0	300	1.8	4*	20*	375*
14–18 yr	1300*	1250	410	5*	3*	1.2	1.3	16	1.3	400	2.4	5*	25*	550*
19–30 yr	1000*	700	400	5*	4*	1.2	1.3	16	1.3	400	2.4	5*	30*	550*
31–50 yr	1000*	700	420	5*	4*	1.2	1.3	16	1.3	400	2.4	5*	30*	550*
51–70 yr	1200*	700	420	10*	4*	1.2	1.3	16	1.7	400	2.4[f]	5*	30*	550*
> 70 yr	1200*	700	420	15*	4*	1.2	1.3	16	1.7	400	2.4[f]	5*	30*	550*
Females														
9–13 yr	1300*	1250	240	5*	2*	0.9	0.9	12	1.0	300	1.8	4*	20*	375*
14–18 yr	1300*	1250	360	5*	3*	1.0	1.0	14	1.2	400[g]	2.4	5*	25*	400*
19–30 yr	1000*	700	310	5*	3*	1.1	1.1	14	1.3	400[g]	2.4	5*	30*	425*
31–50 yr	1000*	700	320	5*	3*	1.1	1.1	14	1.3	400[g]	2.4	5*	30*	425*
51–70 yr	1200*	700	320	10*	3*	1.1	1.1	14	1.5	400[g]	2.4[f]	5*	30*	425*
> 70 yr	1200*	700	320	15*	3*	1.1	1.1	14	1.5	400	2.4[f]	5*	30*	425*
Pregnancy														
≤ 18 yr	1300*	1250	400	5*	3*	1.4	1.4	18	1.9	600[h]	2.6	6*	30*	450*
19–30 yr	1000*	700	350	5*	3*	1.4	1.4	18	1.9	600[h]	2.6	6*	30*	450*
31–50 yr	1000*	700	360	5*	3*	1.4	1.4	18	1.9	600[h]	2.6	6*	30*	450*
Lactation														
≤ 18 yr	1300*	1250	360	5*	3*	1.5	1.6	17	2.0	500	2.8	7*	35*	550*
19–30 yr	1000*	700	310	5*	3*	1.5	1.6	17	2.0	500	2.8	7*	35*	550*
31–50 yr	1000*	700	320	5*	3*	1.5	1.6	17	2.0	500	2.8	7*	35*	550*

NOTE: This table presents recommended dietary allowances (RDAs) and adequate intakes (AIs) followed by an asterisk (*). Both RDAs and AIs may be used as goals for individual intake. RDAs are set to meet the needs of almost all (97 to 98%) individuals in a group. For healthy breastfed infants, the AI is the mean intake. The AI for other life-stage groups is believed to cover their needs, but lack of data or uncertainty in the data prevent clear specification of this coverage.

[a] As cholecalciferol. 1 µg cholecalciferol = 40 IU vitamin D.

[b] In the absence of adequate exposure to sunlight.

[c] As niacin equivalents. 1 mg of niacin = 60 mg of tryptophan; 0–5 months = preformed niacin (not mg NE).

[d] As dietary folate equivalents (DFE). 1 DFE = 1 µg food folate = 0.6 µg of folic acid (from fortified food or supplement) consumed with food = 0.5 µg of synthetic (supplemental) folic acid taken on an empty stomach.

[e] Although AIs have been set for choline, there are few data to assess whether a dietary supply of choline is needed at all stages of the life cycle, and it may be that the choline requirement can be met by endogenous synthesis at some of these stages.

[f] Since 10 to 30% of older people may malabsorb food-bound B$_{12}$, it is advisable for those older than 50 years to meet their RDA mainly by consuming foods fortified with B$_{12}$ or a B$_{12}$-containing supplement.

[g] In view of evidence linking folate intake with neural tube defects in the fetus, it is recommended that all women capable of becoming pregnant consume 400 µg of synthetic folic acid from fortified foods and/or supplements in addition to intake of food folate from a varied diet.

[h] It is assumed that women will continue taking 400 µg of folic acid until their pregnancy is confirmed and they enter prenatal care, which ordinarily occurs after the end of the periconceptional period—the critical time for formation of the neural tube.

Source: Reprinted with permission from *Dietary Reference Intakes*. Copyright 1998 by the National Academy of Sciences. Courtesy of the National Academy Press, Washington, D.C.

Estimated minimum sodium, chloride, and potassium requirements for healthy persons

AGE	WEIGHT (kg)	SODIUM (mg)*†	CHLORIDE (mg)*†	POTASSIUM (mg)‡
Months				
0–5	4.5	120	180	500
6–11	8.9	200	300	700
Years				
1	11	225	350	1000
2–5	16	300	500	1400
6–9	25	400	600	1600
10–18	50	500	750	2000
>18§	70	500	750	2000

*No allowance has been included for large, prolonged losses from the skin through sweat.

†There is no evidence that higher intakes confer any additional health benefit.

‡Desirable intakes of potassium may considerably exceed these values (~3500 mg for adults).

§No allowance has been included for growth. Values given for people under 18 years of age assume a growth rate corresponding to the 50th percentile reported by the National Center for Health Statistics and averaged for males and females.

Estimated safe and adequate daily dietary intakes (ESADDIs) of selected minerals*

CATEGORY	AGE (YEARS)	TRACE ELEMENTS†			
		COPPER (mg)	MANGANESE (mg)	CHROMIUM (µg)	MOLYBDENUM (µg)
Infants	0–0.5	0.4–0.6	0.3–0.6	10–40	15–30
	0.5–1	0.6–0.7	0.6–1	20–60	20–40
Children and adolescents	1–3	0.7–1	1–1.5	20–80	25–50
	4–6	1–1.5	1.5–2	30–120	30–75
	7–10	1–2	2–3	50–200	50–150
	11+	1.5–2.5	2–5	50–200	75–250
Adults		1.5–3	2–5	50–200	75–250

*Because there is less information on which to base recommendations for allowances of minerals, these figures are not given in the main table of RDAs and are provided here in the form of ranges of recommended intakes.

†Because toxic levels for many trace elements may be reached with only several times usual intakes, the upper levels for the trace elements given in this table should not be habitually exceeded.

Canadian Food Guide

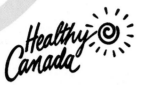

Health and Welfare Canada   Santé et Bien-être social Canada

CANADA'S
Food Guide
TO HEALTHY EATING

Enjoy a variety
of foods from each
group every day.

Choose lower-
fat foods
more often.

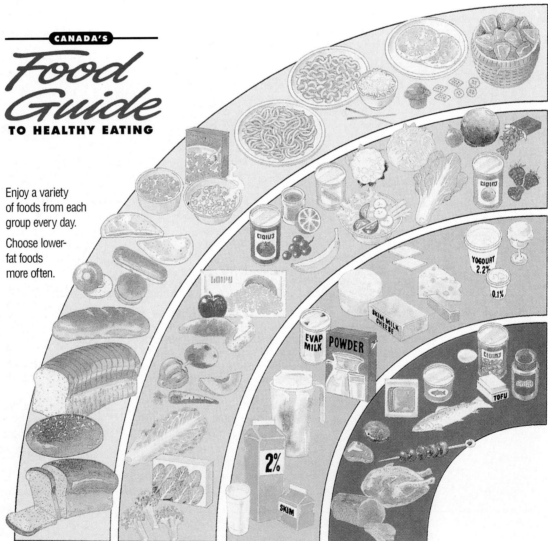

Grain Products
Choose whole-grain
and enriched
products more
often.

Vegetables & Fruit
Choose dark green and
orange vegetables and
orange fruit more often.

Milk Products
Choose lower-fat milk
products more often.

Meat & Alternatives
Choose leaner meats,
poultry and fish, as well
as dried peas, beans, and
lentils more often.

Canada

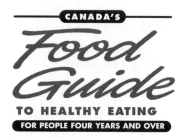

Different People Need Different Amounts of Food

The amount of food you need every day from the 4 food groups and other foods depends on your age, body size, activity level, whether you are male or female and if you are pregnant or breast-feeding. That's why the Food Guide gives a lower and higher number of servings for each food group. For example, young children can choose the lower number of servings, while male teenagers can go to the higher number. Most other people can choose servings somewhere in between.

Grain Products
5–12
SERVINGS PER DAY

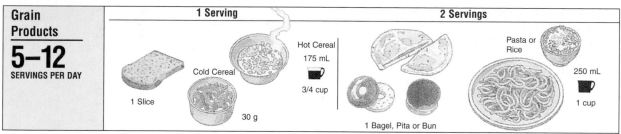

1 Serving
1 Slice
Cold Cereal
30 g
Hot Cereal
175 mL
3/4 cup

2 Servings
1 Bagel, Pita or Bun
Pasta or Rice
250 mL
1 cup

Vegetables & Fruit
5–10
SERVINGS PER DAY

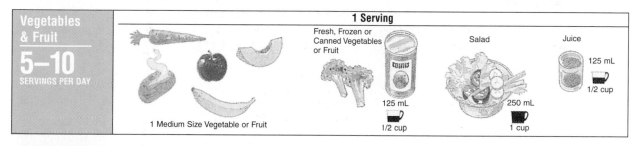

1 Serving
1 Medium Size Vegetable or Fruit
Fresh, Frozen or Canned Vegetables or Fruit
125 mL
1/2 cup
Salad
250 mL
1 cup
Juice
125 mL
1/2 cup

Milk Products
SERVINGS PER DAY
Children 4–9 years: 2-3
Youth 10–16 years: 3–4
Adults: 2-4
Pregnant & Breast-feeding Women: 3-4

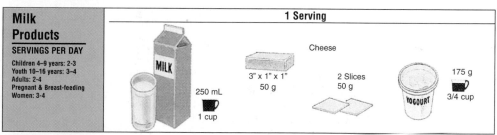

1 Serving
MILK
250 mL
1 cup
Cheese
3" x 1" x 1"
50 g
2 Slices
50 g
YOGOURT
175 g
3/4 cup

Other Foods

Taste and enjoyment can also come from other foods and beverages that are not part of the 4 food groups. Some of these foods are higher in fat or Calories, so use these foods in moderation.

Meat & Alternatives
2–3
SERVINGS PER DAY

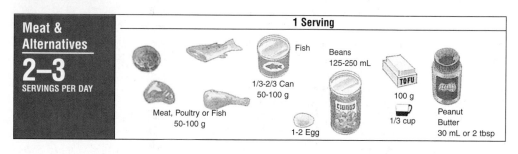

1 Serving
Meat, Poultry or Fish
50-100 g
Fish
1/3-2/3 Can
50-100 g
1-2 Egg
Beans
125-250 mL
TOFU
100 g
1/3 cup
Peanut Butter
30 mL or 2 tbsp

Enjoy eating well, being active and feeling good about yourself. That's 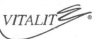 VITALIT®

© Minister of Supply and Services Canada 1992   Cat. No. H39-252 / 1992E   No changes permitted. Reprint permission not required.
ISBN 0-662-19648-1

Nutrient Recommendations for Canadians

TABLE H.1

Recommended nutrient intake

AGE	SEX	WEIGHT (kg)	PROTEIN (g)	VITAMIN A (RE[a])	VITAMIN D (µg)	VITAMIN E (mg)	VITAMIN C (mg)	FOLATE (µg)	VITAMIN B$_{12}$ (µg)	CALCIUM (mg)	PHOSPHORUS (mg)	MAGNESIUM (mg)	IRON (mg)	IODINE (µg)	ZINC (mg)
Months															
0–4	Both	6.0	12[b]	400	10	3	20	25	0.3	250[c]	150	20	0.3[d]	30	2[d]
5–10	Both	9.0	12	400	10	3	20	40	0.4	400	200	32	7	40	3
Years															
1	Both	11	13	400	10	3	20	40	0.5	500	300	40	6	55	4
2–3	Both	14	16	400	5	4	20	50	0.6	550	350	50	6	65	4
4–6	Both	18	19	500	5	5	25	70	0.8	600	400	65	8	85	5
7–9	M	25	26	700	2.5	7	25	90	1.0	700	500	100	8	110	7
	F	25	26	700	2.5	6	25	90	1.0	700	500	100	8	95	7
10–12	M	34	34	800	2.5	8	25	120	1.0	900	700	130	8	125	9
	F	36	36	800	2.5	7	25	130	1.0	1100	800	135	8	110	9
13–15	M	50	49	900	2.5	9	30	175	1.0	1100	900	185	10	160	12
	F	48	46	800	2.5	7	30	170	1.0	1000	850	180	13	160	9
16–18	M	62	58	1000	2.5	10	40[e]	220	1.0	900	1000	230	10	160	12
	F	53	47	800	2.5	7	30[e]	190	1.0	700	850	200	12	160	9
19–24	M	71	61	1000	2.5	10	40[e]	220	1.0	800	1000	240	9	160	12
	F	58	50	800	2.5	7	30[e]	180	1.0	700	850	200	13	160	9
25–49	M	74	64	1000	2.5	9	40[e]	230	1.0	800	1000	250	9	160	12
	F	59	51	800	2.5	6	30[e]	185	1.0	700	850	200	13	160	9
50–74	M	73	63	1000	5	7	40[e]	230	1.0	800	1000	250	9	160	12
	F	63	54	800	5	6	30[e]	195	1.0	800	850	210	8	160	9
75+	M	69	59	1000	5	6	40[e]	215	1.0	800	1000	230	9	160	12
	F	64	55	800	5	5	30[e]	200	1.0	800	850	210	8	160	9
Pregnancy (additional)															
1st trimester			5	0	2.5	2	0	200	0.2	500	200	15	0	25	6
2nd trimester			20	0	2.5	2	10	200	0.2	500	200	45	5	25	6
3rd trimester			24	0	2.5	2	10	200	0.2	500	200	45	10	25	6
Lactation (additional)			20	400	2.5	3	25	100	0.2	500	200	65	0	50	6

[a]Retinol equivalents.
[b]Protein is assumed to be from breast milk and must be adjusted for infant formula.
[c]Infant formula with high phosphorus should contain 375 mg calcium.
[d]Breast milk is assumed to be the source of the mineral.
[e]Smokers should increase vitamin C by 50%.
Source: Scientific Review Committee: *Nutrition Recommendations.* Ottawa, Canada: Health and Welfare, 1990.
Reproduced with permission of the Minister of Supply and Services Canada, 1996.

TABLE H.1

Energy expressed as daily rates

AGE	SEX	ENERGY (cal)	THIAMIN (mg)	RIBOFLAVIN (mg)	NIACIN (NE[b])	n–3 PUFA[a] (g)	n-6 PUFA (g)
Months							
0–4	Both	600	0.3	0.3	4	0.5	3
5–12	Both	900	0.4	0.5	7	0.5	3
Years							
1	Both	1100	0.5	0.6	8	0.6	4
2–3	Both	1300	0.6	0.7	9	0.7	4
4–6	Both	1800	0.7	0.9	13	1.0	6
7–9	M	2200	0.9	1.1	16	1.2	7
	F	1900	0.8	1.0	14	1.0	6
10–12	M	2500	1.0	1.3	18	1.4	8
	F	2200	0.9	1.1	16	1.2	7
13–15	M	2800	1.1	1.4	20	1.5	9
	F	2200	0.9	1.1	16	1.2	7
16–18	M	3200	1.3	1.6	23	1.8	11
	F	2100	0.8	1.1	15	1.2	7
19–24	M	3000	1.2	1.5	22	1.6	10
	F	2100	0.8	1.1	15	1.2	7
25–49	M	2700	1.1	1.4	19	1.5	9
	F	1900	0.8	1.0	14	1.1	7
50–74	M	2300	0.9	1.2	16	1.3	8
	F	1800	0.8[c]	1.0[c]	14[c]	1.1[c]	7[c]
75+	M	2000	0.8	1.0	14	1.1	7
	F[d]	1700	0.8[c]	1.0[c]	14[c]	1.1[c]	7[c]
Pregnancy (additional)							
1st trimester		100	0.1	0.1	1	0.05	0.3
2nd trimester		300	0.1	0.3	2	0.16	0.9
3rd trimester		300	0.1	0.3	2	0.16	0.9
Lactation (additional)		450	0.2	0.4	3	0.25	1.5

[a]PUFA, polyunsaturated fatty acids.
[b]Niacin equivalents.
[c]Level below which intake should not fall.
[d]Assumes moderate physical activity.
Source: Scientific Review Committee. *Nutrition Recommendations*. Ottawa, Canada: Health and Welfare, 1990.
Reproduced with permission of the Minister of Supply and Services Canada, 1996.

β-oxidation: the reactions of the oxidation of FFA molecules to acetyl CoA

17β-estradiol: the most biologically active estrogen steroid hormone that influences lipid metabolism, bone growth, and the development of female secondary sex characteristics; produced by the ovary of the female, and to a lesser extent by the adrenal cortex and testes of the male

3-methylhistidine (3-meth′il-**his**′ti-deen): methylated amino acid that is used as a urine marker for muscle protein catabolism

A

acclimation (a′**kli-ma**′shun): the process of chronic adaptation to an artificially imposed environmental stress

acclimatization (a′**kly**-ma-**ty**-za′shun): the process of chronic adaptation to a given environmental stress

accumulated oxygen deficit: the amount of energy able to be generated by contracting skeletal muscle that did not involve mitochondrial respiration

acetyl CoA: molecule produced from carbohydrate and FFA catabolism that enters into the TCA cycle

acidosis (as′i-**do**′sis): the decrease in pH (increase in free hydrogen ion concentration)

actin (**ac**′tin): a contractile protein of skeletal muscle

action potential: the rapid change in the membrane potential of excitable cells that is conducted along an excitable membrane

acute adaptations: the immediate structural and functional responses to exercise that function to help the body tolerate the exercise or physical activity

acute mountain sickness: the illness that accompanies acute altitude exposure, typically expressed by symptoms of headache and lethargy

adaptation (ad-ap-**ta**′shun): a modification in structure or function that benefits life in a new or altered environment

afterload: the blood pressure exposed to the aortic valve immediately prior to ventricular contraction

aging: a progressive loss of physiological capacities that eventually culminates in death

alpha-gamma coactivation: the interaction between alpha and gamma motor nerves and types I and II afferent nerves of skeletal muscle and muscle spindles that results in smooth and controlled dynamic muscle contractions

alveolar ventilation: the volume of air per unit time that reaches the respiratory zone of the lung (where gas exchange occurs)

amino acids: amine (NH_2)-containing molecules that are the primary components of proteins

amphetamines (am′**fet**-a′meen): drugs that overcome the discomfort and some of the neuromuscular recruitment limitations experienced during intense exercise

anabolic-androgenic steroids: hormones that stimulate growth and the development of secondary sex characteristics

anabolism (a-**nab**′o-lizm): the reactions of the body that increase the size of molecules

anaerobic capacity: the capacity of skeletal muscle to regenerate ATP from nonmitochondrial respiration pathways

anaerobic capacity: the maximal amount of ATP able to be regenerated from creatine phosphate hydrolysis and glycolysis during intense exercise

anatomical dead space: the volume of air within the conducting zone of the lung (not involved in gas exchange)

anemia (a-**ne**′mi-ah): abnormally low erythrocyte content, hemoglobin concentration, or hematocrit of the blood

angina (an′**ji**-na): pain caused by myocardial ischemia, typically confined to the chest or left shoulder, arm, and hand

animal research: research performed with animals as subjects

anthropometery: the study of body and body part dimensions

antidiuretic (an ti-**di** u-**ret**′ik): a substance/condition that causes a decrease in urine volume

antioxidants (an′ti-**ok**′si-dant): substance that provides electrons to reduce free radicals, thus preserving other, more important molecules

applied research: application of pure research findings to further understand exercise

arrhythmia (a′**rith**-me-a): an abnormal cardiac rhythm

arteriosclerosis (ar-tir′eo-**skle**′ro-ses): deterioration, or hardening, of the peripheral arteries, resulting in a decrease in compliance and increase in vascular resistance

asthma (**az**′mah): a condition of the lungs associated with a narrowing of the bronchial airways in response to an irritant

Åstrand-Rhyming nomogram: the nomogram for estimating VO_{2max} from a single bout of cycle ergometry

atherosclerosis (ath-e′ro-**skle**′ro-ses): the narrowing of one or more of the coronary arteries because of a build up of plaque within the vessel lumen

athletic amenorrhea: the absence of a menstrual cycle induced by endocrinological responses from exercise training that inhibit the release of follicle-stimulating hormone from the anterior pituitary gland

atrophy (a-**tro**′fi): the degeneration of muscle, often resulting in a decrease in size and functional capacities

autologous transfusion: the reinfusion of red blood cells that were removed from the same individual

axon (**ak**′son): the long component of a nerve that conducts the action potential from one location to another within the body

B

Bayes's theorem: a mathematical theorem used to estimate the accuracy of predicting coronary artery disease by comparing the pretest probability before an exercise test is performed to the probability of disease after the test

bioelectrical impedance (BIA): the method of determining body fat, fat-free body mass, and total body water by measuring the resistance to current passed through the body

bioenergetics (**bi**′o-en-er-**jet**′iks): the study of energy transfer in chemical reactions within living tissue

biological age: age that is assessed by variables such as maximal oxygen uptake, height, weight, muscle strength, bone development, or flexibility, rather than time

biological control system: a unit within the body that functions to maintain homeostasis

blood: the fluid medium that contains cells that function to transport oxygen and carbon dioxide, cells involved in immunity, certain proteins involved in blood clotting and the transport of nutrients, and electrolytes necessary for optimal cell function

blood doping: the term used for the removal of blood from the body, and its eventual reinfusion at a later date for the purpose of increasing hematocrit and blood oxygen-carrying capacity

blood pressure: the pressure within the cardiovascular system generated by the circulation of blood by the heart

body composition: the science of determining the absolute and relative contributions of specific components of the body

body density: the density of the body when submerged in water, expressed in g/mL

body mass index (BMI): the ratio of [body weight/ (height^2)]

Bohr effect: the decrease in the hemoglobin to oxygen affinity with an increase in temperature, PCO_2, acidosis, and 2,3-BPG

branched-chain amino acids: a subgroup of the large side chain and neutral amino acids that compete with the movement of tryptophan across the blood-brain barrier

buffering capacity: the capacity to remove free hydrogen ions from solution

C

caffeine: a naturally occurring substance that acts as a central nervous system (CNS) stimulant and a competitive antagonist for adenosine receptors in the CNS and periphery

calorimeter (**kal**′o-**rim**′eter): an instrument that measures heat release from the body

calorimetry (**kal**′o-ri-**met**′ri): the measurement of body metabolism from heat release from the body

cardiac catheterization: an invasive procedure where a catheter is advanced to the heart via the femoral artery in order to evaluate the presence and severity of blockages within the coronary arteries

cardiac cycle: the events in a functional heart that occur between successive heart beats

cardiac output: the blood volume pumped by the heart each minute

cardiovascular system: the heart and blood vessels of the body

carnitine (**kar**′ni-teen): a molecule required for the transport of medium- to long-chain fatty acids into the mitochondria

catabolism (ca-**tab**′o-lizm): the reactions of the body that decrease the size of molecules

central fatigue: the term used for the increased perceptions of fatigue during prolonged exercise

chemical energy: energy stored in covalent and noncovalent chemical bonds within molecules

chronic adaptations: changes in body structure and function resulting from repeated exposure to exercise stress that are retained after the exercise is completed

chronological age: age that is based on time (years), and is typically divided into young, middle, and old age

claudication (klaud-e′**ka**-shen): pain confined to the lower extremities during exercise or physical activity because of ischemia resulting from atherosclerosis in the arteries of the limbs, usually the femoral artery

clinical research: research conducted with application to medicine or clinical practice

comparative research: research based on comparing one or more groups of individuals for certain characteristics

complete proteins: proteins that contain all of the essential amino acids

compliance: the ease with which an object can increase volume for a given pressure differential

concentric (**kon-sen**′trik): in reference to skeletal muscle contraction; a contraction involving the shortening of muscle

conducting zone: the zone of the lung where no respiration (gas exchange) occurs

creatine (**cre**-a′tin): the amino acid "backbone" structure of creatine phosphate in skeletal muscle

creatine phosphate: a phosphorylated metabolite that releases a large amount of free energy during dephosphorylation

criterion-referenced fitness standards: fitness standards that are based on an established fitness and health relationship

cross-training: the practice of exercise training with more than one exercise mode

cyclic AMP (cAMP): the second messenger produced by the activation of adenylate cyclase in response to the binding of certain hormones to their cell receptor(s)

D

dehydration: a decreased water content of the body below normal

detraining (de-**tray**′ning): the absence of training, usually occurring after the attainment of training adaptations

diabetes mellitis: a condition characterized by a reduced ability to regulate blood glucose concentrations by means of insulin

diagnostic test: an exercise test performed to diagnose or detect a medical condition

dichloracetate (**di**-klor′o-**ass**′e-tate): an artificially chlorinated derivative of acetyl CoA that stimulates the activity of pyruvate dehydrogenase, reduces lactate accumulation in the blood, and decreases peripheral vascular resistance

diffusion capacity: the capacity of a molecule to move along/down a concentration gradient

diuresis (di u-**re**′sis): an increase in urine volume

dynamometer (di-na-**mom**′e-ter): an instrument for the measurement of muscle force application

E

eccentric (e-**sen**′trik): in reference to skeletal muscle contraction; a contraction involving the lengthening of muscle

economy: the concept pertaining to the oxygen consumption required to perform a given task

effector mechanism: the response resulting from receptor and integrating unit function

efficiency: when applied to exercise, the ratio (expressed as a percentage) between the mechanical energy produced during exercise and the energy cost of the exercise

ejection fraction: the volume of blood pumped by the heart per beat, expressed relative to the end-diastolic volume of the ventricle

electrocardiogram (i-lek-**tro-kard**-e-o-**gram**): a recording from an electrocardiograph

electromyography (e-lek′tro-**mi**′og-ra′fi): study of neuromuscular electrical activity at rest and during muscle contraction

electron transport chain: the series of electron receivers located along the inner mitochondrial membrane that sequentially receive and transfer electrons to the final electron receiver—molecular oxygen

endogenous opioids: hormones released by the anterior pituitary gland that effect a biologic response similar to that of morphine

enzyme: a protein molecule that functions as a biological catalyst

epidemiological research: research using large numbers of subjects that attempts to establish relationships among multiple characteristics

epidemiology (e-pe′**de**-me-′**ol**-e-je): the study of the nature, cause, control, and determinants of the frequency and distribution of disease, disabilities, and death in human populations

EPOC: the abbreviation for excess postexercise oxygen consumption, which refers to the elevated consumption of oxygen, above resting levels, that remains after the end of exercise

ergogenic aid: a physical, mechanical, nutritional, psychological, or pharmacological substance or treatment that either directly improves physiological variables associated with exercise performance or removes subjective restraints which may limit physiological capacity

ergometer (er-**gom**′e-ter): a device used to measure work

ergometry (er-**gom**′e-tree): the science of the measurement of work and power

erythrocyte (e-**rith**′ro-syt): red blood cell

erythrocythemia (e-**rith**′ro-si-the′**mi**-ah): artificially increased red blood cell concentrations in the blood

erythropoietin (e′**rith**-ro-**poy**′e-tin): a hormone released from the kidney that is responsible for stimulating red blood cell production (erythropoiesis)

essential fat: fat and lipid component of the body that comprises cell membranes, bone marrow, intramuscular fat, and so forth

exercise: activity that is performed for the purpose of improving, maintaining, or expressing a particular type(s) of physical fitness

exercise physiology: the study of how exercise alters the structure and function of the human body

exercise training: the repeated use of exercise to improve physical fitness

exercise-induced hypoxemia: a decrease in arterial hemoglobin saturation during exercise

experimental research: research performed that involves the control of a factor, or factors, that will influence an outcome

F

fat-free body mass: the component of the body that is not storage and essential fat

female athlete triad: the syndrome of disordered eating, a cessation of the menstrual cycle, and increased risk for osteoporosis

ferritin (**ferr**′i-tin): the form of iron that is stored in the body

fiber type: a categorization of muscle fibers based on their enzymatic and metabolic characteristics

fibers: muscle cells

Fick equation: the equation based on the Fick principle where, $VO_2 = Q \times a\text{-}vO_2$

fitness: a state of well-being that provides optimal performance

follicular phase: the phase of the menstrual cycle beginning with the onset of menstruation and ending at the start of ovulation, usually 9 to 23 days in duration

free energy: the energy from a reaction that can be used to perform work

free fatty acids: the lipid components of triacylglycerols, which are catabolized in tissues

free radicals: small molecules within the body that have extremely high affinity for electrons

fructose (**fruc**-tos): the form of sugar predominantly found in fruit and honey

functional capacity test: an exercise test performed to assess the functional capacity of an individual

G

gain: the theoretical amount of correction needed, divided by the abnormality remaining after correction

gastric emptying: the emptying of stomach contents into the small intestine

gland: an organ that secretes one or more substances

gluconeogenesis (**glu**′ko-**ne**-o-**jen**′e-sis): formation of glucose from noncarbohydrates, such as amino acids or alcohol

glucose (**glu**-kos): the form of sugar by which carbohydrate is metabolized in animals

glucose polymers: glucose residues connected together to form a chain structure

GLUT4: glucose transporter-4; the predominant glucose transport protein on the sarcolemma of skeletal muscle fibers

glycemic index: a rating of the increase in blood glucose after the ingestion of a standard amount of carbohydrate; based on a comparison of the blood glucose response following the ingestion of an equivalent amount of carbohydrate in the form of white bread

glycerol (**glis**′er-ol): a by-product of glycolysis used in triacylglycerol synthesis; released during the mobilization of fatty acids in lipolysis, and often used as an indirect reflection of the mobilization of fatty acids in blood and adipose tissue

glycogen (**gli**′ko-**jen**): a sugar polysaccharide that is the form of carbohydrate storage in animal tissues

glycogen supercompensation: a regimen of increased carbohydrate ingestion and

modified exercise training that results in maximal storage of glycogen in skeletal muscle

glycogen synthetase: the enzyme catalyzing the addition of glucose residues from UDP-glucose to glycogen

glycogenolysis (**gli**-ko-**jen**-ol-is-is): the removal of glucose units from glycogen, producing glucose-1-phosphate

glycolysis (**gli**-kol′i-sis): reactions involving the catabolism of glucose to pyruvate

glycolytic metabolism: reactions of the glycolytic pathway

growth hormone: a hormone that functions to primarily regulate blood glucose, and secondarily to function in concert with somatomedins to stimulate bone and muscle growth

H

Haldane effect: The decrease in hemoglobin to carbon dioxide affinity with an increase in the partial pressure of oxygen

Haldane transformation: the use of equal inspired and expired nitrogen volumes to solve for either inspired or expired ventilatory volumes

healthy life: the amount of active, robust life that a person has prior to death

heat exhaustion: decreased exercise tolerance due to a combination of dehydration, a reduced plasma volume and cardiovascular compromise, and hyperthermia

heat stroke: the progression from heat exhaustion. When body core temperature increases to values that impair the central nervous system and damages peripheral tissues

helium dilution: the method used to measure the functional residual capacity (FRC) of the lung on the basis of the dilution of a known amount of helium

hematocrit (**hem**′a-to-krit): the ratio of the volume of blood cells and formed elements of blood to total blood volume; usually expressed as a percentage

hemoconcentration (**he**′mo-kon′sen-**tra**′shun): increased hematocrit because of the loss of plasma volume

hemoglobin (**he**′mo-**glo**-bin): the protein on and within red blood cells that contains four heme (iron)-containing groups, each of which can bind oxygen

homeostasis (ho′me-o-**sta**′sis): the maintenance of a constant or unchanging internal environment

homologous transfusion: the reinfusion of red blood cells that were removed from a different individual

hormone: a substance secreted from a tissue or cell that exerts a biological effect on that tissue or cell, or on local or distant cells

human subjects research: research performed with humans as subjects

hydrodensitometry: the method of determining body density by underwater weighing

hyperbaria (hi-per-**bar**′i-ah): increased barometric pressure

hyperemia (hi-per-e′mi-ah): increased blood flow above normal; usually expressed relative to a particular tissue

hyperglycemia (hi per-gli-**se**′me ah): abnormally high blood glucose concentrations (> 5 mmol/L)

hyperhydration (hi′per-**hy**′dra-shun): the increase in body water content above normal values

hyperplasia (hi′per-**pla**′zi-ah): the increase in muscle fiber number in skeletal muscle

hypertension: abnormally high blood pressure ($> 140/90$ mmHg)

hyperthermia (hi′per-**ther**-mi′ah): a body core temperature above $37°C$

hypertrophy (hi-**per**′tro-fi): the increase in size of skeletal muscle because of the increased size of individual muscle fibers

hypobaria (hi-po-**bar**′i-ah): decreased barometric pressure

hypobaric hypoxia: decreased oxygen availability that is due to decreased barometric pressure

hypoglycemia (hi-po-gli-**se**′me-ah): abnormally low blood glucose concentrations (< 35 mmol/L)

hyponatremia (hi′po-na-tre′mi-ah): a decrease in the serum concentration of sodium below 135 mEq/L

hypotension (hi′po-ten′shun): abnormally low blood pressure

hypothermia (hi′po-**ther**-mi′ah): a decreased body temperature below $37°C$

hypoxia (hi-**pok**-se′a): lower than normal oxygen availability

I

incremental exercise: exercise performed at intensities that progressively increase over time

informed consent: a written explanation detailing the risks and benefits of a procedure, such as an exercise test, to be experienced by a human subject

integrating control unit: the component(s) that receive the sensory information from the receptor and redirect information to cause a response

intestinal absorption: the absorption of water and organic and inorganic nutrients from the small intestine

isokinetic: in reference to skeletal muscle contraction, a contraction involving a constant velocity

isometric: in reference to skeletal muscle contraction, a contraction involving no change in the length of muscle

J

journal: a publication that presents results from research

K

Korotkoff sounds: the sounds heard by auscultation during the measurement of blood pressure by sphygmomanometry

kymograph (ki′mo-graf): the rotating drum component of an instrument (e.g., spirometer) that is used to record wave-like modulations (e.g., ventilation)

L

lactate: product of the reduction of pyruvate

lactate paradox: the decreased maximal lactate production by contracting skeletal muscle after chronic altitude exposure

lactate threshold: the term used to denote the intensity of exercise when there is an abrupt increase in lactate accumulation in blood or muscle

lean body mass: the component of the body that is not storage fat

life expectancy: the average, statistically predicted, length of life for an individual

lipolysis (li-**pol**′i-sis): catabolism of triacylglycerols releasing FFA and glycerol

longevity: the duration of life

luteal phase: the phase of the menstrual cycle beginning with the end of ovulation and ending at the start of menstruation, usually 13 days in duration

M

macronutrient: essential food component required in large quantities

maturation (mat-u′ra-shun): the biological and/or behavioral development of a person; not necessarily associated with age

maximal oxygen consumption (VO$_{2max}$): the maximal rate of oxygen consumption by the body

menstrual cycle: the monthly variation in gonadal hormones of the female that result in the release of an ovary and the eventual expulsion of the ovary and developing placenta during menstruation

metabolism: the sum of all reactions of the body

microgravity: conditions of decreased gravitational force

micronutrient: essential food component required only in small quantities

mineral: inorganic micronutrients, essential for normal bodily functions

minute ventilation: the volume of air ventilated in and from the lungs in 1 min

mitochondrial respiration: reactions of the mitochondria that ultimately lead to the consumption of oxygen

mortality: the epidemiological and vital statistic term for death

motor cortex: the cortex region of the precentral gyrus responsible for the origin of the neural processing that instigates most contractions of skeletal muscle

motor unit: an alpha motor nerve and the muscle fibers that it innervates

muscle biopsy: the procedure of removing a sample of skeletal muscle from an individual

muscle power: the mechanical power during dynamic muscle contractions

muscle spindle: the sensory receptor within skeletal muscle that is sensitive to static and dynamic changes in muscle length

muscular strength: the maximal force generated by contracting skeletal muscle for a given contractile velocity

myocardial infarction: injury to the myocardium caused by a lack of blood flow

myocardial ischemia: abnormally low blood flow to the myocardium

myofibrils (mi′o-fi′bril): the longitudinal anatomical unit within skeletal and cardiac muscle fibers that contains the contractile proteins

myoglobin (mi′o-**glo**-bin): intramuscular protein that contains one heme (iron)-containing group that enables the binding of oxygen

myosin (mi′o-sin): the largest of the contractile proteins of skeletal muscle

N

natural life span: the estimated biological life span an individual should expect to achieve, which is suggested to be approximately 85 years of age

negative feedback: responses of a biological control system that oppose the initial stimulus

nerve: the cells of the nervous system that conduct action potentials

neuroendocrinology (nu ro-**en do**-kri-**no′**l o-je): the study of the anatomy and function of the endocrine system and the components of the nervous system that regulate endocrine function

neuromuscular junction: the connection between a branch of an alpha motor nerve and a skeletal muscle fiber

neurotransmitter (**nu′**ro-**trans**-mit′er): a chemical released at a synapse in response to the depolarization of the presynaptic membrane

nitrogen balance: equal nitrogen intake versus excretion from the body

nitrogen washout: an alternative method for measuring the residual volume of the lung

normobaric hypoxia: decreased oxygen availability at normal barometric pressure because of a lowered oxygen fraction of inspired air

nutrients: a food component that can be utilized by the body

nutrition: the science involving the study of food and liquid requirements of the body for optimal function

O

obesity: excess body fat

one repetition maximum (1 RM): the maximum strength from one contraction; typically obtained during dynamic contractions [when the contraction is isometric, this strength measure is termed the maximal voluntary contraction (MVC).]

orthostatic tolerance: the ability to withstand gravitational force in opposing blood flow back to the heart

osmolality (oz′mo-**lal′**i-ti): the number of particles per kilogram of solvent

osmoreceptors (oz′mo-**re-cep′**tors): cells that can generate an action potential in response to changes in blood osmolality

osteoarthritis (**oss**-te-o-**ar**-′thrit-es): a degenerative process caused by the wearing away of the cartilage between two articulating bone surfaces; also called degenerative joint disease

osteoporosis (**oss**-te-o-**por′**o-ses): a decreased bone mineral density, resulting in an increased susceptibility to bone fractures

overfat: a condition of excess body fat as determined from body composition analysis

overload: exposure of the body to stress that it is unaccustomed to

overtraining: training that causes excess overload that the body is unable to adapt to, resulting in decreased exercise performance

overweight: a condition of excess weight based on either a height-weight relationship or computed from body composition analysis

ovulatory phase: the phase of the menstrual cycle involved with ovulation; usually 3 days in duration

oxidative phosphorylation: the production of ATP from the coupled transfer of electrons to the generation of a H^+ gradient between the two mitochondrial membranes

oximetry (ok′sim′e-tri): indirect measurement of the oxygen saturation of hemoglobin in blood

oxygen deficit: the difference between oxygen consumption and the oxygen demand of exercise during non-steady-state exercise conditions

P

peak height velocity: the period of rapid growth during the adolescent period, usually occurring 2 years earlier for girls than boys

phosphagen system: the regeneration of ATP via creatine phosphate hydrolysis and ADP

phosphate loading: the practice of ingesting phosphate for the purpose of improving exercise performance

phosphorous magnetic resonance spectroscopy [(^{31}P)MRS]: the detection of differing frequency sound waves from precessing objects in a magnetic field, the signals from which allow the graphical illustration and quantification of the different signals and their respective intensities

physcial activity: the activity performed by the body for purposes other than the specific development of physical fitness

physical fitness: a state of bodily function that is characterized by the ability to tolerate exercise stress

pneumotachometer (nu′mo-ta-kom′e-ter): an instrument for measuring the instantaneous flow during ventilation

polycythemia (pol′i-**si-the′**mi-ah): above-normal increase in the erythrocyte content of the blood; increased red blood cell concentrations in the blood

pores of Kohn: the holes within alveoli that allow fluid and surfactant to spread across the alveoli membranes

power: the application of force relative to time

predictive value: a measure of how accurately an exercise test identifies an individual with or without coronary artery disease

preload: the load to which a muscle is subjected before shortening; usually explained as the stretch induced on the myocardium by the filling of the ventricles of the heart

profession (pro-fe′shun): an occupation that requires special education and training

progesterone: a steroid hormone synthesized by the developing follicle of the ovary and released during the luteal phase of the menstrual cycle

pubertal growth spurt: the rapid growth of a child associated with puberty

puberty: the period of a child's development when androgen hormones are released and secondary sex characteristics develop

pulmonary edema: accumulation of fluid within and between the tissues of the lungs

pulmonary circulation: the blood and vessels that connect the heart and the lungs

pulmonary transit time: the time it takes for a red blood cell to pass through the respiratory zone of the lung

pure research: research for the purpose of further understanding physiology

Q

quality of life: an individual's ability to perform daily activities (ADLs), such as walking, bathing, dressing, and eating

R

rebound hypoglycemia: the decrease in blood glucose when exercising at least 30 min after the ingestion of carbohydrate

receptor: the integrating control unit

receptors: proteins located within a membrane that are able to bind another molecule (typically a hormone or neurotransmitter)

redox potential: the ratio between NAD^+ and NADH concentrations (NAD^+/NADH)

rehydration: the process of returning fluids to the body during recovery from dehydration

residual volume: the volume remaining in the lungs after a forced maximal exhalation

resistance exercise: muscle contractions performed against a resistance, typically in the form of external loads like those used in weight lifting

respiration: gas exchange

respiratory exchange ratio: the ratio of carbon dioxide production to oxygen consumption, as measured from expired gas analysis indirect calorimetry

respiratory quotient: the ratio of carbon dioxide production to oxygen consumption during metabolism

respiratory zone: the zone of the lung where respiration (gas exchange) occurs

retraining: the process of regaining training adaptations previously lost from a period of detraining

reversibility: the loss of training adaptations when exercise training ceases

rheumatoid arthritis: the pain and joint swelling caused by an inflammation of the membrane surrounding joints

ribosome (ri′bo-som): the cytosolic organelle involved in protein synthesis

risk factors: factors associated with increased risk for acquiring a disease or disability

S

sarcolemma (sar′ko-lem′ah): the cell membrane of a muscle fiber

sarcomere (sar′ko-mere): the smallest contractile unit of skeletal muscle, consisting of the contractile proteins between two Z-lines

second messenger: an intracellular compound that increases in concentration during the amplification response to the binding of a hormone to its receptor

sensitivity: in clinical exercise physiology this term refers to the percentage of individuals with known cardiovascular disease who complete a graded exercise test and have an abnormal (positive) test; the sensitivity of clinically graded exercise testing varies from 50 to 90%

sodium bicarbonate: the molecule in blood that provides the greatest buffer power of acid

specificity: having a fixed relation to a single cause or definite result; in clinical exercise physiology refers to the percentage of individuals with no cardiovascular disease who complete a graded exercise test and have a normal (negative) test with the specificity of clinically graded exercise testing varying from 60 to 90%

spirometer (spi-rom′e-ter): a device used to measure lung volumes

spirometry (spi-rom′e-tri): the measurement of human lung volumes and functional capacities with a spirometer

ST-segment depression: the lowering of the ST segment, usually because of ischemia

steady state: a condition where certain bodily functions have attained dynamic constancy at a level different from homeostasis

storage fat: fat and lipid stored in adipose tissue

stroke (strowk): brain malfunction and damage caused by cerebral ischemia, often resulting from occlusions in the arteries supplying blood to the brain

stroke volume: the volume of blood ejected from the ventricle each beat

surfactant (sur-fak′tant): the lipoprotein molecule found over alveolar membranes that functions to decrease surface tension and improve compliance

synapse (sin′aps): the junction between two nerves

systemic circulation: the vasculature of the body other than the pulmonary circulation

T

taper: a period of reduced training prior to athletic competition

testosterone: a steroid hormone synthesized by the testes, which induces development of male secondary sex characteristics and increased muscle mass

tidal volume: the volume of air ventilated into and out of the lungs with each breath

training (tray′ning): an organized program of exercise designed to stimulated chronic adaptations

transamination (trans-amin′a-shun): the removal of an amino group from one amino acid and its placement on a carbon chain that forms another amino acid

transcription (trans-krip′shun): the duplication of specific DNA regions in the form of RNA

translation: the formation of amino acids from the enzymatic association between ribosomes, RNA, and tRNA

triacylglycerol (tri-as′il-glis′er-ol): a lipid consisting of a glycerol backbone and three free fatty acid molecules, which is the principle form of fat storage in the body

tricarboxylic acid cycle: mitochondrial reactions involving the addition of acetyl CoA to oxaloacetate, and the eventual release of carbon dioxide, electrons, and protons during the reformation of oxaloacetate

tropomyosin (tro′po-my′osin): a contractile protein of striated muscle

troponin (tro′po′nin): the regulatory calcium-binding contractile protein of striated muscle

V

vasoconstriction (vas′o-kon-strik′shun): narrowing of the lumen diameter of blood vessels

vasodilation (vas′o-di-la′shun): widening of the lumen diameter of blood vessels

ventilation: the movement of air into and out of the lungs by bulk flow

ventilatory threshold: the metabolic intensity associated with an increase in the ventilatory equivalent for oxygen (VE/VO_2)

vital capacity: the maximal volume of air that can be exhaled from the lungs in one expiratory effort

vitamins: organic micronutrient of food, essential for normal body functions

VO_{2max}: the maximal rate of oxygen consumption for a given individual

VO_{2peak}: the largest VO_2 during an incremental exercise test where all criteria of VO_{2max} have not been met

voluntary dehydration: the progressive development of dehydration despite the availability of fluid to drink *ad libitum*

W

warm-up: a general term used for practices performed prior to exercise for the purpose of preparing the body for the exercise

water intoxication: excess drinking of fluid (typically plain water) that lowers the concentration of serum sodium, increasing the risk for developing hyponatremia

WBGI: an abbreviation for the wet bulb globe Index, used to rate the relative risk of heat injury associated with given environmental conditions

Wingate test: a 30s all out cycle ergometer test that is used to measure maximal power generation as an indirect reflection of a person's anaerobic capacity

work: the product of an applied force exerted over a known distance against gravity

CREDITS

CHAPTER 3

Fig. 3.4, **p. 30,** Modified from Atkinson, DE: *Cellular energy metabolism and its regulation,* NY: Academic Press, 1977; Fig. 3.9, **p. 35,** From Thibodeau, GA, and Patton, KT: *Anatomy & physiology,* St. Louis: Mosby, 1996; Fig. 3.15, **p. 41,** From Berne, MN: *Physiology,* ed. 3, St. Louis: Mosby, 1993; Fig. 3.16B, **p. 43,** Adapted from Lehninger, AL, et al: *Principles of biochemistry,* NY: Worth, 1993; Fig. 3.22, **p. 48,** From Thibodeau, GA, and Patton, KT: *Anatomy & physiology,* St. Louis: Mosby, 1996 and Rolin Graphics.

CHAPTER 4

Fig. 4.1, **p. 57,** Courtesy Quinton Instrument Co, Bothell, WA; Fig. 4.4B, **p. 60,** Adapted from Costill, DL, et al: *J Swim Res* 2(1): 16-19, 1986; Fig. 4.6, **p. 62,** Adapted from Bursztein, S, et al: *Energy metabolism, indirect calorimetry, and nutrition,* Baltimore: William & Wilkins, 1989; Fig. 4.7, **p. 64,** Adapted from McLean, JA, Tobin, G: *Animal and human calorimetry,* NY: Cambridge University Press, 1987; Fig. 4.8C, **p. 66,** Courtesy Medical Graphics Corp., St. Paul, MN.

CHAPTER 5

Figs. 5.1, 5.2, 5.5, 5.6, 5.8, 5.21 **pp. 78, 79, 82, 84, 98,** From Saladin, KS: *Anatomy and physiology,* Dubuque, IA: WCB/McGraw-Hill, 1998; Fig. 5.4A, **p. 81,** From Desaki, J, and Vehara, Y: *J Neurocytol* 10: 101-110, 1981; Fig. 5.4B, **p. 81,** From Peachey, LD, et al: *Handbook of physiology,* Bethesda, MD: American Physiological Society, 1983; Fig. 5.10, **p. 87,** Modified from Seeley, RR, Stephens, TD, and Tate, P: *Anatomy and physiology,* ed. 4, Dubuque, IA: WCB/McGraw-Hill, 1998, art by Barbara Cousins; Fig. 5.12, **p. 88,** Adapted from Thorstensson, A, Grimby, G, and Karlsson, J: Force-velocity relations and fiber composition in human knee extensor muscles, *J Appl Physiol* 40(1): 12-16, 1976; Fig. 5.13, **p. 89,** From Berne, RM, and Levy, MN: *Physiology,* ed. 3, St. Louis: Mosby, 1993, and data from Gordon, AM, et al: *J Physiol* (London), 184: 170, 1966; Fig. 5.16, **p. 92,** Adapted from Edington, DW,

Edgerton, VR: Muscle fibertype population of human leg muscles, *Histochem J* 7: 259-266, 1975; Fig. 5.22, **p. 100,** Data from Bergh, U, et al: Maximal oxygen uptake and muscle fiber types in trained and untrained humans, *Med Sci Sports* 10:151, 1978; Fig. 5.23, **p. 101,** Data from Gregor, RJ, et al: Torque-velocity relationships and muscle fiber composition in elite female athletes, *J Appl Physiol* 47(2): 388-392, 1979; Fig. 5.24, **p. 103,** Courtesy Therapeutic Technologies, Inc., Dayton, OH.

CHAPTER 6

Fig. 6.3, **p. 113,** Adapted from Saltin, B, and Åstrand, P: Maximal oxygen uptake in athletes, *J Appl Physiol* 25: 353, 1967; Fig. 6.15, **p. 125,** Adapted from references 7, 22, 57, 67, 86, 88, and 118; Fig. 6.18, **p. 128,** Adapted from Arnold, DL, et al: *J Mag Reson Med* 1(3): 307-315, 1984; Fig. 6.22, **p. 133,** Data from Hultman, EH, and Sahlin, K: Acid-base balance during exercise, *Exerc Sport Sci* Rev 7: 41-128, 1980.

CHAPTER 7

Fig. 7.1, **p. 143,** From Thibodeau, GA, and Patton, KT: *Anatomy and physiology,* ed. 3, St. Louis: Mosby, 1996, art by Rolin Graphics; Fig. 7.2, **p. 144,** From Saladin, KS: *Anatomy and physiology,* Dubuque, IA: WCB/McGraw-Hill, 1998; Fig. 7.3, **p. 146,** From Thibodeau, GA, and Patton, KT: *Anatomy and physiology,* ed. 3, St. Louis: Mosby, 1996, art by Christine Oleksyk; Fig. 7.9, **p. 151,** Adapted from Gledhill, ND, et al: Endurance athletes' stroke volume does not plateau: major advantage is diastolic function, *Med Sci Sports Exerc* 26(9): 1116-1121, 1994; Fig. 7.11, **p. 153,** Data from Pendergast, DR: Cardiovascular, respiratory, and metabolic responses to upper body exercise, *Med Sci Sports Exerc* 21(5): S121-S125, 1989.

CHAPTER 8

Figs. 8.1, 8.2, 8.4, **pp. 166, 167, 170,** From Saladin, KS: *Anatomy and physiology,* Dubuque, IA: WCB/McGraw-Hill, 1998; Fig. 8.8, **p. 174,** From Thibodeau, GA, and Patton, KT: *Anatomy*

and physiology, ed. 3, St. Louis: Mosby, 1996; Fig. 8.11, **p. 178,** From Department of Health and Human Services: *Guidelines for diagnoses and management of asthma,* Pub No 91-3042, National Institutes of Health, 1991; Fig. 8.12, **p. 179,** Adapted from Powers, SK, and Williams, J: Exercise-induced hypoxemia in highly trained athletes, *Sports Med* 4: 46-53, 1987.

CHAPTER 9

Fig. 9.1, **p. 187,** From Saladin, KS: *Anatomy and physiology,* Dubuque, IA: WCB/McGraw-Hill, 1998.

CHAPTER 10

Fig. 11.1, **p. 228,** From US Department of Agriculture/US Department of Health and Human Services, August, 1992; Fig. 11.2, **p. 228,** Adapted from Sherman, WM, et al: *Int J Sports Med* 2(2): 114-118, 1981; Fig. 11.3, **p. 229,** Adapted from Costill, DL, et al: *J Appl Physiol* 43: 965-999, 1977; Fig. 11.6, **p. 236,** Adapted from references 24, 34, and 93; Fig. 11.7, **p. 237,** Adapted from Mitchell, JB, et al: *Med Sci Sports Exerc* 21: 269-274, 1989.

CHAPTER 13

Fig. 13.2, **p. 272,** Data from Foster, C, et al: *Am Heart J* 107: 1229-1234, 1984; Fig. 13.3, **p. 273,** Adapted from *The Y's way to physical fitness* with permission of the YMCA of the USA, 101 N.Wacker Drive, Chicago, IL 60606; Fig. 13.4A, **p. 274,** Adapted from Åstrand, P: *Acta Physiologica Scandinavica* 49 (Suppl 169), **p. 51,** 1960; Fig. 13.4B, **p. 275,** Adapted from Legge, BJ, and Bannister, EW: *J Appl Physiol* 61(3): 1203-1209, 1986; Fig. 13.7, **p. 279,** Courtesy Cybex ®, Bay Shore, NY; Table 13.6, **p. 281,** Used with permission of Williams & Wilkins, a Waverly Company.

CHAPTER 14

Fig. 14.4, **p. 291,** Courtesy Warren E. Collins, Braintree, MA.

CHAPTER 15

Table 15.1, **p. 299,** Modified from Metropolitan Life Insurance Company: *1983 height and weight tables announced,* NY: Metropolitan Life Insurance Company, 1983; Fig. 15.4, **p. 305,** Equipment courtesy Life Measurement Instruments, Concord, CA; Table 15.8, **p. 307,** From Jackson, AS, and Pollack, ML: *Phys Sportsmed* 13: 76-90, 1985.

CHAPTER 16

Figs. 16.1, 16.4, **pp. 320, 322,** From Saladin, KS: *Anatomy and physiology,* Dubuque, IA: WCB/McGraw-Hill, 1998; Fig. 16.3, **p. 321,** From Thibodeau, GA, and Patton, KT: *Anatomy and physiology,* ed. 3, St. Louis: Mosby, 1996, art by Network Graphics; Fig. 16.12, **p. 328,** Courtesy The University of New Mexico.

CHAPTER 17

Table 17.1, **p. 342,** From Pate, RR, Shepard, RJ: *Characteristics of physical fitness in youth.* In Lamb, DR, and Gisolfi, CV, (eds): *Perspectives in exercise science and sports medicine,* vol 2, Dubuque, IA: McGraw-Hill, 1989; Tables 17.2, 17.3, **pp. 343-344,** Reprinted with permission from The Cooper Institute for Aerobics Research, Dallas, TX; Fig. 17.1, **p. 345,** Adapted from Ross, JG, et al: *JOPERD,* November/De-

cember, 1987. This figure is redrawn with permission from the *Journal of Physical Education, Recreation, & Dance,* November/December, 1987, **p. 77.** *JOPERD* is a publication of the American Alliance for Health, Physical Education, Recreation, and Dance, 1900 Association Drive, Reston, VA 22091; Fig. 17.3, **p. 346,** Adapted from Gilliam, TB, et al: *Med Sci Sports Exerc* 9(1): 21-25, 1977; Fig. 17.4, **p. 347,** From Malina, RM, Bouchard, C: *Growth, maturation, and physical activity,* Champaign, IL: Human Kinetics, 1991, Copyright 1991 by Robert M. Malina and Claude Bouchard. Reprinted with permission; Fig. 17.5, **p. 348,** Adapted from Tanner, RH, et al: *Arch Dis Child* 41: 454-471; Figs. 17.6, 17.7, **pp. 349-350,** Courtesy, Ross Laboratories; Fig. 17.8, **p. 351,** Reprinted with permission of Macmillan General Reference USA, a division of Simon & Schuster Inc., from Krahenbuhl, GS, et al: *Developmental aspects of maximal aerobic power in children.* In Terjung, RL (ed.): *Exercise and sport sciences reviews,* vol 13, 1985, Copyright © American College of Sports Medicine; Fig. 17.9, **p. 352,** Adapted from Bar-Or, O: *Pediatric sports medicine for the practitioner: from physiological principles to clinical applications,* NY: Springer-Verlag, 1983.

CHAPTER 18

Table 18.4, **p. 367,** Source: American Rheumatism Association.

CHAPTER 19

Fig. 19.11, **p. 391,** Adapted from O'Donnell, TF: *Orthop Clin North Am* 11: 841-855, 1980; Fig. 19.12, **p. 394,** Adapted from Burton, AC, and Edholm, OG: *Monograph of the Physiological Society,* No 2, Bethesda, 1955; Figs. 19.13, 19.14, 19.15, **p. 397,** Courtesy NASA; Fig. 19.16, **p. 398,** Courtesy of the New Mexico Air National Guard.

CHAPTER 20

Fig. 20.3, **p. 413,** Adapted from Griffin, JE, Ojeda, SR: *Textbook of endocrine physiology,* NY: Oxford University Press, 1988.

CHAPTER 21

Fig. 21.3, **p. 428,** Adapted from the Activity Pyramid, Park Nicollet Medical Foundation; Fig. 21.4, **p. 431,** Adapted from the National Center for Health Statistics and the American Heart Association; Focus box 21.3, **p. 433,** Source: Haskell, WL: *Mechanisms by which physical activity may enhance the clinical status of cardiac patients.* In Pollock, ML, Schmidt (eds): *Heart disease and rehabilitation,* 2nd ed, NY: John Wiley & Sons, 1985, **pp. 276-296;** Table 21.4, **p. 436,** Adapted from the National Cholesterol Education Program Committee, *JAMA* 269: 3015-3023, 1993.

INDEX